EMERGING NANOTECHNOLOGIES FOR DIAGNOSTICS, DRUG DELIVERY, AND MEDICAL DEVICES

EMERGING NANOTECHNOLOGIES FOR DIAGNOSTICS, DRUG DELIVERY, AND MEDICAL DEVICES

Edited by

ASHIM K. MITRA
KISHORE CHOLKAR
ABHIRUP MANDAL

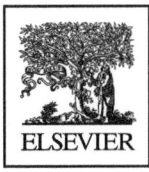

ELSEVIER   elsevier.com

Elsevier
Radarweg 29, PO Box 211, 1000 AE Amsterdam, Netherlands
The Boulevard, Langford Lane, Kidlington, Oxford OX5 1GB, United Kingdom
50 Hampshire Street, 5th Floor, Cambridge, MA 02139, United States

Copyright © 2017 Elsevier Inc. All rights reserved.

No part of this publication may be reproduced or transmitted in any form or by any means, electronic or mechanical, including photocopying, recording, or any information storage and retrieval system, without permission in writing from the publisher. Details on how to seek permission, further information about the Publisher's permissions policies and our arrangements with organizations such as the Copyright Clearance Center and the Copyright Licensing Agency, can be found at our website: www.elsevier.com/permissions.

This book and the individual contributions contained in it are protected under copyright by the Publisher (other than as may be noted herein).

Notices
Knowledge and best practice in this field are constantly changing. As new research and experience broaden our understanding, changes in research methods, professional practices, or medical treatment may become necessary.

Practitioners and researchers must always rely on their own experience and knowledge in evaluating and using any information, methods, compounds, or experiments described herein. In using such information or methods they should be mindful of their own safety and the safety of others, including parties for whom they have a professional responsibility.

To the fullest extent of the law, neither the Publisher nor the authors, contributors, or editors, assume any liability for any injury and/or damage to persons or property as a matter of products liability, negligence or otherwise, or from any use or operation of any methods, products, instructions, or ideas contained in the material herein.

Library of Congress Cataloging-in-Publication Data
A catalog record for this book is available from the Library of Congress

British Library Cataloguing-in-Publication Data
A catalogue record for this book is available from the British Library

ISBN: 978-0-323-42978-8

For information on all Elsevier publications visit our website at https://www.elsevier.com/books-and-journals

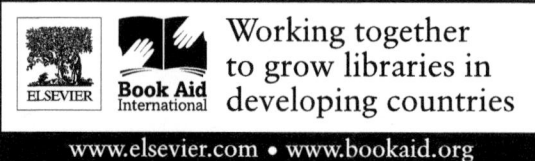

Publisher: Matthew Deans
Acquisition Editor: Simon Holt
Editorial Project Manager: Sabrina Webber
Production Project Manager: Lisa Jones
Designer: Greg Harris

Typeset by TNQ Books and Journals

CONTENTS

List of Contributors   ix
Editor Biographies   xi

1. Therapeutic Applications of Polymeric Materials   1
Kishore Cholkar, Gayathri Acharya, Hoang M. Trinh, Gagandeep Singh

1. Introduction   1
2. Polymers as Drug Delivery Systems   2
3. Polymers in Imaging and Diagnosis   8
4. Conclusion   15
References   15

2. Multifunctional Micro- and Nanoparticles   21
Rubi Mahato

1. Introduction   21
2. Micro- and Nanomaterials in the Synthesis of Multifunctional Carriers   27
3. Types of Functional Moieties   32
4. Functionalization of Micro- and Nanoparticles   35
References   39

3. Nanomicelles in Diagnosis and Drug Delivery   45
Hoang M. Trinh, Mary Joseph, Kishore Cholkar, Ranjana Mitra, Ashim K. Mitra

1. Introduction   45
2. Nanomicelle Preparation   46
3. Application of Nanomicelle in Diagnostics and Imaging   48
4. Application of Nanomicelles in Drug Delivery   50
5. Conclusion   53
References   54

4. Diagnosis and Drug Delivery to the Brain: Novel Strategies   59
Abhirup Mandal, Rohit Bisht, Dhananjay Pal, Ashim K. Mitra

1. Introduction   60
2. Barriers for Brain Drug Delivery   60
3. Physiology of the Blood—Brain Barrier   60
4. Invasive Drug Delivery Approaches   62
5. Noninvasive Drug Delivery Approaches   64

6.	Nanotechnology Approaches	67
7.	Active Blood–Brain Barrier Targeting Strategies	69
8.	Novel Nanoplatforms and Delivery Vehicles for BBB Targeting	73
9.	Development of Neurodiagnostic Nanoimaging Platforms	74
10.	Conclusion	77
	Acknowledgment	79
	References	79

5. Emerging Nanotechnology for Stem Cell Therapy 85

Varun Khurana, Deep Kwatra, Sujay Shah, Abhirup Mandal, Ashim K. Mitra

1.	Introduction	85
2.	Application of Nanoparticles in Isolation of Stem Cells	86
3.	Application of Nanoparticles in Stem Cell Tracking	89
4.	Role of Nanotechnology in Regulating Microenvironment of Stem Cells: Potential Roles in Tissue Engineering	93
5.	Nanoparticles as Macromolecular Delivery Systems for Stem Cells	96
6.	Future Prospects and Challenges Facing the Field	100
	References	100

6. Nanoparticulate Systems for Therapeutic and Diagnostic Applications 105

Rajashekar Kammari, Nandita G. Das, Sudip K. Das

1.	Introduction	105
2.	Why Nanotechnology and Nanomedicine?	106
3.	Types of Nanoparticles in Drug Delivery	108
4.	Conclusion	138
	References	138

7. Peptide and Protein-Based Therapeutic Agents 145

Mary Joseph, Hoang M. Trinh, Ashim K. Mitra

1.	Introduction	146
2.	Challenges With Peptide and Protein Therapeutics	147
3.	Chemical Modifications	147
4.	Micro- and Nanotechnology for Biologics in Drug Delivery	150
5.	Protein- and Peptide-Based Therapeutics	155
6.	Conclusion	161
	References	161

8. Nanotechnology in Intracellular Trafficking, Imaging, and Delivery of Therapeutic Agents 169

Animikh Ray, Ashim K. Mitra

1.	Introduction	169
2.	Mechanisms	171

3.	Macropinocytosis	173
4.	Conclusion	185
	References	185

9. Electrospun Nanofibers in Drug Delivery: Fabrication, Advances, and Biomedical Applications — 189

Vibhuti Agrahari, Vivek Agrahari, Jianing Meng, Ashim K. Mitra

1.	Introduction	190
2.	Stimuli-Responsive Nanofibers in Drug Delivery Applications	195
3.	Applications of Electrospun Nanofibers	201
4.	Conclusion	210
	References	211

10. Nanosystems for Diagnostic Imaging, Biodetectors, and Biosensors — 217

Gayathri Acharya, Ashim K. Mitra, Kishore Cholkar

1.	Introduction	217
2.	Nanosystems as Platforms for Advanced Diagnostic Imaging	218
3.	Diagnostic Imaging With Nanosystems	226
4.	Biological Sensors	232
5.	Conclusions	244
	References	244

11. Micro- and Nanotechnology-Based Implantable Devices and Bionics — 249

Rohit Bisht, Abhirup Mandal, Ashim K. Mitra

1.	Introduction	249
2.	Biocompatibility Issues of Implants	252
3.	Microtechnology-Based Implantable Devices and Bionics	258
4.	Nanotechnology-Based Implantable Devices and Bionics	272
5.	Conclusions and Future Perspectives	280
	References	281

12. Solid Lipid Nanoparticles in Drug Delivery: Opportunities and Challenges — 291

Ameya Deshpande, Majrad Mohamed, Saloni B. Daftardar, Meghavi Patel, Sai H.S. Boddu, Jerry Nesamony

1.	Introduction	292
2.	Components of Solid Lipid Nanoparticles	293
3.	Solid Lipid Nanoparticle Production Techniques	295
4.	Drug-Loading Capacity of Solid Lipid Nanoparticles	298
5.	Drug Incorporation Models of Solid Lipid Nanoparticles	299
6.	Drug Release From Solid Lipid Nanoparticles	300
7.	Applications of Solid Lipid Nanoparticles for Drug Delivery	302
8.	Stability Concerns of Solid Lipid Nanoparticles	310

9. Toxicity Aspects of Solid Lipid Nanoparticles	319
10. Diagnostic Applications of Solid Lipid Nanoparticles	320
11. In Vivo Fate of Solid Lipid Nanoparticles	321
12. Conclusions	322
References	323

13. Microneedles in Drug Delivery — 331

Rubi Mahato

1. Introduction	331
2. Skin Structure and Barrier to Transdermal Delivery	331
3. Microneedles	333
4. Selection of Microneedle Designs for Applications	346
5. Commercial Microneedle Devices	346
References	349

14. Nanotechnology-Based Medical and Biomedical Imaging for Diagnostics — 355

Kishore Cholkar, Nupoor D. Hirani, Chandramouli Natarajan

1. Introduction	355
2. Fluorescence-Based Imaging and Diagnostics	356
3. Nanocarriers in Biological Imaging	359
4. Photoacoustic and Ultrasound Imaging	367
5. Conclusions	369
References	370

15. Drug and Gene Delivery Materials and Devices — 375

Ann-Marie Ako-Adounvo, Beatriz Marabesi, Rayssa Costa Lemos, Ayuk Patricia, Pradeep K. Karla

1. Introduction	375
2. Advances in Delivery Systems	376
3. Gene Delivery	383
4. Gene Therapy Products	385
5. Conclusion and Future Direction	385
Acknowledgment	386
References	386

Index — 393

LIST OF CONTRIBUTORS

Gayathri Acharya
GlaxoSmithKline, Collegeville, PA, United States

Vibhuti Agrahari
University of Missouri—Kansas City, Kansas City, MO, United States

Vivek Agrahari
University of Missouri—Kansas City, Kansas City, MO, United States

Ann-Marie Ako-Adounvo
Howard University, Washington, DC, United States

Rohit Bisht
University of Auckland, Auckland, New Zealand

Sai H.S. Boddu
The University of Toledo Health Science Campus, Toledo, OH, United States

Kishore Cholkar
Ingenus Pharmaceuticals/RiconPharma LLC, Denville, NJ, United States

Saloni B. Daftardar
The University of Toledo Health Science Campus, Toledo, OH, United States

Nandita G. Das
Butler University, Indianapolis, IN, United States

Sudip K. Das
Butler University, Indianapolis, IN, United States

Ameya Deshpande
The University of Toledo Health Science Campus, Toledo, OH, United States

Nupoor D. Hirani
Ingenus Pharmaceuticals/RiconPharma LLC, Denville, NJ, United States

Mary Joseph
University of Missouri—Kansas City, Kansas City, MO, United States

Rajashekar Kammari
Butler University, Indianapolis, IN, United States

Pradeep K. Karla
Howard University, Washington, DC, United States

Varun Khurana
Nevakar LLC, Bridgewater, NJ, United States

Deep Kwatra
University of Missouri—Kansas City, Kansas City, MO, United States

Rayssa Costa Lemos
Howard University, Washington, DC, United States

Rubi Mahato
Fairleigh Dickinson University, Florham Park, NJ, United States

Abhirup Mandal
University of Missouri—Kansas City, Kansas City, MO, United States

Beatriz Marabesi
Howard University, Washington, DC, United States

Jianing Meng
University of Missouri—Kansas City, Kansas City, MO, United States

Ashim K. Mitra
University of Missouri—Kansas City, Kansas City, MO, United States

Ranjana Mitra
University of Missouri—Kansas City, Kansas City, MO, United States

Majrad Mohamed
The University of Toledo Health Science Campus, Toledo, OH, United States

Chandramouli Natarajan
University of Missouri—Kansas City, Kansas City, MO, United States

Jerry Nesamony
The University of Toledo Health Science Campus, Toledo, OH, United States

Dhananjay Pal
University of Missouri—Kansas City, Kansas City, MO, United States

Meghavi Patel
The University of Toledo Health Science Campus, Toledo, OH, United States

Ayuk Patricia
Howard University, Washington, DC, United States

Animikh Ray
University of Missouri—Kansas City, Kansas City, MO, United States

Sujay Shah
INSYS Therapeutics Inc, Chandler, AZ, United States

Gagandeep Singh
College of Staten Island, Staten Island, NY, United States

Hoang M. Trinh
University of Missouri—Kansas City, Kansas City, MO, United States

EDITOR BIOGRAPHIES

Ashim K. Mitra is a professor and chair of Pharmaceutical Sciences at the University of Missouri—Kansas City, USA. He was named one of the two recipients for the 2007 ARVO/Pfizer Ophthalmics Translational Research Award. He is the vice provost for Interdisciplinary Research for the University of Missouri—Kansas City, and director of Translational Research at UMKC School of Medicine. He is also the University of Missouri Curators' Professor of Pharmacy and UMKC's Chairman of Pharmaceutical Sciences. He is the author and coauthor of over 250 research articles, book chapters, and review papers. Professor Mitra is the recipient of a number of research awards from the National Institutes of Health, the American Association of Pharmaceutical Scientists, the American Association of Colleges of Pharmacy, and numerous other pharmaceutical organizations. He is the recipient of the University Trustee's Faculty Research Award in 1999 from the University of Missouri and National Collegiate Inventor of the Year Award in 1992 from the National Invention Center and the BF Goodrich Corporation. He has served as the editor of Ophthalmic Drug Delivery Systems (CRC Press), which is currently in its second edition, and a coeditor of Advanced Drug Delivery Reviews (Wiley).

Dr. Kishore Cholkar completed his PhD from University of Missouri—Kansas City, USA. During his academic career he was awarded with several travel awards. He is an active member of American Association of Pharmaceutical Scientists (AAPS), Association of Research in Vision and Ophthalmology (ARVO), Pharmaceutical Sciences Graduate Student Association (PSGSA), and United States Pharmacopeia and Ophthalmology group (OMICS). Moreover, Dr. Cholkar received the First Best Poster Award from Ophthalmology group in 2014 at Ophthalmology-2014 Conference, Baltimore, USA. He is the first author of more than 10 scholarly articles in peer-reviewed journals. One article, of which he was the first author, "Novel strategies for anterior segment ocular drug delivery" in the Journal of Ocular Pharmacology and Therapeutics, was in the top 10% of papers in Pharmacology and Toxicology of 2013 with approximately 50 independent citations. Another article of Dr. Cholkar's work is "Development and validation of a fast and sensitive bioanalytical method for the quantitative determination of glucocorticoids—quantitative measurement of dexamethasone in rabbit ocular matrices by liquid chromatography tandem mass spectrometry" in the Journal of Pharmaceutical and Biomedical Analysis of 2010 with 37 independent citations. "Ocular drug delivery systems: An overview" has been independently cited 75 times since its 2013 publication in World Journal of Pharmacology. Dr. Cholkar has more than 300 citations for his work with h index of 9 and i10 index of 9. In addition, Dr. Cholkar actively participates in manuscript reviews of new research submissions for leading academic journals and actively participates in research and development. At present, he is working as a Sr. Product Development Scientist at Ingenus Pharmaceuticals LLC/RiconPharma LLC, Denville, New Jersey, USA. Most of his work focuses on development of specialty products for topical application.

Abhirup Mandal is currently a PhD candidate at University of Missouri—Kansas City School of Pharmacy. He is also a pharmacist by training, with a Bachelors of Pharmacy degree from the Manipal College of Pharmaceutical Sciences, India. Abhirup has worked extensively in improving drug development and delivery strategies with comprehensive knowledge in analytical techniques, formulation of small molecule— and macromolecule-based nanocarriers, in vitro 3-D cell culture models, uptake and transport experiments, and brain and ocular microdialysis techniques. His research accomplishments include transporter-targeted drug delivery, prodrug development, and formulation approaches for improving brain and ocular drug absorption. He has published more than 13 peer-reviewed scientific research and review articles in reputed international journals including Advanced Drug Delivery Reviews and Journal of Controlled Release. He is an active member of American Association of Pharmaceutical Scientists (AAPS) and has presented more than 10 abstracts in various scientific meetings. He was awarded the Graduate Student Research Award in Drug Discovery and Development Interface at the AAPS 2016 annual meeting.

CHAPTER 1

Therapeutic Applications of Polymeric Materials

Kishore Cholkar[1], Gayathri Acharya[2], Hoang M. Trinh[3], Gagandeep Singh[4]

[1]Ingenus Pharmaceuticals/RiconPharma LLC, Denville, NJ, United States; [2]GlaxoSmithKline, Collegeville, PA, United States; [3]University of Missouri—Kansas City, Kansas City, MO, United States; [4]College of Staten Island, Staten Island, NY, United States

Contents

1. Introduction	1
2. Polymers as Drug Delivery Systems	2
2.1 Polymer—Drug Conjugates	5
2.2 Polymers in Ocular Drug Delivery	6
2.3 Polymers in Tissue Engineering	7
3. Polymers in Imaging and Diagnosis	8
4. Conclusion	15
References	15

1. INTRODUCTION

Polymers are one of the most important agents in pharmaceuticals. Polymers provide a wide range of applications in diverse biomedical fields such as, but not limited to, drug delivery, tissue engineering, implants, prostheses, ophthalmology, dental materials, and bone repair [1,2]. For better understanding, polymers may be broadly classified as biodegradable and nonbiodegradable. Biodegradable polymers represent a most important class due to their biocompatibility with biological fluids (blood/serum), tissues, and cells with minimal/no toxicity [3]. Moreover, such polymers degrade over time due to hydrolysis and therefore require no surgical procedure for their removal. Examples include polylactic acid (PLA), polyglycolic acid (PGA), polylactic glycolic acid (PLGA), and polycaprolactones (PCL). Nonbiodegradable polymers can achieve long-term near-zero-order drug release kinetics. Examples of such polymers include polyvinyl alcohol (PVA), ethylene vinyl acetate, and polysulfone capillary fiber. Although biocompatible, these polymers are not biodegradable polymers. On the other hand, various natural and synthetic polymers have applications in drug delivery, imaging, and diagnosis. Examples include polyesters, polyamides, poly(amino acids), polyorthoesters, polyurethanes, and polyacrylamides [4]. Among them, thermoplastic aliphatic polyesters like poly(lactic acid) (PLA), poly(glycolic acid) (PGA), and especially their copolymer poly(lactic-*co*-glycolic acid) (PLGA) are of significant interest due to their biocompatibility, process ability, and biodegradability.

Other most common and extensively studied biodegradable polymers include poly(E-caprolactone) (PCL), chitosan, gelatin, and poly(alkyl cyanoacrylates).

Early studies by Duncan et al., reported the development of first polymer—drug conjugates with applications for biomedical field [2,5]. Since then, several polymer—drug conjugates have been developed and commercialized. Polymeric systems may offer advantages such as improved drug stability, reduced toxicity, and enhanced targetability. Moreover, these polymers have been introduced in medical practice [6]. Biocompatible, biodegradable polymers and copolymers have demonstrated therapeutic potential in three major areas: (1) diagnostic applications, (2) therapeutic delivery, and (3) theranostics [6].

Polymer-based diagnostic agents are employed in diagnostic techniques such as fluorescence, imaging, magnetic resonance imaging (MRI), positron emission tomography (PET), single photon emission computed tomography (SPECT), and ultrasound diagnosis [6]. Moreover, polymeric systems have been intensively investigated as carrier systems for active pharmaceutical ingredient/s [2]. Polymeric systems may offer protection and improve the half-life for highly unstable drugs such as resolvins [7]. Moreover, half-lives for biologics such as DNA and RNA and protein stability may be enhanced. Moreover, it can provide protection against in vivo degradation and premature inactivation [2]. Several stimuli (pH and temperature)-responsive smart polymeric drug delivery vehicles have been designed to achieve targeted drug delivery. Such polymeric systems exhibit improved efficacy and aid in optimizing the dose. Current investigations are being focused on applications of polymers in therapeutics [2]. For example, polymer synthesis methods allow designing the polymer architecture, which in turn plays an important role in biological activity [8,9]. Various ligands can be conjugated to polymer backbone, which may result in targeting a specific receptor and transporter site.

A drug delivery system must release the drug at or into the target as well as maintain therapeutic drug levels for a desired duration [10] in blood stream, allowing for distribution to tissues by the enhanced permeability and retention (EPR) effect. Additionally, active targeting may be achieved by the polymer carrier, a polymer—drug conjugate, or the drug [10].

2. POLYMERS AS DRUG DELIVERY SYSTEMS

In recent years, various engineered nanoscale materials have been developed or are currently under investigation for drug delivery applications. Polymer blends are of significant interest in the biomedical field due to its wide variety of applications [11—14]. Compatibility of the copolymers and their interaction with the active pharmaceutical ingredient (API) play an important role in deciding the phase separation of the blend, which in turn plays an important role in the release behavior of the drug from the blend. The release rate may be tailored by varying ratio of the polymers in the copolymers blend [15]. Biocompatible and biodegradable nanomicelles based on block copolymer (BCP) are certainly one of the most promising nanostructures, for controlled delivery of poorly water-soluble drugs such as doxorubicin (DOX), paclitaxel, and clofazimine. These micellar drug formulations offer various advantages such as increased circulation time, improved water solubility, and tumor tissue targeting via the enhanced permeation and retention (EPR) effect [16]. The EPR effect exploits the increased porosity of the vasculature immediately surrounding a tumor. Polymeric nanomicelles (diameters 10−100 nm) can enter the tumor cells through endothelial cell lining of healthy capillary walls and can be retained in the lymphatic system [16]. In spite of these advantages, progress in the development of these systems have been hampered by slow and incomplete drug release (degradation times ranging from days to months) [17,18]. Extensive research is going on at present to overcome slow drug release, enhancing therapeutic efficacy and responding to changes in the environmental condition.

In particular, degradation in response to external stimuli is highly advantageous due to enhanced release of encapsulated drug molecules at the target site. Stimuli-responsive polymers are defined as polymers that undergo physical or chemical changes in response to surrounding environment [19].

Incorporating disulfide bond at the junctions of hydrophobic and hydrophilic blocks has emerged as a unique pathway to control the intracellular drug release. In particular, reductive-sensitive shedding nanomicellar systems are of great interest due to a high imbalance of glutathione (GSH) level between intracellular and extracellular environments [20,21]. The presence of a high redox potential difference between the oxidizing extracellular space and reducing intracellular space makes the disulfide bond a potential candidate as intracellular drug delivery tool [22]. Furthermore, the tumor tissues are reducing and hypoxic rendering disulfide-containing BCP specifically suitable for anticancer drug delivery. The other common strategy is to include disulfide linkage thereby cross-linking through S−S bonds. Fig. 1.1 illustrates doxorubicin incorporated into spherical nanomicelles. It is composed of polyethylene glycol (PEG)-SS-PCL, which permeates the tumor cell through the leaky vasculature and releasing the drug S−S cleavage by GSH intracellularly. Polymer properties may be tuned by changing the polymer architecture from linear or cross-linked to a partially or highly branched structure [6]. Owing to the unique properties, hyperbranched polymers (HBPs) with biocompatible and biodegradable polymers have demonstrated great potential for therapeutic applications [23−26].

The drug product, genetic segment, or the diagnostic agent may be encapsulated or conjugated with HBPs [6]. Zhu et al. synthesized a hyperbranched poly-(((S-(4-vinyl) benzyl S'-propyltrithiocarbonate)-co-(poly(ethylene glycol) methacrylate)) (poly(VBPT-co-PEGMA)) with multiple thiol groups via SCVP-RAFT (self-condensing vinyl polymerization-reversible addition-fragmentation chain transfer polymerization) copolymerization (Fig. 1.4) [27,28]. The authors demonstrated that thiol-containing anticancer drugs may be conjugated to this biocompatible HBP via disulfide linkages after aminolysis reaction to achieve a redox-responsive drug release (Fig. 1.2).

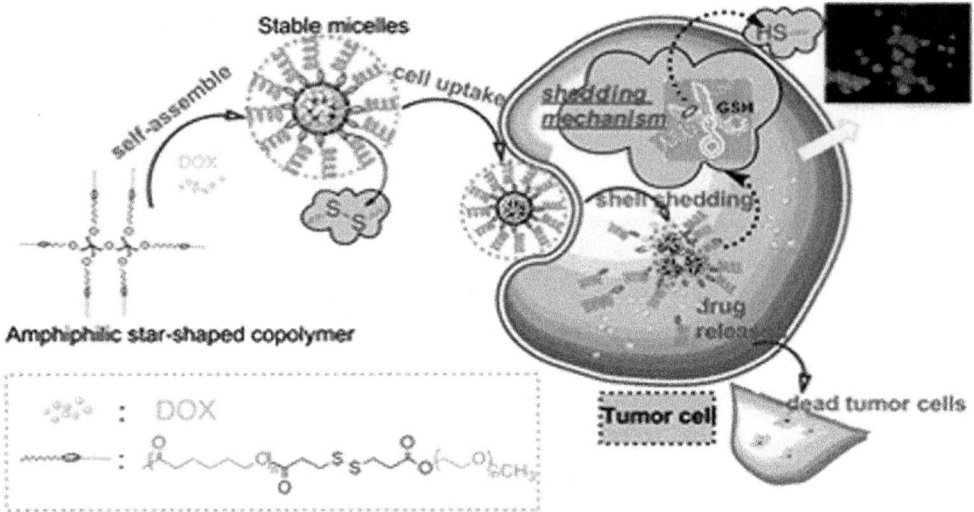

Figure 1.1 Scheme illustrating the spherical micelles based on polyethylene glycol–SS–polycaprolactone incorporating drug [doxorubicin (DOX)] and entering tumor cell through the leaky vasculature and releasing the drug on shedding triggered by glutathione (GSH) inside the cell. *(Reprinted with permission from Royal Society of Chemistry. Tian-Bin Ren YF, Zhang Z-H, Li L, Li Y-Y. Shell-sheddable micelles based on star-shaped poly(ε-caprolactone)-SS-poly(ethyl glycol) copolymer for intracellular drug release. Soft Matter 2011;7:2329—31.)*

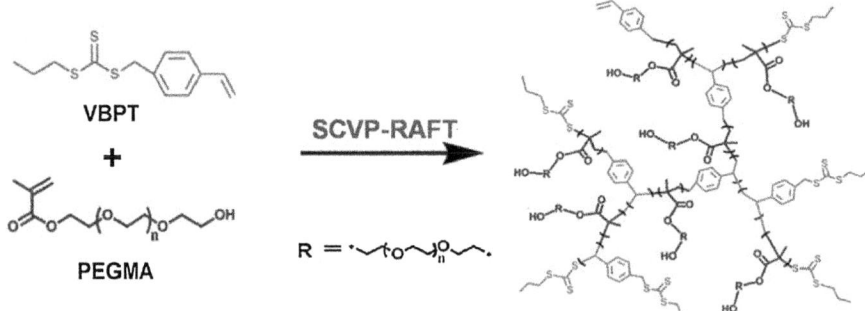

Figure 1.2 A schematic illustration of hyperbranched poly-(S-(4-vinyl) benzyl S′-propyltrithiocarbonate)-co-(poly(ethylene glycol) methacrylate)) (poly(VBPT-co-PEGMA)) constructed by SCVP-RAFT (self-condensing vinyl polymerization-reversible addition-fragmentation chain transfer polymerization) using VBPT and PEGMA monomers. *(Reproduced from Zhuang Y, et al. Facile fabrication of redox-responsive thiol-containing drug delivery system via RAFT polymerization. Biomacromolecules 2014;15(4):1408—18. Copyright 2014 American Chemical Society.)*

PEG–based HBP has also been explored for drug delivery as these systems may exhibit enhanced encapsulation efficiency and controlled drug release. This technology also offers postpolymerization modification, which may add stimuli-responsive features depending upon the functionality. Ji and coworkers have synthesized photoresponsive,

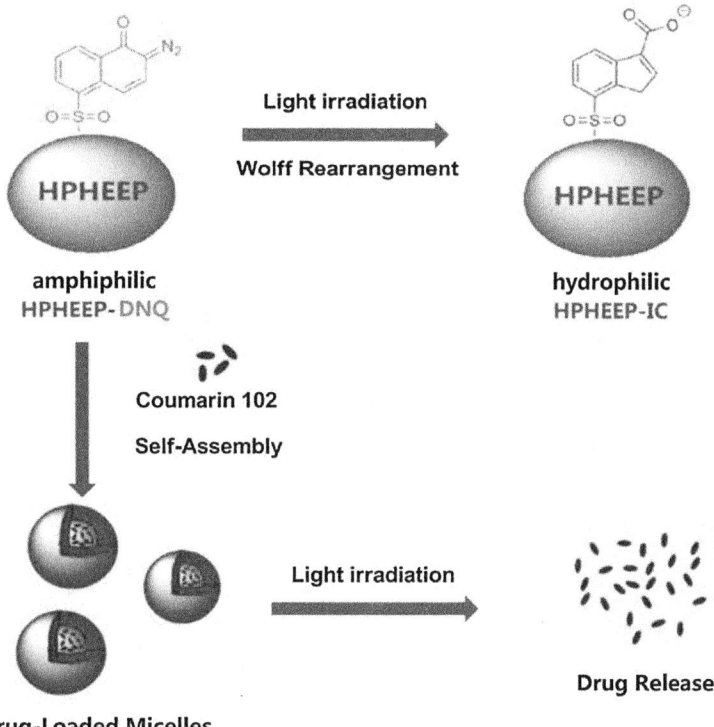

Figure 1.3 Photoresponsive behavior of hyperbranched polyphosphate (HPHEEP)—2-diazo-1,2-naphthoquinone-5-sulfonyl chloride (DNQ) and schematic illustration of the self-assembly and light-triggered drug release behavior of HPHEEP-DNQ micelles. *(Reproduced with permission from Chaojian Chen GL, Liu X, Pang S, Zhu C, Lv L, Ji J. Photo-responsive, biocompatible polymeric micelles self-assembled from hyperbranched polyphosphate-based polymers. Polym Chem 2011;2:1389—97.)*

biocompatible, and biodegradable hyperbranched polyphosphate (HPHEEP) via terminal modification, hydrophobic 2-diazo-1,2-naphthoquinone-5-sulfonyl chloride (DNQ) [29]. The resulting polymer can self-assemble into nanomicelles in water. The photochemical reaction of DNQ moieties under ultraviolet exposure results in destabilization of the nanomicelles to achieve photoresponsive drug release (Fig. 1.3) [6].

2.1 Polymer—Drug Conjugates

Another extensively studied nanoscale material for drug delivery is polymer—drug conjugates [12]. Small-molecule therapeutic agents, especially anticancer drugs, have the following disadvantages. They have poor aqueous solubility, short circulation half-life, may cause embolism, and off-target distribution, resulting in toxicity to normal cells [30]. The conjugation of small-molecule drugs to polymeric nanocarriers can overcome these problems. Polymer—drug conjugates can extend the in vivo circulation time and reduce cellular uptake to the endocytic route. The initial clinical trials with PEG were carried out in the early 1990s [31]. It can improve the plasma stability and solubility of the drug while reducing immunogenicity. Various PEGylated drugs are in clinical practice. For example, Adagen (PEG—adenosine deaminase) is indicated in immunodeficiency disease; Pegasys (PEG—a-interferon 2a) is prescribed to treat hepatitis B and C infections; and Oncaspar (PEG—L-asparaginase) can be recommended to treat acute lymphoblastic leukemia [30]. Besides PEG, other linear polymers that have also been studied as polymeric drug delivery carriers include polyglutamic acid, polysaccharide, and poly(allylamine hydrochloride).

2.2 Polymers in Ocular Drug Delivery

Natural and synthetic polymers have been introduced in ocular drug delivery. Natural polymers include starch, sodium alginate, sodium hyaluronate, xanthan gum, gelatin, gellan gum, guar gum, collagen, chitosan, and albumin. On the other hand, synthetic polymers include, but not limited to, hydroxypropyl methyl cellulose, hydroxypropyl cellulose, poly(acrylic acid), carbomers, sodium hyaluronose, chitosan, cyclodextrins, polygalacturonic acid, xyloglucan, xanthan gum, gellan gum, poly(ortho esters), hydroxyl ethyl cellulose, PVA, PGA, PLA, PCL, and poly(lactide-co-glycolide). These polymers may be straight chain or branched. Moreover, such polymers may be blended to achieve the desired drug release profile from the polymeric matrix. Mostly, such polymers are designed to encapsulate the active pharmaceutical ingredient for sustained or controlled drug release. In general, block copolymers may include diblock or triblock. However, Mitra et al. synthesized pentablock copolymers with different ratios of polymer block in the polymeric chain [32]. Such polymers may be custom tailored with respect to API to achieve desired drug loading and release. Moreover, these polymers can be applied in the preparation of nanoparticles and thermosensitive hydrogels. Nanoparticles prepared with pentablock copolymers encapsulated both small and large molecules. Thermosensitive polymers exhibit liquid or solution properties at room temperature (25°C) and transition to gel at physiological temperatures (34—37°C). Such a polymer can be applied to encapsulate drug-loaded nanoparticles for sustained drug release. In vivo studies were conducted in New Zealand albino rabbits to demonstrate biocompatibility and biodegradability. This study reveals that pentablock copolymer turns into a gel depot followed by slow degradation (Fig. 1.6). Interestingly, pentablock hydrogel encapsulating pentablock blank nanoparticles injected into rabbit eye demonstrate a depot over 90 days. Moreover, the depot did not appear to interfere with the field of vision.

Other amphiphilic polymers such as vitamin E tocopheryl polyethylene glycol (Vit. E. TPGS), octoxynol-40, and hydrogenated castor oil-40/60 have been evaluated for ocular drug delivery. These polymers have the ability to spontaneously generate nanomicelles in aqueous environment. Studies were conducted to encapsulate hydrophobic drugs such as voclosporin, rapamycin, dexamethasone, resolvin analog, acyclovir derivatives and peptides like cyclosporine [7,33—39]. Results indicated that solubility of these highly hydrophobic drugs was significantly improved in aqueous solution because of the drug encapsulation in the polymeric nanomicelles. The hydrophilic corona of nanomicelles aids in solubility. Hydrophobic interactions of the drug within the nanomicelle core stabilize and improves drug solubility. Biocompatibility studies on ocular cell lines demonstrated the delivery system to be safe and well tolerated.

In vivo studies conducted in New Zealand albino rabbits demonstrated that nanomicelles carried the drug to deeper anterior ocular tissues. Interestingly, the drug was detected in the back of the eye tissues (retina/choroid) with topical drop administration. These results indicate that nanomicelles follow conjunctival–scleral pathway to reach retina from topical dosing [34,35,38,39]. Such a technology can offer a platform for delivery of small and macromolecular drugs to posterior ocular tissues.

2.3 Polymers in Tissue Engineering

Tissue engineering/regeneration hypothesizes that a progenitor cell is recruited or delivered at an injured site to regenerate the damaged tissue. A synthetic porous three-dimensional polymeric scaffold has been engineered that enhances functional tissue regeneration by facilitating progenitor cell migration, proliferation, and differentiation. Such scaffolds may be prepared from natural or synthetic polymers. Natural polymers such as chitin, gelatin, elastin, fibrinogen, silk fibroin, and collagen have been utilized as scaffolds in tissue engineering. These polymers can be molded to scaffolds like hydrogel scaffolds (Fig. 1.4), PET grafts, and electrospun PCL mats (Fig. 1.5). Chitin is a biopolymer (N-acetyl-glucosamine monomer) extracted from shellfish. Depending upon the processing method N-acetyl-glucosamine and N-glucosamine units may be randomly or block distributed throughout the biopolymer chain. In a biopolymer if the fraction of N-acetyl-glucosamine units is higher than 50%, the biopolymer is called chitin. Chitin and its derivatives have applications as wound dressing materials, drug delivery systems, and candidates for tissue engineering. Hydroxyapatite (HA) or other calcium-containing materials amalgamated with chitin are commonly referred as "composite." These materials have application in orthopedics and periodontics. For example, a combination of polymer with HA provided maximum osteoconductive behavior of HA in vivo. The matrix progressively resorbs and allows bone growth to occur inside the implant [40,41]. nHA [$Ca_{10}(PO_4)_6(OH)_2$] displays high surface area to volume ratio and mimics apatite like structure and composition of hard tissues like bone, dentine, and enamel [42–44]. This material is nontoxic, noninflammatory, nonimmunogenic, nondecomposable, osteoconductive. Moreover, it demonstrates stability in body fluids and forms chemical bonds with surrounding hard tissues [45,46]. β-Chitin/HA and α-chitin/HA nanocomposite scaffolds were synthesized from a mixture of β-chitin hydrogel and nHA by freeze-drying technique [47,48]. Biocompatibility for such nanocomposite scaffolds was studied with MG

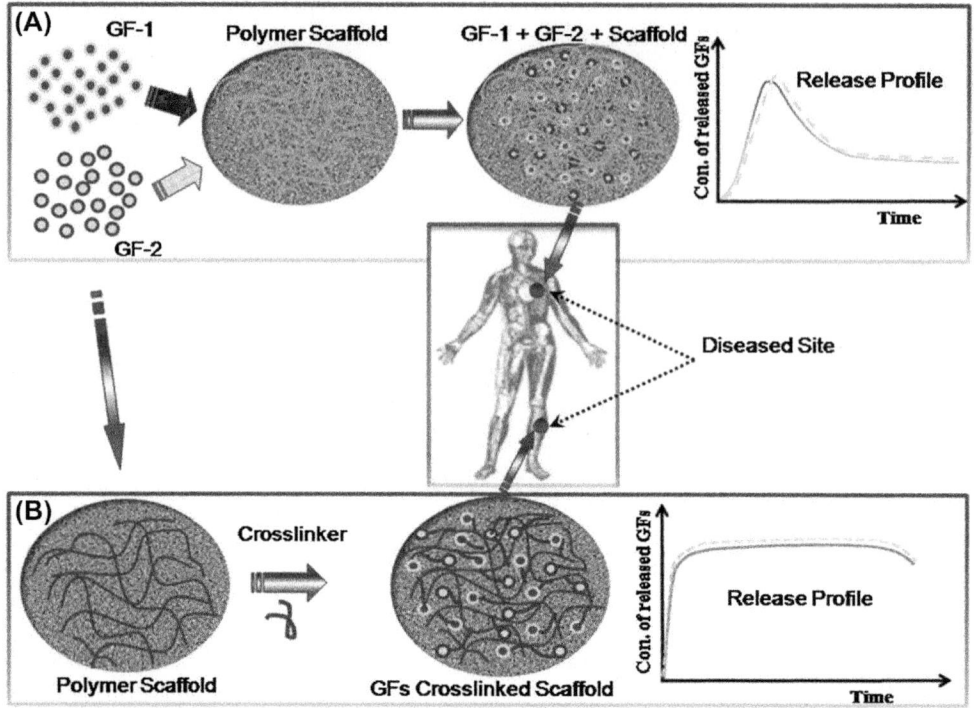

Figure 1.4 Schematic illustration of methods for immobilization of bioactive factor molecules [growth factors (GFs)] into hydrogels scaffolds. (A) Noncovalent immobilization of two different types of GFs loaded into hydrogels directly via entrapment before implantation and their expected release profile. (B) Covalent immobilization of two types of GFs modified and thereafter covalently cross-linked to the hydrogels via cross-linkers before implantation to the diseased site and their sustained release profile. *(Reproduced from Shuai X, et al. Micellar carriers based on block copolymers of poly(epsilon-caprolactone) and poly(ethylene glycol) for doxorubicin delivery. J Control Release 2004;98(3):415−26.)*

63 cells. The results indicated that cells were viable and exhibited enhanced attachment and proliferation onto the nanocomposite scaffolds. This result essentially signifies that nanocomposite scaffolds may serve as potential candidates for bone tissue engineering. Natural polymers, synthetic polymers, combination or blend of polymers and their application in tissue engineering are presented in Table 1.1.

3. POLYMERS IN IMAGING AND DIAGNOSIS

Polymers consist of multiple similar units bonded together and have been widely employed in therapeutic and diagnostic applications. Based on the monomer units, the polymers display various physical and chemical properties. Because of the mechanical and functional properties, many biological and synthetic polymers have become the important materials for medical applications such as vascular or urinary catheters, vascular

Polymers in Diagnosis, Imaging and Drug Delivery   9

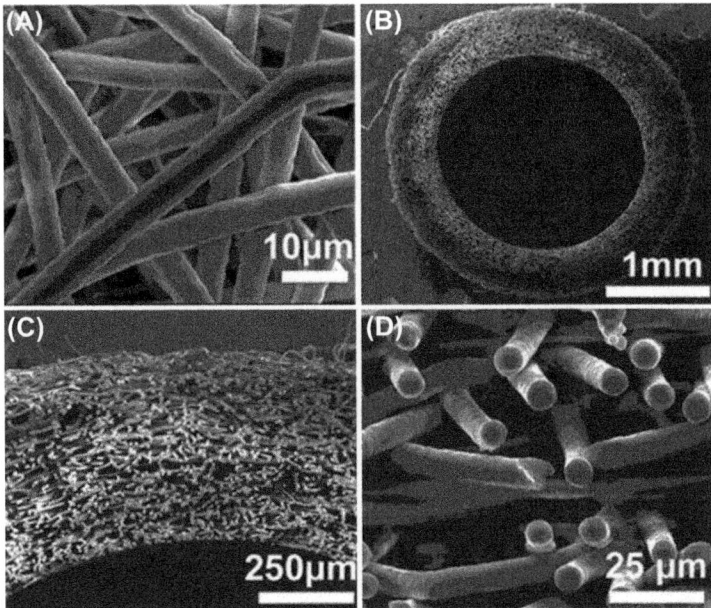

Figure 1.5 Scanning electron microscope images of electrospun polycaprolactone mats with thicker fibers (A) and cross-sections of the tubular thicker fiber grafts (B–D). *(Reproduced with permission from Wang Z, et al. The effect of thick fibers and large pores of electrospun poly(epsilon-caprolactone) vascular grafts on macrophage polarization and arterial regeneration. Biomaterials 2014;35(22):5700–10. Copyright 2014, Elsevier.)*

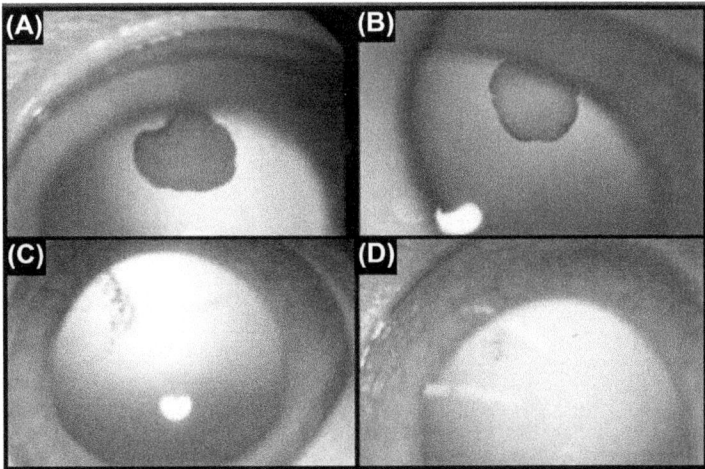

Figure 1.6 Gel forming pentablock copolymer; depot formation after intravitreal injection into rabbit eye. Images taken on (A) day 1, (B) day 21, (C) day 42, and (D) day 49 show the gel biodegrading over time.

Table 1.1 List of natural polymer scaffolds and their applications

Polymer	Application	Remarks/conclusions	References
Gelatin/poly(lactic acid-co-glycolic acid) (PLGA) bilayered nanofibers	Fabrication of meniscal tissue engineering scaffold	In vitro, the meniscal cells derived from New Zealand white rabbits menisci seeded in the scaffolds demonstrated cell proliferation. The bilayered gelatin/PLGA scaffold revealed concurrent effects of mechanics and cytocompatibility. Moreover, such scaffold appears to be a promising scaffold for future meniscal repair strategies	[84]
Collagen-BDDGE (1,4-butanediol diglycidyl ether)-elastin core-shell scaffold	Tendon regeneration	A prototype of the core module implanted in a rat tendon lesion model demonstrated safety, biocompatibility, and ability of the scaffold to induce tendon regeneration. Results indicate that such a device may support and induce in situ tendon regeneration	[85]
Fibrinogen-based nanofibers	Differentiation of human mesenchymal stem cells for cartilage development	Human adipose-derived mesenchymal stem cells established significant chondrogenic differentiation and may generate quality cartilage when cultured on 2D and randomly oriented fibrinogen/poly-lactic acid nanofibers relative to 3D sandwich-like environments. The adhering cells demonstrated well-developed focal adhesion complexes and actin cytoskeleton arrangements. This confirms proper cellular interaction with either random or aligned nanofibers	[86]
Electrospun fibrinogen-PLA nanofibers	Vascular tissue engineering	Development of a new type of hybrid fibrinogen-polylactic acid (FBG-PLA) nanofibers with improved stiffness, combining the good mechanical properties of PLA with the excellent cell recognition properties of native FBG	[87]
Silk fibroin nanofibrous scaffold	Bone tissue engineering application	Results confirm the positive correlation of alkaline phosphatase activity, alizarin staining, and expression of runt-related transcription factor 2, osteocalcin, and type 1 collagen representing the biomimetic property of the scaffolds. Developed composite demonstrated to be a potential scaffold for bone tissue engineering application	[88]

Agarose/silk fibroin blended hydrogel	In vitro cartilage tissue engineering	The hydrogels demonstrated immunocompatibility, which was evidenced by minimal in vitro secretion of tumor necrosis factor-α (TNF-α) by murine macrophages. Results suggest promising attributes of blended hydrogels and nonmulberry silk fibroin–agarose blends as alternative biomaterial for cartilage tissue engineering	[89]
Electrospun silk–fibroin nanofiber	Skin tissue engineering	Histologic findings in only electrospun SF scaffolds evidenced significant proliferation of fibroblasts in deeper layer and more differentiation of keratinocytes in superficial layer. Results suggest that 3D electrospun SF scaffolds may be suitable for skin tissue engineering	[90]
In situ cross-linking and mineralization of electrospun collagen scaffolds	Bone tissue	Among the catecholamines, matrix containing norepinephrine displayed superior mechanical, photoluminescence, and biological properties than matrix loaded with dopamine. Such smart multifunctional scaffolds may potentially be utilized to repair and regenerate bone defects and injuries	[91]
Thermosensitive collagen hydrogel	Constructing tissue engineering complex	Thermosensitive collagen hydrogel–poly-L-lactic acid fiber joint-constructed complex extracellular matrix had good biocompatibility and dynamic culture. Such construct may promote the distribution of bone marrow-derived mesenchymal stem cells on the surface and inside the structure, thus promoting cell proliferation, so it could be used for the in vitro construction of tissue engineering complex	[92]
Acellular collagen scaffold	Urethral regeneration	Spontaneous repopulation of urothelial and smooth muscle cells on all grafts was demonstrated. Cellular organization increased with time; however, 20% of both fistula and stenosis could be observed postoperatively. This off-the-shelf scaffold with a promising urethral regeneration has a potential for clinical application	[93]

Continued

Table 1.1 List of natural polymer scaffolds and their applications—cont'd

Polymer	Application	Remarks/conclusions	References
Biomimetic porous PLGA scaffolds	Kidney tissue regeneration	Results suggest that the tissue-engineering techniques can be an effective alternative method for treatment of kidney diseases. Moreover, the extracellular matrix incorporated poly(lactic-co-glycolic acid) scaffolds may be one of the promising materials for biomedical applications including tissue engineered scaffolds and biodegradable implants	[94]
Cell-free methacrylated hyaluronic acid/poly(lactide-co-glycolide) (HA-MA/PLGA) scaffolds	Regeneration of full-thickness cartilage defects	Expression of inflammatory factor interleukin-1β was downregulated, although TNF-α is remarkably upregulated. With the anti-inflammatory, bioactive properties and good restoration of full-thickness cartilage defect in vivo, the oriented macroporous HA-MA/PLGA hybrid scaffold has a great potential for practical application in in situ cartilage regeneration	[95]
Nanohydroxyapatite/poly(L-lactic acid) (HA/PLLA) spindle composites	Bone tissue engineering	The in vitro tests indicate that HA/PLLA biocomposites have good biodegradability and bioactivity when immersed in simulated body fluid solutions. All the results suggested that HA/PLLA nanobiocomposites are appropriate to be applied as bone substitute in bone tissue engineering	[96]

or ureteral stents, and surgical or cosmetic implant materials [49–51]. Due to the flexibility of the characteristic backbone, polymers may be modified or conjugated with imaging or diagnosis agents and delivered into patients. In this section, polymer-based materials in diagnosis will be discussed. The instruments for diagnosis include MRI, fluorescence, PET, and SPECT.

1. **MRI:** Under strong radio-frequency pulses MRI detects the alteration of hydrogen nuclei (^{1}H) in the tissues. Differentiation between various tissues is computed to diagnose the disease. Gd^{3+} chelates are the most useful contrast agent and have been in use currently because of relaxation and high paramagnetism [52]. To improve the signal or sensitivity of MRI, different polymer-based nanomaterial platforms have been utilized to carry Gd^{3+} chelates including dendrimers [53–55], polymers [54,56–58], nanoparticles [59], and nanomicelles [60,61]. Many studies have demonstrated that nanocarriers can carry enhanced loading, produce longer circulation time, and improve pharmacokinetic and tissue sensitivity [54,62–64]. Rudovsky et al. have developed the polyamidoamine (PAMAM) dendrimer conjugated to Gd-DOTA (DOTA = 1,4,7,10-tetraazacyclododecane-1,4,7,10-tetraacetic acid) and suggested that the overall relaxivity was significantly improved [53]. Different generations of dendrimer (G1, G2, and G4) were conjugated with chelate by the thiourea linker to form G1-(Gd-DO3A-P$^{BnN\{CS\}}$)$_8$, G2-(Gd-DO3A-P$^{BnN\{CS\}}$)$_{16}$, and G4-(Gd-DO3A-P$^{BnN\{CS\}}$)$_{59}$. The relaxivity and water residence life-time were compared along with the electrostatic interactions. The G1-(Gd-DO3A-P$^{BnN\{CS\}}$)$_8$ increased relaxivity 1.8-fold. The authors concluded that the water exchange process had not affected the relaxivity, but adduct formation reduces the internal motion of the dendrimer. In another study, Gd^{3+}-1,4,7,10-tetraazacyclododecane-1,4,7-triacetic-2-hydroxypropyl-β-cyclodextrin/pluronic (polyrotaxane) dendrimers conjugated with Gd^{3+} chelates have generated a 30-min longer circulation time and were significantly higher in payload with high sensitivity [52]. Nongadolinium contrast agent such as manganese (II) also has been included to enhance the imaging diagnosis with MRI [56]. Zhen Ye et al. have synthesized polydisulfide manganese (II)-based biodegradable macromolecular MRI contrast agents and evaluated the effectiveness in MDA-MB-231 breast cancer mice xenografts model [56]. The authors concluded that polydisulfide Mn(II) complexes and polydisulfide Gd(III) complexes have the same r1 relaxivity, with significant myocardium and tumor enhancement. Hence, manganese should be an alternative nongadolinium contrast agent.

2. **Fluorescence diagnosis:** Fluorescence is another technique widely indicated in imaging and diagnosis. It has been applied to study the phenotypic intracellular organelle changes and targeted drug delivery [65,66]. Olson et al. have developed MRI and fluorescence of dendrimeric nanoparticles [67]. Cy5- and gadolinium-labeled cell-penetrating peptides (ACPPs) conjugated to PAMAM dendrimer

were examined in the HT-1080 tumor mice model. Following tail-vein injection, MRI and fluorescence of dendrimeric nanoparticles (size 200 μm) produced 4- to 15-fold higher uptake in tumor than unconjugated ACPPs. It also increased the florescence intensity and relaxivity [67]. Moreover, after the surgery tumor-free survival was significantly improved in both short term (8 weeks) and long term (24 weeks) melanoma B16F10 model treated groups [68]. These result indicates that there is a significant potential for MRI and fluorescence imaging with dendrimeric nanoparticles to drastically improve tumor diagnosis and provide better treatment.

3. **PET:** PET is an advanced imaging technique that offers picomolar sensitivity with quantitative or semiquantitative imaging modalities. PET imaging detects radiolabeled compounds such as ^{64}Cu, ^{18}F, ^{68}Ga, or ^{89}Zr in the body [69]. Polymer-based carriers have been studied as carrier for such compounds. This technology opens a new vista for PET image—guided drug delivery. It has allowed drug delivery to specific targets thereby producing maximum therapeutic efficacy [70]. Multifunctional polymeric carriers such as liposomes, nanoparticles, nanomicelles, and dendrimers have been studied [71—75]. Paudyal et al. have developed a complex, bevacizumab with the bifunctional chelator radiolabeled with ^{64}Cu and DOTA [74] and examined in colorectal cancer xenografts [74]. The results show higher tumor accumulation of the complex, about 22.7 ± 1.0%ID/g (injected dose/gram) at 24 h, 24 ± 0.2%ID/g at 48 h, and 19.0 ± 2.5%ID/g at 72 h. In another study, Xiao et al. also prepared DOX-loaded multifunctional nanomicelles with tumor targeting, pH-control release, and PET imaging conjugates. The carriers composed of amphiphilic BCP, H40-poly(L-glutamate-hydrazone-doxorubicin)-b-poly(ethylene glycol), cyclo(Arg-Gly-Asp-D-Phe-Cys) peptides, and macrocyclic chelators (1,4,7-triazacyclononane-N,N',N''-triacetic acid [NOTA], for (64)Cu-labeling and PET imaging known as H40-DOX-cRGD [76]. This carrier is prepared by PEG conjugation with peptide (NOTA for PET, represents imaging and pH-sensitive hydrazine for control release) for controlled release. Those modifications have caused higher cellular uptake in U87MG human glioblastoma tumor model. Maximum tumor targeting was achieved while minimizing side effects of DOX.

4. **SPECT:** SPECT is a nuclear imaging technique where radioisotopes such as ^{99m}Tc, ^{123}I, ^{111}In, ^{188}Re, ^{166}Ho, ^{177}Lu, and ^{67}Ga are employed [77,78]. Similar to other imaging techniques, SPECT has been widely applied as an image-guided drug delivery system. Such a system was of significant help in diagnosis and effective treatment of cancer [79]. Polymeric carriers such as liposome, dendrimer, nanomicelles, and nanoparticles have been investigated and studied as a multifunctional carrier for therapeutics and imaging agents with targeting moieties [80]. Cheng et al. have developed glucose-regulated protein 78 binding peptide (GRP78) guided by ^{111}In-labeled poly (ethylene glycol)—poly(ε-caprolactone) in polymeric nanomicelles to treat

gastric cancer [81]. The results indicated a statistically significant higher radioactive intensity with targeted nanomicelle accumulation in tumor compared with untargeted. ^{111}In-labeled micelles in tumor xenograft model. In another study, polymer polyglutamic acid was conjugated with DOX and labeled with ^{99m}Tc for diagnosis and treatment of HER2-positive human mammary carcinoma model (BT-474) [82]. This imaging and targeted carrier can deliver active agents in specific target regions. It has also shown higher survival in mice model while reducing toxicity.

4. CONCLUSION

Polymers have become extremely important carriers for biomedical application such as diagnosis, imaging, and drug delivery. Extensive evaluation of natural and synthetic polymers has been conducted in the past decade. Such polymeric materials are also utilized to prepare microparticles, nanoparticles, neosomes, nanomicelles, and implants/scaffolds. A significant research has been conducted to evaluate these polymers with preclinical evaluations such that these materials can make into clinics. These polymers are being applied in diseases such as, but not limited to, cancer and ocular delivery and to translocate blood—brain barrier to achieve therapeutic levels in the central nervous system (CNS). In the near future, such polymers may aid in reducing the frequency of drug administration. In conclusion, biocompatible, biodegradable, and patient compliant drug delivery, imaging, and diagnostic systems have revolutionized CNS, cancer, and other disease treatment.

REFERENCES

[1] Saravanabhavan SS, Dharmalingam S. Fabrication of polysulphone/hydroxyapatite nanofiber composite implant and evaluation of their in vitro bioactivity and biocompatibility towards the post-surgical therapy of gastric cancer. Chem Eng J 2013;234:380—8.
[2] Liu S, Maheshwari R, Kiick KL. Polymer-based therapeutics. Macromolecules 2009;42(1):3—13.
[3] Pandey SK, Haldar C, Patel DK, Maiti P. Biodegradable polymers for potential delivery systems for therapeutics. Adv Polym Sci 2013;254:169—202.
[4] Bachelder EM, et al. Acetal-derivatized dextran: an acid-responsive biodegradable material for therapeutic applications. J Am Chem Soc 2008;130(32):10494—5.
[5] Duncan R. Polymer conjugates as anticancer nanomedicines. Nat Rev Cancer 2006;6(9):688—701.
[6] Huang Y, et al. Synthesis and therapeutic applications of biocompatible or biodegradable hyperbranched polymers. Polym Chem 2015;6:2794—812.
[7] Cholkar K, Gilger BC, Mitra AK. Topical delivery of aqueous micellar resolvin E1 analog (RX-10045). Int J Pharm 2016;498(1—2):326—34.
[8] Toshinobu Higashimura MS. Living polymerization and selective dimerization: two extremes of the polymer synthesis by cationic polymerization. Adv Polym Sci 2005;62:49—94.
[9] Yoshihiko Ito TM, Suginome M. Structural modification of living polymers: synthesis of helical block copolymers from a single monomer via palladium-mediated aromatizing polymerization of 1,2-diisocyanobenzenes. Macromolecules 2000;33(11):4034—8.
[10] Liechty WB, et al. Polymers for drug delivery systems. Annu Rev Chem Biomol Eng 2010;1:149—73.
[11] Cascone MG, Sim B, Downes S. Blends of synthetic and natural polymers as drug delivery systems for growth hormone. Biomaterials 1995;16(7):569—74.

[12] Park TG, C S, Langer RS. Controlled drug delivery using polymer/pluronic blends. Google patents. 1994 (USA).
[13] Marks JA, et al. Pairwise polymer blends for oral drug delivery. J Pharm Sci 2014;103(9):2871–83.
[14] Munj HR, et al. Biocompatible electrospun polymer blends for biomedical applications. J Biomed Mater Res B Appl Biomater 2014;102(7):1517–27.
[15] Tipduangta P, et al. Electrospun polymer blend nanofibers for tunable drug delivery: the role of transformative phase separation on controlling the release rate. Mol Pharm 2016;13(1):25–39.
[16] Tian-Bin Ren YF, Zhang Z-H, Li L, Li Y-Y. Shell-sheddable micelles based on star-shaped poly(ε-caprolactone)-SS-poly(ethyl glycol) copolymer for intracellular drug release. Soft Matter 2011;7: 2329–31.
[17] Shuai X, et al. Micellar carriers based on block copolymers of poly(epsilon-caprolactone) and poly(ethylene glycol) for doxorubicin delivery. J Control Release 2004;98(3):415–26.
[18] Ikada Y, Tsuji H. Biodegradable polyesters for medical and ecological applications. Macromol Rapid Commun 2000;21(3):117–32.
[19] Binauld S, Stenzel MH. Acid-degradable polymers for drug delivery: a decade of innovation. Chem Commun 2013;49:2082–102.
[20] Boomer JA, Inerowicz HD, Zhang Z-Y, Bergstrand N, Edwards K, Kim J-M, Thompson DH. Acid-triggered release from sterically stabilized fusogenic liposomes via a hydrolytic dePEGylation strategy. Langmuir 2003;19(16):6408–15.
[21] Takae S, et al. PEG-detachable polyplex micelles based on disulfide-linked block catiomers as bioresponsive nonviral gene vectors. J Am Chem Soc 2008;130(18):6001–9.
[22] Saito G, Swanson JA, Lee KD. Drug delivery strategy utilizing conjugation via reversible disulfide linkages: role and site of cellular reducing activities. Adv Drug Deliv Rev 2003;55(2):199–215.
[23] Jin H, et al. Biocompatible or biodegradable hyperbranched polymers: from self-assembly to cytomimetic applications. Chem Soc Rev 2012;41(18):5986–97.
[24] Wang D, et al. Bioapplications of hyperbranched polymers. Chem Soc Rev 2015;44(12):4023–71.
[25] Calderon M, et al. Dendritic polyglycerols for biomedical applications. Adv Mater 2010;22(2): 190–218.
[26] Qi Zhu FQ, Zhu B, Zhu X. Hyperbranched polymers for bioimaging. R Chem Soc Adv 2013;3: 2071–83.
[27] Yuanyuan Zhuang QZ, Tu C, Wang D, Wu J, Xia Y, Tong G, He L, Zhu B, Yan D, Zhu X. Protein resistant properties of polymers with different branched architecture on a gold surface. J Mater Chem 2012;22:23852–60.
[28] Zhuang Y, et al. Facile fabrication of redox-responsive thiol-containing drug delivery system via RAFT polymerization. Biomacromolecules 2014;15(4):1408–18.
[29] Chen C, Liu G, Liu X, Pang S, Zhu C, Lv L, Ji J. Photo-responsive, biocompatible polymeric micelles self-assembled from hyperbranched polyphosphate-based polymers. Polym Chem 2011;2:1389–97.
[30] Zhang L, Gu FX, Chan JM, Wang AZ, Langer RS, Farokhzad OC. Nanoparticles in medicine: therapeutic applications and developments. Clin Pharmacol Ther 2008;83(5):761–9.
[31] Davis FF. Peptide and protein pegylation. Adv Drug Deliv Rev 2002;54(4):457–8.
[32] Mitra AK, M GP. Pentablock polymers. Google patents. 2010 (USA).
[33] Cholkar K, Gilger BC, Mitra AK. Corrigendum to "topical delivery of aqueous micellar resolvin E1 analog (RX-10045)". Int. J. Pharm. 498 (2016) 326–334 Int J Pharm 2016;509(1–2):528.
[34] Cholkar K, Gilger BC, Mitra AK. Topical, aqueous, clear cyclosporine formulation design for anterior and posterior ocular delivery. Transl Vis Sci Technol 2015;4(3):1.
[35] Cholkar K, et al. Nanomicellar topical aqueous drop formulation of rapamycin for back-of-the-eye delivery. AAPS PharmSciTech 2015;16(3):610–22.
[36] Cholkar K, et al. Optimization of dexamethasone mixed nanomicellar formulation. AAPS PharmSciTech 2014;15(6):1454–67.
[37] Vadlapudi AD, et al. Aqueous nanomicellar formulation for topical delivery of biotinylated lipid prodrug of acyclovir: formulation development and ocular biocompatibility. J Ocul Pharmacol Ther 2014;30(1):49–58.

[38] Earla R, et al. Bioanalytical method validation of rapamycin in ocular matrix by QTRAP LC-MS/MS: application to rabbit anterior tissue distribution by topical administration of rapamycin nanomicellar formulation. J Chromatogr B Anal Technol Biomed Life Sci 2012;908:76—86.

[39] Earla R, et al. Development and validation of a fast and sensitive bioanalytical method for the quantitative determination of glucocorticoids — quantitative measurement of dexamethasone in rabbit ocular matrices by liquid chromatography tandem mass spectrometry. J Pharm Biomed Anal 2010; 52(4):525—33.

[40] Ito M. In vitro properties of a chitosan-bonded hydroxyapatite bone-filling paste. Biomaterials 1991; 12(1):41—5.

[41] Higashi S, et al. Polymer-hydroxyapatite composites for biodegradable bone fillers. Biomaterials 1986; 7(3):183—7.

[42] Ge Z, et al. Hydroxyapatite-chitin materials as potential tissue engineered bone substitutes. Biomaterials 2004;25(6):1049—58.

[43] Tokura S, Tamura H. O-carboxymethyl-chitin concentration in granulocytes during bone repair. Biomacromolecules 2001;2(2):417—21.

[44] Farzadi A, Solati-Hashjin M, Bakhshi F, Aminian A. Synthesis and characterization of hydroxyapatite/β-tricalcium phosphate nanocomposites using microwave irradiation. Ceram Int 2011;37(1):65—71.

[45] Murugan R, Ramakrishna S. Bioresorbable composite bone paste using polysaccharide based nano hydroxyapatite. Biomaterials 2004;25(17):3829—35.

[46] Chen F, Wang Z-C, Lin C-J. Preparation and characterization of nanosized hydroxyapatite particles and hydroxyapatite/chitosan nanocomposite for use in biomedical materials. Mater Lett 2002;57: 858—61.

[47] Sudheesh Kumar PT, Srinivasan S, Lakshmanan V-K, Tamura H, Nair SV, Jayakumar R. β-Chitin hydrogel/nano hydroxyapatite composite scaffolds for tissue engineering applications. Carbohydr Polym 2011;85(3):584—91.

[48] Kumar PT, et al. Synthesis, characterization and cytocompatibility studies of alpha-chitin hydrogel/nano hydroxyapatite composite scaffolds. Int J Biol Macromol 2011;49(1):20—31.

[49] Ulery BD, Nair LS, Laurencin CT. Biomedical applications of biodegradable polymers. J Polym Sci B Polym Phys 2011;49(12):832—64.

[50] Maitz MF. Applications of synthetic polymers in clinical medicine. Biosurface Biotribol 2015;1(3): 161—76.

[51] Wang Y-J, Larsson M, Huanga W-T, Chiouc S-H, Nichollsd SJ, Chaoe J-I, Liu D-M. The use of polymer-based nanoparticles and nanostructured materials in treatment and diagnosis of cardiovascular diseases: recent advances and emerging designs. Prog Polym Sci 2016;57:153—78.

[52] Zhou Z, et al. Gd^{3+}-1,4,7,10-Tetraazacyclododecane-1,4,7-triacetic-2-hydroxypropyl-beta-cyclodex trin/pluronic polyrotaxane as a long circulating high relaxivity MRI contrast agent. ACS Appl Mater Interfaces 2015;7(40):22272—6.

[53] Rudovsky J, et al. PAMAM dendrimeric conjugates with a Gd-DOTA phosphinate derivative and their adducts with polyaminoacids: the interplay of global motion, internal rotation, and fast water exchange. Bioconjug Chem 2006;17(4):975—87.

[54] Xu R, et al. Synthesis and evaluation of nanoglobule-cystamine-(Gd-DO3A), a biodegradable nanosized magnetic resonance contrast agent for dynamic contrast-enhanced magnetic resonance urography. Int J Nanomed 2010;5:707—13.

[55] Laus S, et al. Rotational dynamics account for pH-dependent relaxivities of PAMAM dendrimeric, Gd-based potential MRI contrast agents. Chemistry 2005;11(10):3064—76.

[56] Ye Z, et al. Polydisulfide manganese(II) complexes as non-gadolinium biodegradable macromolecular MRI contrast agents. J Magn Reson Imaging 2012;35(3):737—44.

[57] Rowe MD, et al. Tuning the magnetic resonance imaging properties of positive contrast agent nanoparticles by surface modification with RAFT polymers. Langmuir 2009;25(16):9487—99.

[58] Cheng KT, Lu ZR, Kaneshiro T. Gd-DTPA l-Cystine bispropyl amide copolymers. In: Molecular Imaging and Contrast Agent Database (MICAD); 2004. Bethesda (MD).

[59] Chen KJ, et al. A small MRI contrast agent library of gadolinium(III)-encapsulated supramolecular nanoparticles for improved relaxivity and sensitivity. Biomaterials 2011;32(8):2160—5.

[60] Hu J, et al. Drug-loaded and superparamagnetic iron oxide nanoparticle surface-embedded amphiphilic block copolymer micelles for integrated chemotherapeutic drug delivery and MR imaging. Langmuir 2012;28(4):2073–82.
[61] Li X, et al. Amphiphilic multiarm star block copolymer-based multifunctional unimolecular micelles for cancer targeted drug delivery and MR imaging. Biomaterials 2011;32(27):6595–605.
[62] Lu ZR, et al. Polydisulfide Gd(III) chelates as biodegradable macromolecular magnetic resonance imaging contrast agents. Int J Nanomed 2006;1(1):31–40.
[63] Mohs AM, Lu ZR. Gadolinium(III)-based blood-pool contrast agents for magnetic resonance imaging: status and clinical potential. Expert Opin Drug Deliv 2007;4(2):149–64.
[64] Zong Y, et al. Contrast-enhanced MRI with new biodegradable macromolecular Gd(III) complexes in tumor-bearing mice. Magn Reson Med 2005;53(4):835–42.
[65] Chowdhury SR, et al. Simultaneous evaluation of substrate-dependent oxygen consumption rates and mitochondrial membrane potential by TMRM and safranin in cortical mitochondria. Biosci Rep 2016;36(1):e00286.
[66] Graef F, Gordon S, Lehr CM. Anti-infectives in drug delivery-overcoming the gram-negative bacterial cell envelope. Curr Top Microbiol Immunol 2016;398:475–96.
[67] Olson ES, et al. Activatable cell penetrating peptides linked to nanoparticles as dual probes for in vivo fluorescence and MR imaging of proteases. Proc Natl Acad Sci USA 2010;107(9):4311–6.
[68] Nguyen QT, et al. Surgery with molecular fluorescence imaging using activatable cell-penetrating peptides decreases residual cancer and improves survival. Proc Natl Acad Sci USA 2010;107(9): 4317–22.
[69] Ametamey SM, Honer M, Schubiger PA. Molecular imaging with PET. Chem Rev 2008;108(5): 1501–16.
[70] Chakravarty R, Hong H, Cai W. Positron emission tomography image-guided drug delivery: current status and future perspectives. Mol Pharm 2014;11(11):3777–97.
[71] Lammers T, et al. Nanotheranostics and image-guided drug delivery: current concepts and future directions. Mol Pharm 2010;7(6):1899–912.
[72] Rossin R, et al. In vivo imaging of ^{64}Cu-labeled polymer nanoparticles targeted to the lung endothelium. J Nucl Med 2008;49(1):103–11.
[73] Liu S, et al. PET imaging of colorectal and breast cancer by targeting EphB4 receptor with ^{64}Cu-labeled hAb47 and hAb131 antibodies. J Nucl Med 2013;54(7):1094–100.
[74] Paudyal B, et al. Positron emission tomography imaging and biodistribution of vascular endothelial growth factor with ^{64}Cu-labeled bevacizumab in colorectal cancer xenografts. Cancer Sci 2011; 102(1):117–21.
[75] Jensen AI, et al. Positron emission tomography based analysis of long-circulating cross-linked triblock polymeric micelles in a U87MG mouse xenograft model and comparison of DOTA and CB-TE2A as chelators of copper-64. Biomacromolecules 2014;15(5):1625–33.
[76] Xiao Y, et al. Multifunctional unimolecular micelles for cancer-targeted drug delivery and positron emission tomography imaging. Biomaterials 2012;33(11):3071–82.
[77] Mariani G, et al. A review on the clinical uses of SPECT/CT. Eur J Nucl Med Mol Imaging 2010; 37(10):1959–85.
[78] Chakravarty R, Hong H, Cai W. Image-guided drug delivery with single-photon emission computed tomography: a review of literature. Curr Drug Targets 2015;16(6):592–609.
[79] Brandon D, et al. The role of single-photon emission computed tomography and SPECT/computed tomography in oncologic imaging. Semin Oncol 2011;38(1):87–108.
[80] Patil V, et al. Imaging small human prostate cancer xenografts after pretargeting with bispecific bombesin–antibody complexes and targeting with high specific radioactivity labeled polymer–drug conjugates. Eur J Nucl Med Mol Imaging 2012;39(5):824–39.
[81] Cheng CC, et al. Novel targeted nuclear imaging agent for gastric cancer diagnosis: glucose-regulated protein 78 binding peptide-guided ^{111}In-labeled polymeric micelles. Int J Nanomed 2013;8:1385–91.
[82] Khaw BA, et al. Bispecific antibody complex pre-targeting and targeted delivery of polymer drug conjugates for imaging and therapy in dual human mammary cancer xenografts: targeted polymer drug conjugates for cancer diagnosis and therapy. Eur J Nucl Med Mol Imaging 2014;41(8):1603–16.

[83] Wang Z, et al. The effect of thick fibers and large pores of electrospun poly(epsilon-caprolactone) vascular grafts on macrophage polarization and arterial regeneration. Biomaterials 2014;35(22):5700–10.

[84] Li P, et al. Applying electrospun gelatin/poly(lactic acid-*co*-glycolic acid) bilayered nanofibers to fabrication of meniscal tissue engineering scaffold. J Nanosci Nanotechnol 2016;16(5):4718–26.

[85] Sandri M, et al. Fabrication and pilot in vivo study of a collagen-BDDGE-elastin core-shell scaffold for tendon regeneration. Front Bioeng Biotechnol 2016;4:52.

[86] Forget J, et al. Differentiation of human mesenchymal stem cells toward quality cartilage using fibrinogen-based nanofibers. Macromol Biosci 2016.

[87] Gugutkov D, et al. Electrospun fibrinogen-PLA nanofibres for vascular tissue engineering. J Tissue Eng Regen Med 2016. http://dx.doi.org/10.1002/term.2172.

[88] Singh BN, et al. Carboxymethyl cellulose enables silk fibroin nanofibrous scaffold with enhanced biomimetic potential for bone tissue engineering application. Carbohydr Polym 2016;151:335–47.

[89] Singh YP, Bhardwaj N, Mandal BB. Potential of agarose/silk fibroin blended hydrogel for in vitro cartilage tissue engineering. ACS Appl Mater Interfaces 2016.

[90] Park YR, et al. Three-dimensional electrospun silk-fibroin nanofiber for skin tissue engineering. Int J Biol Macromol 93(Pt B), December 2016:1567–74.

[91] Dhand C, et al. Bio-inspired in situ crosslinking and mineralization of electrospun collagen scaffolds for bone tissue engineering. Biomaterials October 2016;104:323–38.

[92] Huang L, et al. Morphological study of dynamic culture of thermosensitive collagen hydrogel in constructing tissue engineering complex. Bioengineered 2016;7(4):266–73.

[93] Pinnagoda K, et al. Engineered acellular collagen scaffold for endogenous cell guidance, a novel approach in urethral regeneration. Acta Biomater 2016.

[94] Lih E, et al. Biomimetic porous PLGA scaffolds incorporating decellularized extracellular matrix for kidney tissue regeneration. ACS Appl Mater Interfaces August 24, 2016;8(33):21145–54.

[95] Dai Y, et al. Cell-free HA-MA/PLGA scaffolds with radially oriented pores for in situ inductive regeneration of full thickness cartilage defects. Macromol Biosci November 2016;16(11):1632–42.

[96] Yan W, et al. In vitro investigation of nanohydroxyapatite/poly(L-lactic acid) spindle composites used for bone tissue engineering. J Mater Sci Mater Med 2016;27(8):130.

CHAPTER 2

Multifunctional Micro- and Nanoparticles

Rubi Mahato
Fairleigh Dickinson University, Florham Park, NJ, United States

Contents

1. Introduction	21
1.1 Microparticles	22
1.2 Nanoparticles	25
1.3 Trojan Microparticles	26
1.4 Multifunctional Micro- and Nanoparticles	26
2. Micro- and Nanomaterials in the Synthesis of Multifunctional Carriers	27
2.1 Lipid-Based Micro/Nanocarriers	28
2.1.1 Liposome	*28*
2.1.2 Microemulsions	*29*
2.1.3 Solid-Lipid Nanoparticles	*29*
2.2 Polymeric Micro/Nanocarriers	30
2.2.1 Natural Polymers	*30*
2.2.2 Synthetic Polymers	*30*
2.3 Inorganic Micro/Nanocarriers	31
2.3.1 Quantum Dots	*31*
2.3.2 Magnetic Nanoparticles	*32*
2.3.3 Gold Nanoparticles	*32*
3. Types of Functional Moieties	32
3.1 Peptides	32
3.2 Proteins and Antibodies	33
3.3 Nucleic Acids	33
3.4 Carbohydrates	34
3.5 Fluorescent Dyes	34
4. Functionalization of Micro- and Nanoparticles	35
4.1 Methods of Conjugating Functional Moieties to Micro- and Nanoparticles	35
References	39

1. INTRODUCTION

In the past two decades (between 1995–2015) particulate drug delivery systems have grown from their novice stage to the development of micro- and nanoparticle-based products for diagnostic and therapeutic purposes. Some of these technologies have been approved for clinical application, and many more have advanced to clinical trial.

Currently micro- and nanotechnology is actively pursued in various areas of scientific research, and the area has attracted many scientists from multidisciplinary scientific field. By definition, microparticles are particulate dispersion or solid particles with a size in the range of 1–1000 µm, whereas nanoparticles represent solid particles in the size range of 1–1000 nm. However, a majority of the microparticles and nanoparticles are smaller than 100 µm and 200 nm, respectively. A difference in the size between micro- and nanoparticles elicits various effects in terms of morphology and behavior. Nanoparticles show better penetration through the biological tissues, barriers, and cellular membranes. However, they do possess some disadvantages such as smaller retention time in tissues, body cavities, and blood circulation. On the other hand, microparticles may not penetrate very deep into tissue, and can deliver cargo into cells that are phagocytic in nature, but display longer retention time [1]. In terms of pharmaceutical applications micro- and nanoparticles have been widely employed in medicine, biochemistry, and aerosol research. Micro- and nanoparticles offer a number of advantages over the conventional dosage form, the most useful of which is that these particles can be formulated into solid, liquid, and semisolid dosage forms. As a solid dosage form the particles can be formulated as dry powder, which can be applied for pulmonary delivery by inhalation. As a liquid dosage form these particles can be injected into tissue as well as blood circulation. As a semisolid dosage form the drug can be incorporated into a suitable vehicle and can be formulated for topical application. Micro- and nanoparticle formulations can be administered through various routes such as oral, parenteral, pulmonary, nasal, ocular, and transdermal [2]. The dosages can be self-administered or be integrated into the microneedle device [3]. In addition, microparticles and nanoparticles (NPs) can be formulated to deliver poorly soluble drugs, to protect the drug from chemical and proteolytic degradation, and to reduce the dose. The particles tend to accumulate in inflamed tissue, which in turn improves the efficacy and reduces toxicity. Moreover, such particles can be designed as extended release dosage form to improve patient compliance [4,5]. Besides, the particles can be modified with specific ligands to target cell, tissue, or organ, along with a fluorescent dye for imaging. Such modified particulates are known as multifunctional micro-nanoparticles. Multifunctional micro- and nanoparticle systems can integrate targeting, imaging, and treatment modalities on the surface and core of the particulate structure, resulting in more effective treatment in various diseased tissues [6]. Table 2.1 summarizes a number of nanoparticle-based drug and delivery systems that have been approved or are undergoing clinic trials.

1.1 Microparticles

In general microparticles fall in the size range of 1–1000 µm; such forms are commercially available in a wide variety of materials including ceramics, glass, polymers, and metals. These are small particles made of solid or small liquid droplets surrounded by a

Table 2.1 Nanoparticle-based medicines already approved by the FDA or undergoing clinic trial

Commercial name	Platform	Targeting ligand	Active pharmaceutical ingredient	Indication	Status	References
Nanoparticle systems without targeting ligand						
DaunoXome	Liposome		Daunorubicin	Kaposi sarcoma	Approved	[8]
Myocet	Liposome		Doxorubicin	Combinational therapy of recurrent breast and ovarian cancer	Approved	[9]
Doxil/Caelyx	PEG-liposome		Doxorubicin	Refractory Kaposi sarcoma, recurrent breast and ovarian cancer	Approved	[10]
Onco TCS	Liposome		Vincristine	Relapsed aggressive non-Hodgkin lymphoma	Approved	[11]
Abraxane	Albumin-bound paclitaxel NP		Paclitaxel	Metastatic breast cancer	Approved	[12]
Genexol-PM	PLA-PEG micelle		Paclitaxel	Metastatic breast cancer	Approved	[13]
Nanoparticle systems with targeting ligands						
CALAA-01	Cyclodextrin-containing polymeric NP	Transferrin	siRNA	Solid tumor	Phase I	[14]
MBP-426	Liposome	Transferrin	Oxaliplatin	Gastric, esophageal, gastric-esophageal adenocarcinoma	Phase Ib/II	[15]
MCC-465	Liposome	F(ab')$_2$ fragment of human Ab GAH	Doxorubicin	Metastatic stomach cancer	Phase I (not continued)	[16]
BIND-014	PLGA-PEG NP	PSMA-specific peptide	Docetaxel	Solid tumor	Phase I	[17]
SGT53-01	Liposome	Transferrin receptor-specific scAb	p53 gene	Solid tumor	Phase I	[18]

FDA, Food and Drug Administration; *GAH*, goat anti human; *NP*, nanoparticle; *PEG*, poly(ethylene glycol); *PLGA*, poly(D,L-lactic-co-glycolic acid); *PLA*, poly (lactic acid); *PSMA*, prostate specific membrane antigen; *siRNA*, small interfering RNA.
Adapted and modified from Yu MK, Park J, Jon S. Targeting strategies for multifunctional nanoparticles in cancer imaging and therapy. Theranostics 2012;2(1):3. http://www.thno.org/v02p0003.htm.

membrane of natural or synthetic polymer film of varying thickness and permeability. The film also acts as a release rate controlling substance [19]. Microparticles are usually encountered in daily life including pollen, flour, powdered sugar, sand, and dust. Microparticles carry a much larger surface area-to-volume ratio than the macro forms. Thus their behavior can be different. For example, metal microparticles can be explosive in air.

In biological systems, however, microparticles refer to small membrane-bound vesicles that are released from the cell surface by the process of outward budding. These microparticles are therefore composed of fragments of parent cell, which comprises the plasma membrane proteins, as well as nucleic and cytoplasmic constituents of the parent cell [20,21]. Once the microparticles bud off from the parent cells the particles are released into the systemic circulation, and can deliver the cargo to the recipient cells [22].

In this chapter we focus on the general types of unmodified microparticles and multifunctional microparticles. Microparticles are formed by entrapping or encapsulating an agent in the form of solid, liquid, or gas, into a polymeric matrix or shell. Depending on the method of preparation these microcarriers can be developed as microparticles, microcapsules, or microspheres. In a microparticle, the drug is physically and uniformly dispersed, whereas microcapsules are micrometric reservoirs containing the drug in the core completely surrounded by a polymeric shell. Microspheres sometimes are also referred to as microbeads or monolithic spheres, where the therapeutic agent is either homogenously dissolved or dispersed in a polymeric matrix (Fig. 2.1) [4].

Microparticles may be prepared as free-flowing powders in various shapes (e.g., globular, spherical, elliptical, kidney-shaped, rice grain-shaped), flocculent and massive, collected as dry aggregates, or suspended directly in a vehicle for administration. The active ingredient may be dispersed in a protective matrix or it may be surrounded by a coating, shell, or membrane. The thickness of the membrane is generally within the range of 0.2 µm to several micrometers. The release of active ingredient from the core material across the surrounding shell is controlled by various mechanisms, such as mechanical rupture of the shell wall or gradual degradation (e.g., dissolution, diffusion, chemically triggered, or biodegradation) [23,24].

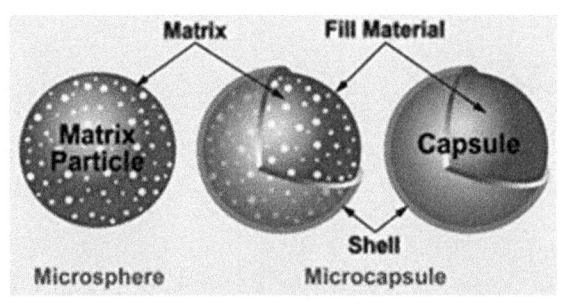

Figure 2.1 Microparticle structures. *(Reprinted with permission from Manjanna K, Shivakumar B., Kumar TP. Microencapsulation: an acclaimed novel drug-delivery system for NSAIDs in arthritis. Crit Rev Ther Drug Carr Syst 2010;27(6). (Copyright 2010 Begell House.))*

1.2 Nanoparticles

Nanoscale carriers range in size from 1 nm to less than 1000 nm, which falls in the range of colloidal dispersion. Fig. 2.2 depicts examples of different nanomedicines and their approximate sizes. NPs can easily penetrate through the tissue and cell membrane. Therefore drug absorption is significantly increased at the site of administration. In spite of these advantages, NPs face the challenge of efficient administration and transport to the absorption sites, such as pulmonary alveoli, intestinal mucosa, and ocular and CNS barriers. This is especially true in the case of pulmonary administration. Due to their size, the dose can be cleared rapidly from the system. Another limitation of nanoparticles includes the chances of particle–particle aggregation due to small size and large surface area, which may lead to limited drug loading and burst release. In addition, only the NP of appropriate size and modified surface chemistry can escape the immediate recognition by the immune system, thereby increasing the circulation time [25,26]. Nevertheless,

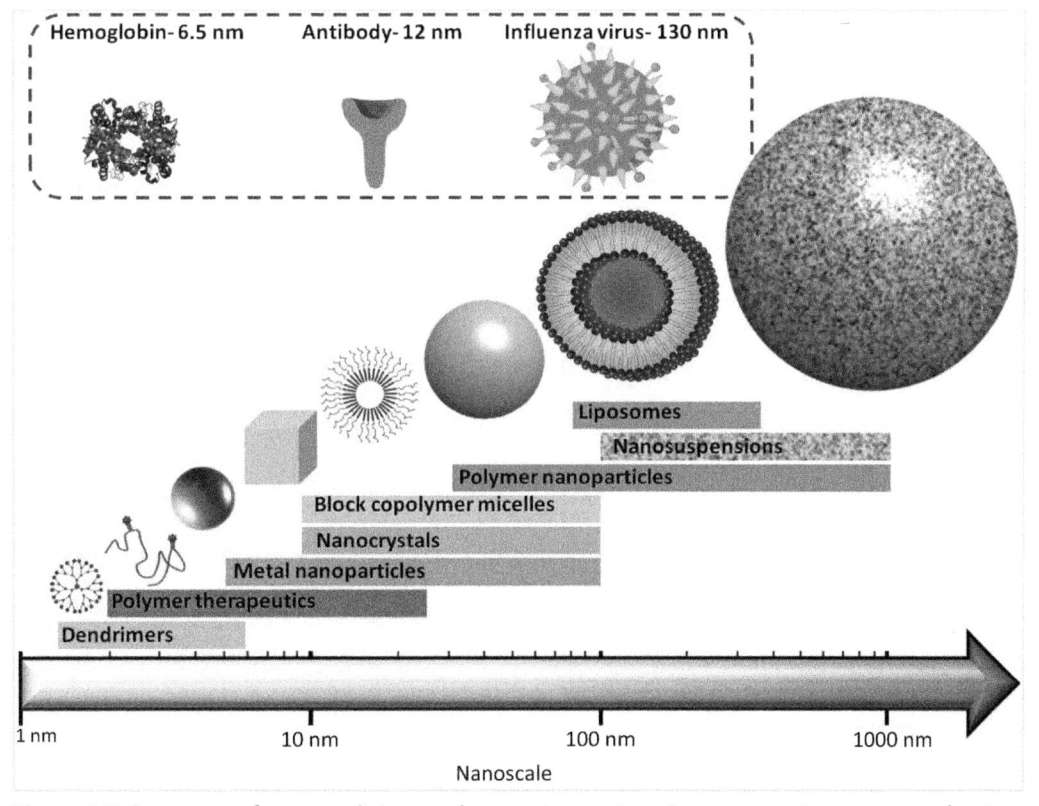

Figure 2.2 Structures of nanomedicines and approximate sizes. For comparative purposes, the sizes of biological nanostructures are shown at the top of the figure. *(Reproduced with permission from the British Society for nanomedicine web page (www.BritishSocietyNanomedicine.org).)*

the unique optical properties, appropriate size scale, ease of synthesis, and facile surface chemistry of nanoparticles can overcome these drawbacks. Additionally, nanoparticles can be designed to tailor drug release kinetics due to internal environment such as pH or external stimuli such as ultrasound, heat, and magnet. An advantage of controlled release may be the unlikeliness of premature dissociation of the drug from the NP before it reaches the target site, thereby the system can minimize drug accumulation in healthy tissues and organs, lowering systemic toxicity [6].

1.3 Trojan Microparticles

A disadvantage of nanoparticles is that their size range is too small to ensure retention in the deep lung. The particles can be inhaled, but these constructs are totally expelled during exhalation. The larger microparticles in micron size ensure their retention into the system for a longer period, but the constructs poorly penetrate cell and tissue relative to nanoparticles. The ideal particle sizes for pulmonary administration are between 2 and 5 μm, corresponding to the typical size of microparticles. Therefore such microparticles may be the optimal system for targeting the pulmonary alveoli. However, these particles are too large to diffuse and allow an efficient administration. This problem can be solved by combining the properties of micro- and nanoparticles through encapsulation of nanoparticles in microparticles. The multiscale nano-in-microparticle systems are known as Trojan particles [27]. Such particles as taken up by the target site can be retained for a fairly long time, especially in the pulmonary alveoli, and then the NPs are released, which can diffuse through the barriers.

1.4 Multifunctional Micro- and Nanoparticles

The horizon of micro-nanoparticles is rapidly expanding. Researchers in this field have developed newer fabrication techniques from engineering perspective to develop complex multifunctional particles. Such multifunctional particles can accomplish multiple tasks, such as imaging, diagnostics, and therapy. It can also perform a single advanced function by incorporating multiple units. Multifunctional micro- or nanoparticles enable simultaneous delivery of multiple therapeutic agents, such as gene silencing and drug delivery. Moreover, imaging agent (for diagnostic purpose) and drug targeting can be combined. In contrast to monofunctional micro/nanoparticles that deliver only a single payload of an active agent, multifunctional micro/nanoparticles can integrate various functionalities inside the core of the particle or on the surface to synergistically achieve maximal therapeutic effect (Fig. 2.3). Currently many clinical trials are being conducted with various combinations of micro- and nanoparticles to achieve the optimal result [28–30]. Micro-nanoparticles have been successfully and effectively modified to target cancer cells [6] and to deliver insulin across skin, intestinal wall, or other mucosae [31]. It can also incorporate stimuli-responsive elements for releasing the drug in an

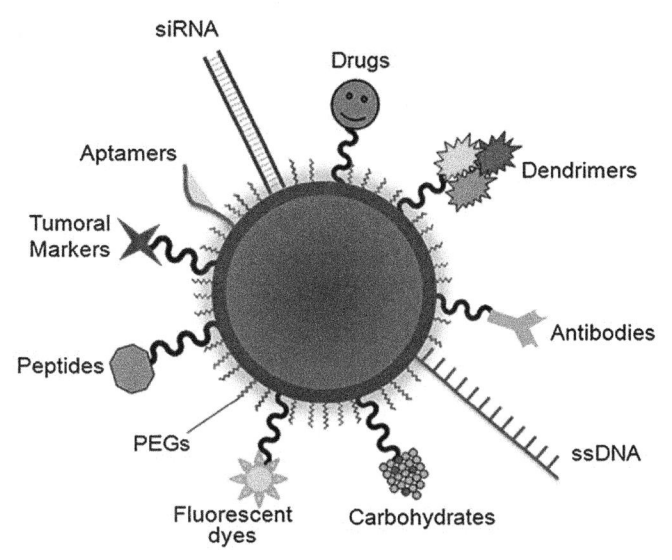

Figure 2.3 *Schematic representation of a multifunctional micro/nanocarrier.* Micro- and nanoparticles contain nucleic acids such as RNA and DNA for gene silencing and colorimetric assays. Aptamers and anticancer agents can also be modified for delivery to the target tissue. Carbohydrates may be included as sensitive colorimetric probes. Polyethyleneglycol can improve solubility and lower immunogenicity. Responsive nanocarriers can also trigger reactions due to external stimuli. Tumor markers, peptides, carbohydrates, polymers, and antibodies (Abs) can be included to improve micro- and nanocarrier residence time, effectiveness, and selectivity. Multifunctional systems can also carry fluorescent dyes that can act as reporter molecules tethered to particle surfaces and employed as tracking and/or contrast agents [32]. *(Adapted from Conde J, et al. Revisiting 30 years of biofunctionalization and surface chemistry of inorganic nanoparticles for nanomedicine. Front Chem, 2014;2:48. http://dx.doi.org/10.3389/fchem.2014.00048.)*

on-demand manner. In this chapter, multifunctional micro-nanoparticle systems featuring a variety of targeting moieties for in vitro and/or in vivo imaging and therapy are discussed.

2. MICRO- AND NANOMATERIALS IN THE SYNTHESIS OF MULTIFUNCTIONAL CARRIERS

Micro- and nanoparticles are prepared with a number of organic and inorganic materials. Multifunctional micro-nanoparticles are fabricated by conjugating or integrating one or more of functionalization units, such as targeting ligands, therapeutic, imaging, and delivering agents. Organic micro-nanoparticles, such as liposomes, dendrimers, polymeric micelles, and micro/nanogels are attractive building blocks for multifunctional micro/nanoparticles due to their versatile surface and core chemistry, high degree of biodegradability, effective endocytosis by the target cell, and high payload efficiency [33]. Organic micro/nanoparticles can be divided into lipid-based carriers and polymeric carriers. Lipid-based carriers include liposome, microemulsion, and solid-lipid micro-nanoparticles, whereas polymeric carriers include linear chain of polymer, solid micro/nanoparticle, micro/nanogel, nanomicelle, layer-by-layer carriers, dendrimer, and polymersome. On the other hand, inorganic carriers include gold nanoparticles, silica nanoparticles, magnetic particles, and quantum dots (QDs) (Fig. 2.4).

2.1 Lipid-Based Micro/Nanocarriers
2.1.1 Liposome
Liposomes are lipid bilayer spherical vesicles (50–100 nm) made of phospholipids, cholesterol, or other similar lipid molecules. Such vesicles display similar structures to biological membranes with an internal aqueous phase. Based on size and number of layers liposomes can be classified into unilamellar, multilammelar, and oligolamellar [34]. Their amphiphilic nature enables liposomes to transport hydrophilic drugs such as small

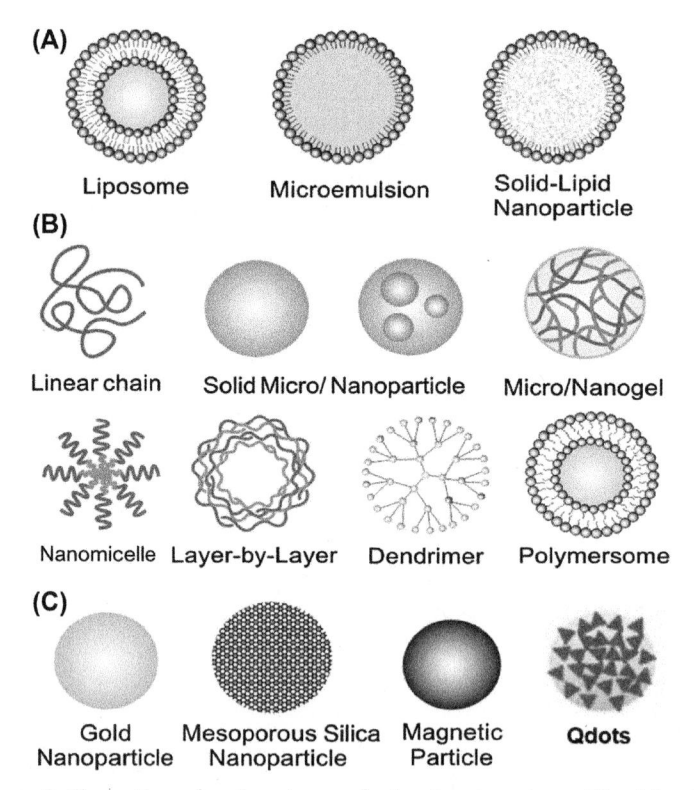

Figure 2.4 Schematic illustration of various types of micro/nanocarriers utilized for drug delivery. (A) Lipid-based carriers. (B) Polymeric carriers. (C) Inorganic carriers. *(Reprinted and modified with permission from Mo R, et al. Emerging micro-and nanotechnology based synthetic approaches for insulin delivery. Chem Soc Rev 2014;43(10):3595–629. (Copyright 2014; Royal Society of Chemistry.))*

interfering RNA (siRNA), microRNA (miRNA), plasmid DNA, and insulin entrapped within the aqueous interior [31,35], whereas hydrophobic drugs are trapped into the lipid membrane. Physicochemical properties of liposomes render excellent circulation, penetration, and diffusion. Moreover, the liposome surface can be modified with ligands and/or polymers to increase cell specificity [36]. pH- and enzyme-sensitive drugs such as insulin entrapped in the liposomes can be effectively protected from pH variation, enzymatic attack, and immune recognition. Moreover, liposome surface coating and ligand modification can improve drug stability in the gastrointestinal lumen. Liposomes can be coated with poly(ethylene glycol) (PEG-lipid) or sugar chain derived from mucin (mucin-lipid) or chitosan (CS; chitosan-lipid) to increase the oral delivery and stability of drug payloads and improve circulation time of the liposome [31].

2.1.2 Microemulsions
The term microemulsion in self-microemulsifying drug delivery systems refers to small particles or droplets with the actual size less than 250 nm. These droplets exhibit high flexibility [37,38]. Unlike emulsions, lipid-based micro/nanoemulsions are single optically isotropic and thermodynamically stable solutions. Such transparent solutions are composed of water as a dispersed phase and oil as an external dispersion phase stabilized by surfactant or cosurfactant with the hydrophilic block around the aqueous core and the hydrophobic tails in the oil phase [39,40].

These micro- and nanoemulsions also display enhanced drug permeation across the intestinal wall, thereby significantly increasing oral drug bioavailability [41,42]. Microemulsions have been extensively utilized to enhance permeation of small as well as large molecules such as plasmid DNA [3]. The advantages of microemulsion over other formulations are that it is easy to prepare, scale up, and there is almost 100% drug entrapment. In addition, because of thermodynamic stability it remains stable over a long period.

2.1.3 Solid-Lipid Nanoparticles
Solid-lipid nanoparticles (SLNs) are submicron colloidal carriers composed of a single lipid core matrix that is solid at body temperature, and is coated with a surfactant acting as stabilizer [43–45]. These structures are more stable than liposomes or emulsions. As a result of the relatively inflexible core lipids that are solid at body temperature, SLNs are rigid and can have either positive or negative charge, with average sizes ranging between 50 and 1000 nm [38]. Biodegradable, biocompatible, and physiological lipids are generally utilized to prepare these nanoparticles, hence toxicity associated with the polymeric nanoparticles are minimized. Oral absorption and bioavailability of several drugs have been improved by formulating them into drug-loaded SLN particles [46]. SLNs can be functionalized with various materials, such as CS to improve oral bioavailability of insulin [47]; apolipoprotein E, which is recognized by low-density lipoprotein receptors on blood–brain barrier for targeted drug delivery into the brain [48]; polylysine–heparin for

tenofovir (vaginal microbicide) delivery for human immunodeficiency virus (HIV) prevention [49]; and anti-CD64 antibody that specifically targets macrophages in rheumatoid arthritis along with in vivo imaging [50].

2.2 Polymeric Micro/Nanocarriers

Polymeric micro/nanocarriers are drug carriers of natural, semisynthetic, and synthetic polymers within the nano- to microscale range. These carriers may include polymeric micro/nanospheres and micro/nanocapsules. The former consists of polymeric particle matrices, whereas the latter denotes vesicles (generally oily) covered with polymers [51]. Polymeric particles provide stability and protection of macromolecular drugs such as proteins, peptides, or DNA molecules from various environmental hazards such as pH, temperature, and enzymatic degradation [52–55]. Polymeric NPs have been extensively applied to oral, transdermal, and ocular delivery systems.

2.2.1 Natural Polymers

This class of polymers consists of CS, alginate, albumin, hyaluronic acid (HA), collagen, and gelatin. The natural polymers have been extensively used to prepare micro- and nanoparticles. Among them, CS has been frequently utilized in the preparation of NPs with different routes of delivery.

2.2.1.1 Chitosan-Based Micro/nanoparticles

CS is a natural cationic polysaccharide composed of glucosamine and N-acetylglucosamine units, which impart properties such as biocompatibility, biodegradability, and nontoxicity [56]. The physicochemical properties of CS are remarkably dependent on the degree of deacetylation, molecular weight, and surrounding pH value. CS is extensively utilized for superior mucoadhesive property and penetration-enhancing effect, which can increase drug bioavailability [57,58]. CS-based micro/nanoparticles have been successfully used to deliver drugs by different routes, including oral [58], topical [59], pulmonary [60], and nasal [61].

2.2.2 Synthetic Polymers

Synthetic polymers can be structured into two different groups: biodegradables and nonbiodegradables. Poly(D,L-lactic-co-glycolic acid) (PLGA) is the most commonly selected biodegradable polymer, whereas polyacrylamide and polystyrene are considered as nondegradable polymers for the preparation of micro- and nanoparticles.

2.2.2.1 Dendrimers

Dendrimers are highly branched synthetic polymers with a diameter less than 15 nm. The polymers possess layered architectures constituting a central core, an internal region, and numerous terminal groups that determine dendrimer properties. Dendrimers can accommodate multiple functionalities at the terminal groups. A dendrimer can be prepared by multiple types of chemistry, the nature of which defines the dendrimer solubility and biological activity. Dendritic molecules, such as polyamidoamine, poly(propylene imine) polyamide, polyglycerol, and triazine, are synthesized by assembling monomeric subunits. The aggregates form uniform tree-like structures that allow for encapsulation of drug payload in the internal star structures. The branches and terminal groups can be complexed with functionalities, such as targeting ligands, imaging and diagnostic agents, as well as other drug molecules [62,63].

2.2.2.2 Nanomicelles
Nanomicelles are self-assembling nanosized (10–100 nm) colloidal dispersions with a core and shell structure [64]. The structures are constructed with amphiphilic blocks with the core made up of hydrophobic blocks, such as propylene oxide, L-lysine, aspartic acid, D,L-lactic acid, PLGA, and spermine, whereas the outer shell consists of hydrophilic blocks, such as PEG, polyethyleneimine, poly(N-vinyl-2-pyrrolidone), and poly(vinyl alcohol) [65,66]. Nanomicelles can encapsulate hydrophobic drugs and imaging agents in the core, thus circumventing the need for toxic organic solvents. These nanomicelles can deliver drugs by systemic, ocular, transdermal, and oral routes.

2.2.2.3 Micro/Nanogel
Polymeric micro/nanogels are fabricated by cross-linking polymer chains to create an inner porous space that can accommodate a large volume of payload, and therefore are conducive for simultaneous delivery of multiple treatment modalities [67].

2.3 Inorganic Micro/Nanocarriers

Inorganic micro- and nanoparticles, such as QDs, polystyrene, magnetic, ceramic, and metallic nanoparticles, contain a central core composed of inorganic materials that define their fluorescent, magnetic, electronic, and optical properties [34]. Carbon nanotubes and fullerene may be categorized as inorganic nanoparticles. The rigid outer surface and the durable core of these inorganic carriers can be complexed with a variety of drug/active agent payloads.

2.3.1 Quantum Dots
QDs are colloidal fluorescent semiconductor nanocrystals (2–10 nm) with narrow emission and a broad range of absorption bands. This material is predominantly used in fabricating imaging probes [68]. The central core of QDs consists of combinations of elements from groups II–VI of the periodic system (CdSe, CdTe, CdS, PbSe, ZnS, and ZnSe) or III–V (GaAs, GaN, InP, and InAs), which are "overcoated" with a layer of ZnS. QDs are photostable, and resistant to photobleaching. These dots show exceptional resistance to

photo and chemical degradation. These properties render QDs excellent contrast agents for imaging and labels for bioassays [69].

2.3.2 Magnetic Nanoparticles
Magnetic nanoparticles are iron derivative spherical nanocrystals of 10—20 nm size with a Fe^{2+} and Fe^{3+} core surrounded by dextran or PEG molecules. Due to magnetic properties these particles can be employed to label biomolecules in bioassays, as well as magnetic resonance imaging (MRI) and image contrast for the diagnosis of tumor and other diseases [70,71]. Magnetic nanoparticles can be applied in magnetic-assisted drug delivery, targeting, hyperthermia treatment of tumors, and magnetic transfection of cells [72].

2.3.3 Gold Nanoparticles
Gold nanoparticles can be considered as a type of metallic nanoparticle; others are made of Ni, Pt, and TiO_2 nanoparticles. Gold nanoparticles (AuNPs), also known as colloidal gold, constitute a suspension of submicrometer-sized gold metal particle in a fluid and can be obtained with diameters between 3 and 200 nm [73]. Gold nanoparticles (<50 nm) can be prepared with different geometries, such as nanospheres, nanoshells, nanorods, or nanocages. These particles show localized surface plasmon resonant properties, i.e., under irradiation they absorb light and emit photons with the same frequency in all directions. Gold nanoparticles possess extraordinary optical and electronic properties with high stability and biocompatibility, which render these particles excellent label as biosensors for imaging and diagnostic purposes [73,74]. AuNPs are fabricated along with the organic polymers (liposome) to form hybrid systems. This construct can integrate diagnostic and therapeutic agents for effective delivery accompanied by real-time monitoring of treatment response and tumor growth [75].

3. TYPES OF FUNCTIONAL MOIETIES
3.1 Peptides
Peptides have the potential for stabilization and functionalization of micro- and nanoparticles. Wang et al. demonstrated that multiple functional peptide can stabilize AuNPs with a one-step surface coating procedure. The surface functionalities can be selectively addressed on a microarray [76]. The stability conferred by peptide ligands usually depends on their length, hydrophobicity, and charge. Biofunctional peptide sequences, such as "membrane translocation signals" like the HIV-TAT peptide sequence [77], are capable of transporting nanoscale materials across cell membranes. "Nuclear localization signals" could be used for further intracellular targeting [78].

Peptides have been utilized to fabricate multifunctional nanoparticles for targeted cancer imaging and therapy. Medarova et al. synthesized a breast tumor—targeted nanodrug designed to specifically shuttle siRNA to human breast cancer. Simultaneously the construct allows noninvasive monitoring of the siRNA delivery process [79].

3.2 Proteins and Antibodies

Specific functions of proteins such as antigen—antibody detection may be very useful in targeted delivery. The primary advantage of Abs or their fragments is that the antigen-binding region is highly specific as well as different among Abs [80]. Therefore different specificities can be imparted with distinct Abs. However, attachment of Abs to the surface of micro- and nanoparticles can impair this function if the antigen-binding sites are sterically blocked due to conjugation.

The presence of two epitope-binding sites in a single Ab offers an exceedingly high selectivity and binding affinity for the target of interest. Rituximab (Rituxan) for non-Hodgkin lymphoma treatment, trastuzumab (Herceptin) for breast cancer treatment, bevacizumab (Avastin) designed to inhibit angiogenesis, and cetuximab (Erbitux) for advanced colorectal cancer treatment have been developed and approved by the Food and Drug Administration for use as therapeutic Abs [7]. Abs can be utilized as whole molecules or a small fragment consisting binding sites such as scfv or fab fragments [81—83]. AuNP-cetuximab Ab conjugate [84] and QD-antibody conjugates [85,86] have also been widely indicated as bioconjugated nanocarriers for simultaneous tumor detection, inhibition, and in vitro bioassay applications, respectively. Moreover, immunoliposomes (antibody-conjugated liposomes) can be utilized for targeted delivery of hydrophilic as well as hydrophobic agents because of liposome's ability to encapsulate both. Wu et al. employed anti-c-Met scFv antibody-conjugated PEGylated liposomes for efficient delivery of doxorubicin to c-Met overexpressing lung cancer cells as well as xenograft model [87]. These constructs enhanced cellular uptake and tumor accumulation of the drug, thereby antitumor activity.

3.3 Nucleic Acids

By modifying a nucleic acid with a thiol group in either the $5'$ or $3'$ end it is possible to assemble DNA onto the AuNP surface [88]. The reaction variables such as salt concentration, oligo/NP ratio or micro- and nanoparticle size can be controlled. This property can be used for AuNP modification with DNAs, which can be applied in biosensing or as DNA probe for diagnosis [89]. Conde et al. reported the potential of a single molecular nanoconjugate to intersect with all the RNA pathways: from gene-specific downregulation to silencing, i.e., siRNA and miRNA pathways, by gold nanobeacons. These nanoconjugates functionalized with a fluorophore labeled hairpin-DNA are capable of efficiently silencing single gene expression, exogenous siRNA, and an endogenous miRNA while yielding a quantifiable fluorescence signal directly proportional to the level of silencing [90].

Park et al. developed reducible HA—siRNA conjugate for target-specific systemic delivery of siRNA to the liver. The conjugation of anionic HA to siRNA enhanced the charge density of siRNA, enabling the formation of nanocomplex with linear polyethyleneimine (LPEI). This construct enhanced the in vivo gene silencing efficiency by 60% relative to naked siRNA/LPEI complex [91]. In addition, QDs have also been functionalized with nucleic acids and extensively applied as DNA sensors [92,93]. On the other hand, magnetic NPs have been functionalized with plasmid DNA and siRNA and are employed as tools for enhanced delivery of nucleic acids under an external magnetic field [94,95].

3.4 Carbohydrates

The unique physical, chemical, and optical properties of the carbohydrate-coated micro and nanocarriers offer a series of advantages that range from ensuring water solubility, biocompatibility, and stability to targeting [96]. Smaller carbohydrates, such as lactose, glucose, and mannose [97—100] can be thiolated for attachment to AuNPs via ligand exchange. These nanoparticles may be useful as sensitive colorimetric probes for a variety of metal ions. Mannose and lactose have also been added for the reduction of gold salts and stabilization of the nanoparticles. Carbohydrates can also be included to target different cells and/or enhance the cellular uptake of NPs in a highly specific mechanism. For instance, Moros et al. functionalized magnetic NPs with glucose and galactose and studied their interactions with Vero cells in vitro [101]. Although these monosaccharides share the same chemical formula, except for the spatial conformation of the hydroxyl group in C-4, the cell entrance pattern was completely different with their modification. Although magnetic NPs-glucose entered throughout the cell, magnetic NPs-galactose remained predominantly in the cell periphery.

Carbohydrates have also been conjugated to QDs [102—104]. For example, Kikkeri et al. synthesized PEGylated QDs capped with D-mannose, D-galactose, and D-galactosamine to study specific carbohydrate—protein interactions by in vitro imaging and in vivo liver targeting [102].

3.5 Fluorescent Dyes

Fluorescent dyes are often conjugated with the micro- and nanocarriers for bioassays, imaging and diagnostic purposes, as well as monitoring drug delivery to the target tissues. Several studies have reported the use of fluorescent quenching methods for detection of DNA and proteins. Ray et al. reported the fluorophore labeled single-stranded DNA (ssDNA) adsorbed onto AuNPs for DNA detection, where the presence of a complementary target triggers desorption of the newly formed double-stranded DNA (dsDNA) from the nanostructures due to electrostatic variation between ssDNA and dsDNA, and fluorescence emission is restored [105]. Proteins have also been probed through NP fluorescence-mediated systems, especially for protein detection via quenching, through the interaction with fluorescent AuNPs [106,107].

The inclusion of dyes onto magnetic NPs allows the creation of multifunctional NPs, which might be applied for MRI and optical imaging. Medarova et al. reported the synthesis of a multifunctional magnetic NP that included near-infrared optical imaging dye, peptides for membrane translocation, and synthetic siRNA targeting a specific gene [108]. The in vivo accumulation of those NPs and silencing efficiency of siRNA could be simultaneously assessed by MRI and optical imaging.

4. FUNCTIONALIZATION OF MICRO- AND NANOPARTICLES

Functionalization is carried out to improve the performance of micro- and nanoparticles by attaching on the surface or integrating within the structure one or more functional groups. Some basic components of functionalization in the field of biomedicine include diagnostic agent, targeting ligand, spacer group, and imaging and therapeutic agents.

Micro- and nanocarriers have been functionalized with various chemical functional groups such as thiols, disulfides, amines, nitriles, carboxylic acids, phosphines and biomacromolecules [109–114]. Surface functionalization of micro- and nanoparticles can occur by two ways, one is functionalization with biological (macro) molecules such as peptides, carbohydrates, lipids, fatty acids, proteins, and nucleic acids (genes, oligomers, aptamers, and ribozymes/DNAzymes) and the other is functionalization with specific ligands such as mono- or oligosaccharides (carbohydrates), folate receptor, Abs, and biotin [51].

4.1 Methods of Conjugating Functional Moieties to Micro- and Nanoparticles

A broad spectrum of chemical approaches such as adsorption, emulsification, polymerization, covalent bonding, and bioconjugation have been undertaken to conjugate targeting moieties, therapeutic molecules, or contrast agents to micro- and nanoparticle surfaces. These methods can be categorized as conventional bioconjugation strategies (direct conjugation, linker chemistry, physical interactions), click chemistry, or hybridization methods (Table 2.2) [7]. The primary goal of targeted ligand conjugation is to bind a targeting moiety without losing its functionality after attachment to the nanoparticle. For example, binding of an antibody to a micro- or nanoparticle must not shield the functional region that is essential for its recognition. Similarly, conjugation of therapeutic agents such as drugs and siRNA must be designed to release from an NP system after cellular uptake to produce therapeutic effects [7]. While selecting a coupling strategy for functional moiety one must consider the stability of the micro/nanoparticle, the functional groups, the bioconjugation conditions (pH, temperature, ionic strength, solvent, and structure of the surfactant) and the biomolecule to attach, among others [32]. For detailed conjugation methods please see Refs. [7] and [32].

Table 2.2 Methods of conjugating functional moieties during nanoparticle fabrication [7]

Conventional bioconjugation strategies
Direct conjugation; suitable for the conjugation of fluorescence dyes, chelators, and drugs.

Nanoparticle	functional moiety		conjugate
Amine-functionalized nanoparticle	Succinimidyl ester	→	
	Isothiocyanate	→	
Aldehyde-functionalized nanoparticle	Hydrazide	Schiff-base condensation →	
Active hydrogen-functionalized nanoparticle	Amine	Mannich reaction →	
Maleimide-functionalized liposome	Sulfhydryl	→	
Gold nanoparticle	Sulfhydryl	→	

Table 2.2 Methods of conjugating functional moieties during nanoparticle fabrication [7]—cont'd

Linker chemistry; suitable for the attachment of targeting ligands.

Nanoparticle	linker	functional moiety	conjugate
Amine-functionalized nanoparticle +	SMCC	Sulfhydryl	
	NHS-PEG-MAL	Sulfhydryl	
	SPDP	Sulfhydryl	
	SIA	SATA-activated Sulfhydryl	
Carboxyl-functionalized nanoparticle +	NHS ester Intermediate (EDC/NHS activation)	Amine	

Continued

Table 2.2 Methods of conjugating functional moieties during nanoparticle fabrication [7]—cont'd

Physical interaction; suitable for the assembly of therapeutic agents onto the nanoparticles.

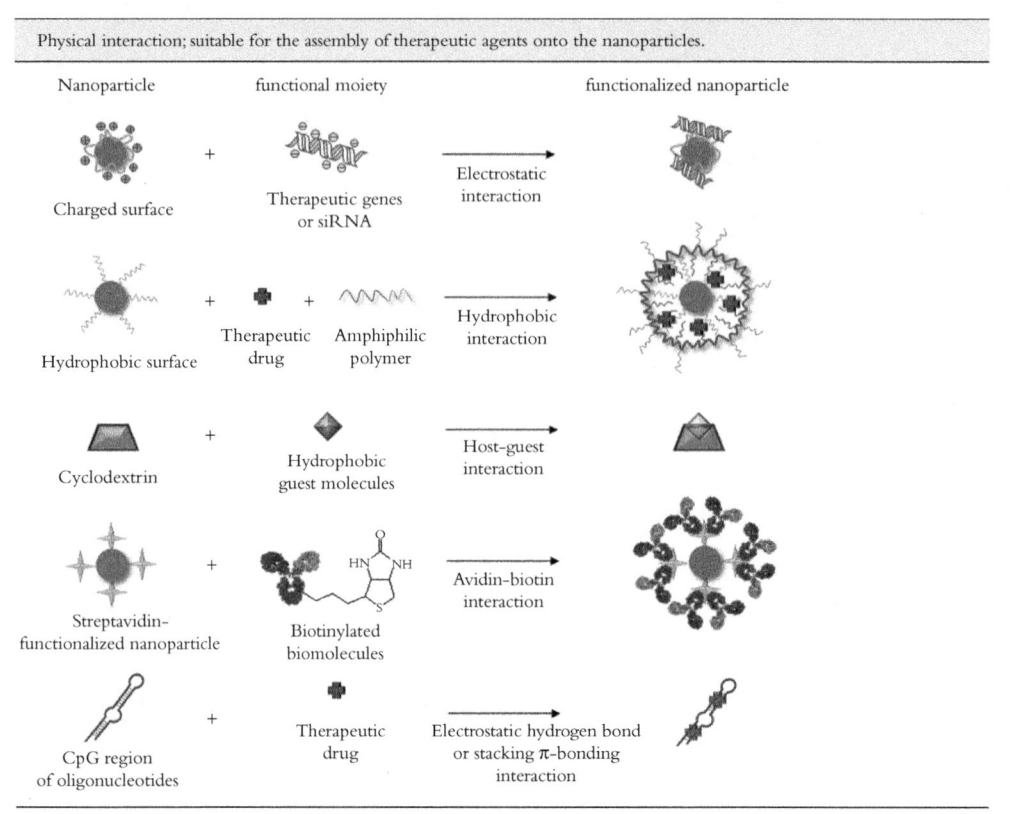

Nanoparticle	functional moiety		functionalized nanoparticle
Charged surface	Therapeutic genes or siRNA	Electrostatic interaction	
Hydrophobic surface	Therapeutic drug + Amphiphilic polymer	Hydrophobic interaction	
Cyclodextrin	Hydrophobic guest molecules	Host-guest interaction	
Streptavidin-functionalized nanoparticle	Biotinylated biomolecules	Avidin-biotin interaction	
CpG region of oligonucleotides	Therapeutic drug	Electrostatic hydrogen bond or stacking π-bonding interaction	

Click chemistry; suitable for the conjugation of targeting ligands

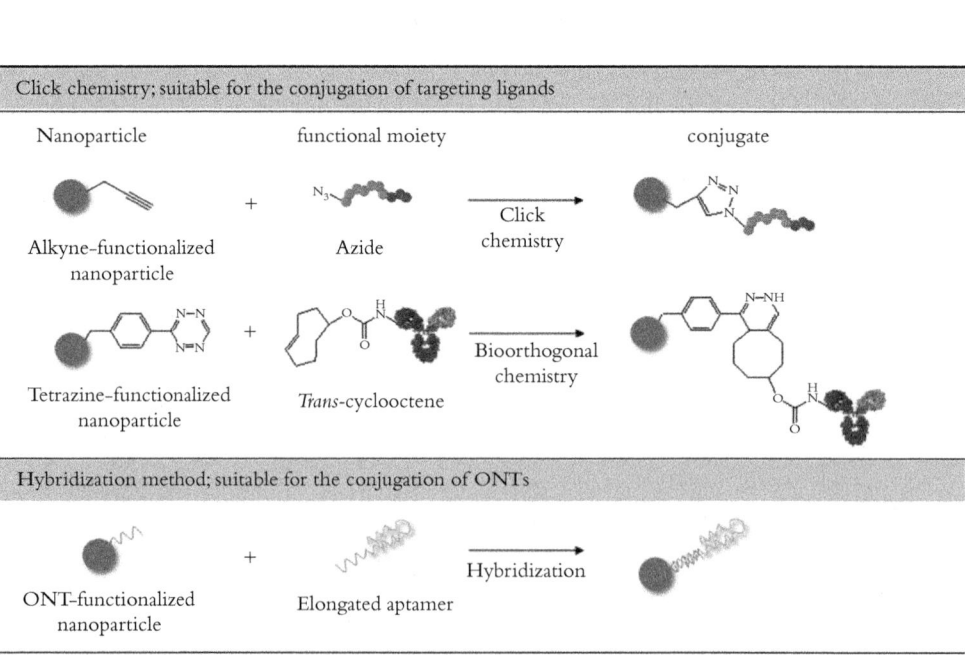

Nanoparticle	functional moiety		conjugate
Alkyne-functionalized nanoparticle	Azide	Click chemistry	
Tetrazine-functionalized nanoparticle	*Trans*-cyclooctene	Bioorthogonal chemistry	

Hybridization method; suitable for the conjugation of ONTs

ONT-functionalized nanoparticle	Elongated aptamer	Hybridization	

EDC, 1-ethyl-3-(3-(dimethylamino)-propyl) carbodiimide; *NHS*, N-hydroxysuccinimide; *NHS-PEG-MAL*, N-succinimidyl-poly(ethylene glycol)-maleimide; *SATA*, N-succinimidyl-S-acetylthioacetate; *SIA*, N-succinimidyl iodoacetate; *SMCC*, succinimidyl-4-(N-maleimidomethyl) cyclo-hexane-1-carboxylate; *SPDP*, N-succinimidyl 3-(2-pyridyldithio) propionate.
Adapted from Yu MK, Park J, Jon S. Targeting strategies for multifunctional nanoparticles in cancer imaging and therapy. Theranostics 2012;2(1):3. http://www.thno.org/v02p0003.htm.

REFERENCES

[1] Kohane DS. Microparticles and nanoparticles for drug delivery. Biotechnol Bioeng 2007;96(2): 203—9.
[2] Kumar CS. Nanomaterials for medical diagnosis and therapy, vol. 10. John Wiley & Sons; 2007.
[3] Larrañeta E, et al. Microneedles: a new frontier in nanomedicine delivery. Pharm Res 2016;33(5): 1055—73.
[4] Sharma P. Microparticles drug delivery system: a review 2016.
[5] Prow TW, et al. Nanoparticles and microparticles for skin drug delivery. Adv Drug Deliv Rev 2011; 63(6):470—91.
[6] Srinivasan M, Rajabi M, Mousa SA. Multifunctional nanomaterials and their applications in drug delivery and cancer therapy. Nanomaterials 2015;5(4):1690—703.
[7] Yu MK, Park J, Jon S. Targeting strategies for multifunctional nanoparticles in cancer imaging and therapy. Theranostics 2012;2(1):3.
[8] Peer D, et al. Nanocarriers as an emerging platform for cancer therapy. Nat Nanotechnol 2007;2(12): 751—60.
[9] Pastan I, et al. Immunotoxin therapy of cancer. Nat Rev Cancer 2006;6(7):559—65.
[10] Shi J, et al. Self-assembled targeted nanoparticles: evolution of technologies and bench to bedside translation. Acc Chem Res 2011;44(10):1123—34.
[11] Krown SE, et al. Use of liposomal anthracyclines in Kaposi's sarcoma. In: Seminars in oncology. Elsevier; 2004.
[12] Mrozek E, et al. Phase I trial of liposomal encapsulated doxorubicin (Myocet™; D-99) and weekly docetaxel in advanced breast cancer patients. Ann Oncol 2005;16(7):1087—93.
[13] O'brien M, et al. Reduced cardiotoxicity and comparable efficacy in a phase III trial of pegylated liposomal doxorubicin HCl (CAELYX™/Doxil®) versus conventional doxorubicin for first-line treatment of metastatic breast cancer. Ann Oncol 2004;15(3):440—9.
[14] Sarris A, et al. Liposomal vincristine in relapsed non-Hodgkin's lymphomas: early results of an ongoing phase II trial. Ann Oncol 2000;11(1):69—72.
[15] Petrelli F, Borgonovo K, Barni S. Targeted delivery for breast cancer therapy: the history of nanoparticle-albumin-bound paclitaxel. Expert Opin Pharmacother 2010;11(8):1413—32.
[16] Lim W, et al. Phase I pharmacokinetic study of a weekly liposomal paclitaxel formulation (Genexol®-PM) in patients with solid tumors. Ann Oncol 2009. http://dx.doi.org/10.1093/annonc/mdp315.
[17] Davis ME. The first targeted delivery of siRNA in humans via a self-assembling, cyclodextrin polymer-based nanoparticle: from concept to clinic. Mol Pharm 2009;6(3):659—68.
[18] Sankhala K, et al. A phase I pharmacokinetic (PK) study of MBP-426, a novel liposome encapsulated oxaliplatin. J Clin Oncol 2009;27(15S):2535.
[19] Wise DL. Handbook of pharmaceutical controlled release technology. CRC Press; 2000.
[20] Hugel B, et al. Membrane microparticles: two sides of the coin. Physiology 2005;20(1):22—7.
[21] Andaloussi SE, et al. Extracellular vesicles: biology and emerging therapeutic opportunities. Nat Rev Drug Discov 2013;12(5):347—57.
[22] Montoro-García S, et al. Circulating microparticles: new insights into the biochemical basis of microparticle release and activity. Basic Res Cardiol 2011;106(6):911—23.
[23] Manjanna K, Shivakumar B, Kumar TP. Microencapsulation: an acclaimed novel drug-delivery system for NSAIDs in arthritis. Crit Rev Ther Drug Carr Syst 2010;27(6).
[24] Venkatesan P, Manavalan R, Valliappan K. Microencapsulation: a vital technique in novel drug delivery system. J Pharm Sci Res 2009;1(4):26—35.
[25] Shvedova AA, Kagan VE, Fadeel B. Close encounters of the small kind: adverse effects of man-made materials interfacing with the nano-cosmos of biological systems. Annu Rev Pharmacol Toxicol 2010;50:63—88.
[26] Gil PR, Parak WJ. Composite nanoparticles take aim at cancer. ACS Nano 2008;2(11):2200—5.
[27] Anton N, Jakhmola A, Vandamme TF. Trojan microparticles for drug delivery. Pharmaceutics 2012; 4(1):1—25.
[28] Megerdichian C, Olimpiadi Y, Hurvitz SA. nab-Paclitaxel in combination with biologically targeted agents for early and metastatic breast cancer. Cancer Treat Rev 2014;40(5):614—25.

[29] Hrkach J, et al. Preclinical development and clinical translation of a PSMA-targeted docetaxel nanoparticle with a differentiated pharmacological profile. Sci Transl Med 2012;4(128):128ra39.
[30] Kim BY, Rutka JT, Chan WC. Nanomedicine. N Engl J Med 2010;363(25):2434–43.
[31] Mo R, et al. Emerging micro-and nanotechnology based synthetic approaches for insulin delivery. Chem Soc Rev 2014;43(10):3595–629.
[32] Conde J, et al. Revisiting 30 years of biofunctionalization and surface chemistry of inorganic nanoparticles for nanomedicine. Front Chem 2014;2:48.
[33] Jia F, et al. Multifunctional nanoparticles for targeted delivery of immune activating and cancer therapeutic agents. J Control Release 2013;172(3):1020–34.
[34] Sanvicens N, Marco MP. Multifunctional nanoparticles—properties and prospects for their use in human medicine. Trends Biotechnol 2008;26(8):425–33.
[35] Lin Y-Y, et al. Tumor burden talks in cancer treatment with PEGylated liposomal drugs. PLoS One 2013;8(5):e63078.
[36] Torchilin VP. Recent advances with liposomes as pharmaceutical carriers. Nat Rev Drug Discov 2005;4(2):145–60.
[37] Serajuddin AT. Enhanced microemulsion formation in lipid-based drug delivery systems by combining mono-esters of medium-chain fatty acids with di-or tri-esters. J Excip Food Chem 2012;3(2):29–44.
[38] Baroli B. Penetration of nanoparticles and nanomaterials in the skin: fiction or reality? J Pharm Sci 2010;99(1):21–50.
[39] Ghosh PK, et al. Design and development of microemulsion drug delivery system of acyclovir for improvement of oral bioavailability. AAPS PharmSciTech 2006;7(3):E172–7.
[40] Lawrence MJ, Rees GD. Microemulsion-based media as novel drug delivery systems. Adv Drug Deliv Rev 2000;45(1):89–121.
[41] Thakkar H, et al. Formulation and characterization of lipid-based drug delivery system of raloxifene-microemulsion and self-microemulsifying drug delivery system. J Pharm Bioallied Sci 2011;3(3):442.
[42] Sharma G, et al. Microemulsions for oral delivery of insulin: design, development and evaluation in streptozotocin induced diabetic rats. Eur J Pharm Biopharm 2010;76(2):159–69.
[43] Müller RH, Radtke M, Wissing SA. Solid lipid nanoparticles (SLN) and nanostructured lipid carriers (NLC) in cosmetic and dermatological preparations. Adv Drug Deliv Rev 2002;54:S131–55.
[44] Wissing S, Kayser O, Müller R. Solid lipid nanoparticles for parenteral drug delivery. Adv Drug Deliv Rev 2004;56(9):1257–72.
[45] Mehnert W, Mäder K. Solid lipid nanoparticles: production, characterization and applications. Adv Drug Deliv Rev 2001;47(2):165–96.
[46] Das S, Chaudhury A. Recent advances in lipid nanoparticle formulations with solid matrix for oral drug delivery. AAPS PharmSciTech 2011;12(1):62–76.
[47] Fonte P, et al. Chitosan-coated solid lipid nanoparticles enhance the oral absorption of insulin. Drug Deliv Transl Res 2011;1(4):299–308.
[48] Neves AR, Queiroz JF, Reis S. Brain-targeted delivery of resveratrol using solid lipid nanoparticles functionalized with apolipoprotein E. J Nanobiotechnol 2016;14(1):1.
[49] Alukda D, Sturgis T, Youan BBC. Formulation of tenofovir-loaded functionalized solid lipid nanoparticles intended for HIV prevention. J Pharm Sci 2011;100(8):3345–56.
[50] Albuquerque J, et al. Solid lipid nanoparticles: a potential multifunctional approach towards rheumatoid arthritis theranostics. Molecules 2015;20(6):11103–18.
[51] Bennet D, Kim S. Polymer nanoparticles for smart drug delivery 2014 [chapter].
[52] Soppimath KS, et al. Biodegradable polymeric nanoparticles as drug delivery devices. J Control Release 2001;70(1):1–20.
[53] Panyam J, Labhasetwar V. Biodegradable nanoparticles for drug and gene delivery to cells and tissue. Adv Drug Deliv Rev 2003;55(3):329–47.
[54] Cui Z, Mumper RJ. Plasmid DNA-entrapped nanoparticles engineered from microemulsion precursors: in vitro and in vivo evaluation. Bioconjugate Chem 2002;13(6):1319–27.

[55] Chen M-C, et al. A review of the prospects for polymeric nanoparticle platforms in oral insulin delivery. Biomaterials 2011;32(36):9826–38.
[56] Halim AS, et al. Biocompatibility and biodegradation of chitosan and derivatives. In: Chitosan-based systems for biopharmaceuticals: delivery, targeting and polymer therapeutics; 2012. p. 57–73.
[57] Zhang X, et al. Preparation and characterization of insulin-loaded bioadhesive PLGA nanoparticles for oral administration. Eur J Pharm Sci 2012;45(5):632–8.
[58] Yeh T-H, et al. Mechanism and consequence of chitosan-mediated reversible epithelial tight junction opening. Biomaterials 2011;32(26):6164–73.
[59] Zhang Z, et al. Polymeric nanoparticles-based topical delivery systems for the treatment of dermatological diseases. Wiley Interdiscip Rev Nanomed Nanobiotechnol 2013;5(3):205–18.
[60] Yamamoto H, et al. Surface-modified PLGA nanosphere with chitosan improved pulmonary delivery of calcitonin by mucoadhesion and opening of the intercellular tight junctions. J Control Release 2005;102(2):373–81.
[61] Illum L, Farraj NF, Davis SS. Chitosan as a novel nasal delivery system for peptide drugs. Pharm Res 1994;11(8):1186–9.
[62] Kojima C, et al. Synthesis of polyamidoamine dendrimers having poly(ethylene glycol) grafts and their ability to encapsulate anticancer drugs. Bioconjugate Chem 2000;11(6):910–7.
[63] Lee CC, et al. Designing dendrimers for biological applications. Nat Biotechnol 2005;23(12): 1517–26.
[64] Trivedi R, Kompella UB. Nanomicellar formulations for sustained drug delivery: strategies and underlying principles. Nanomedicine 2010;5(3):485–505.
[65] Felber AE, Dufresne M-H, Leroux J-C. pH-sensitive vesicles, polymeric micelles, and nanospheres prepared with polycarboxylates. Adv Drug Deliv Rev 2012;64(11):979–92.
[66] Hong CA, Nam YS. Functional nanostructures for effective delivery of small interfering RNA therapeutics. Theranostics 2014;4(12):1211–32.
[67] Chacko RT, et al. Polymer nanogels: a versatile nanoscopic drug delivery platform. Adv Drug Deliv Rev 2012;64(9):836–51.
[68] Huang H-C, et al. Inorganic nanoparticles for cancer imaging and therapy. J Control Release 2011; 155(3):344–57.
[69] Medintz IL, et al. Quantum dot bioconjugates for imaging, labelling and sensing. Nat Mater 2005; 4(6):435–46.
[70] Lu AH, Salabas EeL, Schüth F. Magnetic nanoparticles: synthesis, protection, functionalization, and application. Angew Chem Int Ed 2007;46(8):1222–44.
[71] Kievit FM, Zhang M. Surface engineering of iron oxide nanoparticles for targeted cancer therapy. Acc Chem Res 2011;44(10):853–62.
[72] Donnelly RF, Singh TRR. Novel delivery systems for transdermal and intradermal drug delivery. John Wiley & Sons; 2015.
[73] Sperling RA, et al. Biological applications of gold nanoparticles. Chem Soc Rev 2008;37(9):1896–908.
[74] Huang X, et al. Gold nanoparticles: interesting optical properties and recent applications in cancer diagnostics and therapy 2007.
[75] Bao Q-Y, et al. The enhanced longevity and liver targetability of Paclitaxel by hybrid liposomes encapsulating Paclitaxel-conjugated gold nanoparticles. Int J Pharm 2014;477(1):408–15.
[76] Wang Z, et al. The peptide route to multifunctional gold nanoparticles. Bioconjugate Chem 2005; 16(3):497–500.
[77] Conde J, et al. Design of multifunctional gold nanoparticles for in vitro and in vivo gene silencing. ACS Nano 2012;6(9):8316–24.
[78] Chithrani DB. Intracellular uptake, transport, and processing of gold nanostructures. Mol Membr Biol 2010;27(7):299–311.
[79] Kumar M, et al. Image-guided breast tumor therapy using a small interfering RNA nanodrug. Cancer Res 2010;70(19):7553–61.
[80] Arruebo M, Valladares M, González-Fernández Á. Antibody-conjugated nanoparticles for biomedical applications. J Nanomater 2009;2009:37.

[81] Albanell J, Baselga J. Trastuzumab, a humanized anti-HER2 monoclonal antibody, for the treatment of breast cancer. Drugs Today (Barc) 1999;35(12):931–46.
[82] Ferrara N. VEGF as a therapeutic target in cancer. Oncology 2005;69(Suppl. 3):11–6.
[83] Que-Gewirth N, Sullenger B. Gene therapy progress and prospects: RNA aptamers. Gene Ther 2007;14(4):283–91.
[84] Conde J, et al. Antibody–drug gold nanoantennas with Raman spectroscopic fingerprints for in vivo tumour theranostics. J Control Release 2014;183:87–93.
[85] East DA, et al. QD-antibody conjugates via carbodiimide-mediated coupling: a detailed study of the variables involved and a possible new mechanism for the coupling reaction under basic aqueous conditions. Langmuir 2011;27(22):13888–96.
[86] Tan WB, Jiang S, Zhang Y. Quantum-dot based nanoparticles for targeted silencing of HER2/neu gene via RNA interference. Biomaterials 2007;28(8):1565–71.
[87] Lu R-M, et al. Single chain anti-c-Met antibody conjugated nanoparticles for in vivo tumor-targeted imaging and drug delivery. Biomaterials 2011;32(12):3265–74.
[88] Hurst SJ, Lytton-Jean AK, Mirkin CA. Maximizing DNA loading on a range of gold nanoparticle sizes. Anal Chem 2006;78(24):8313–8.
[89] Cao YC, et al. A two-color-change, nanoparticle-based method for DNA detection. Talanta 2005;67(3):449–55.
[90] Conde J, Rosa J, Baptista P. Gold-nanobeacons as a theranostic system for the detection and inhibition of specific genes. Protoc Exch 2013;10.
[91] Park K, et al. Reducible hyaluronic acid–siRNA conjugate for target specific gene silencing. Bioconjugate Chem 2013;24(7):1201–9.
[92] Crut A, et al. Detection of single DNA molecules by multicolor quantum-dot end-labeling. Nucleic Acids Res 2005;33(11):e98.
[93] Zhang C-y, Hu J. Single quantum dot-based nanosensor for multiple DNA detection. Anal Chem 2010;82(5):1921–7.
[94] Dobson J. Gene therapy progress and prospects: magnetic nanoparticle-based gene delivery. Gene Ther 2006;13(4):283–7.
[95] Plank C, Zelphati O, Mykhaylyk O. Magnetically enhanced nucleic acid delivery. Ten years of magnetofection—progress and prospects. Adv Drug Deliv Rev 2011;63(14):1300–31.
[96] García I, Marradi M, Penadés S. Glyconanoparticles: multifunctional nanomaterials for biomedical applications. Nanomedicine 2010;5(5):777–92.
[97] Otsuka H, et al. Quantitative and reversible lectin-induced association of gold nanoparticles modified with α-lactosyl-ω-mercapto-poly(ethylene glycol). J Am Chem Soc 2001;123(34):8226–30.
[98] Reynolds AJ, Haines AH, Russell DA. Gold glyconanoparticles for mimics and measurement of metal ion-mediated carbohydrate-carbohydrate interactions. Langmuir 2006;22(3):1156–63.
[99] Martínez-Ávila O, et al. Gold manno-glyconanoparticles: multivalent systems to block HIV-1 gp120 binding to the lectin DC-SIGN. Chemistry–A Eur J 2009;15(38):9874–88.
[100] Schofield CL, Field RA, Russell DA. Glyconanoparticles for the colorimetric detection of cholera toxin. Anal Chem 2007;79(4):1356–61.
[101] Moros M, et al. Monosaccharides versus PEG-functionalized NPs: influence in the cellular uptake. ACS Nano 2012;6(2):1565–77.
[102] Kikkeri R, et al. In vitro imaging and in vivo liver targeting with carbohydrate capped quantum dots. J Am Chem Soc 2009;131(6):2110–2.
[103] Cai X, et al. Galactose decorated acid-labile nanoparticles encapsulating quantum dots for enhanced cellular uptake and subcellular localization. Pharm Res 2012;29(8):2167–79.
[104] Yang Y, et al. Study of carbohydrate–protein interactions using glyco-QDs with different fluorescence emission wavelengths. Carbohydr Res 2012;361:189–94.
[105] Ray PC, Fortner A, Darbha GK. Gold nanoparticle based FRET assay for the detection of DNA cleavage. J Phys Chem B 2006;110(42):20745–8.
[106] Mayilo S, et al. Long-range fluorescence quenching by gold nanoparticles in a sandwich immunoassay for cardiac troponin T. Nano Lett 2009;9(12):4558–63.

[107] He X, et al. Near-infrared fluorescent nanoprobes for cancer molecular imaging: status and challenges. Trends Mol Med 2010;16(12):574—83.
[108] Medarova Z, et al. In vivo imaging of siRNA delivery and silencing in tumors. Nat Med 2007;13(3): 372—7.
[109] Roux S, et al. Synthesis, characterization of dihydrolipoic acid capped gold nanoparticles, and functionalization by the electroluminescent luminol. Langmuir 2005;21(6):2526—36.
[110] Zayats M, et al. Reconstitution of apo-glucose dehydrogenase on pyrroloquinoline quinone-functionalized Au nanoparticles yields an electrically contacted biocatalyst. J Am Chem Soc 2005; 127(35):12400—6.
[111] Ulman A. Formation and structure of self-assembled monolayers. Chem Rev 1996;96(4):1533—54.
[112] Fan H, et al. Synthesis of organo-silane functionalized nanocrystal micelles and their self-assembly. J Am Chem Soc 2005;127(40):13746—7.
[113] Ramirez E, et al. Influence of organic ligands on the stabilization of palladium nanoparticles. J Organomet Chem 2004;689(24):4601—10.
[114] Woehrle GH, Hutchison JE. Thiol-functionalized undecagold clusters by ligand exchange: synthesis, mechanism, and properties. Inorg Chem 2005;44(18):6149—58.

CHAPTER 3

Nanomicelles in Diagnosis and Drug Delivery*

Hoang M. Trinh[1], Mary Joseph[1], Kishore Cholkar[2], Ranjana Mitra[1], Ashim K. Mitra[1]

[1]University of Missouri—Kansas City, Kansas City, MO, United States; [2]Ingenus Pharmaceuticals/RiconPharma LLC, Denville, NJ, United States

Contents

1. Introduction	45
2. Nanomicelle Preparation	46
3. Application of Nanomicelle in Diagnostics and Imaging	48
3.1 Computed Tomography	48
3.2 Magnetic Resonance Imaging	49
3.3 Near-Infrared Fluorescent Imaging	49
4. Application of Nanomicelles in Drug Delivery	50
4.1 Solubilize Poorly Water-Soluble Drugs	50
4.2 Targeted Nanomicelles	52
4.3 Stimuli-Responsive Nanomicelles	52
4.3.1 pH Sensitive	52
4.3.2 Temperature Sensitive	52
4.3.3 Light Sensitive	53
4.3.4 Ultrasound Responsive	53
4.3.5 Others	53
4.4 Multifunctional Nanomicelle Carrier	53
5. Conclusion	53
References	54

Objectives

- To provide an overview about nanomicelle-based delivery system.
- To elucidate various chemical compositions and methods of nanomicelle preparation.
- To describe the application of nanomicelles in diagnosis.
- To summarize various drug delivery applications of nanomicelles.

1. INTRODUCTION

Nanomicelles are colloidal constructs (5—100 nm) formed from amphiphilic monomers (surface active agents) that self-aggregate above the critical micelle concentration in

*All authors have equally contributed to the chapter.

aqueous systems. The concentration at which monomers start to self-aggregate is referred to "critical micellar concentration (CMC)." In general, such monomer molecules have two distinct structural segments, a small hydrophobic head and a long hydrophilic tail. Depending on the concentration (low to high) monomers exist in three different phases in aqueous solution: (1) monomers, (2) an arranged monolayer of amphiphiles at the air—solvent interphase, and (3) nanomicelles. Constructs formed from amphiphilic monomers offer unique advantages such as improved solubility of sparingly soluble compounds, stability, reproducibility and ease of scale up at pilot and bulk scale, and ease of sterilization. Lipophilic molecules are embraced inside the hydrophobic core of micelles formed by van der Walls forces [1]. On the other hand, the outer hydrophilic corona (1) provides steric stability by forming hydrogen bonding with the surrounding aqueous medium [1,2], (2) protects the construct from being recognized and engulfed by the reticuloendothelial system (RES) thereby providing longer circulation time, (3) is amenable to conjugation with a ligand for active targeting, (4) renders the encapsulated molecule nondetectable by analytical methods such as nuclear magnetic resonance and UV—visible spectroscopy, and (5) generates clear solutions [3—6]. Micellar constructs may comprise pH- and temperature-sensitive polymers releasing the cargo in response to stimuli. However, nanomicellar constructs may present limitations such as premature release of cargo, lack of controlled/sustained drug release, and inability to encapsulate hydrophilic molecules. Nanomicellar shape is largely dependent on the size of the head and/or tail of the amphiphilic monomer. If the monomer head segments have rod structure, the nanomicelles have lamellae shape and reverse results in spherical construct [7].

2. NANOMICELLE PREPARATION

Nanomicelles may be prepared from surface active agents like surfactants and synthetic block copolymers. Amphiphilic monomers exist as ionic, nonionic, and zwitterionic forms. Ionic surfactants may carry a charge (anion or cation). Anionic and cationic surfactants include sodium dodecyl sulfate and dodecyltrimethyl ammonium bromide, respectively [8]. Nonionic surfactants such as *n*-dodecyl tetra (ethylene oxide) are neutral. On the other hand, zwitterionic surfactants such as dioctanoyl phosphatydyl choline carry both positive and negative charges. Amphiphilic block copolymers can be synthesized from biocompatible and biodegradable polyoxyl, polyester, or polypeptide derivatives. Polymer blocks may be arranged as linear diblock, triblock, pentablock (A-B, A-B-A, or A-A-B-A-A type), and branched types. In block copolymer arrangements, A and B represent any of the polymers such as, but are not limited to, poly(lactic acid)—poly(ethylene glycol) (PEG)—poly(L-lysine) (PLL), poly ethylene oxide, poly(D,L-lactic acid), polypropylene oxide, poly glycolic acid, poly(aspartic acid), poly(glutamic acid), poly(L-lysine), and poly-(histidine). In most of the copolymer blocks polyethylene glycol (PEG) is commonly inserted in the polymer chain as the hydrophilic segment because of advantages such as high water solubility, low toxicity, avoidance of reticuloendothelial recognition, biocompatibility, and steric stability [9].

Nanomicelles can be prepared by different protocols depending upon the physicochemical properties of the polymer chain length and monomer property. The method of nanomicelle preparation may be divided into two categories, namely, (1) direct dissolution and (2) solvent casting. Direct dissolution aka simple equilibrium method is employed for block copolymers that are moderately hydrophobic. Examples include poloxamers and poly(butyl acrylate) block copolymers with hydrophilic end synthesized from one anionic, one cationic, and four nonionic hydrophilic blocks [10]. In this method, drug and copolymer are simultaneously dissolved in aqueous solution. Nanomicelle formation is initiated by heating the aqueous solution. Application of heat allows dehydration of the micellar core resulting in nanomicellar structure. An appropriate drug-to-copolymer ratio and thermal application can induce nanomicelle formation in aqueous solution.

Solvent casting procedures may be further divided into four methods: (1) dialysis, (2) oil in water (o/w) emulsion, (3) solution casting, and (4) freeze drying. The dialysis method requires application of high boiling point, water-soluble organic solvents such as dimethyl sulfoxide, *N,N*-dimethylformamide, tetrahydrofuran, dimethylacetamide, and ethanol. This method is suitable to prepare block copolymers that are not readily soluble in aqueous medium. In this method, copolymers and drug are separately dissolved in water-soluble organic solvents. An organic solvent with copolymer and drug in solution are loaded into a dialysis membrane bag and dialyzed against water for more than 12 h with subsequent replacement of water at predetermined time points. This process involves slow removal of water-soluble organic solvent that triggers nanomicelle formation leading to drug encapsulation. However, such method has limitations such as low encapsulation efficiency and drug loss during the dialysis process. However, the o/w emulsion method involves physical entrapping of molecules. In this process, lipophilic organic solvents such as dichloromethane, ethyl acetate, and acetone are used. The encapsulation process involves dissolving the copolymer and drug in organic solvent with a small amount of water. The organic solvent is removed by continuous stirring of the solvent mixture. In this method, evaporation of the organic solvent triggers nanomicelle formation with simultaneous physical entrapment of the hydrophobic drug in the core of the micelles [11]. A solvent casting method involves both organic and aqueous solvents. In this method, both drug and polymer/s are dissolved in organic solvent such as ethanol to obtain a clear solution. The organic solution is removed under high vacuum, which results in a thin film. Evaporation of organic solvent favors polymer—drug interactions. Rehydration of this thin film with aqueous solvent spontaneously develops drug-loaded nanomicelles [3—6]. The final method of preparation is a one-step freeze drying process. The copolymers and drugs are dissolved in *tert*-butanol. The mixture (drug and copolymer in water/*tert*-butanol) is subjected to freeze drying or lyophilization. During this process, *tert*-butanol induces the formation of fine ice crystals that rapidly sublime leaving behind the freeze-thawed cake. Rehydration of this cake spontaneously develops drug-loaded nanomicelles [12].

3. APPLICATION OF NANOMICELLE IN DIAGNOSTICS AND IMAGING

Medical imaging plays a very important role in early detection, diagnostics, and treatment of various diseases to improve public health [13–16]. Currently medical imaging has significantly improved the longevity of patients with cancer preventing tumor metastasis because of early detection [17–19]. Imaging not only aids in detection but also allows follow-up during treatment [20,21]. Many imaging tools have been developed including computed tomography (CT) imaging, magnetic resonance imaging (MRI), nuclear medicine imaging, mammography, ultrasound, and X-ray imaging. Nanoparticles and nanomicelles have been developed for medical imaging [22] combined with drug delivery system due to various advantages. (1) Nanomicelles are in low nanometer ranges and can be introduced as intravenous injections. The vesicles reduce the risk of blood vessel blockage, and enhance accumulation in tissues through enhanced permeability and retention (EPR) [23,24]. (2) Polymeric nanomicelles improve the solubility of hydrophobic drugs or dyes and (3) impart high stability and bioavailability and (4) are nontoxic [25,26]. These properties of nanomicelles allow potential pharmaceutical applications. The following section provides some descriptions of established nanomicellar medical imaging applications.

3.1 Computed Tomography

CT is an imaging procedure that utilizes special X-ray equipment to take images from different angles. Multiple images create cross-sectional (tomographic) scans of parts of the body and generate detailed images of the diseased tissue areas in the body. The image processes X-ray absorption, allowing for the discrimination of differences among tissues, while generating separate images for specific organs. CT provides three-dimensional images that can detect the impairment of tissues or organ and are a valuable tool for diagnosis. To provide higher quality of CT scan or visualize the vascular structure, contrast materials such as iodine may be injected to patients. In cancer, cardiology, and other diseases, the intravascular space (blood pool imaging) shows the current blood flow or vascular system state, which is very helpful in diagnosis or in evaluating disease stages. Irregular or new blood vessels represent very small and fragile structure. Therefore the smaller sized and targeted carriers to deliver contrast agents are highly effective. Moreover, the carriers need to avoid phagocytosis in blood circulation. Certainly, nanomicelles have met all the requirements for diagnosis and drug delivery. Torchilin et al. have developed a long-circulating, iodine-loading micelles [27,28]. The iodine-loaded PLL-PEG nanomicelle with a size of 80 nm enhanced the heart, liver, spleen, and blood pool after 3 h administration in rat. Patil et al. also compared the pharmacokinetic profile of polyethylene glycol-*b*-polyphosphoramidate (PEG-*b*-PPA)/DNA micellar nanoparticles following various routes of administration using single photon emission computed tomography/CT [29]. This article reported that intrabiliary infusion is the most effective route for DNA liver-targeted delivery. Several CT imaging techniques have been investigated and some show better blood circulation residence time summarized in the review [30].

3.2 Magnetic Resonance Imaging

MRI detects the alteration of hydrogen nuclei (^{1}H) in the body under strong applications of radiofrequency pulses. In MRI the action of radiofrequency signal can be modified by paramagnetic metals such as manganese (Mn), gadolinium (Gd), or dysprosium (Dy) and iron oxide [25]. Those metallic agents have been conjugated with diethylenetriaminepentaacetic acid (DTPA) to form hydrophilic chelated metal cations. To encapsulate inside the nanomicelle hydrophobic core, the amphiphilic chelating complex has been synthesized such as methoxy poly(ethylene glycol)-b-poly(L-lactic acid). Along with amphiphilic copolymers such as methoxy poly(ethylene glycol)-b-poly(L-histidine) (PEG-p(L-His)), the amphiphilic chelating complex aggregates to form nanomicelles, which display a higher effect of MR positive (T1) contrast agents [31]. Torchilin et al. have reported antibody modification of poly-L-lysine (PLL) where DTPA polymer generated better image in animals with a short period of time. In another study, Gd (indium 111)-DTPA–phosphatidylethanolamine (PE) and indium 111-DTPA–stearylamine (SA) into PEG (5 kDa)–PE nanomicelles showed more local lymphatics and higher accumulation in lymph nodes relative to indium 111-PEG–liposomes [32]. Gadolinium-labeled phosphorescent polymeric nanomicelles have showed higher tumor localization in head and neck tumor [33]. Also, Song et al. have successfully developed the PEGylated Fe$_3$O$_4$ nanomicelles, which can escape RES uptake. Therefore this technology can provide in tumor targeting diagnosis by MRI [34]. Moreover, several studies have considered the combination of diagnosis and therapy using gold nanoshells [35–37].

3.3 Near-Infrared Fluorescent Imaging

Near-infrared fluorescent (NIRF) imaging is a novel imaging modality for early cancer detection with high sensitivity and deep tissue penetration. It is a promising technique to improve patient life by enhancing cancer theranostics. NIRF dyes draw intensive and fluorescence emission. This technique plays an important role in imaging quality. Dyes are hydrophobic in nature with poor photostability and weak fluorescence emission properties in vivo [38]. Several attempts have been made to overcome those limitations such as encapsulating hydrophobic dyes in nanoparticles, and nanomicelles [39–43]. NIRF dyes are categorized into several types such as phthalocyanines, cyanines, squaraines, 4,4-difluoro-4-bora-3a,4a-diaza-s-indacene (BODIPYs), rhodamine analogs, and porphyrin derivatives [38]. A small number of native NIRF dyes have the self-capability to target tumors such as heptamethine indocyanine IR-780 iodide dyes, IR-783, and porphyrin derivatives Pz 247 [44]. However, most of these dyes need a target moiety or carrier to penetrate across tissues to generate tumor accumulation. For example, carbocyanine dye such as indocyanine green (ICG) is hydrophobic and can be encapsulated into the nanomicellar core [45–49]. Polymeric nanomicelle has improved the fluorescent stability, cellular uptake, and tumor targeting ability of chemotherapeutics. Hong Yang et al. have developed monomethoxy poly(ethylene glycol) and alkylamine-grafted poly(L-aspartic acid) carbocyanine-loaded nanomicelles for subcutaneous injections [50]. Nanomicelles can enhance tumor accumulation of carbocyanine. These constructs may offer better photostability and higher signal to noise ratio. Therefore the retention of NIRF signals lasts up to 8 days in both hypo- and hypervascular tumors with negligible noise at normal tissues in mice. In addition, Wu et al. also demonstrated that ICG-loaded hybrid polypeptide nanomicelles poly(ethylene glycol)-b-poly(L-lysine)-b-poly(L-leucine) (PEG-PLL-PLLeu) have produced significant improvement in quantum yield as well as fluorescent stability [46]. This system generated better tumor targeting capability and longer circulation time.

4. APPLICATION OF NANOMICELLES IN DRUG DELIVERY

As discussed earlier, nanomicelles offer several advantages as drug delivery carriers, including (1) small size (10–50 nm), (2) structural stability, (3) avoidance of RES uptake, (4) enhance EPR effect, (5) less toxic, (6) ability to entrap large amounts of hydrophobic drugs and solubilize in water, and (7) conjugation with target ligand. Several successful drug-loaded nanomicelle carriers have been studied in clinical trials, which are summarized in Table 3.1 [FDA-approval (Genexol-PM) of clinical trial in patients with breast cancer]. This section will be divided into three main nanomicelle applications in drug delivery.

4.1 Solubilize Poorly Water-Soluble Drugs

Drugs with poor water solubility are classified as class II and IV compounds according to the Biopharmaceutics Classification System [51]. It is challenging for scientists to deliver hydrophobic drugs and diagnostic agents at therapeutic levels. Nanomicelles can be considered as promising carriers to solubilize hydrophobic drugs [52,53]. Since nanomicelles are amphiphilic molecules the hydrophobic core can accommodate the hydrophobic drugs and the corona being highly hydrophilic produces a clear aqueous solution. This approach has demonstrated that nanomicelles can significantly increase the solubility of lipophilic drugs several fold (10- to 8400-fold) [4–6,54,55]. For example, efavirenz, an antiretroviral, is poorly water soluble (about 4 μg/mL). Polymeric nanomicelles of efavirenz increased the solubility up to 34 mg/mL (8400-fold). The pharmacokinetic (PK) profile of the drug has been evaluated in Wistar rats [54]. PK parameters such as Cmax increase three times for all doses ranging between 20 and 80 mg/kg. A clear, aqueous nanomicellar topical eye drop contains 0.1% (1.0 mg/mL) cyclosporine (CsA), whereas CsA has a solubility of only 12 ng/mL (patent # 20150202150).

Table 3.1 Different micelles in clinical trial

Nanomicelles	Drug	Block copolymer	Indication	Clinical phase	References
NK105	Paclitaxel	poly(ethylene glycol) (PEG)-poly(aspartate)	Metastatic or recurrent breast cancer	III	[88,89] https://clinicaltrials.gov/ct2/show/NCT01644890
NK012	Sn-38	PEG-PGlu(SN-38)	Metastatic triple negative breast cancer	II	[90] https://clinicaltrials.gov/ct2/show/NCT00951054
NK911	Doxorubicin	PEG-poly(aspartate)	Solid tumors	II	[91]
NC-6300/K 912	Epirubicin	PEG-poly(aspartate)	Hepatocellular carcinoma	I	[92]
NC-6004	Cisplatin	PEG-poly(glutamic acid)	Solid tumors	I/II/III	[93] https://clinicaltrials.gov/ct2/show/NCT02043288 https://clinicaltrials.gov/ct2/show/NCT00910741 https://clinicaltrials.gov/ct2/show/NCT02240238
NC-4016	Oxaliplatin	PEG-poly(glutamic acid)	Solid tumors (lymphoma)	I	https://clinicaltrials.gov/ct2/show/NCT01999491
SP1049 C	Doxorubicin	Pluronic L61 and F127	Adenocarcinoma of esophagus Gastroesophageal	III	[94,95]
Genexol-PM	Paclitaxel	PEG-poly(D,L-lactic acid)	Breast, lung, ovarian cancer	III/approved in South Korea	https://clinicaltrials.gov/ct2/show/NCT01770795 https://clinicaltrials.gov/ct2/show/NCT01426126
Paclical	Paclitaxel	XR-17	Ovarian cancer	III	https://clinicaltrials.gov/ct2/show/NCT00989131

CsA nanomicelles delivered the drug to back-of-the-eye tissues such as retina/choroid with high level (53.7 ng/g tissue) following the topical eye drop administration.

4.2 Targeted Nanomicelles

To maximize delivery and minimize side effects, target moieties can be conjugated to create active targeting nanomicelles. Such nanomicelle constructs can target cells based on (1) interactions with specific biological targets such as cell surface receptors, transporters and (2) conjugation with locally applied signal protein (phage fusion proteins) [56]. Tao Wang et al. have developed paclitaxel-loaded phosphatidyl ethanolamine (PEG-PE) micelles, which were modified with MCF-7-specific phage fusion proteins targeting cancer cells [57]. The targeted phage nanomicelles expressed higher tumor selectivity in cancer cells over normal cells. Such targeting may enhance the anticancer effect of paclitaxel in xenograft mice model. Several target ligands have been exploited including monoclonal antibody [58–60], peptides [61–65], and aptamer [66,67]. Ahn et al. have prepared an antibody fragment conjugated nanomicelles loaded with platinum to target pancreatic cancer on tumor xenografts [59]. Compared with the nontargeted micelles, Fab′-nanomicelles exhibit 15-fold higher in vitro cellular uptake and significant antitumor effect for more than 40 days in pancreatic tumor xenografts.

4.3 Stimuli-Responsive Nanomicelles

4.3.1 pH Sensitive

The pH of tumor environment is acidic (6.5–7.2) compared with normal tissues (7.4). These differences in pH have been exploited to cleave the pH-sensitive ligands to release drugs from the micelles carriers. In a nutshell, under physiological condition (pH 7.4) drug molecules are entrapped inside nanomicelles. Therapeutic agents can be released selectively under acidic conditions such as tumor cell, endosomes, or lysosomes. Several pH-sensitive nanomicelles have been developed. The construct generated low toxicity and higher selectivity [68–72]. Anionic groups (poly acrylic acid, poly methacrylic acid, poly glutamic acid) and cationic groups (dimethylamino ethyl methacrylate, poly histidine) are common pH-sensitive components. For example, Bae et al. have prepared pH-sensitive poly(ethylene glycol)-poly(aspartate hydrazone adriamycin)–loaded nanomicelles, which release selectively in the low pH environment due to acid-sensitive hydrazine linker [73].

4.3.2 Temperature Sensitive

Temperature difference of the environment may have an effect on the CMC. The most common polymer is poly(N-isopropylacrylamide), which transforms to a hydrophobic insoluble polymer from hydrophilic polymer around 32°C. Soga et al. have developed another thermosensitive polymeric micelles [74–77].

4.3.3 Light Sensitive

A few studies indicate that hydrophobicity and hydrophilicity of nanomicelles can be shifted under light exposure. Briefly, nanomicelles can be disrupted or reversed by light. This property can be utilized to trigger drug release and delivery [78,79]. Andrew et al. have reported that the micellar system is very sensitive to infrared light causing release of fluorescence probe such as Nile red [80].

4.3.4 Ultrasound Responsive

Ultrasound can generate a frequency around 20 kHz or more, which can be utilized to enhance tumor drug uptake. Ultrasound has enhanced drug delivery by inducing (1) deeper tissue penetration, (2) perturbation of normal and tumor cell membrane, and (3) drug release from nanomicelle [81–85]. Marin et al. have studied the release and intracellular uptake of doxorubicin (Dox) from pluronic micelles, the most common ultrasound-sensitive nanomicelles. Higher Dox release from pluronic micelles was observed under high-frequency ultrasound [86].

4.3.5 Others

Other stimuli-responsive nanomicelle systems have been studied including enzyme- and redox-responsive systems. Enzymes are known to overexpresses in tumor cells. The oxidative and reductive enzyme expressions vary between intracellular and extracellular environments. Those differences are utilized in developing nanomicelle carrier to deliver drugs to the target.

4.4 Multifunctional Nanomicelle Carrier

Multifunctional nanomicelle comprises at least two ligands. Multifunctional micelles could enhance the hydrophobic drug delivery to specific target. Moreover, it can carry imaging agents that enable nanomicelle tracking released by pH-sensitive polymer or ultrasound exposure. Li et al. have developed acid-sensitive nanomicelle for both targeted drug delivery and MRI in liver cancer cells [87]. Doxorubicin and superparamagnetic iron oxide nanoparticles (imaging agents) were encapsulated inside poly(ethylene glycol)-*b*-poly(*N*-(*N'*,*N'*-diisopropylaminoethyl) glutamine) (PEG-P(GA-DIP)) and surface modified with folate acid for targeting. This multifunctional nanomicelle facilitated specific tumor targeting and enhanced therapeutic effect as well as MRI diagnosis.

5. CONCLUSION

Nanomicelles can be very effective in nanomedicine. Several nanomicelle formulations have now been developed and some are in clinical trials. Nanomicellar constructs can offer many advantages such as size, drug loading of both hydrophobic and hydrophilic agents, circulation time, safety, easy to conjugate target moiety for tumor uptake,

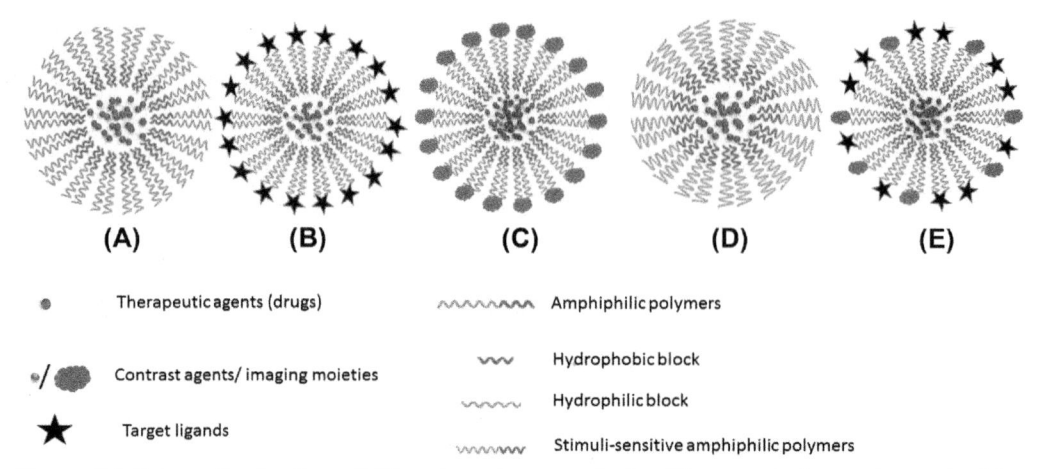

Figure 3.1 Schematic drawing of (A) polymeric nanomicelle, (B) nanomicelle conjugated with a targeting ligands, (C) nanomicelle incorporating contrast agents or imaging moieties, (D) stimuli-sensitive polymeric nanomicelles (thermo/pH/light/ultrasound sensitive), and (E) multifunctional nanomicelles with targeting ligands, contrast agents, imaging moieties, and therapeutic agents.

imaging, and triggered release. These properties offer opportunity for pharmaceutical scientists to develop appropriate formulations that maximize therapeutic efficacy and minimize side effects.

REFERENCES

[1] Torchilin VP. Micellar nanocarriers: pharmaceutical perspectives. Pharm Res 2007;24(1):1–16.
[2] Jones M, Leroux J. Polymeric micelles – a new generation of colloidal drug carriers. Eur J Pharm Biopharm 1999;48(2):101–11.
[3] Cholkar K, Gilger BC, Mitra AK. Topical delivery of aqueous micellar resolvin E1 analog (RX-10045). Int J Pharm 2016;498(1–2):326–34.
[4] Cholkar K, Gilger BC, Mitra AK. Topical, aqueous, clear cyclosporine formulation design for anterior and posterior ocular delivery. Transl Vis Sci Technol 2015;4(3):1.
[5] Cholkar K, et al. Nanomicellar topical aqueous drop formulation of rapamycin for back-of-the-eye delivery. AAPS PharmSciTech 2015;16(3):610–22.
[6] Cholkar K, et al. Optimization of dexamethasone mixed nanomicellar formulation. AAPS PharmSciTech 2014;15(6):1454–67.
[7] Cai S, et al. Micelles of different morphologies—advantages of worm-like filomicelles of PEO-PCL in paclitaxel delivery. Pharm Res 2007;24(11):2099–109.
[8] Sammalkorpi M, Karttunen M, Haataja M. Ionic surfactant aggregates in saline solutions: sodium dodecyl sulfate (SDS) in the presence of excess sodium chloride (NaCl) or calcium chloride (CaCl(2)). J Phys Chem B 2009;113(17):5863–70.
[9] Koo OM, Rubinstein I, Onyuksel H. Camptothecin in sterically stabilized phospholipid micelles: a novel nanomedicine. Nanomedicine 2005;1(1):77–84.
[10] Garnier S, Laschewsky A. New amphiphilic diblock copolymers: surfactant properties and solubilization in their micelles. Langmuir 2006;22(9):4044–53.

[11] La SB, Okano T, Kataoka K. Preparation and characterization of the micelle-forming polymeric drug indomethacin-incorporated poly(ethylene oxide)-poly(beta-benzyl L-aspartate) block copolymer micelles. J Pharm Sci 1996;85(1):85—90.
[12] Dufresne MHFF, Jones MC, Rnager M, Leroux JC. Block copolymer micelles-engineering versatile carriers for drugs and biomacromolecules. In: Challenges in drug delivery for the new millenium bulletin technique gattefosse. France: Z. Swiss Federal Institute of Technology; 2003. p. 87—102.
[13] Dean Deyle G. The role of MRI in musculoskeletal practice: a clinical perspective. J Man Manip Ther 2011;19(3):152—61.
[14] Alvarez Moreno E, Jimenez de la Pena M, Cano Alonso R. Role of new functional MRI techniques in the diagnosis, staging, and follow-up of gynecological cancer: comparison with PET-CT. Radiol Res Pract 2012;2012:219546.
[15] Agdeppa ED, Spilker ME. A review of imaging agent development. AAPS J 2009;11(2):286—99.
[16] Nieciecki M, Cacko M, Krolicki L. The role of ultrasound and nuclear medicine methods in the preoperative diagnostics of primary hyperparathyroidism. J Ultrason 2015;15(63):398—409.
[17] Daly C, et al. Patterns of diagnostic imaging and associated radiation exposure among long-term survivors of young adult cancer: a population-based cohort study. BMC Cancer 2015;15:612.
[18] Linet MS, et al. Cancer risks associated with external radiation from diagnostic imaging procedures. CA Cancer J Clin 2012;62(2):75—100.
[19] Vercher-Conejero JL, et al. Positron emission tomography in breast cancer. Diagn (Basel) 2015;5(1): 61—83.
[20] Hennedige T, Venkatesh SK. Imaging of hepatocellular carcinoma: diagnosis, staging and treatment monitoring. Cancer Imaging 2013;12:530—47.
[21] Flores LG, et al. Detection of pancreatic carcinomas by imaging lactose-binding protein expression in peritumoral pancreas using [18F]fluoroethyl-deoxylactose PET/CT. PLoS One 2009;4(11):e7977.
[22] Toy R, et al. Targeted nanotechnology for cancer imaging. Adv Drug Deliv Rev 2014;76:79—97.
[23] Kwon GS. Polymeric micelles for delivery of poorly water-soluble compounds. Crit Rev Ther Drug Carr Syst 2003;20(5):357—403.
[24] Fang J, Nakamura H, Maeda H. The EPR effect: unique features of tumor blood vessels for drug delivery, factors involved, and limitations and augmentation of the effect. Adv Drug Deliv Rev 2011;63(3):136—51.
[25] Torchilin VP. PEG-based micelles as carriers of contrast agents for different imaging modalities. Adv Drug Deliv Rev 2002;54(2):235—52.
[26] Torchilin VP. Polymer-coated long-circulating microparticulate pharmaceuticals. J Microencapsul 1998;15(1):1—19.
[27] Torchilin VP, Frank-Kamenetsky MD, Wolf GL. CT visualization of blood pool in rats by using long-circulating, iodine-containing micelles. Acad Radiol 1999;6(1):61—5.
[28] Trubetskoy VS, et al. Block-copolymer of polyethylene glycol and polylysine as a carrier of organic iodine: design of long-circulating particulate contrast medium for X-ray computed tomography. J Drug Target 1997;4(6):381—8.
[29] Patil RR, et al. Probing in vivo trafficking of polymer/DNA micellar nanoparticles using SPECT/CT imaging. Mol Ther 2011;19(9):1626—35.
[30] Lusic H, Grinstaff MW. X-ray-computed tomography contrast agents. Chem Rev 2013;113(3): 1641—66.
[31] Torchilin VP. Polymeric contrast agents for medical imaging. Curr Pharm Biotechnol 2000;1(2): 183—215.
[32] Trubetskoy VS, et al. Stable polymeric micelles: lymphangiographic contrast media for gamma scintigraphy and magnetic resonance imaging. Acad Radiol 1996;3(3):232—8.
[33] Kumar R, et al. Combined magnetic resonance and optical imaging of head and neck tumor xenografts using gadolinium-labelled phosphorescent polymeric nanomicelles. Head Neck Oncol 2010; 2:35.
[34] Song L, et al. Effective PEGylation of Fe_3O_4 nanomicelles for in vivo MR imaging. J Nanosci Nanotechnol 2015;15(6):4111—8.

[35] Li Y, et al. Light-triggered concomitant enhancement of magnetic resonance imaging contrast performance and drug release rate of functionalized amphiphilic diblock copolymer micelles. Biomacromolecules 2012;13(11):3877—86.

[36] Hu J, et al. Drug-loaded and superparamagnetic iron oxide nanoparticle surface-embedded amphiphilic block copolymer micelles for integrated chemotherapeutic drug delivery and MR imaging. Langmuir 2012;28(4):2073—82.

[37] Li X, et al. Amphiphilic multiarm star block copolymer-based multifunctional unimolecular micelles for cancer targeted drug delivery and MR imaging. Biomaterials 2011;32(27):6595—605.

[38] Yi X, et al. Near-infrared fluorescent probes in cancer imaging and therapy: an emerging field. Int J Nanomed 2014;9:1347—65.

[39] Wu J, Pan D, Chung LW. Near-infrared fluorescence and nuclear imaging and targeting of prostate cancer. Transl Androl Urol 2013;2(3):254—64.

[40] Luo S, et al. A review of NIR dyes in cancer targeting and imaging. Biomaterials 2011;32(29):7127—38.

[41] Miki K, et al. High-contrast fluorescence imaging of tumors in vivo using nanoparticles of amphiphilic brush-like copolymers produced by ROMP. Angew Chem Int Ed Engl 2011;50(29):6567—70.

[42] Escobedo JO, et al. NIR dyes for bioimaging applications. Curr Opin Chem Biol 2010;14(1):64—70.

[43] Kirchherr AK, Briel A, Mader K. Stabilization of indocyanine green by encapsulation within micellar systems. Mol Pharm 2009;6(2):480—91.

[44] Yang X, et al. Near IR heptamethine cyanine dye-mediated cancer imaging. Clin Cancer Res 2010;16(10):2833—44.

[45] Wang H, et al. In vivo photoacoustic molecular imaging of breast carcinoma with folate receptor-targeted indocyanine green nanoprobes. Nanoscale 2014;6(23):14270—9.

[46] Wu L, et al. Hybrid polypeptide micelles loading indocyanine green for tumor imaging and photothermal effect study. Biomacromolecules 2013;14(9):3027—33.

[47] Zheng C, et al. Indocyanine green-loaded biodegradable tumor targeting nanoprobes for in vitro and in vivo imaging. Biomaterials 2012;33(22):5603—9.

[48] Zheng X, et al. Enhanced tumor treatment using biofunctional indocyanine green-containing nanostructure by intratumoral or intravenous injection. Mol Pharm 2012;9(3):514—22.

[49] Shafirstein G, et al. Indocyanine green enhanced near-infrared laser treatment of murine mammary carcinoma. Int J Cancer 2012;130(5):1208—15.

[50] Yang H, et al. Micelles assembled with carbocyanine dyes for theranostic near-infrared fluorescent cancer imaging and photothermal therapy. Biomaterials 2013;34(36):9124—33.

[51] Wu CY, Benet LZ. Predicting drug disposition via application of BCS: transport/absorption/elimination interplay and development of a biopharmaceutics drug disposition classification system. Pharm Res 2005;22(1):11—23.

[52] Dian L, et al. Enhancing oral bioavailability of quercetin using novel soluplus polymeric micelles. Nanoscale Res Lett 2014;9(1):2406.

[53] Xu W, Ling P, Zhang T. Polymeric micelles, a promising drug delivery system to enhance bioavailability of poorly water-soluble drugs. J Drug Deliv 2013;2013:340315.

[54] Chiappetta DA, et al. Oral pharmacokinetics of the anti-HIV efavirenz encapsulated within polymeric micelles. Biomaterials 2011;32(9):2379—87.

[55] Savic R, Eisenberg A, Maysinger D. Block copolymer micelles as delivery vehicles of hydrophobic drugs: micelle-cell interactions. J Drug Target 2006;14(6):343—55.

[56] Sutton D, et al. Functionalized micellar systems for cancer targeted drug delivery. Pharm Res 2007;24(6):1029—46.

[57] Wang T, et al. Paclitaxel-loaded PEG-PE-based micellar nanopreparations targeted with tumor-specific landscape phage fusion protein enhance apoptosis and efficiently reduce tumors. Mol Cancer Ther 2014;13(12):2864—75.

[58] Torchilin VP, et al. Immunomicelles: targeted pharmaceutical carriers for poorly soluble drugs. Proc Natl Acad Sci USA 2003;100(10):6039—44.

[59] Ahn J, et al. Antibody fragment-conjugated polymeric micelles incorporating platinum drugs for targeted therapy of pancreatic cancer. Biomaterials 2015;39:23—30.

[60] Lu ZR, Kopeckova P, Kopecek J. Polymerizable Fab' antibody fragments for targeting of anticancer drugs. Nat Biotechnol 1999;17(11):1101—4.

[61] Sarisozen C, Abouzeid AH, Torchilin VP. The effect of co-delivery of paclitaxel and curcumin by transferrin-targeted PEG-PE-based mixed micelles on resistant ovarian cancer in 3-D spheroids and in vivo tumors. Eur J Pharm Biopharm 2014;88(2):539—50.

[62] Sawant RR, et al. Targeted transferrin-modified polymeric micelles: enhanced efficacy in vitro and in vivo in ovarian carcinoma. Mol Pharm 2014;11(2):375—81.

[63] Danhier F, Le Breton A, Preat V. RGD-based strategies to target alpha(v) beta(3) integrin in cancer therapy and diagnosis. Mol Pharm 2012;9(11):2961—73.

[64] Xiao K, et al. "OA02" peptide facilitates the precise targeting of paclitaxel-loaded micellar nanoparticles to ovarian cancer in vivo. Cancer Res 2012;72(8):2100—10.

[65] Zhan C, et al. Cyclic RGD conjugated poly(ethylene glycol)-*co*-poly(lactic acid) micelle enhances paclitaxel anti-glioblastoma effect. J Control Release 2010;143(1):136—42.

[66] Li X, et al. Targeted delivery of anticancer drugs by aptamer AS1411 mediated Pluronic F127/cyclodextrin-linked polymer composite micelles. Nanomedicine 2015;11(1):175—84.

[67] Mu C, et al. Solubilization of flurbiprofen into aptamer-modified PEG-PLA micelles for targeted delivery to brain-derived endothelial cells in vitro. J Microencapsul 2013;30(7):701—8.

[68] Wang XQ, Zhang Q. pH-sensitive polymeric nanoparticles to improve oral bioavailability of peptide/protein drugs and poorly water-soluble drugs. Eur J Pharm Biopharm 2012;82(2):219—29.

[69] Wu XL, et al. Tumor-targeting peptide conjugated pH-responsive micelles as a potential drug carrier for cancer therapy. Bioconjugate Chem 2010;21(2):208—13.

[70] Kim D, et al. Doxorubicin loaded pH-sensitive micelle: antitumoral efficacy against ovarian A2780/DOXR tumor. Pharm Res 2008;25(9):2074—82.

[71] Bae Y, Nishiyama N, Kataoka K. In vivo antitumor activity of the folate-conjugated pH-sensitive polymeric micelle selectively releasing adriamycin in the intracellular acidic compartments. Bioconjugate Chem 2007;18(4):1131—9.

[72] Lee ES, Na K, Bae YH. Doxorubicin loaded pH-sensitive polymeric micelles for reversal of resistant MCF-7 tumor. J Control Release 2005;103(2):405—18.

[73] Bae Y, et al. Preparation and biological characterization of polymeric micelle drug carriers with intracellular pH-triggered drug release property: tumor permeability, controlled subcellular drug distribution, and enhanced in vivo antitumor efficacy. Bioconjugate Chem 2005;16(1):122—30.

[74] Soga O, van Nostrum CF, Hennink WE. Thermosensitive and biodegradable polymeric micelles with transient stability. J Control Release 2005;101(1—3):383—5.

[75] Soga O, et al. Thermosensitive and biodegradable polymeric micelles for paclitaxel delivery. J Control Release 2005;103(2):341—53.

[76] Soga O, et al. Physicochemical characterization of degradable thermosensitive polymeric micelles. Langmuir 2004;20(21):9388—95.

[77] Soga O, van Nostrum CF, Hennink WE. Poly(*N*-(2-hydroxypropyl) methacrylamide mono/di lactate): a new class of biodegradable polymers with tunable thermosensitivity. Biomacromolecules 2004;5(3):818—21.

[78] Lin HM, et al. Light-sensitive intelligent drug delivery systems of coumarin-modified mesoporous bioactive glass. Acta Biomater 2010;6(8):3256—63.

[79] Alvarez-Lorenzo C, Bromberg L, Concheiro A. Light-sensitive intelligent drug delivery systems. Photochem Photobiol 2009;85(4):848—60.

[80] Goodwin AP, et al. Synthetic micelle sensitive to IR light via a two-photon process. J Am Chem Soc 2005;127(28):9952—3.

[81] Xia H, Zhao Y, Tong R. Ultrasound-mediated polymeric micelle drug delivery. Adv Exp Med Biol 2016;880:365—84.

[82] Husseini GA, Pitt WG, Martins AM. Ultrasonically triggered drug delivery: breaking the barrier. Colloids Surf B Biointerfaces 2014;123:364—86.

[83] Ahmed SE, Martins AM, Husseini GA. The use of ultrasound to release chemotherapeutic drugs from micelles and liposomes. J Drug Target 2015;23(1):16—42.

[84] Husseini GA, Pitt WG. Ultrasonic-activated micellar drug delivery for cancer treatment. J Pharm Sci 2009;98(3):795—811.

[85] Marin A, Muniruzzaman M, Rapoport N. Mechanism of the ultrasonic activation of micellar drug delivery. J Control Release 2001;75(1−2):69−81.
[86] Marin A, et al. Drug delivery in pluronic micelles: effect of high-frequency ultrasound on drug release from micelles and intracellular uptake. J Control Release 2002;84(1−2):39−47.
[87] Li X, et al. Acid-triggered core cross-linked nanomicelles for targeted drug delivery and magnetic resonance imaging in liver cancer cells. Int J Nanomed 2013;8:3019−31.
[88] Matsumura Y. The drug discovery by nanomedicine and its clinical experience. Jpn J Clin Oncol 2014;44(6):515−25.
[89] Kato K, et al. Phase II study of NK105, a paclitaxel-incorporating micellar nanoparticle, for previously treated advanced or recurrent gastric cancer. Invest New Drugs 2012;30(4):1621−7.
[90] Matsumura Y. Preclinical and clinical studies of NK012, an SN-38-incorporating polymeric micelles, which is designed based on EPR effect. Adv Drug Deliv Rev 2011;63(3):184−92.
[91] Matsumura Y, et al. Phase I clinical trial and pharmacokinetic evaluation of NK911, a micelle-encapsulated doxorubicin. Br J Cancer 2004;91(10):1775−81.
[92] Takahashi A, et al. NC-6300, an epirubicin-incorporating micelle, extends the antitumor effect and reduces the cardiotoxicity of epirubicin. Cancer Sci 2013;104(7):920−5.
[93] Plummer R, et al. A Phase I clinical study of cisplatin-incorporated polymeric micelles (NC-6004) in patients with solid tumours. Br J Cancer 2011;104(4):593−8.
[94] Alakhova DY, et al. Effect of doxorubicin/pluronic SP1049C on tumorigenicity, aggressiveness, DNA methylation and stem cell markers in murine leukemia. PLoS One 2013;8(8):e72238.
[95] Valle JW, et al. A phase 2 study of SP1049C, doxorubicin in P-glycoprotein-targeting pluronics, in patients with advanced adenocarcinoma of the esophagus and gastroesophageal junction. Invest New Drugs 2011;29(5):1029−37.

CHAPTER 4

Diagnosis and Drug Delivery to the Brain: Novel Strategies

Abhirup Mandal[1], Rohit Bisht[2], Dhananjay Pal[1], Ashim K. Mitra[1]
[1]University of Missouri—Kansas City, Kansas City, MO, United States; [2]University of Auckland, Auckland, New Zealand

Contents

1. Introduction	60
2. Barriers for Brain Drug Delivery	60
3. Physiology of the Blood—Brain Barrier	60
3.1 Conventional Strategies for Brain Drug Delivery	62
4. Invasive Drug Delivery Approaches	62
4.1 Convection Enhanced Drug Delivery	62
4.2 BBB Permeability Modulation	62
4.3 Ultrasound-Mediated BBB Disruption	63
4.4 Optical Modulation of Vascular Permeability	63
5. Noninvasive Drug Delivery Approaches	64
5.1 Chemical Derivatization	64
5.2 Prodrug Lipidization	65
5.3 Transporter-Targeted Prodrugs	65
5.4 Intranasal Drug Delivery	66
6. Nanotechnology Approaches	67
6.1 Nanoparticles	67
6.2 Polymeric Nanoparticles	67
6.3 Lipid Nanoparticles	68
6.4 Magnetic Nanoparticles	69
7. Active Blood—Brain Barrier Targeting Strategies	69
7.1 Absorptive-Mediated Transcytosis	70
7.2 Transporter-Mediated Transcytosis	71
7.3 Receptor-Mediated Transcytosis	71
7.4 Blood—Brain Tumor Barrier Targeting Strategies	72
8. Novel Nanoplatforms and Delivery Vehicles for BBB Targeting	73
8.1 Mesenchymal Stem Cells	73
8.2 Macrophages	73
8.3 Exosomes	74
9. Development of Neurodiagnostic Nanoimaging Platforms	74
9.1 Conventional Imaging Modalities	74
9.2 Optical Imaging	76
9.3 Hybrid Imaging Using Optical Contrast	77
10. Conclusion	77
Acknowledgment	79
References	79

Emerging Nanotechnologies for Diagnostics, Drug Delivery, and Medical Devices
ISBN 978-0-323-42978-8

1. INTRODUCTION

Improved methods for diagnosis and treatment of neurodegenerative disorders, human immunodeficiency virus (HIV) infection, glioblastoma multiforme (GBM), and other malignant tumors in the brain are desperately needed [1,2]. Despite the application of combination therapy, surgery, chemotherapy, and radiotherapy, brain disorders present an immense challenge due to rapid development and poor prognosis. Statistics published by the United Nations Programme on HIV/AIDS, World Health Organization, and United Nations Children's Fund in 2014 reported approximately 37 million people living with HIV/AIDS [3]. Additionally, more than 15,000 new cases of malignant gliomas are diagnosed in the United States every year. A major hurdle for treatment of HIV, GBM, and other CNS disorders is drug penetration into the brain parenchyma [4].

The CNS is a complex and delicate system surrounded by a natural protective barrier, called the blood—brain barrier (BBB). BBB limits entry of toxic substances such as bacteria and viruses while also preventing adequate brain availability of drugs and xenobiotics. Additionally, brain tumors exhibit many distinctive characteristics relative to other tumors in peripheral tissues such as a complicated anatomical structure and the nature of oncogenesis. All these factors add to the complexity and subsequent failure of currently available therapeutic regimens [5].

The foremost challenge of CNS therapy is the delivery of therapeutics to target the brain with minimal effects on other tissues. First-pass metabolism of orally administered drugs and efflux pumps expressed on the BBB diminish the delivery of therapeutics to the brain [6]. This chapter primarily emphasizes on targeted delivery and diagnostic strategies as well as combination strategies to overcome these factors. This chapter will also serve as a valuable reference to researchers interested in learning the fundamental function of the BBB, in vivo monitoring and imaging of therapeutics, and improving brain drug delivery via targeted approaches.

2. BARRIERS FOR BRAIN DRUG DELIVERY

Drug delivery to the brain poses a significant challenge. Despite the brain being a highly perfused organ, physiological barriers control the transfer of various substances including nutrients to the brain. The two main barriers contributing to the low brain bioavailability are BBB and blood—cerebrospinal fluid (BCSF) barrier [7]. Besides these barriers preventing therapeutic levels in the brain, the oncogenesis of gliomas is even more complicated [8]. Understanding the morphology and properties of these barriers is essential to successfully deliver drugs to the brain.

3. PHYSIOLOGY OF THE BLOOD—BRAIN BARRIER

The BBB acts as a neuroprotective shield by filtering harmful substances back into the blood stream and supplying brain tissues with nutrients. The BBB is composed of mainly three layers: an inner endothelial cell layer that forms the wall of brain capillaries, a basement membrane, and end feet processes of astrocytes and pericytes. The endothelial cells comprising the BBB express extensive tight junctions (TJs), have sparse pinocytic vesicular transport, and lack fenestrations unlike other endothelial cells [9]. These cells are mainly responsible for regulating the passage of drugs across the brain, leukocyte migration, and maintaining brain homeostasis crucial for neuronal activity. Pericytes and astrocytic/glial foot processes surround the brain capillary endothelial cells (BCECs). These cells provide trophic, metabolic, and structural support to the brain. TJs are responsible for limiting paracellular transport of hydrophilic molecules across the BBB due to high trans-endothelial electrical resistance of 1500–2000 Ω cm^2 [10]. TJs also possess an intricate structure of transmembrane proteins including junctional adhesion molecule-1, occludin, and claudin. Moreover, cytoplasmic accessory proteins (zonula occludens-1 and -2, cingulin, AF-6, and 7H6) are also involved. Fig. 4.1 illustrates an overview of the BBB and BCSF barrier [10a,10b]. In addition to BBB and BCSF, there are other barriers such as the blood–brain tumor barrier (BBTB) [1].

The BCSF barrier is the second most important CNS barrier next to BBB. It is formed by the epithelial cells of the choroid plexus. It mainly controls the transport of molecules within the interstitial fluid of the brain parenchyma by regulating the flow between blood and CSF. Facilitated diffusion, active transport, and efflux from blood into the CSF are the mechanisms for molecular transport via the choroid plexus [11].

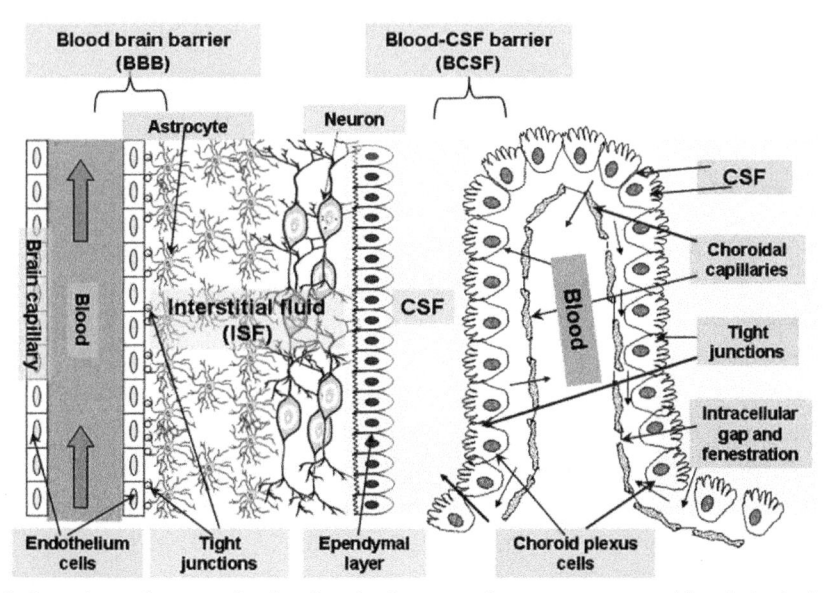

Figure 4.1 Overview of two major barriers in the central nervous system: blood–brain barrier and blood–cerebrospinal fluid barrier. *(Adapted from Pardridge WM. Why is the global CNS pharmaceutical market so under-penetrated? Drug Discov Today 2002;7(1):5–7 and Bradbury M, Begley DJ, Kreuter J, editors. The blood-brain barrier and drug delivery to the CNS. USA: Informa Healthcare; 2000.)*

3.1 Conventional Strategies for Brain Drug Delivery

Drug delivery to the CNS is highly challenging. Various drug delivery strategies have been employed to improve patient compliance, prolong drug half-life, minimize healthcare costs, and improve pharmacokinetics of degradable peptides and proteins. These strategies may be classified into two broad categories based on the method of drug delivery used. Invasive methods utilize direct delivery of therapeutic agents into the brain parenchyma or by disrupting the BBB. On the other hand, noninvasive methods take advantage of endogenous pathways to achieve therapeutic concentrations in the CNS [12].

4. INVASIVE DRUG DELIVERY APPROACHES

Invasive drug delivery approaches aim at maximizing the amount of a therapeutic agent at the target site through surgical methods or BBB disruption. Although invasive strategies can be aggressive, such procedures can prevent drugs from entering the systemic circulation thereby minimizing peripheral side effects. Transcranial injections, including intracerebral or intracerebroventricular techniques, are considered to be the gold standard for invasive brain drug delivery [13]. This process includes direct injection into the CNS through a cannula or insertion of a probe at the target site.

4.1 Convection Enhanced Drug Delivery

Convection enhanced drug delivery (CED) utilizes direct intracerebral injection with positive hydrostatic pressure for drug infusion. The hydrostatic pressure helps the drug to penetrate the brain tissues, and generates a fluid pressure gradient that causes the drug to further penetrate into the target site. Unlike other invasive techniques that utilize direct diffusion-dependent drug injections, CED uses bulk flow to achieve uniform drug distribution throughout the target site. Drugs, peptides, small interfering RNA (siRNA), and other macromolecules have been delivered to brain tissues with CED [14].

CED involves an image-guided insertion of a small catheter into the brain tissue. Various imaging techniques such as ultrasound are applied to guide the placement of the catheter. Positive pressure generated by the infusion pump allows the drug to be actively pumped into the brain. Studies suggest that the amount of drug reaching the target site is equivalent to the amount of drug being infused indicating high delivery efficiency via CED. In addition, it is always recommended to select a small catheter for the infusion purpose since it can damage the structural integrity of the brain parenchyma. Preclinical and clinical studies have found CED to be a promising strategy for the treatment of neurological disorders including brain tumors, epilepsy, and stroke [15–17].

4.2 BBB Permeability Modulation

Modulation of vascular permeability by transient disruption of brain capillary endothelial cells allows macromolecules to permeate into the CNS. These techniques may allow specific spatial delivery thus reducing side effects on surrounding normal tissues. Moreover, temporal specificity may also be achieved by transient opening of the BBB, which is restored after drug treatment [18—20]. Osmotic disruption of the BBB is another technique for increasing BBB permeability. It is performed by introducing high concentrations of mannitol into the carotid artery [21,22]. However, a major drawback of this technique is the lack of spatial as well as temporal specificity. New techniques are being aimed at disrupting the BBB without compromising the transient and spatial specificity wherein tissue recovery is rapid causing no permanent damage to the BBB and surrounding tissues.

4.3 Ultrasound-Mediated BBB Disruption

Ultrasound-mediated drug delivery (USMD) is a transient technique for delivering therapeutic agents into the CNS by disrupting the BBB. USMD employs ultrasound-activated microbubbles to exert mechanical force on the BBB, thus disrupting its integrity. This temporary disruption allows the therapeutic agent to leak into the target tissues in the CNS. Microbubbles are small (typically 1—8 μm in diameter) gas-filled, lipid- or protein-shelled microspheres that promote irreversible disruption of the BBB. Therapeutic agents along with a measured volume of microbubbles are initially injected intravenously. Once microbubbles and therapeutic agents have distributed throughout the blood stream, an ultrasound beam is focused on the target site of the BBB. The beam causes the microbubbles to oscillate, thus exerting and disrupting the TJs of the BBB through mechanical forces. This process leads to leakage of therapeutic agents into the target tissue. Ultrasound energy may hereby be confined within a smaller area (a few millimeters), leading to localized drug delivery and reducing possible side effects. Studies have demonstrated negligible capillary rupture and normal selective permeability is achieved within a few hours of treatment. This therapy renders USMD an ideal candidate for the treatment of tumors particularly glioblastoma, which requires aggressive chemotherapy [23].

However, USMD has not yet been applied clinically. Preclinical studies have demonstrated that elevated concentrations of microbubbles in the systemic circulation led to the disruption of capillaries for extended periods of time or even permanently resulting in an influx of blood proteins and also toxic substances such as bacteria and antibodies from the blood into the CNS. Due to these concerns, USMD is still in preclinical stages and the procedure needs further improvement and optimization for clinical application [24—27].

4.4 Optical Modulation of Vascular Permeability

Optical modulation of BBB permeability is attained by applying a femtosecond near-infrared pulsed laser. This technique is employed to induce leakage of blood plasma out of the BBB. Short pulsed lasers cause deep tissue penetration with minimal scattering and localized nonlinear absorption. With minimal invasive optical modulation, short pulsed lasers have performed as one of the most powerful techniques for in vivo imaging and subcellular organelle disruption [13,28]. Once the laser irradiation is discontinued, targeted blood vessels fully recover with minimal perturbation of BBB integrity contributing to the reversible nature of this method. Monoclonal antibodies, recombinant proteins, peptides, and trans-activating transcriptional activator (TAT) are the potential therapies that could be delivered with this technique. However, a major constraint of this technique is limited tissue penetration of the laser energy. Short pulsed lasers are only capable of penetrating approximately 1 nm deep into the tissue, which is not deep enough for adequate brain drug delivery. Additionally, near-infrared lasers can lead to generation of reactive oxygen species within the cell, leading to membrane dysfunction and DNA fragmentation ultimately causing cell apoptosis. Due to these limitations, optical modulation of the BBB is unlikely to be appropriate for clinical studies. However, further improvements in optical resolution and laser technology may be beneficial for future drug delivery applications [29,30].

5. NONINVASIVE DRUG DELIVERY APPROACHES

Although invasive methods can provide maximal drug delivery to the brain target site, these approaches cannot be translated to chronic disorders that require long-term intervention such as neurodegenerative disorders. Invasive strategies involve surgery and hospitalization. In contrast, noninvasive drug delivery strategies exploit various endogenous mechanisms to penetrate or bypass the BBB. These include nanocarriers such as custom lipids or peptides to transport therapeutic agents into the CNS. Such noninvasive strategies could also involve chemical derivatizations that utilize structural modification and prodrug synthesis to target and enhance transport into the CNS. Moreover, intranasal delivery may directly deliver drugs to the CNS via the olfactory pathway [31].

5.1 Chemical Derivatization

Low-molecular-weight lipophilic drugs (MW < 400 Da) are capable of penetrating the BBB through simple diffusion [32]. However, the majority of drugs lacking these properties are unable to enter the CNS. In such cases, a prodrug strategy can be a viable approach for CNS drug delivery. Various physiochemical properties such as molecular weight, solubility, stability, and permeability may be modified to improve CNS delivery. Other factors such as affinity toward influx and efflux transporters, protein binding, and metabolism by various enzymes and other tissues also need to be considered while designing a prodrug [33].

Albert first introduced the concept of prodrugs in 1985 and defined a prodrug as an inactive form of drug that undergoes bioconversion to the active parent form, by either chemical or enzymatic transformation in vivo [34]. The prodrug is converted to the active parent drug to exert its therapeutic effect only after crossing the BBB. Thus the active drug cannot diffuse back into circulation, forming a "locked-in" system. This is the primary feature of the prodrug approach for drug delivery to the CNS [35].

5.2 Prodrug Lipidization

The most common and simplest way of delivering CNS drugs across the BBB is by converting polar functional groups into a lipophilic prodrug. By increasing lipophilicity, it is anticipated that the prodrug will exhibit better permeation across the BBB [36]. A classic example of prodrug lipidization is heroin, a deacetylated derivative of morphine. The parent drug morphine is reported to exhibit lower brain uptake. However, O-acetylation of morphine generates heroin, which is capable of crossing the BBB approximately 100-fold higher than morphine [37].

One of the challenges for the prodrug strategy is site-specific delivery. Although, many prodrugs have achieved enhanced penetration into cells through the lipid bilayer of the plasma membrane, they experienced unfavorable bioconversion leading to lower concentrations of the active drug at the target site. Moreover, the rate of metabolism by cytochrome P-450 and other metabolizing enzymes accelerate with lipophilicity. All these limitations have dampened the practicality of this approach. In fact, there are only a few CNS prodrugs that have been modified by simple lipidization of polar groups in a molecule [38].

5.3 Transporter-Targeted Prodrugs

Site-specific transport can be achieved by targeting prodrugs to endogenous transporters. Two major endogenous transport mechanisms utilized in CNS drug delivery are receptor-mediated transport (RMT) and carrier-mediated transport [39]. These mechanisms will be discussed in detail in a later section.

The L-amino acid transporter (LAT) is highly expressed on the BBB. It is a type of membrane transport protein that is responsible for importing large neutral amino acids such as L-tyrosine and L-leucine in a Na^+-independent manner. Of the various amino acid transporters, LAT-1 is the most abundantly expressed influx transporter on the BBB [40]. This transporter plays a prime role in transporting naturally occurring amino acids as well as amino acid—related products such as L-3,4-dihydroxyphenylalanine (L-DOPA) and gabapentin. Table 4.1 depicts various carriers available for BBB transport by prodrug derivatization.

L-DOPA, a precursor of dopamine, is indicated in Parkinson disease. Carboxylation of dopamine generates L-DOPA, which acts as a pseudonutrient substrate for LAT-1 [41]. Once L-DOPA penetrates into the brain through LAT-1, a decarboxylase enzyme induces decarboxylation of L-DOPA, thus delivering dopamine into the CNS. However, to prevent the premature bioconversion of L-DOPA, patients with Parkinson disease are administered a combination of carbidopa and L-DOPA (Sinemet). Carbidopa acts as a

Table 4.1 Examples of endogenous transporters on brain capillary endothelial cells that can be exploited by carrier-mediated transport systems

Carrier type	Carrier	Representative substrate
LAT1	Neutral amino acid	L-Phenylalanine
GLUT1	Hexose	Glucose
MCT1	Monocarboxylic acid	Lactic acid
CAT1	Cationic amino acid	Arginine
CNT2	Nucleoside	Adenosine
SVCT2	Ascorbic acid	Vitamin C
SMVT	Multivitamin	Biotin

decarboxylase inhibitor and prevents peripheral conversion of L-DOPA to dopamine thus eliminating the risks of side effects. A current research study focused on developing a new hybrid glutathione-methionine peptidomimetic prodrug of L-DOPA to avoid its oxidative degradation in gastric fluid [42].

The broad specificities of various transporters and receptors have opened a wide array of drug modifications by chemical derivatization. Although several endogenous transporter substrate derivatives have been developed and studied extensively, one of the major challenges remains whether the drug is able to maintain its activity in the brain after crossing the BBB. Other issues with this strategy might be complications with the dosing regimens since transporter expression may vary from patient to patient.

5.4 Intranasal Drug Delivery

Intravenously administered drugs may undergo metabolism by the liver and other tissues in conjunction with absorption by peripheral tissues after reaching systemic circulation leading to undesirable side effects. In contrast, intranasal drug delivery represents a safe and effective technique for the delivery of therapeutics into the CNS by a pathway bypassing the BBB [43].

The olfactory epithelium in the nasal cavity is hereby utilized for direct delivery of therapeutic agents into the CNS. The primary mechanism of intranasal absorption is entry of the drug into the olfactory bulb through the olfactory epithelium. Once the drug reaches the olfactory bulb, it diffuses through the olfactory and trigeminal nerves thus effectively distributing the drug throughout the brain. One of the prime advantages of intranasal delivery is that the therapeutic agent can be administered in form of a liquid or aerosol even in an outpatient setting [44].

Intranasal drug delivery appears to be a safe and effective method for drug transport into the CNS. This method has several applications in preclinical as well as clinical setups. Intranasal delivery of insulin in clinical trials has shown to improve cognitive functions [45]. An improvement from deficient to normal insulin levels in the CNS of patients with Alzheimer disease was also demonstrated. Additionally, intranasal oxytocin was shown to improve social and emotional functions in patients with autism spectrum disorder suggesting the effectiveness of intranasal drug delivery [46,47].

Several approaches including mucoadhesive microparticle carriers are being developed to enhance adhesion and retention time of therapeutic agents in the olfactory epithelium. Application of these mucoadhesive carriers resulted in controlled release of dopamine into the CNS suggesting a possible role in the treatment of diseases such as Parkinson. However, only a small fraction of dose is able to diffuse through the olfactory epithelium [48,49]. Therefore research is now focused on other delivery strategies that can enhance diffusion across the olfactory epithelium.

6. NANOTECHNOLOGY APPROACHES
6.1 Nanoparticles

Nanotechnology has brought new possibilities in the development of various delivery systems such as systemic CNS delivery. Nanotechnology has been applied in the production of materials, devices, and electronic biosensors with sizes ranging from low to high nanometers. Nanotechnology-based products are being extensively used in clinics, drug delivery, and diagnosis [50]. Nanocarriers are designed for specific targeting of therapeutic agents to specific tissues and organs while also minimizing exposure of healthy tissues to toxic insults. Poorly distributed drugs can be easily loaded into a nanocarrier, and can thus deliver therapeutic concentrations into the brain. Nanoparticles being small in size pass through BBB capillaries and diffuse into the target tissues, releasing the loaded drug directly at the site of action [51].

Despite the advances and breakthroughs, nanotechnology-based strategies and approaches are not very effective in treating CNS disorders including GBM, HIV, and Alzheimer disease. Keeping in mind the dearth of currently available therapies for such debilitating disorders, targeting of drugs to the CNS will be the mainstay for the future development of nanotechnology-based therapeutics. Functionalization of nanocarriers will perhaps be the foremost step toward nanoscale CNS drug delivery systems.

Nanocarriers are colloidal systems in which the drug is either entrapped within the colloidal matrix of the nanoparticle or coated on the particle surface via conjugation or adsorption. Various nanocarriers have been developed and examined for delivery and diagnostic purposes such as polymeric, lipid-based, magnetic, and dendritic nanocarriers [52]. Other types of nanocarriers include micelles, nanogels, nanoemulsions, nanosuspensions, and ceramic as well as metal-based nanocarriers [53,54].

6.2 Polymeric Nanoparticles

Polymeric nanoparticles are the most widely studied nanocarriers. These constructs are commonly composed of acrylics such as poly butyl cyanoacrylate (PBCA) or polyesters. Rapid degradation of acrylic polymers prevents accumulation in the CNS and consequently

Table 4.2 Nanoparticle-conjugated platforms for delivery across the BBB [1]

Nanoparticle platform	Therapeutic agents (and effect)
PBCA NP coated with polysorbate 80	Dalargin (analgesic)
PBCA NP coated with polysorbate 80	Doxorubicin (antitumor antibiotic)
PBCA NP coated with polysorbate 80	Kytorphin (analgesic)
PBCA NP	NMDA receptor antagonist MRZ 2/576 (antagonist)
PBCA NP coated with polysorbate 80	Tubocurarine (increased BBB permeability)
PEG-PHDCA	PrPres specific drug in prion disease
PBCA NP coated with polysorbate 80	Tacrine (anti-Alzheimer drug)
PBCA NP coated with polysorbate 80	Rivastigmine (anti-Alzheimer drug)
PBCA NP coated with polysorbate 80	Gemcitabine (antiglioma drug)
DMAEMA/HEMA (pH sensitive)	Paclitaxel
LDC-polysorbate 80 NPs	Diminazene (anti—human African trypanosomiasis)
DO-FUdR-SLN	5-Fluoro-2′-deoxyuridine (very efficient in brain targeting)
PBCA NPs, MMA-SPM NPs, and SLNs	Stavudine (D4T), delavirdine, and saquinavir (anti-HIV agents and enhanced BBB permeability)
PBCA NPs coated with apolipoprotein B and E	Loperamide and dalargin (increased BBB permeability)

BBB, blood—brain barrier; *DMAEMA*, poly (N, N-dimethylaminoethyl methacrylate); *DO-FUdR*, 3′,5′-dioctanoyl-5-fluoro-2'-deoxyuridine; *HEMA*, 2-hydroxyethyl methacrylate; *HIV*, human immunodeficiency virus; *LDC*, lipid drug conjugate; *MMA-SPM*, methylmethacrylate-sulfopropylmethacrylate; *NMDA*, N-methyl-D-aspartate; *NP*, nanoparticle; *PBCA*, poly butyl cyanoacrylate; *PEG*, polyethylene glycol; *PHDCA*, polycyanoacrylate; *SLN*, solid lipid nanoparticle.

reduces adverse side effects. On the other hand, polyester nanoparticles degrade into water and carbon dioxide rendering these materials safer in comparison to acrylic polymers [55,56].

One primary barrier to the penetration of therapeutic agents into the CNS are the efflux pumps, which include several multidrug resistance proteins [permeability glycoprotein (P-gp), multidrug resistance-associated protein (MRP), and breast cancer resistance protein (BCRP)]. These efflux proteins actively export molecules out of the CNS. Polymeric nanoparticles have the potential to circumvent these efflux systems. Additionally, polymeric nanocarriers are capable of surface modifications such as PEGylation. This process improves nanoparticle selectivity and targetability in the CNS. Antiretroviral drugs including nucleoside reverse transcriptase inhibitors such as lamivudine and zidovudine may be successfully delivered into the CNS using lipophilic PBCA-based polymeric nanoparticles [57,58]. Nanoparticle-conjugated platforms utilized for CNS delivery are presented in Table 4.2.

6.3 Lipid Nanoparticles

Solid lipid nanoparticles (SLNs) primarily consist of fatty acids or mono-, di-, or triglycerides. Such lipid matrices remain in the solid state at normal body temperature. The highly lipophilic nature of SLNs renders these particles to facilitate BBB transport.

Advantages of SLNs include good tolerance, high bioavailability, CNS targeting, and biodegradability without formation of any toxic degradation product [59].

SLNs have been extensively used for the delivery of chemotherapeutic agents into the CNS. In fact, surface-modified polyethylene glycol (PEG)-coated SLNs apart from evading efflux pumps, prevent detection by the reticuloendothelial system thus imparting a stealth-like property [60]. DNA-loaded surface-modified SLNs have shown to exhibit high gene expression in vivo relative to control [61].

6.4 Magnetic Nanoparticles

Magnetic nanoparticles (MNPs) have gained interest in the field of drug delivery. These magnetic particles have the ability to target specific cells thus lowering systemic exposure of cytotoxic compounds. Magnetic nanoparticles are prepared from stable colloidal suspensions of MNPs in liquid carriers. The most commonly used liquid carriers are composed of iron oxides. Such nanocarriers exhibit superparamagnetic behavior at room temperature under the influence of a magnetic field [62].

The mechanism of MNP-mediated drug delivery is based on binding of therapeutic agents to the magnetic fluids. Surface-bound therapeutics are injected into the systemic circulation and are localized at the target site under an external magnetic field. However, MNPs may agglomerate and form clusters, which can be prevented by surface modifications. Such surface modifications render MNPs more stable. It can also eliminate remnant magnetization once the external field is removed, while also rendering MNPs more biostable, biodegradable, and nontoxic. A major limitation of MNPs is the size dependency. Although MNPs with a diameter larger than 200 nm are sequestered by the spleen, those smaller than 10 nm are easily removed by renal clearance [63].

MNPs integrated with other technologies offer an effective mechanism to treat multiple brain tumors such as gliomas. Higher drug concentrations are observed at the tumor site with magnetic nanoparticle [64]. However, several concerns with MNPs are noticed such as poor degradation leading to accumulation in normal tissues. Chronic inflammatory reactions, hemolysis, rise in reactive oxygen species leading to mitochondrial damage and cell death have been reported [65].

7. ACTIVE BLOOD–BRAIN BARRIER TARGETING STRATEGIES

The BBB acts as a natural defensive layer to protect the brain from various toxic substances while providing the brain with necessary nutrients for proper functioning [66]. Capillary endothelial cells are partially covered by pericytes, basement membrane, and almost fully covered by astrocytic/glial foot processes, which render the BBB a highly efficient barrier. Approximately 98% of small molecules and nearly 100% of large molecules including genes and proteins are prevented from entering the brain [67]. Fig. 4.2 illustrates various structural components of the BBB.

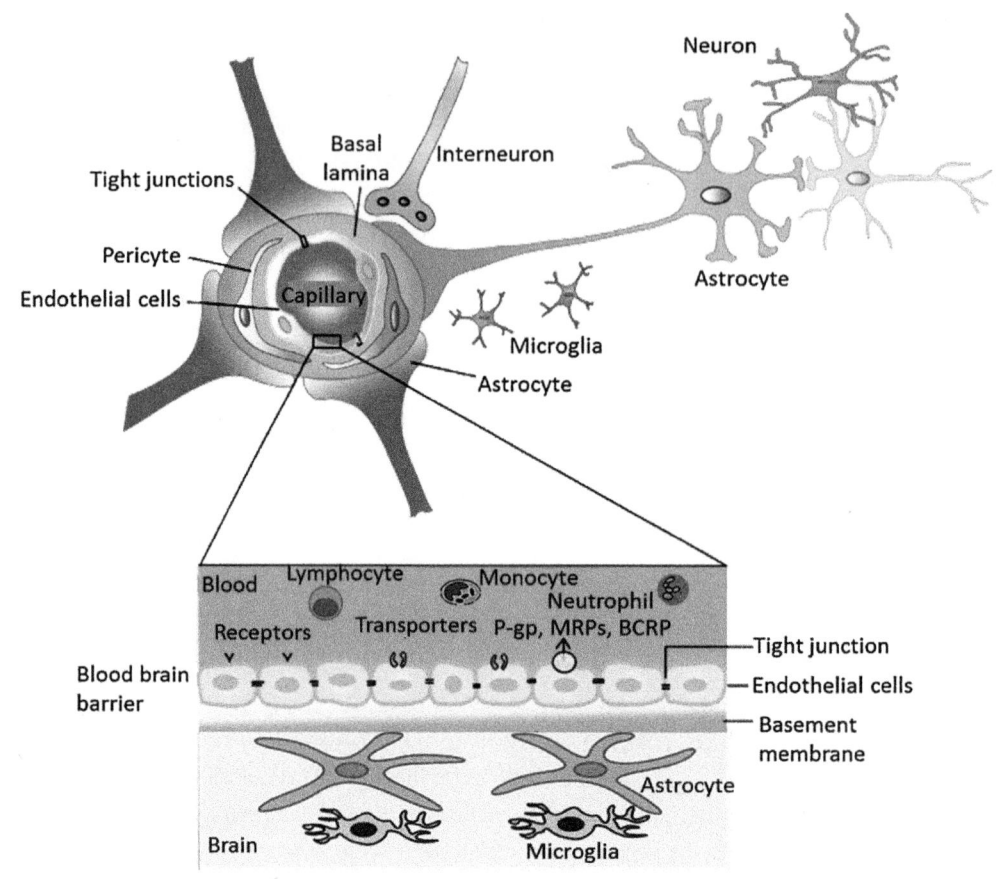

Figure 4.2 Structural components of the blood—brain barrier. *(Republished with permission of Nanda K, Mandava, Patel M, Mitra AK. Advanced Drug Delivery to the Brain: John Wiley and Sons Inc. 2013 [chapter 21], permission conveyed through Copyright Clearance Center, Inc.)*

To overcome this challenge, many active targeting strategies have been adopted, which are mainly divided into absorptive-mediated transcytosis (AMT), transporter-mediated transcytosis (TMT), and receptor-mediated endocytosis (RMT) [68].

7.1 Absorptive-Mediated Transcytosis

AMT can facilitate drug transport across the BBB through cationic proteins or cell-penetrating peptides (CPPs) [68]. The mechanism is primarily based on electrostatic interactions between positively charged protein moieties and negatively charged brain endothelial cells. For example, cationic bovine serum albumin—conjugated PEGylated nanoparticles (CBSA-NP) exhibited 7.76 times higher permeability relative to plain BSA-NP across BBB [69]. Similarly, aclarubicin (ACL)-loaded bovine serum albumin—conjugated PEGylated nanoparticles (CBSA-NP-ACL) exhibited prolonged survival of a glioblastoma-bearing mice [70].

Furthermore, CPP-based drug delivery systems have shown potential in enhanced BBB transport. Delivery of cargoes including peptides, proteins, DNA/RNA, antibodies, imaging agents, and nanodrug carriers such as liposomes and micelles has become possible by overcoming lipophilic barriers of cellular membrane with CPPs. These peptides are typically a chain of cationic amino acids such as lysine or arginine or sequences containing polar/charged and nonpolar, hydrophobic amino acids in an alternating pattern [71]. CPPs are derived from natural proteins including TAT, penetratin, and the Syn-B vectors. Among these, TAT is the most frequently used. Several studies have shown the potential of TAT-modified nanodrug carrier transport into the brain for diagnosis and treatment of CNS disorders. For instance, TAT (AYGRKKRRQRRR) was covalently conjugated with cholesterol to prepare doxorubicin-loaded liposomes for glioma therapy. Higher brain concentrations of doxorubicin were achieved resulting in higher survival rates of glioma-bearing rats. These studies show that AMT can be utilized as a potential strategy for targeting BBB [72].

7.2 Transporter-Mediated Transcytosis

Influx transporters are expressed on the cerebral endothelium. These proteins are primarily responsible for the transport of nutrients and endogenous substances into the brain. TMT utilizes these transport systems for various BBB-targeting strategies. It is a substrate-selective process where the drugs closely mimicking the endogenous substrates will be transported into the brain [11].

Glucose transporters (GLUT) are known to facilitate transport of glucose from blood to the brain. It was observed that when a mannose derivative was incorporated onto a liposome, the delivery system exhibited better penetration across the BBB via the glucose transporter (GLUT1) into the mouse brain [71]. Choline transporters are another group of transport systems responsible for binding with positively charged quaternary ammonium groups or simple cations. Sixty nanometer size particles coated with quaternary ammonium ligands have shown enhanced penetrability across an in vitro BBB model (bovine BCEC) [73]. Histidine/peptide (peptide/histidine transporter), large neutral amino acid transporter (LAT1), and vitamin transporters [sodium-dependent multivitamin transporter (SMVT) and sodium-dependent vitamin C transporter (SVCT)] are some of the influx transporters that have gained attention [74—76]. These transporters are being studied extensively for targeted drug delivery to the brain.

7.3 Receptor-Mediated Transcytosis

AMT strategies have the potential in treating CNS disorders. However, poor specificity and high toxicity due to unspecific binding with any negatively charged cell membrane constituents limit their utility. Additionally, TMT is highly specific and recognizes only those constructs that closely mimic endogenous carrier substrates leading to low selectivity. Receptor-mediated transcytosis is one of the promising strategies for targeted delivery across the BBB with high specificity, selectivity, and affinity [77]. However, there might be a possibility of competition between endogenous substrates and drug ligands for the same receptor leading to reduced targeting efficiency. Receptors expressed on the brain capillary endothelium include transferrin receptor (TfR) [78], low-density lipoprotein receptor [79], insulin, and nicotinic acetylcholine receptors [80,81]. Targeting with endogenous ligands as well as ligands based on phage display or structure-guided design can be exploited for receptor-mediated transcytosis.

The TfR, highly expressed on brain capillary endothelial cells, is one of the most widely characterized targets for drug delivery to the brain. Highly selective brain targeting efficiencies and antiglioma activities were exhibited by transferrin-conjugated paclitaxel-loaded polyphosphoester hybrid micelles [82]. However, transferrin may compete with natural ligands reducing its efficacy. As an alternative to this strategy, a mouse monoclonal antibody (Mab) against rat TfR (OX26) was studied. Immunoliposome-based drug delivery systems including OX26 coupled with liposomes have shown very high drug levels in rat brain [83].

Another commonly selected target is the low-density lipoprotein receptor—related protein (LRP). It has been utilized to facilitate transport of ligand-conjugated nanocarriers across the BBB. Aprotinin, an LRP ligand, exhibited at least 10-fold greater transcytosis across bovine brain capillary endothelial cells relative to holo-transferrin [84]. Angiopep, derived from aprotinin, has generated even higher transcytosis capacity and parenchymal accumulation, rendering it a promising candidate for targeted drug delivery against glioma and other CNS disorders [85].

Among these receptors, nicotinic acetylcholine receptors are expressed highly on brain capillary endothelial cells [85]. These ligand-gated ion channels can bind with loop II of snake toxin with high affinity and specificity. Several studies indicated that these receptors can be targeted for siRNA delivery to the brain. Results obtained from these studies indicate its safe and noninvasive nature for intracranial drug transport [86,86a].

7.4 Blood—Brain Tumor Barrier Targeting Strategies

Similar to BBB, the BBTB is located between the brain tumor tissue and microvessels formed by brain capillary endothelial cells. As the brain tumor grows in size, it invades the normal surrounding brain tissues. Once tumor cells grow to a certain size/volume, the BBB is damaged and BBTB is formed. The blood—tumor barrier of solid malignant tumor cells growing in the peripheral tissues are more permeable compared with the BBTB of similar malignant tumors growing in the brain [87]. The gradual deterioration of the BBB as well as angiogenesis renders BBTB a highly inaccessible barrier even for nanodrug carriers. Although the integrity of the BBB is compromised in malignant gliomas, the infiltrating gliomas exploit the brain vasculature thus limiting the transport of chemotherapeutic agents into gliomas. At this stage targeting various receptors present on the BBB/BBTB may offer a chance for treating malignant gliomas. These receptors mainly involve epidermal growth factor receptors and integrin [88].

The adhesion receptor integrin, particularly integrin $\alpha v \beta 3$, is highly expressed on malignant gliomas but not on normal brain cells. Cyclic arginine-glycine-aspartic acid peptide and its analogs are ligands for integrin, which can be targeted for drug delivery to malignant gliomas [89]. Another receptor, endothelial growth factor receptor (EGFR), is a transmembrane tyrosine kinase normally expressed in epithelial, mesenchymal, and neuronal tissues. However, it is highly expressed on BBTB, which can serve as a potential target for glioma therapy. Endothelial growth factor and anti-EGFR monoclonal antibodies are the most common EGFR ligands for this purpose [90].

8. NOVEL NANOPLATFORMS AND DELIVERY VEHICLES FOR BBB TARGETING

8.1 Mesenchymal Stem Cells

The brain homeostasis is tightly maintained by the BBB, circulating immunocytes such as macrophages, and distinct subsets of lymphocytes. These immunocytes utilize specialized mechanisms to penetrate the BBB without compromising its structural integrity. Stem cells, particularly mesenchymal stem cells, can also penetrate the BBB. These cells show tropism for brain tumors in animal models. However, their transmigration mechanism across the BBB is poorly understood. In fact, potential for teratogenicity is a major concern [91].

8.2 Macrophages

Macrophages have numerous advantages as a brain delivery tool. They appear to be the natural choice as a cellular/biological vehicle for the delivery of nanoparticles into the CNS for a variety of reasons. First, to maintain brain homeostasis, routine trafficking of macrophages occurs through BBB. However, during neuroinflammatory conditions, a high turnover rate of macrophages ensues (30% in 90 days) leading to higher uptake into the CNS. Second, under normal physiological conditions, monocytes/macrophages can traverse the BBB through highly regulated paracellular diapedesis and also through less well-defined transcellular diapedesis. It is a process of movement by which leukocytes escape out of the circulatory system and travel toward the site of tissue damage or infection. Such transmigration of macrophages occurs into the brain without any structural damage to the BBB. Third, macrophages are attracted and infiltrated into the brain during inflammation and tumor growth. This mechanism can render them as potential delivery vehicle carrying therapeutic nanoparticles for the treatment of CNS disorders including malignant gliomas. Finally, macrophages are responsible for carrying out the natural function of phagocytosis of foreign bodies. This property enables macrophages to entrap a variety of nanocarriers including therapeutic, diagnostic, and imaging agents, which are otherwise restricted by the BBB [92–94].

8.3 Exosomes

Exosomes represent another type of biological vehicle. Exosomes are gaining popularity for the delivery of therapeutic agents. These are cell-derived vesicles that are present in biological fluids including blood and urine under physiological and pathological conditions. These extracellular vesicles range between 30 and 120 nm in size. These vesicles are involved in intercellular trafficking of cell-specific cargo such as peptides and proteins. The surface architecture of exosomes enables efficient fusion with target cells, thereby delivering the cargo into the cells. Incorporation of neuron-specific peptides on macrophages or exosomes by chemical conjugation or simple adsorption to facilitate trafficking into the brain should be explored in the future. These strategies may provide maximum therapeutic concentrations in the brain for the treatment of various CNS disorders [95–97]. Fig. 4.3 illustrates cell-mediated transcytosis by monocytes/macrophages and exosomes for active BBB targeting.

9. DEVELOPMENT OF NEURODIAGNOSTIC NANOIMAGING PLATFORMS

The field of brain imaging has made significant progress with the advent of multifunctional nanoparticles. Monitoring events at molecular levels and at the same time tracking development of neurological diseases and tumor formation are now possible. Several well-established imaging platforms like positron emission tomography (PET) [98], single photon emission computed tomography (SPECT) [99], magnetic resonance imaging (MRI) [100], computerized tomography (CT) [101], and optical contrast-based imagining techniques such as bioluminescence imaging [102], fluorescence molecular tomography (FMT) [103], and optoacoustic tomography [104] have gained tremendous popularity and applicability in neurological research.

9.1 Conventional Imaging Modalities

Over the last three decades, X-ray CT, MRI, and PET are the common methods that are being utilized for visualization and imaging of drug transport and therapeutic effects. X-ray CT has emerged as one of the most promising visualization techniques for imaging drug distribution and treatment efficacy. It is mainly based on indirect tracking of morphological changes. Several studies have been performed for in vivo imaging of various tissue vasculatures with nanocarriers loaded with CT imaging agents. Altogether, application of X-ray CT imaging may have a significant impact on human health care system. Additionally, micro-CT and hybrid systems combining PET and SPECT with X-ray CT are gaining significant interest in preclinical as well as clinical settings.

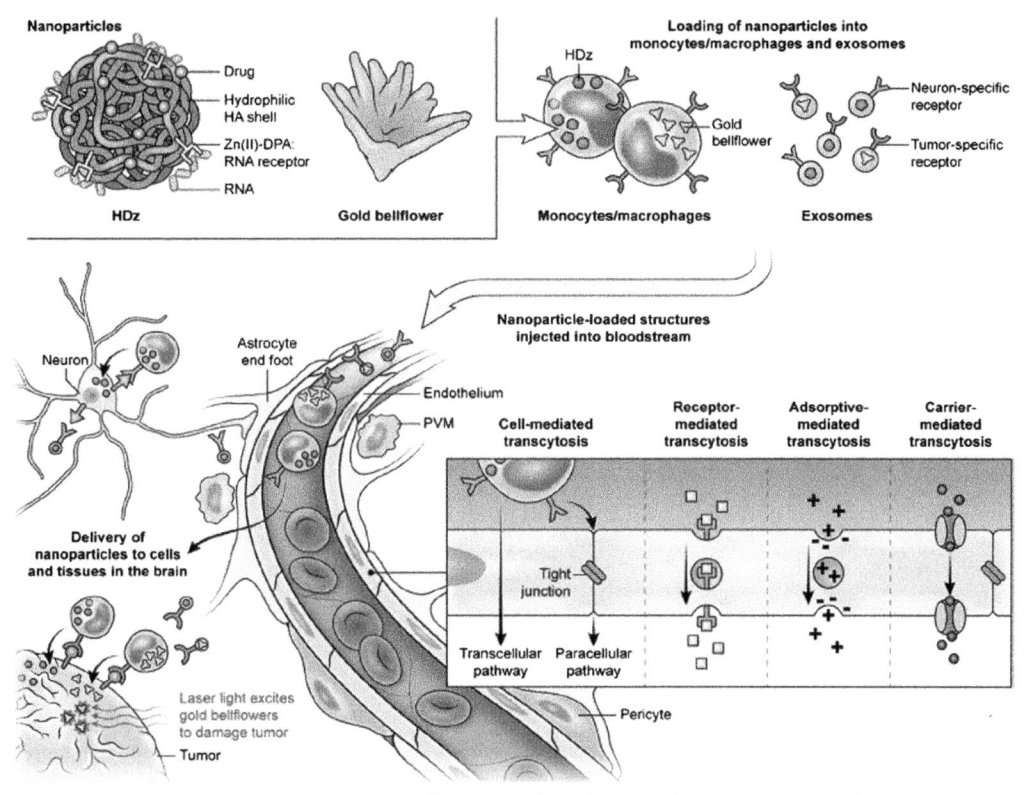

Figure 4.3 Major transport mechanisms for active blood–brain barrier targeting, focusing on cell-mediated transcytosis by monocytes/macrophages and exosomes. *HA*, hyaluronic acid; *HDz*, hyaluronic acid nanoparticles; *PVM*, perivascular macrophages. *(Reprinted with permission from Ali IU, Chen X. Penetrating the blood–brain barrier: promise of novel nanoplatforms and delivery vehicles. ACS Nano 2015;9(10):9470–4. Copyright 2015 American Chemical Society.)*

Commonly used CT contrast agents are based on small molecules that effectively absorb X-rays. However, nonspecific distribution, short half-life, and low sensitivity have limited their use and performance [105].

MRI has emerged as a tool in oncology and CNS disorders because of its distinct functional imaging potential as well as better contrast among soft tissues in comparison with CT. However, MRI displays low sensitivity to exogenous agents. Manganese has shown promising results as a T1 contrast neutral tracer for MRI [106]. MNPs are also of considerable interest as contrast agents for MRI. In fact, multifunctional platforms including superparamagnetic iron oxide NPs, paramagnetic contrast agent (gadolinium), or perfluorocarbons have been extensively exploited for their potential role in tracking single or clusters of labeled cells within target tissues [107].

PET is another noninvasive imaging technology that enables tracking of distribution of positron emitter-labeled compounds. The high sensitivity of PET renders it exceptionally superior in comparison with CT and MRI. Since its introduction in the late 1970s, PET has become a powerful tool for imaging and detection of molecular tracers and is currently being employed for diagnosis, monitoring, and imaging gene expressions with diverse probes. However, high costs, low sensitivity, and low spatial resolution are some of the drawbacks that limit its application [108,109].

9.2 Optical Imaging

Simplicity, low cost, and small size of equipment allow optical imaging with unique capabilities. Visible and near-infrared wavelengths extend many probing mechanisms with highly specific contrast approaches in this technique. The use of this approach extends from detection of intrinsic functional information on blood oxygenation to molecular sensing. Nonionizing properties of light radiation may allow repeated doses to animal or patients without any harm or side effects. Easy differentiation between soft tissues and ability to gather functional information by specific absorption with natural chromophores are the advantages of optical contrast methods over other imaging modalities. Furthermore, application of extrinsically administered "switchable" and "tumor-selective" fluorescent optical agents can advance the application of optical contrast methods in imaging at both cellular and subcellular levels [110].

Various fluorogenic-substrate-sensitive fluorochromes are commercially available and are extensively applied as fluorescent probes/markers for biological imaging. So far, these optical methods represent a highly effective technique in clinical as well as preclinical studies such as tissue hemodynamics, gene expression profiling, cancer growth, inflammation-mediated protease upregulation detection, and monitoring efficacy of anticancer treatments [111]. A combination of recently developed near-infrared probes with optical imaging may add to this highly sensitive technology for in vivo and real-time imaging. Expression patterns of various enzymes involved in tumor development and metastasis can also be monitored. Despite several advantages, optical imaging is limited by scattering. Thick tissues absorb and diffuse light significantly leading to degradation of spatial resolution, penetration capabilities, and overall image qualities.

Diffuse optical tomography methods have been recently developed. This technique is capable of providing volumetric optical contrast images of the entire human brain. The applications range from real-time functional neuroimaging to detection of gliomas [112].

FMT is an advanced method that illuminates samples at multiple projections and exploits mathematical models of photon propagation in tissues. Based on the distribution of fluorescent molecular probes or proteins, the underlying imaging contrast is reconstructed in three dimensions. Fig. 4.4 depicts a state-of-the-art free-space FMT scanner for in vivo tomographic imaging. So far, FMT has been successfully employed in molecular imaging studies of CNS disorders. Several studies have demonstrated the ability of FMT to resolve three-dimensional fluorochromes to quantify tissues and analyze response over time [113,114].

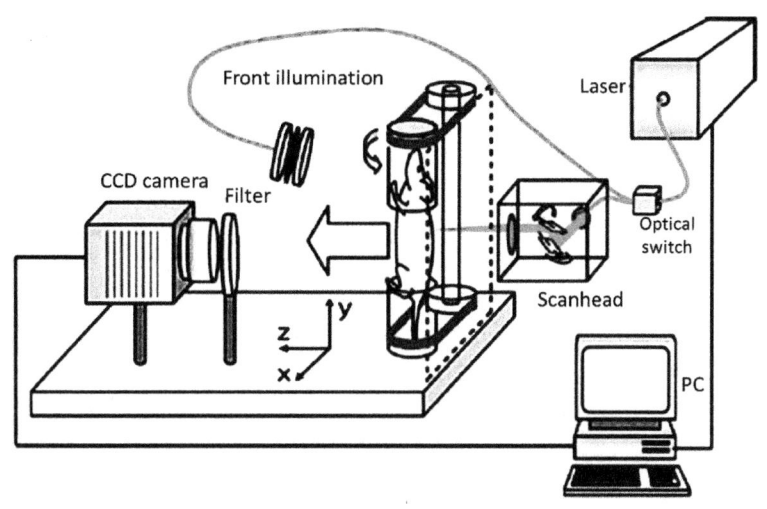

Figure 4.4 Schematic of a free-space 360 degrees projection fluorescence molecular tomography imaging system. *CCD*, charge-coupled device; *PC*, personal computer. *(Reprinted with permission from Macmillan Publishers Ltd: Nature Medicine, Ntziachristos V, et al. Fluorescence molecular tomography resolves protease activity in-vivo. Nat Med 2002;8(7):757–60, copyright (2002).)*

9.3 Hybrid Imaging Using Optical Contrast

Optoacoustic (or photoacoustic) tomography is an alternative hybrid imaging method that has been recently developed. This method is based on the detection of ultrasonic signals induced by absorption of pulsed light. It leads to high optical contrast images combined with good spatial resolution not limited by light scattering in tissues [115]. Multispectral optoacoustic tomography is one of the hybrid imaging methods that is still in its infancy with respect to development and application. However, it is one of the rapidly emerging fields in imaging sciences that can overcome barriers of optical imaging retaining its contrast, resolution, and sensitivity [116,117]. Table 4.3 describes various techniques for CNS imaging.

10. CONCLUSION

The BBB presents a formidable barrier for brain transport of therapeutic agents from the systemic circulation to the brain. Complex TJs and efflux systems expressed on capillary endothelial cells significantly limit brain permeation of therapeutic agents. This inability of adequate drug transport to the brain parenchyma led to the development of several advanced methods for brain targeting and drug delivery. Such approaches involve modulation of the BBB permeability, chemical derivatization, prodrug lipidization, intranasal drug delivery, and nanotechnology approaches such as nanoparticles and micelles. Moreover, active BBB targeting strategies through various transcytosis mechanisms are

Table 4.3 A list of different techniques for depth-resolved imaging of the CNS [1]

Imaging method	Anatomical contrast	Molecular/functional contrast	Sensitivity to contrast agents	Spatial resolution*	Penetration depth	Cost	Safety	Applicability
X-ray CT	Medium	Poor	μmol (10^{-6})	10–500 μm scalable	Whole body	Medium	Medium	Preclinical/clinical
MRI	Good	Medium	nmol (10^{-9})	30–500 μm scalable	Whole body	High	Good	Preclinical/clinical
PET/SPECT	Poor	Good	fmol (10^{-14})	1–5 mm	Whole body	High	Medium	Preclinical/clinical
3D light microscopy	Good	Good	fmol (10^{-14})	0.2–10 μm	Superficial (<1 mm)	Medium	Good	Preclinical/clinical
FMT	Poor	Good	pmol (10^{-12})	1–2 mm	~20 mm	Low	Good	Preclinical/clinical
MSOT microscopy/tomography	Good	Good	pmol (10^{-12})	5–200 μm scalable	~30 mm	Low	Good	Preclinical/clinical

CT, computerized tomography; *FMT*, fluorescence molecular tomography; *MRI*, magnetic resonance imaging; *MSOT*, multispectral optoacoustic tomography; *PET*, positron emission tomography; *SPECT*, single photon emission computed tomography.
* Spatial resolution usually depends on the overall size of the imaged object/area; therefore a range has been provided.

promising approaches that are currently being developed. Novel nanoplatforms with biological materials such as mesenchymal stem cells, macrophages, and exosomes as delivery vehicles are the latest advancements in the field of brain-targeted drug delivery. Additionally, MNPs and modern hybrid imaging technologies have opened up the field of diagnosis and drug delivery to the CNS. However, further efforts are needed for targeted drug delivery as well as brain imaging to improve therapies for CNS disorders.

ACKNOWLEDGMENT

This work was supported by NIH grant R01 AI071199. We would also like to thank Dr. Ilva D. Rupenthal for her valuable help and guidance.

REFERENCES

[1] Bhaskar S, et al. Multifunctional nanocarriers for diagnostics, drug delivery and targeted treatment across blood—brain barrier: perspectives on tracking and neuroimaging. Part Fibre Toxicol 2010;7:3.
[2] Carlsson SK, Brothers SP, Wahlestedt C. Emerging treatment strategies for glioblastoma multiforme. EMBO Mol Med 2014;6(11):1359—70.
[3] Fettig J, et al. Global epidemiology of HIV. Infect Dis Clin North Am 2014;28(3):323—37.
[4] Zhou J, et al. Novel delivery strategies for glioblastoma. Cancer J 2012;18(1):89—99.
[5] Abbott NJ, et al. Structure and function of the blood—brain barrier. Neurobiol Dis 2010;37(1):13—25.
[6] Laquintana V, et al. New strategies to deliver anticancer drugs to brain tumors. Expert Opin Drug Deliv 2009;6(10):1017—32.
[7] Nau R, Sorgel F, Eiffert H. Penetration of drugs through the blood-cerebrospinal fluid/blood—brain barrier for treatment of central nervous system infections. Clin Microbiol Rev 2010;23(4):858—83.
[8] Nakada M, et al. Aberrant signaling pathways in glioma. Cancers (Basel) 2011;3(3):3242—78.
[9] McCaffrey G, Davis TP. Physiology and pathophysiology of the blood—brain barrier: *P*-glycoprotein and occludin trafficking as therapeutic targets to optimize central nervous system drug delivery. J Investig Med 2012;60(8):1131—40.
[10] Wong AD, et al. The blood—brain barrier: an engineering perspective. Front Neuroeng 2013;6:7.
[10a] Pardridge WM. Why is the global CNS pharmaceutical market so under-penetrated? Drug Discov Today 2002;7(1):5—7.
[10b] Bradbury M, Begley DJ, Kreuter J, editors. The blood-brain barrier and drug delivery to the CNS. USA: Informa Healthcare; 2000.
[11] Sanchez-Covarrubias L, et al. Transporters at CNS barrier sites: obstacles or opportunities for drug delivery? Curr Pharm Des 2014;20(10):1422—49.
[12] de Boer AG, Gaillard PJ. Strategies to improve drug delivery across the blood—brain barrier. Clin Pharmacokinet 2007;46(7):553—76.
[13] Choi M, et al. Minimally invasive molecular delivery into the brain using optical modulation of vascular permeability. Proc Natl Acad Sci USA 2011;108(22):9256—61.
[14] Barua NU, Gill SS, Love S. Convection-enhanced drug delivery to the brain: therapeutic potential and neuropathological considerations. Brain Pathol 2014;24(2):117—27.
[15] Debinski W, Tatter SB. Convection-enhanced delivery for the treatment of brain tumors. Expert Rev Neurother 2009;9(10):1519—27.
[16] Ferguson S, Lesniak MS. Convection enhanced drug delivery of novel therapeutic agents to malignant brain tumors. Curr Drug Deliv 2007;4(2):169—80.
[17] Healy AT, Vogelbaum MA. Convection-enhanced drug delivery for gliomas. Surg Neurol Int 2015;6(Suppl 1):S59—67.
[18] Abbott NJ. Inflammatory mediators and modulation of blood—brain barrier permeability. Cell Mol Neurobiol 2000;20(2):131—47.
[19] Rapoport SI. Modulation of blood—brain barrier permeability. J Drug Target 1996;3(6):417—25.
[20] Gjedde A, Crone C. Biochemical modulation of blood—brain barrier permeability. Acta Neuropathol Suppl 1983;8:59—74.

[21] Neuwelt EA, et al. Osmotic blood—brain barrier disruption: pharmacodynamic studies in dogs and a clinical phase I trial in patients with malignant brain tumors. Cancer Treat Rep 1981;65(Suppl. 2): 39—43.
[22] Neuwelt EA, et al. Effect of osmotic blood—brain barrier disruption on methotrexate pharmacokinetics in the dog. Neurosurgery 1980;7(1):36—43.
[23] Bae MJ, et al. Utilizing ultrasound to transiently increase blood—brain barrier permeability, modulate of the tight junction proteins, and alter cytoskeletal structure. Curr Neurovasc Res 2015;12(4): 375—83.
[24] Aryal M, et al. Ultrasound-mediated blood—brain barrier disruption for targeted drug delivery in the central nervous system. Adv Drug Deliv Rev 2014;72:94—109.
[25] Burgess A, et al. Focused ultrasound-mediated drug delivery through the blood—brain barrier. Expert Rev Neurother 2015;15(5):477—91.
[26] Etame AB, et al. Focused ultrasound disruption of the blood—brain barrier: a new frontier for therapeutic delivery in molecular neurooncology. Neurosurg Focus 2012;32(1):E3.
[27] Jalali S, et al. Focused ultrasound-mediated BBB disruption is associated with an increase in activation of AKT: experimental study in rats. BMC Neurol 2010;10:114.
[28] Curry FR, Adamson RH. Vascular permeability modulation at the cell, microvessel, or whole organ level: towards closing gaps in our knowledge. Cardiovasc Res 2010;87(2):218—29.
[29] Melancon MP, et al. Near-infrared light modulated photothermal effect increases vascular perfusion and enhances polymeric drug delivery. J Control Release 2011;156(2):265—72.
[30] Zhang F, Xu CL, Liu CM. Drug delivery strategies to enhance the permeability of the blood—brain barrier for treatment of glioma. Drug Des Dev Ther 2015;9:2089—100.
[31] Pardridge WM. Non-invasive drug delivery to the human brain using endogenous blood—brain barrier transport systems. Pharm Sci Technol Today 1999;2(2):49—59.
[32] Alavijeh MS, et al. Drug metabolism and pharmacokinetics, the blood—brain barrier, and central nervous system drug discovery. NeuroRx 2005;2(4):554—71.
[33] Rautio J, et al. Prodrug approaches for CNS delivery. AAPS J 2008;10(1):92—102.
[34] Albert A. Chemical aspects of selective toxicity. Nature 1958;182(4633):421—2.
[35] Han HK, Amidon GL. Targeted prodrug design to optimize drug delivery. AAPS PharmSci 2000; 2(1):E6.
[36] Pavan B, Dalpiaz A. Prodrugs and endogenous transporters: are they suitable tools for drug targeting into the central nervous system? Curr Pharm Des 2011;17(32):3560—76.
[37] Pardridge WM. Drug transport across the blood—brain barrier. J Cereb Blood Flow Metab 2012; 32(11):1959—72.
[38] Zhu BT. On the general mechanism of selective induction of cytochrome P450 enzymes by chemicals: some theoretical considerations. Expert Opin Drug Metab Toxicol 2010;6(4):483—94.
[39] Upadhyay RK. Drug delivery systems, CNS protection, and the blood—brain barrier. Biomed Res Int 2014;2014:869269.
[40] Boado RJ, et al. Selective expression of the large neutral amino acid transporter at the blood—brain barrier. Proc Natl Acad Sci USA 1999;96(21):12079—84.
[41] Barbeau A. L-dopa therapy in Parkinson's disease: a critical review of nine years' experience. Can Med Assoc J 1969;101(13):59—68.
[42] Katzenschlager R, Lees AJ. Treatment of Parkinson's disease: levodopa as the first choice. J Neurol 2002;249(Suppl. 2):II19—24.
[43] Miyake MM, Bleier BS. The blood—brain barrier and nasal drug delivery to the central nervous system. Am J Rhinol Allergy 2015;29(2):124—7.
[44] Gizurarson S. Anatomical and histological factors affecting intranasal drug and vaccine delivery. Curr Drug Deliv 2012;9(6):566—82.
[45] Hamidovic A. Position on zinc delivery to olfactory nerves in intranasal insulin phase I—III clinical trials. Contemp Clin Trials 2015;45(Pt B):277—80.
[46] Morris JK, Burns JM. Insulin: an emerging treatment for Alzheimer's disease dementia? Curr Neurol Neurosci Rep 2012;12(5):520—7.

[47] Freiherr J, et al. Intranasal insulin as a treatment for Alzheimer's disease: a review of basic research and clinical evidence. CNS Drugs 2013;27(7):505—14.
[48] During MJ, et al. Controlled release of dopamine from a polymeric brain implant: in vivo characterization. Ann Neurol 1989;25(4):351—6.
[49] Tiwari G, et al. Drug delivery systems: an updated review. Int J Pharm Investig 2012;2(1):2—11.
[50] De Jong WH, Borm PJ. Drug delivery and nanoparticles:applications and hazards. Int J Nanomed 2008;3(2):133—49.
[51] Wohlfart S, Gelperina S, Kreuter J. Transport of drugs across the blood—brain barrier by nanoparticles. J Control Release 2012;161(2):264—73.
[52] Micheli MR, et al. Lipid-based nanocarriers for CNS-targeted drug delivery. Recent Pat CNS Drug Discov 2012;7(1):71—86.
[53] Wong HL, Wu XY, Bendayan R. Nanotechnological advances for the delivery of CNS therapeutics. Adv Drug Deliv Rev 2012;64(7):686—700.
[54] Gomes MJ, Neves J, Sarmento B. Nanoparticle-based drug delivery to improve the efficacy of antiretroviral therapy in the central nervous system. Int J Nanomed 2014;9:1757—69.
[55] Tosi G, et al. Polymeric nanoparticles for the drug delivery to the central nervous system. Expert Opin Drug Deliv 2008;5(2):155—74.
[56] Patel T, et al. Polymeric nanoparticles for drug delivery to the central nervous system. Adv Drug Deliv Rev 2012;64(7):701—5.
[57] Sagar V, et al. Towards nanomedicines for neuroAIDS. Rev Med Virol 2014;24(2):103—24.
[58] Dwibhashyam VS, Nagappa AN. Strategies for enhanced drug delivery to the central nervous system. Indian J Pharm Sci 2008;70(2):145—53.
[59] Cacciatore I, et al. Solid lipid nanoparticles as a drug delivery system for the treatment of neurodegenerative diseases. Expert Opin Drug Deliv 2016:1—11.
[60] Li SD, Huang L. Nanoparticles evading the reticuloendothelial system: role of the supported bilayer. Biochim Biophys Acta 2009;1788(10):2259—66.
[61] Zhang Y, Satterlee A, Huang L. In vivo gene delivery by nonviral vectors: overcoming hurdles? Mol Ther 2012;20(7):1298—304.
[62] Dilnawaz F, Sahoo SK. Therapeutic approaches of magnetic nanoparticles for the central nervous system. Drug Discov Today 2015;20(10):1256—64.
[63] Singh D, et al. Bench-to-bedside translation of magnetic nanoparticles. Nanomedicine (Lond) 2014;9(4):501—16.
[64] Peng XH, et al. Targeted magnetic iron oxide nanoparticles for tumor imaging and therapy. Int J Nanomed 2008;3(3):311—21.
[65] Ran Q, et al. Eryptosis indices as a novel predictive parameter for biocompatibility of Fe_3O_4 magnetic nanoparticles on erythrocytes. Sci Rep 2015;5:16209.
[66] Zheng W, Aschner M, Ghersi-Egea JF. Brain barrier systems: a new frontier in metal neurotoxicological research. Toxicol Appl Pharmacol 2003;192(1):1—11.
[67] Pardridge WM. The blood—brain barrier: bottleneck in brain drug development. NeuroRx 2005;2(1):3—14.
[68] Herve F, Ghinea N, Scherrmann JM. CNS delivery via adsorptive transcytosis. AAPS J 2008;10(3):455—72.
[69] Lu W, et al. Cationic albumin conjugated pegylated nanoparticle with its transcytosis ability and little toxicity against blood—brain barrier. Int J Pharm 2005;295(1—2):247—60.
[70] Lu W, et al. Aclarubicin-loaded cationic albumin-conjugated pegylated nanoparticle for glioma chemotherapy in rats. Int J Cancer 2007;120(2):420—31.
[71] Wei X, et al. Brain tumor-targeted drug delivery strategies. Acta Pharm Sin B 2014;4(3):193—201.
[72] Qin Y, et al. Liposome formulated with TAT-modified cholesterol for improving brain delivery and therapeutic efficacy on brain glioma in animals. Int J Pharm 2011;420(2):304—12.
[73] Gil ES, et al. Quaternary ammonium beta-cyclodextrin nanoparticles for enhancing doxorubicin permeability across the in vitro blood—brain barrier. Biomacromolecules 2009;10(3):505—16.

[74] Uchida Y, et al. Major involvement of Na(+) − dependent multivitamin transporter (SLC5A6/SMVT) in uptake of biotin and pantothenic acid by human brain capillary endothelial cells. J Neurochem 2015;134(1):97−112.

[75] Bhardwaj RK, et al. The functional evaluation of human peptide/histidine transporter 1 (hPHT1) in transiently transfected COS-7 cells. Eur J Pharm Sci 2006;27(5):533−42.

[76] Castro M, et al. High-affinity sodium-vitamin C co-transporters (SVCT) expression in embryonic mouse neurons. J Neurochem 2001;78(4):815−23.

[77] Xu S, et al. Targeting receptor-mediated endocytotic pathways with nanoparticles: rationale and advances. Adv Drug Deliv Rev 2013;65(1):121−38.

[78] Pardridge WM, Eisenberg J, Yang J. Human blood−brain barrier transferrin receptor. Metabolism 1987;36(9):892−5.

[79] Ueno M, et al. The expression of LDL receptor in vessels with blood−brain barrier impairment in a stroke-prone hypertensive model. Histochem Cell Biol 2010;133(6):669−76.

[80] Vu CU, et al. Nicotinic acetylcholine receptors in glucose homeostasis: the acute hyperglycemic and chronic insulin-sensitive effects of nicotine suggest dual opposing roles of the receptors in male mice. Endocrinology 2014;155(10):3793−805.

[81] Pardridge WM, Eisenberg J, Yang J. Human blood−brain barrier insulin receptor. J Neurochem 1985;44(6):1771−8.

[82] Zhang P, et al. Transferrin-modified c[RGDfK]-paclitaxel loaded hybrid micelle for sequential blood−brain barrier penetration and glioma targeting therapy. Mol Pharm 2012;9(6):1590−8.

[83] Jones AR, Shusta EV. Blood−brain barrier transport of therapeutics via receptor-mediation. Pharm Res 2007;24(9):1759−71.

[84] Georgieva JV, Hoekstra D, Zuhorn IS. Smuggling drugs into the brain: an overview of ligands targeting transcytosis for drug delivery across the blood−brain barrier. Pharmaceutics 2014;6(4):557−83.

[85] Orthmann A, et al. Improved treatment of MT-3 breast cancer and brain metastases in a mouse xenograft by LRP-targeted oxaliplatin liposomes. J Biomed Nanotechnol 2016;12(1):56−68.

[86] Gasanov SE, Dagda RK, Rael ED. Snake venom cytotoxins, phospholipase A$_2$s, and Zn^{2+}-dependent metalloproteinases: mechanisms of action and pharmacological relevance. J Clin Toxicol 2014;4(1):1000181.

[86a] Kumar P, et al. Transvascular delivery of small interfering RNA to the central nervous system. Nature 2007;448(7149):39−43.

[87] van Tellingen O, et al. Overcoming the blood−brain tumor barrier for effective glioblastoma treatment. Drug Resist Updates 2015;19:1−12.

[88] Deguchi Y, Kurihara A, Pardridge WM. Retention of biologic activity of human epidermal growth factor following conjugation to a blood−brain barrier drug delivery vector via an extended poly(ethylene glycol) linker. Bioconjugate Chem 1999;10(1):32−7.

[89] Reardon DA, et al. Cilengitide: an integrin-targeting arginine-glycine-aspartic acid peptide with promising activity for glioblastoma multiforme. Expert Opin Investig Drugs 2008;17(8):1225−35.

[90] Taylor TE, Furnari FB, Cavenee WK. Targeting EGFR for treatment of glioblastoma: molecular basis to overcome resistance. Curr Cancer Drug Targets 2012;12(3):197−209.

[91] Choi SA, et al. Human adipose tissue-derived mesenchymal stem cells target brain tumor-initiating cells. PLoS One 2015;10(6):e0129292.

[92] Biju K, et al. Macrophage-mediated GDNF delivery protects against dopaminergic neurodegeneration: a therapeutic strategy for Parkinson's disease. Mol Ther 2010;18(8):1536−44.

[93] Tong HI, et al. Physiological function and inflamed-brain migration of mouse monocyte-derived macrophages following cellular uptake of superparamagnetic iron oxide nanoparticles-implication of macrophage-based drug delivery into the central nervous system. Int J Pharm 2016;505(1−2):271−82.

[94] Ali IU, Chen X. Penetrating the blood−brain barrier: promise of novel nanoplatforms and delivery vehicles. ACS Nano 2015;9(10):9470−4.

[95] Katakowski M, Chopp M. Exosomes as tools to suppress primary brain tumor. Cell Mol Neurobiol 2016;36(3):343−52.

[96] Nazarenko I, Rupp AK, Altevogt P. Exosomes as a potential tool for a specific delivery of functional molecules. Methods Mol Biol 2013;1049:495−511.

[97] Liu Y, et al. Targeted exosome-mediated delivery of opioid receptor mu siRNA for the treatment of morphine relapse. Sci Rep 2015;5:17543.
[98] Vallabhajosula S. Positron emission tomography radiopharmaceuticals for imaging brain beta-amyloid. Semin Nucl Med 2011;41(4):283—99.
[99] Amen DG, et al. Brain SPECT imaging in complex psychiatric cases: an evidence-based, underutilized tool. Open Neuroimag J 2011;5:40—8.
[100] Nelson CA. Incidental findings in magnetic resonance imaging (MRI) brain research. J Law Med Ethics 2008;36(2). p. 315—9, 213.
[101] Sharif-Alhoseini M, et al. Indications for brain computed tomography scan after minor head injury. J Emerg Trauma Shock 2011;4(4):472—6.
[102] Hochgrafe K, Mandelkow EM. Making the brain glow: in vivo bioluminescence imaging to study neurodegeneration. Mol Neurobiol 2013;47(3):868—82.
[103] Deliolanis NC, Ntziachristos V. Fluorescence molecular tomography of brain tumors in mice. Cold Spring Harb Protoc 2013;2013(5):438—43.
[104] Burton NC, et al. Multispectral opto-acoustic tomography (MSOT) of the brain and glioblastoma characterization. Neuroimage 2013;65:522—8.
[105] Lee B, Newberg A. Neuroimaging in traumatic brain imaging. NeuroRx 2005;2(2):372—83.
[106] Pan D, et al. Manganese-based MRI contrast agents: past, present and future. Tetrahedron 2011;67(44):8431—44.
[107] Brasch RC, et al. Brain nuclear magnetic resonance imaging enhanced by a paramagnetic nitroxide contrast agent: preliminary report. Am J Roentgenol 1983;141(5):1019—23.
[108] Politis M, Piccini P. Positron emission tomography imaging in neurological disorders. J Neurol 2012;259(9):1769—80.
[109] Nelson LD, et al. Positron emission tomography of brain beta-amyloid and tau levels in adults with down syndrome. Arch Neurol 2011;68(6):768—74.
[110] Taber KH, Hillman EM, Hurley RA. Optical imaging: a new window to the adult brain. J Neuropsychiatry Clin Neurosci 2010;22(4). p. iv, 357-360.
[111] Galban CJ, et al. Applications of molecular imaging. Prog Mol Biol Transl Sci 2010;95:237—98.
[112] Culver JP, et al. Diffuse optical tomography of cerebral blood flow, oxygenation, and metabolism in rat during focal ischemia. J Cereb Blood Flow Metab 2003;23(8):911—24.
[113] Lu FM, Yuan Z. PET/SPECT molecular imaging in clinical neuroscience: recent advances in the investigation of CNS diseases. Quant Imaging Med Surg 2015;5(3):433—47.
[114] Ntziachristos V, et al. Fluorescence molecular tomography resolves protease activity in vivo. Nat Med 2002;8(7):757—60.
[115] Xia J, Yao J, Wang LV. Photoacoustic tomography: principles and advances. Electromagn Waves (Camb) 2014;147:1—22.
[116] Attia AB, et al. Multispectral optoacoustic and MRI coregistration for molecular imaging of orthotopic model of human glioblastoma. J Biophot 2016;9(7):701—8.
[117] Nahrendorf M, et al. Hybrid PET-optical imaging using targeted probes. Proc Natl Acad Sci USA 2010;107(17):7910—5.

CHAPTER 5

Emerging Nanotechnology for Stem Cell Therapy

Varun Khurana[1], Deep Kwatra[3], Sujay Shah[2], Abhirup Mandal[3], Ashim K. Mitra[3]

[1]Nevakar LLC, Bridgewater, NJ, United States; [2]INSYS Therapeutics Inc, Chandler, AZ, United States; [3]University of Missouri—Kansas City, Kansas City, MO, United States

Contents

1. Introduction	85
2. Application of Nanoparticles in Isolation of Stem Cells	86
3. Application of Nanoparticles in Stem Cell Tracking	89
4. Role of Nanotechnology in Regulating Microenvironment of Stem Cells: Potential Roles in Tissue Engineering	93
5. Nanoparticles as Macromolecular Delivery Systems for Stem Cells	96
6. Future Prospects and Challenges Facing the Field	100
References	100

1. INTRODUCTION

Stem cells are specialized cells within tissues that possess two distinct properties of self-renewal and also the ability to differentiate into a wide variety of cell types with specialized lineages [1]. Their ability to divide into a progenitor cell that does not differentiate further, while simultaneously generating another cell that either differentiates or multiplies into specialized cells gives these cells their "Stem"ness [2]. Stem cells can display different properties depending on their source and timing of collection, and their capabilities to generate different lineages (pluripotent vs. multipotent). Broadly, these cells can be classified as embryonic stem cells and adult stem cells [3]. Embryonic stem cells are usually derived from early animal or human embryos. In a culture with the right conditions, they are capable of multiplying indefinitely and are pluripotent, i.e., giving rise to specialized cells. Adult stem cells or somatic stem cells, on the other hand, are generally multipotent, and capable of generating only a subset of lineages, which are usually restricted to the tissue from which these cells derived.

The capability of stem cells to differentiate into different lineages render these cells attractive candidates in multiple therapies such as injury repairs, tissue regeneration, neurodegeneration, cardiac diseases, osteoarthritis, rheumatoid arthritis, and diabetes. These properties also render these cells candidate for pharmacological and toxicological tests, as well as drug screening tools. Although stem cells hold a lot of promise in the field of regenerative medicine, there are a number of obstacles that limit their utility. Some of these limitations are moral, ethical, and legal, based on the origin of these stem cells particularly, in the case of embryonic stem cells. Some of these issues can be addressed by utilizing induced pluripotent stem cells, derived from somatic cells possessing characteristics similar to embryonic stem cells [4,5]. There are technical limitations, such as the lack of suitable techniques to efficiently understand and control microenvironment of the stem cells. The signals lead to orderly transduction of targeted transplanted stem cells [5,6]. This retention and short survival rate of transplanted cells in the damaged tissues result in limited utility [7]. Table 5.1 provides a list of stem cells and their scope for the targeted delivery of anticancer therapeutics. Nanotechnology has led to several advancements in stem cell therapy by addressing some of these issues [8].

Nanotechnology refers to the engineering and development of materials, carrier systems, or devices at molecular scale primarily between 1 and 1000 nm in diameter. Although there have been multiple applications of nanotechnology in drug delivery, implants, and medical devices, its utilization in stem cell—based therapies is more recent. With the advent of improved and safer nanomaterials such systems can be applied to medical applications. Simultaneously, there have been advances in the application of stem cells in regenerative medicine along with improvement in techniques for isolation and maintenance of stem cells. As both these technologies have advanced, a better synergy has appeared between the two leading to enhanced nanotechnology-based stem cell therapies [9]. One of the major applications of nanotechnology in the area of stem cell research involves tracking the movement of stem cells that have been transplanted. Another major application of nanotechnology is an improved delivery and targeting of stem cells. Stems cells transplanted by nanocarriers have improved survival rates since these cells are established in safer microenvironment through the release of survival-enhancing biomolecules. A mechanism by which nanoparticles can provide a suitable microenvironment for stem cells is to serve as carriers or cocarriers for biologically active molecules, such as adhesion factors and growth factors. Moreover, nanostructures can improve stem cell transplantation and differentiation. Furthermore, nanoparticle delivery systems can be designed for intra—stem cell delivery of DNA, RNA, siRNA, proteins, peptides, or drug molecules capable of regulating stem cell differentiation [9,10].

In this chapter, we discuss how advances in nanotechnology played a role in enhancing stem cell research, mainly in the terms of application in the isolation and traces of stem cells. Moreover, regulation of proliferation/differentiation of stem cells, intracellular delivery of macro- or micromolecules in stem cells, and their application in tissue engineering and regeneration are described in this chapter.

2. APPLICATION OF NANOPARTICLES IN ISOLATION OF STEM CELLS

Isolation of stem cells from a pool of differentiated cells is a critical step for eventual utilization in any biomedical work. An ideal isolation technique should be quick and easy to

Table 5.1 Stem cells (SCs) sources [16]

Name	Sources	Advantages	Disadvantages
Embryonic SCs	Inner cell mass of the mammalian blastocyst	Pluripotent, enabling them to form derivatives of all three germ layers	• Results destruction of the embryo, making them an ethically controversial source • Form teratomas when transplanted in vivo, limiting their current clinical value
Hematopoietic SCs	• Bone marrow, umbilical cord, blood, and peripheral blood • Embryonic SCs • Induced pluripotent SCs	• Multipotent, can form lymphoid and myeloid blood cells • Extracted in high yields • Readily cryopreserved • Intrinsic tumor-tropic properties	Limited differentiation potential
Mesenchymal SCs	• Fetal origins (Wharton jelly and cord blood) • Developing tooth bud of the mandibular third molar • Adult tissues such as bone marrow and adipose tissue • embryonic SCs • Induced pluripotent SCs	• Differentiate into mesenchymal lineages that make up bone, cartilage, fat, and muscle • Readily cryopreserved • Many types are tumor-tropic • Readily genetically manipulated	• Limited differentiation potential • Limited yield depending on source
Neural SCs	• Brain, spinal cord, and retina • Embryonic SCs • Induced pluripotent SCs	• Multipotent, can give rise to neurons, astrocytes, and oligodendrocytes • Tumor-tropic properties • Readily genetically manipulated	• Limited differentiation potential • Difficult to source

Continued

Table 5.1 Stem cells (SCs) sources [16]—cont'd

Name	Sources	Advantages	Disadvantages
Endothelial SCs	• Bone marrow • Embryonic SCs • Induced pluripotent SCs	• Multipotent, give rise to endothelial precursor cells, which form blood and lymphoid vessels • Readily cryopreserved • Readily genetically manipulated	Limited differentiation potential
Induced SCs	Derived from somatic cells using reprogramming technologies	• Can be driven into many different cell types • Creation of patient-specific cell types • Can be made using various viral and nonviral methods	• Tumorigenicity poses a considerable clinical hurdle • Heterogeneity in final induced SC population • Technically challenging • Low efficiency of conversion

perform to isolate the stem cells from an assortment of cellular mixtures in a cost-effective manner. Stem cells express unique biomarkers that can be utilized to isolate and purify these cells. Magnetic nanoparticles, including superparamagnetic iron oxide (SPIO) nanoparticles, are most utilized for isolation of stem cells. SPIO nanoparticles, approved for human use by the US Food and Drug Administration, have also been utilized in magnetic resonance imaging (MRI) for enhancing the contrast of cellular targets. These nanoparticles have also been extensively utilized in other biomedical applications, such as isolation and separation of cells and sample preparation [11,12], immunological assays [13], delivery of drugs and genetic material to cells and tissues [14], as well as diseases such as hyperthermia [8].

For isolation of stem cells with magnetic nanoparticles, stem cells first need to be labeled with the nanoparticles. The cells can be labeled either by attaching magnetic nanoparticles to the cell surface, or by internalizing the nanoparticles. The labeled nanoparticles can then be isolated with a combination of flow cytometry and magnetic separation. Magnetic nanoparticles in combination with CD34 antibody have been successfully applied to isolate and enrich peripheral blood progenitor cells from human. Jing et al. [15] reported conjugation of SPIO with CD34 antibody to label CD34$^+$ stem cells. These cells are then isolated from fresh and cryopreserved clinical leukapheresis samples of human blood with a continuous quadrupole magnetic flow sorter (QMS) system. The QMS consists of a flow channel and a quadrupole magnet for cell sorting.

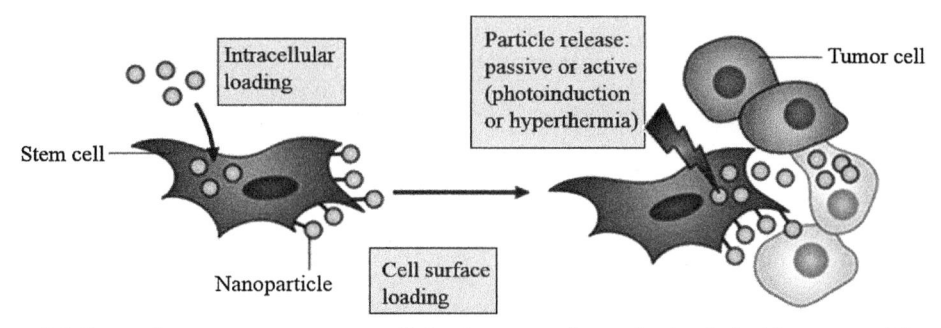

Figure 5.1 Strategies to promote tumor cell death: stem cells can be loaded with nanoparticles containing chemotherapy or imaging agents that are released in the vicinity of the tumor, either passively or in response to external stimuli.

The efficacy of this technique has been examined with seven different commercial progenitor cell labeling kits. High cell recovery and enrichment up to 60–69% purity could be obtained. Fig. 5.1 demonstrates strategies for cell-surface or intracellular loading of nanoparticles for stem cell therapy [16].

3. APPLICATION OF NANOPARTICLES IN STEM CELL TRACKING

Traditionally, the transplanted stem cells are labeled in vitro by various techniques and then visualized by immunohistochemistry after tissue extraction. Such invasive techniques have limited application. There is a constant demand for a better and more effective noninvasive technique for long-term stem cell imaging and tracking of transplanted stem cells. This technique should monitor survival, migration, and differentiation. Considerable research has been conducted with various types of nanoparticles, including magnetic nanoparticles, silica nanoparticles, quantum dots, and gold nanoparticles as vehicles for stem cell delivery [17]. Various types of nanoparticles show variable effects on stem cell viability, proliferation, differentiation, cytotoxicity, and ability to track the stem cells. Hence, each technique has its own advantages and limitations.

SPIO nanoparticles have been utilized to label stem cells, as previously mentioned. Magnetic nanoparticle-labeled stem cells can then be visualized noninvasively by utilizing MRI. These iron oxide nanoparticles are often coated with polymeric materials, such as dextran or carboxydextran, to prevent aggregation and to enhance solubility [18]. SPIO nanoparticles are typically internalized into the stem cells during in vitro processing, with or without the use of transfection agents [19]. These nanoparticles can be derivatized with internalizing peptides, such as the activating transcriptional activator peptide. SPIO can further be labeled for tracking. It can be isolated by conjugation with other probes, such as fluorescent molecules. Such modification instances allow for better tracking, as well as sorting and purification of stem cells [20]. Jendelová et al. utilized MRI for the tracking of transplanted bone marrow and embryonic stem cells, labeled by iron oxide nanoparticles in rat brain and spinal cord. To differentiate between the two stem cell populations, the authors labeled the rat bone marrow stromal cells with bromodeoxyuridine (BrdU) and transfected embryonic stem cells with promoter-driven enhanced green fluorescent protein (pEGFP-C1) to introduce the expression of green fluorescence protein. The authors were able to demonstrate that grafted mesenchymal and embryonic stem cells labeled with iron oxide nanoparticles migrate into the injured CNS and could be tracked noninvasively for 50 days. This migration was further confirmed by histological staining with fluorophores [21]. Jin et al. utilized a similar approach for tracking the survival, migration, and differentiation of magnetically labeled seed cells-bone marrow-derived mesenchymal stem cells. These cells were injected into the intra-articular space of knee joints in rabbits. These colabeled stem cells with SPIO and BrdU were then utilized in combination with Prussian blue staining and transmission electron microscopy to observe the intracellular iron. Such images were able to track the cells noninvasively for 12 weeks. Again combining with immunohistochemical staining these processes were able to confirm the tracking of the stem cells reaching the defect site [22].

Cell tracking with iron oxide nanoparticles has been well established in MRI. However, in experimental animal models, the readout can often be unreliable as the intrinsic iron signal derived from erythrocytes sometimes masks the labeled cells. Interference can also be observed because of postoperative local signal voids such as metal, hemorrhage, or air. These shortcomings in this technique are often overcome by gadolinium-based contrast agents, which have an advantage over regular iron oxide—based SIPO. Such nanoparticles provide a positive contrast on T1-weighted images, which are less prone to interference. Shen et al. utilized MRI of mesenchymal stem cells labeled with dual agents (magnetic and fluorescence) in rat spinal cord injury. In this study stem cell from the marrow were paramagnetically and fluorescently labeled with a complex of gadolinium-diethylene triamine pentaacetic acid (Gd-DTPA) with rhodamine-conjugated polyethylenimine (PEI)-FluoR. The rats implanted with labeled stem cells were successfully observed and tracked by serial MRI. The images are correlated with fluorescent microscopy. The rats treated with mesenchymal stem cells achieved significantly higher Basso—Beattie—Bresnahan locomotors test scores than controls [23]. Similarly, Liu et al. evaluated cell tracking effects of transplanted mesenchymal stem cells with jetPEI/Gd-DTPA complexes in animal models of hemorrhagic spinal cord injury. In their study, first the mesenchymal stem cells were labeled with jetPEI/Gd-DTPA particles and examined for transfection efficiency by MRI in vitro. Differentiation assays were also carried out to confirm that the gedunin labeling did not alter the differentiation ability of the stem cells. The labeled cells were then transplanted into rat spinal cord injury and monitored by MRI in vivo and confirmed with fluorescence images. The results also confirmed the applicability of gedunin-based contrast agents in stem cell tracking [24].

Quantum dots are another type of nanoparticles that have been extensively applied in cellular imaging and tracking due to their unique spectral, physical, and chemical properties. These advantages allow for concurrent monitoring of several intercellular and intracellular interactions in live cells over short and long periods. Quantum dots delivered to cytoplasm result in intense and stable fluorescence that can be easily tracked and imaged. Furthermore, these images are not known to alter the differentiation potential of stem cells, as demonstrated in rat pancreatic stem cells [25]. Quantum dots have also been applied in vivo to view mouse embryonic stem cells labeled with Qtracker through multiplex imaging [26]. Lin et al. reported murine embryonic stem cells that were labeled with six different quantum dots. None affected the viability, proliferation, and differentiation of the stem cells adversely. The authors were able to view cells that were injected subcutaneously onto the backs of athymic nude mice with good contrast. Although it was not suitable for deep tissue imaging, it could be utilized as a proof-of-concept study for viewing labeled stem cells in vivo [26].

Quantum dots also have been bioconjugated to enhance their internalization, targeting, as well as tracking. Barnett et al. reported a conjugate of high quantum efficiency photostable and multispectral quantum dot nanocrystals with fluorescent tracer, 1,1′-dioctadecyl-3,3,3′,3′-tetramethylindocarbo cyanine perchlorate-labeled acetylated LDL. The nanocrystals can be applied for long-term tracking of endothelial progenitor cell subpopulations in ocular angiogenesis with improved signal-to-noise ratio [27]. Shah et al. further utilized quantum dot bioconjugates for labeling and imaging of human mesenchymal stem cells during proliferation and osteogenic differentiation. In this study, the researchers utilized a specialized peptide CGGGRGD, which was cross-linked onto the CdSe—ZnS quantum dots coated with carboxyl groups utilizing amine groups. The peptide causes the quantum dots to bind with selected integrins on the membrane of human mesenchymal stem cells, which allowed for long-term labeling [28]. Quantum dots—based multifunctional nanoparticles were also developed by Li et al. for effective differentiation and long-term tracking of human mesenchymal stem cells. These investigators modified the quantum dots with β-cyclodextrin and CKKRGD peptide (Cys-Lys-Lys-Arg-Gly-Asp), which resulted in enhanced cellular uptake of nanoparticles as well as siRNA, which regulates differentiation. Such combination provides a powerful tool to simultaneously enhance differentiation and long-term tracking of stem cells, both in vitro and in vivo [29].

Due to the inert and biocompatible characteristics of gold, nanotracers or gold nanoparticles have also been prepared as labeling and tracking agents for stem cells. The inherent properties of gold make it nonreactive to any biological material. Studies have shown that gold nanoparticles do not interfere with the viability or cellular functioning of stem cells, making them useful candidates for long-term imaging and tracking of stem cells in vivo [30]. Nam et al. utilized gold nanotracers for in vivo ultrasound and photoacoustic monitoring of mesenchymal stem cells. The gold nanotracer-labeled mesenchymal stem cells injected intramuscularly in the lower limb of the Lewis rat were detected with ultrasound-guided photoacoustic imaging. High detection sensitivity, spatial resolution, and greater penetration depth render it as useful techniques [31].

Choi et al. utilized a polydopamine-coated gold core-shell nanoprobe for long-term intracellular detection of differentiation in human mesenchymal stem cells by targeting specific microRNA (miRNA). The polydopamine shell was utilized to immobilize the fluorescently labeled hairpin DNA strands on the nanoparticles, which were capable of targeting specific miRNA (miR-29b and miR-31). The gold core and polydopamine shell were able to quench the fluorescence of the immobilized hairpin DNA. Once internalized, the nanoprobes target the miRNA that are present only within the differentiating stem cells. Interaction of the hairpin DNA with miRNAs within the cells leads to dissociation of the miRNA from the gold-polydopamine nanoparticles and thus enables recovery of the fluorescence signal. This technique allows for identification, isolation, and tracking of specific types of stem cells within a diverse population [32]. In a different study, a dual gold nanoparticle system for mesenchymal stem cell tracking was developed. This construct is capable of monitoring both delivered stem cells and infiltrating macrophages by photoacoustic imaging. Macrophages play an important role in wound healing and vascular regeneration. These cells also interact with stem cells, due to phagocytosis. The dual gold nanoparticle system enables monitoring of macrophage infiltration and endocytosis of stem cells. Two separate contrast agent nanoparticles were needed. This technique is based on transfer of contrast agents from stem cells to macrophages as a result of internalization. Gold nanorods (absorbance in the near-infrared region) labeled with mesenchymal stem cells and gold nanospheres (absorbance in the visible light region) were applied to label macrophages. Nanosphere endocytosis leads to peak broadening due to plasmon coupling, thus allowing two different cell types as well as interaction monitoring [33].

Silica nanoparticles were also studied for stem cell labeling with multiple imaging techniques. Photostable cyanine dye—loaded fluorescent silica nanoparticles can improve optical imaging of human mesenchymal stem cells, which aids in the direct discrimination between live and early-stage apoptotic cells. With this nanoparticle technology, the labeled cells can be visualized by flow cytometry, confocal and transmission electron microscopy. Dye-loaded silica nanoparticles also known as IRIS Dots are capable of discriminating between live and early-stage apoptotic stem cells through a distinct external cell surface distribution [34]. Engineered silica nanoparticles, due to resistance to degradation and ease of functionalization, have been utilized as contrast agents for labeling stem cells in multiple disease conditions. Gallina et al. developed fluorescent, amorphous 50-nm silica nanoparticles. This group examined the effects on viability and function of human bone marrow—derived mesenchymal stem cells in a beating heart model. The bright fluorescence emitted by the internalized nanoparticles made them optimal candidates for stem cell tracking inside heart tissue [35]. Fig. 5.2 shows improved results of stem cell therapy by guiding this growth in the right direction through nanoscale scaffolds.

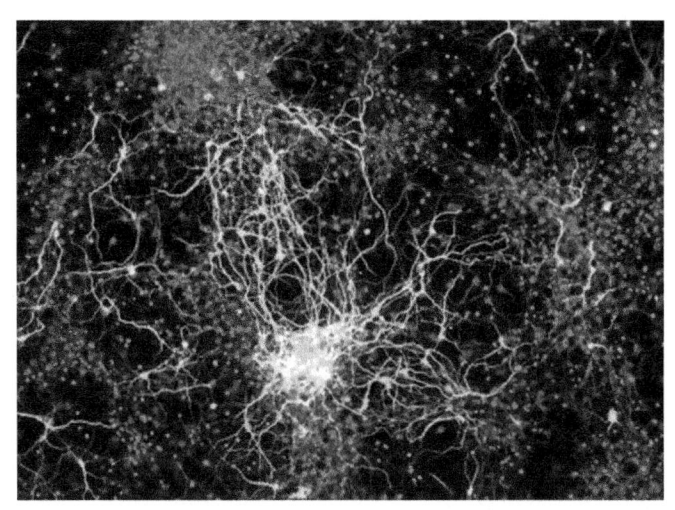

Figure 5.2 Stem cells can be used to regrow damaged tissue in many areas of the body. Nanoscale scaffolds can improve results of stem cell therapy by guiding this growth in the right direction. *(Image credit: National Eye Institute.)*

Silica nanoparticles can be combined with multiple technologies to form multifunctional tracking agents. Jokerst et al. developed a multimodal, silica-based nanoparticlulate system that can serve multiple functions, such as cell sorting through fluorescence, guided cell implantation in real time with ultrasound, and high-resolution long-term monitoring by MRI. This technology can be very useful for improving stem cell therapy by improving delivery and preventing death of implanted stem cells in ischemia, inflammation, or immune response [36]. Cobalt zinc ferrite nanoparticles encapsulated by amorphous silica have been developed as a contrast agent. It can also act as magnetic label for tracking transplanted stem cells within an organism using MRI [37]. Similarly fluorescein isothiocyanate (FITC)-incorporated silica-coated magnetic nanoparticles have been developed for specific labeling of neurogenic, endothelial, and myogenic differentiated cells derived from human amniotic fluid stem cells [38]. The multiple mechanisms for tracking the cells in vivo provide a more precise and confirmatory scientific technique allowing for more accurate determination of stem cell health and activity.

4. ROLE OF NANOTECHNOLOGY IN REGULATING MICROENVIRONMENT OF STEM CELLS: POTENTIAL ROLES IN TISSUE ENGINEERING

Stem cells are usually found in the living organisms in specific anatomical locations called as a niche in a highly controlled and specific microenvironment. Such expressions allow for the stem cell to have specific interactions necessary for proper regulation. These niches play specialized roles of regulating stem cells due to the presence of other specialized cells. The presence of noncellular materials such as extracellular matrices as well as biomolecules can generate tissue matrices. Cells around the stem cells within the niche produce matrix biomolecules such as fibronectin, laminin, collagen, elastins, and proteoglycans that produce specialized structures that are necessary for the growth and maintenance of stem cells. The nanostructures formed by these biomolecules serve as anchorage points, facilitating cell adhesion molecules to bind as well as immobilization of soluble factors. The extracellular proteins on the stem cell surfaces interact with amino acids expressed on the extracellular matrices or specialized three-dimensional (3D) structures to activate/deactivate a cascade of signaling pathways within the cells. These structures end up regulating adhesion, proliferation, migration, and cell differentiation [9,39]. Other microenvironmental factors that control stem cell localization, proliferation, and differentiation are mineral components, i.e., calcium. Calcium sensors expressed on the hematopoietic stem cell surface allow them to find their niche and translocate from the fetal liver to the bone marrow [40]. Reproducing the structural complexities of nanostructures present in the extracellular matrices has significantly improved our understanding of the stem cell—matrix interactions. It has delineated interactions and regulation of various processes within the stem cells. This knowledge has also helped us better regulate the bioactive remodeling of the stem cells [41]. The biometric scaffolds made through nanotechnology satisfy the essential characteristic requirements of biocompatibility and biodegradability. It also provides appropriate bimolecular signaling to allow for proper proliferation and differentiation of the stem cells.

How the structure and properties of nanomaterials may impact the proliferation and differentiation of stem cells has in itself become a new scientific frontier especially in the field of regenerative medicine. Most of the early studies on the role of the microenvironment in stem cell differentiation were carried out with two-dimensional (2D) biomaterial structures. Two-dimensional approaches have their advantages such as low cost, high throughput, and capability of delineating multiple interactions at once. True interactions of the stem cells in vivo are 3D in nature [42]. Hence new investigation has been directed to nanofabrication to develop 3D biodegradable scaffolds. These constructs are designed to catalyze stem cells to differentiate into specific cells of the organ/tissue required [43,44]. The biodegradable matrices and nanoscaffolds allow the transplanted cells to eventually take the 3D structure of the tissue as the scaffold eventually disappears [45,46].

Giri et al. studied the telomerase activity of rat embryonic liver progenitor cells in nanoscaffold-coated model bioreactor. This protein is known to control cellular processes such as proliferation, differentiation, immortalization, cell injury, and aging [47]. The investigators cultured a rat embryonal liver progenitor cell line RLC-18 in a self-assembly nanostructured scaffold-coated bioreactor. The researchers compared this to 2D models of collagen-coated plates and uncoated plates. These studies reported low telomerase activity and limited cell proliferation. Scaffold interaction may play a significant role in controlling critical cellular functions in the bioartificial liver construction. Self-assembling peptide nanoscaffold has also been examined to study the influence of electrical stimulation on 3D cultures of adipose tissue—derived progenitor cells [48]. Studies revealed that the process of electrostimulation along with 3D scaffolding may eventually lead to development of effective cardiac cells. Tam et al. utilized a nanoscaffold impregnated with mesenchymal stem cells derived from the Wharton jelly of human umbilical cords. These investigators suggested that this system improves wound healing [49]. The authors utilized an aloe vera (due to its antibacterial properties) polycaprolactone nanoscaffold impregnated with green fluorescent protein—labeled stem cells for healing of excisional and diabetic wounds. The excisional and diabetic wounds in mice showed rapid wound closure, reepithelialization, and increased numbers of sebaceous glands and hair follicles compared with controls suggesting that the combination of stem cells with nanoscaffolding provide synergistic benefits in wound healing.

Other material examined as a nanoscaffold for potential bone tissue engineering is graphene. Elkhenany et al. contemplated the use of graphene as a nanoscaffold for goat mesenchymal stem cells. The researchers reported the effect of this material on the proliferation and differentiation of bone progenitor cells and compared it with polystyrene-coated tissue culture plates [50]. The results suggested that oxidized graphene films support in vitro proliferation and osteogenic differentiation even in medium containing fetal bovine serum without the addition of any glucocorticoid or specific growth factors. It has been suggested that graphene scaffold and goat mesenchymal stem cell combination may be a promising potential construct for bone tissue engineering. Mousavi et al. studied the expansion of human umbilical cord blood hematopoietic stem/progenitor cells in 3D polycaprolactone nanoscaffold coated with fibronectin to overcome the major obstacle of limited cell dose [51]. These studies suggested that 3D scaffold can result in greater expansion of total cells (58-fold expansion) compared with 2D cultures (38-fold expansion). More importantly, the $CD34^+$ (stem cell marker) cells are also significantly higher in 3D scaffolds (40-fold) relative to 2D cell culture (2.66-fold). PuraMatrix hydrogel [52] and gelatin [53] are some of the other materials employed to generate nanoscaffolds for tissue engineering. Neural stem/progenitor cells cultured in PuraMatrix hydrogel following transplantation in rat brain injury resulted in significant reduction in lesion volume, lowering in neurological deficits, and higher cell survival, which may be another promising approach toward in reengineering.

Another method for controlling growth and differentiation of stem cells is to grow the stem cells on a lab-on-a-chip. It is a tool that incorporates numerous laboratory tasks onto a small device, usually only millimeters or centimeters in size [54]. Some of these chips contain nanoreservoirs. Each chip surface containing thousands of reservoir cavities with radius in the nanometer range. The reservoir can be filled with biomaterials such that a stem cell may be exposed to in a niche, including lipid bilayers as well as voltage-gated channels. The chip technology allows for electrical exposure at specific time points to specific cells under chemical environment in a controlled manner. Such controlled environment renders the stem cell to differentiate in a correct manner. It also allows the cells to grow in layers making a complex tissue. These microfluidics-based technologies create a new path forward both for further development in regenerative medicine as well as for the development of high-throughput screening platforms. Sciancalepore et al. generated a renal microdevice that resembles in vivo structure of a kidney proximal tubule by embedding a population of tubular adult renal stem cells into a microsystem. The stem cells were exposed to fluid shear stress in the chip, which led to the correct polarization of the cells. It is in contrast to static cultures resulting in an ideal platform for testing agents for therapeutic and toxicological responses [55]. Similar technologies have been utilized to develop other organs on a chip such as heart-on-a-chip platform for cardiac drug screening as well as heart regeneration [56,57]. Li et al. utilized custom-built microfluidic perfusion bioreactors. This apparatus was integrated with ultrasound standing wave traps for cartilage tissue engineering. This system involved the use of sweeping acoustic drive frequencies (890—910 kHz) along with continuous perfusion of chondrogenic culture medium at a low-shear flow rate. This technique provides improved mechanical stimulation and mass transfer rates. This process induced the generation of 3D agglomerates of human articular chondrocytes, which resulted in enhanced cartilage formation [58]. Similarly, Mooney et al. have reported unique properties of carbon nanotubes (CNTs) in synergy with human mesenchymal stem cells (hMSCs). By using a fluorescent dye, single-walled nanotubes (SWNTs) were found to migrate through the cell wall to a nuclear location after 24 h. In addition, SWNTs had no significant effect on adipogenesis, osteogenesis, or chondrogenesis. This indicates CNTs had no adverse effects on hMSC biocompatibility, proliferation, or differentiation and have tremendous potential for future approaches in tissue repair/regeneration (Fig. 5.3) [59].

5. NANOPARTICLES AS MACROMOLECULAR DELIVERY SYSTEMS FOR STEM CELLS

As mentioned throughout this chapter, a major challenge in stem cell therapeutics is to find a suitable way of controlling their proliferation and differentiation. Multiple biomolecules such as DNA, RNA, peptides, or proteins are capable of regulating stem cell differentiation. However, these macromolecules need to be delivered efficiently into the stem cells to be effective. Conventional methods of macromolecular delivery are generally not efficient with many limitations. Physical methods, such as electroporation and nucleofection, can efficiently deliver biomolecules into the cells, but these techniques, by design, cause damage to the cells. Various types of viral vectors can also be related to transfection agents. However, such vectors suffer from risk of toxicity and mutagenesis, as well as immunogenic responses. Chemical transfection agents also suffer from limited

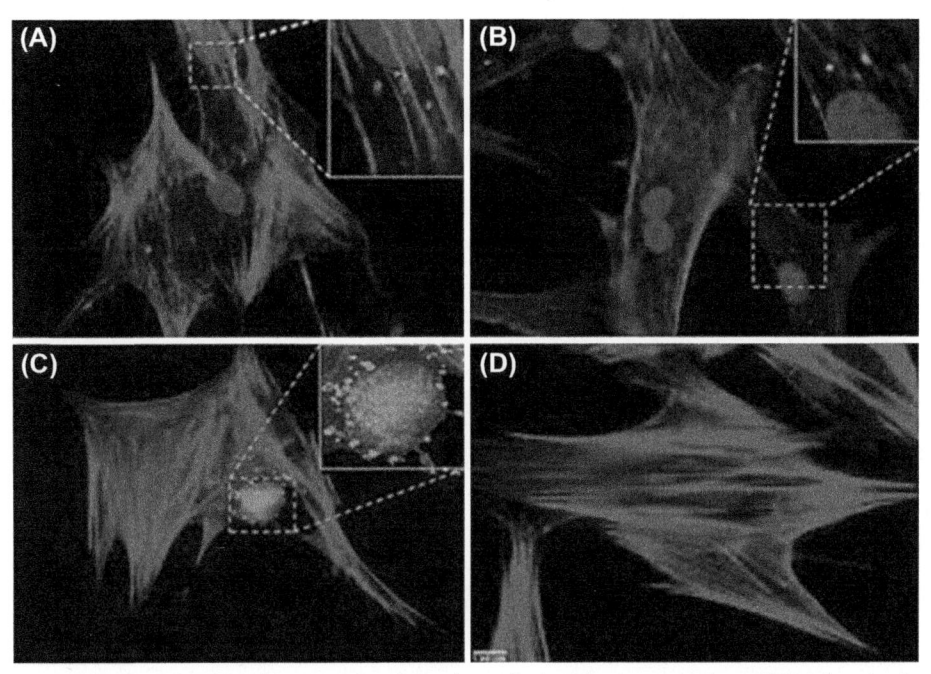

Figure 5.3 Uptake of COOH-functionalized single-walled carbon nanotubes (CNTs) by the human mesenchymal stem cells (hMSCs). Fluorescent images of biotinylated CNT within the cell after (A) 24 h, (B) 48 h, and (C) 6 days and (D) hMSC alone (scale bar 130 μm). *(Reprinted with permission from Mooney E, et al. Carbon nanotubes and mesenchymal stem cells: biocompatibility, proliferation and differentiation. Nano Lett 2008;8(8):2137−43. Copyright (2008) American Chemical Society.)*

transfection efficacy and poor toxicity profile. Nanoparticle delivery systems on the other hand have multiple advantages. Not only are these carriers suitable for the biomolecules but these systems can also be surface modified to attach targeting moieties. This strategy can help deliver the cargo to the intended cells thereby limiting potential toxicities or unintended consequences. The nanoparticles can be made of polymeric materials that are biocompatible, biodegradable, and safe.

Nanoparticles of various shapes, designs and building blocks have been prepared as carriers to deliver small and large biomolecules to stem cells. Zhu et al. reprogrammed mouse embryonic fibroblasts to pluripotency. An arginine-terminated polyamidoamine nanoparticle-based nonviral gene delivery system was developed using a single plasmid construct carrying OSKM (pOSKM) [60]. These studies suggest that nanoparticles not only result in successful generation of induced pluripotent cells but also provide significantly higher transfection efficiency than conventional transfection reagents. Sohn et al. also worked on the induction of pluripotency within the bone marrow mononuclear cells utilizing an acid-sensitive polyketal (PK3)-based nanoparticle system. This construct was delivered to mature embryonic stem cell−specific miRNAs [61].

The results showed that a polyketal-miRNA delivery system can successfully generate various reprogrammed cells without permanent genetic manipulation. Mesoporous silica nanoparticles, because of their multifunctional properties, have also been utilized for nonviral cell labeling and as differentiation agents for induced pluripotent stem cells [62]. Chen et al. evaluated the feasibility and efficiency of FITC-conjugated mesoporous silica nanoparticles for labeling of induced pluripotent stem cells. The researchers also showed that FITC-conjugated mesoporous silica nanoparticles of various surface charges are efficiently internalized by the induced pluripotent stem cells with minimal cytotoxicity. Cationic nanoparticles were selected to deliver hepatocyte nuclear factor 3β in a plasmid. It improved the mRNA expression levels of liver-specific genes in stem cells rendering quick differentiation into hepatocyte-like cells with mature functions.

Throughout this chapter we have mainly focused on embryonic and mesenchymal stem cells but there is another type of stem cells utilized for originating, maintaining, and progressing cancers with cancer stem cells [63,64]. These cells have been identified as a vital obstacle in cancer therapy due to higher expression of drug resistance proteins, as well as slower proliferation relative to other cancer cells [65,66]. Expression of specific proteins unique to cancer stem cells can be targeted by nanoparticles. Hence, multifunctional nanoparticles have played a key role in cancer stem cell therapies [67,68]. Specific genes and micro- and siRNAs have been delivered to cancer stem cells to render them more sensitive to conventional chemotherapies. One such miRNA, miR-200c, functions as an effective cancer stem cell inhibitor that can restore sensitivity to microtubule-targeting drugs [69]. In this work, Liu et al. utilized the intelligent gelatinases-stimuli nanoparticles to codeliver miR-200c and chemotherapeutic docetaxel to cancer stem cells and conventional cancer cells and test their synergy [70]. The nanoparticles can provide efficient delivery of the miRNA into the tumor cells thereby achieving sustained miR-200c expression. A cotherapeutic loaded nanoparticles significantly enhanced cytotoxicity of docetaxel. A lowering in class III beta-tubulin level and reversal of epithelial to mesenchymal transition were noted. The residual posttreatment tumors were retransplanted into nude mice. This process showed slower growth relative to originally seeded cells probably due to efficient targeting of cancer stem cells. Another miRNA, miR-182, is known to express antitumor activity through repression of Bcl2-like12, c-Met, and hypoxia-inducible factor 2α [71]. The miRNA miR-182 is also known to enhance sensitivity to chemotherapy, lower glioma-initiating cell (glioblastoma stem cells) sphere size, expansion, and stemness in vitro [72]. Kauri et al. synthesized miR-182-based spherical nucleic acids, which were basically gold nanoparticles covalently functionalized with mature miR-182 duplexes. The construct was intravenously administered into orthotopic glioblastoma multiforme xenografts. These studies revealed that these spherical nucleic acids penetrated the blood−brain/blood−tumor barrier, which resulted in reduced tumor burden and longer animal survival.

Shah et al. developed a targeted nanomedicine for suppression of CD44 with cell death induction in ovarian cancer. Overexpression of the CD44 membrane receptor is known to induce cancer stem cell–specific progression of tumor initiation, growth, migration, development of drug resistance, and metastases. Hence, these scientists designed a polypropylenimine dendrimer-based nanoscale targeted drug delivery system for the delivery of CD44 siRNA and anticancer drug paclitaxel. Targeted nanomedicine for ovarian cancer was achieved with a synthetic analog of luteinizing hormone-releasing hormone peptide. A highly optimized targeted delivery system in ovarian cancer cells isolated from patients with malignant ascites resulted in the reduction of CD44 mRNA and protein. The therapy effectively caused tumor shrinkage through the induction of cell death. It also provided prevention of adverse reactions on healthy tissue. CD44 has also been targeted with nanoparticles in other cancers, such as leukemia [73] using polymeric nanoparticle-mediated silencing of CD44 and hyaluronic acid–based self-assembling nanosystems for siRNA delivery in lung cancer [74]. One more gene that has been targeted in cancer therapy is c-Myc, which is known to play a key role in glioma cancer stem cell propagation. Ma et al. prepared and evaluated methoxy-poly-(ethylene-glycol)-poly-(lactide-co-glycolide) nanoparticles loaded with plasmid DNA inserted with three types of siRNA fragments capable of targeting c-Myc gene. This carrier system showed a high encapsulation capacity, as well as transfection efficiency, resulting in significant apoptosis. Tangudu et al. also utilized c-Myc-conjugated nanoparticles to deliver small oligos (anti-miRs and mimics) and larger DNAs (encoding short hairpin RNAs), which suppressed breast and colorectal cancer tumor growth arrest and increased survival in animal models [75].

Introduction of wild-type p53 gene in glioblastoma cells has been shown to lower resistance to temozolomide through downregulation of O(6)-methylguanine-DNA methyltransferase. However, it has been difficult to utilize p53-based therapies in glioblastoma due to lack of efficient delivering of the gene into the brain across the blood–brain barrier (BBB). Kim et al. developed a systemic nanodelivery platform composed of self-assembling nanocomplex capable of crossing the BBB. This construct can efficiently target glioblastoma as well as the stem cells [76]. This study suggested that systemic delivery of the p53 nanoparticles downregulated the methyltransferase expression, induced apoptosis in intracranial glioblastoma xenografts, as well as sensitized the overall glioblastoma cell population (stem as well as bulk tumor cells). Another combination study was reported by Gomez-Cabrero and Reisfeld where IMD-0354 (inhibitor of nuclear factor κB) was targeted by cancer stem cells. It was combined with doxorubicin and encapsulated in targeted nanoparticles [77]. In these studies, targeting was performed with a legumain inhibitor. This construct enhances drug delivery under hypoxia, which is present within the tumor microenvironment. However, under normoxia, reducing potential causes toxic effects. The efficiency of this formulation can be raised by reduction of ATP-binding cassette (ABC) transporter expression and activity. Moreover, a decrease in expression of stem cell markers Oct4, Nanog, and Sox2 was observed in the breast cancer cells.

6. FUTURE PROSPECTS AND CHALLENGES FACING THE FIELD

Thousands of basic research and clinical studies are being carried out currently involving the use of stem cells. The success of a lot of these studies depends on the availability of technologies capable of isolating, tracking, targeting, delivering, and regulating the stem cells. These cells need to be tagged, imaged, and tracked for efficient stem cell–based properties in which nanotechnology can play a key role. The current tracking and imaging techniques suffer from eventual loss of signal. Inefficient techniques for whole body tracking with multiple nanotechnology approaches (some of which were described in this chapter) can provide significant improved cancer stem cell therapy.

Regulation of stem cell differentiation is a very important part of successful stem cell–based therapy, especially in regenerative medicine. This regulation often requires delivery of highly specialized biomolecules within the stem cells at specific times. Nanotechnology has generated highly biocompatible and targeted delivery systems with high internalization efficiency. But these delivery systems still have to cross multiple biological barriers before these constructs can reach stem cells. Further progress is needed to improve their translocation into the target cells. Nanotechnology has also helped regulation of the stem cell differentiation by acting as scaffolds that can provide temporary 3D matrices for the stem cells to receive signals from and guide in tissue formation. These nanoscaffolds can act as matrix support, biomolecule delivery systems, and tracking agents, thus serving multiple purposes in stem cell–based therapy. However, these technologies are far from perfect. Further studies are needed to investigate how the stem cells interact with various scaffold structures. This information can help us to create the ideal nanoscale composites for particular cancer cell being targeted.

Stem cell therapy and nanotechnology are both bourgeoning fields in oncology. Both strategies have not reached their full potential. Nanotechnology is playing an important role in expanding our current knowledge of stem cells and helping us design more targeted and highly effective anticancer therapy.

REFERENCES

[1] Gomes MJ, Neves J, Sarmento B. Nanoparticle-based drug delivery to improve the efficacy of antiretroviral therapy in the central nervous system. Int J Nanomedicine 2014;9:1757–69.
[2] Orkin SH, Morrison SJ. Stem-cell competition. Nature 2002;418(6893):25–7.
[3] Jiang Y, et al. Pluripotency of mesenchymal stem cells derived from adult marrow. Nature 2002;418(6893):41–9.
[4] Spitalieri P, et al. Human induced pluripotent stem cells for monogenic disease modelling and therapy. World J Stem Cells 2016;8(4):118–35.
[5] Liu SV. iPS cells: a more critical review. Stem Cells Dev 2008;17(3):391–7.
[6] Metcalf D. Concise review: hematopoietic stem cells and tissue stem cells: current concepts and unanswered questions. Stem Cells 2007;25(10):2390–5.
[7] Calin M, Stan D, Simion V. Stem cell regenerative potential combined with nanotechnology and tissue engineering for myocardial regeneration. Curr Stem Cell Res Ther 2013;8(4):292–303.

[8] Wang Z, Ruan J, Cui D. Advances and prospect of nanotechnology in stem cells. Nanoscale Res Lett 2009;4(7):593−605.
[9] Ferreira L, et al. New opportunities: the use of nanotechnologies to manipulate and track stem cells. Cell Stem Cell 2008;3(2):136−46.
[10] Moghimi SM, Hunter AC, Murray JC. Nanomedicine: current status and future prospects. FASEB J 2005;19(3):311−30.
[11] Bhana S, Wang Y, Huang X. Nanotechnology for enrichment and detection of circulating tumor cells. Nanomedicine 2015;10(12):1973−90.
[12] He J, et al. Magnetic separation techniques in sample preparation for biological analysis: a review. J Pharm Biomed Anal 2014;101:84−101.
[13] Chandra S, Nigam S, Bahadur D. Combining unique properties of dendrimers and magnetic nanoparticles towards cancer theranostics. J Biomed Nanotechnol 2014;10(1):32−49.
[14] Wang R, et al. Well-defined Peapod-like magnetic nanoparticles and their controlled modification for effective imaging guided gene therapy. ACS Appl Mater Interfaces 2016;8(18):11298−308.
[15] Jing Y, et al. Blood progenitor cell separation from clinical leukapheresis product by magnetic nanoparticle binding and magnetophoresis. Biotechnol Bioeng 2007;96(6):1139−54.
[16] Stuckey DW, Shah K. Stem cell-based therapies for cancer treatment: separating hope from hype. Nat Rev Cancer 2014;14(10):683−91.
[17] Patel S, Lee KB. Probing stem cell behavior using nanoparticle-based approaches. Wiley Interdiscip Rev Nanomed Nanobiotechnol 2015;7(6):759−78.
[18] Reimer P, Balzer T. Ferucarbotran (Resovist): a new clinically approved RES-specific contrast agent for contrast-enhanced MRI of the liver: properties, clinical development, and applications. Eur Radiol 2003;13(6):1266−76.
[19] Hsiao JK, et al. Magnetic nanoparticle labeling of mesenchymal stem cells without transfection agent: cellular behavior and capability of detection with clinical 1.5 T magnetic resonance at the single cell level. Magn Reson Med 2007;58(4):717−24.
[20] Murahari MS, Yergeri MC. Identification and usage of fluorescent probes as nanoparticle contrast agents in detecting cancer. Curr Pharm Des 2013;19(25):4622−40.
[21] Jendelová P, et al. Magnetic resonance tracking of transplanted bone marrow and embryonic stem cells labeled by iron oxide nanoparticles in rat brain and spinal cord. J Neurosci Res 2004;76(2):232−43.
[22] Jin XH, et al. In vivo MR imaging tracking of supermagnetic iron-oxide nanoparticle-labeled bone marrow mesenchymal stem cells injected into intra-articular space of knee joints: experiment with rabbit. Zhonghua Yi Xue Za Zhi 2007;87(45):3213−8.
[23] Shen J, et al. Magnetic resonance imaging of mesenchymal stem cells labeled with dual (MR and fluorescence) agents in rat spinal cord injury. Acad Radiol 2009;16(9):1142−54.
[24] Liu Y, et al. Evaluation of cell tracking effects for transplanted mesenchymal stem cells with jetPEI/Gd-DTPA complexes in animal models of hemorrhagic spinal cord injury. Brain Res 2011;1391:24−35.
[25] Danner S, et al. Quantum dots do not alter the differentiation potential of pancreatic stem cells and are distributed randomly among daughter cells. Int J Cell Biol 2013;2013, 918242.
[26] Lin S, et al. Quantum dot imaging for embryonic stem cells. BMC Biotechnol 2007;7:67.
[27] Barnett JM, Penn JS, Jayagopal A. Imaging of endothelial progenitor cell subpopulations in angiogenesis using quantum dot nanocrystals. Methods Mol Biol 2013;1026:45−56.
[28] Shah B, et al. Labeling and imaging of human mesenchymal stem cells with quantum dot bioconjugates during proliferation and osteogenic differentiation in long term. Conf Proc IEEE Eng Med Biol Soc 2006;1:1470−3.
[29] Li J, et al. Multifunctional quantum dot nanoparticles for effective differentiation and long-term tracking of human mesenchymal stem cells in vitro and in vivo. Adv Healthc Mater 2016;5(9):1049−57.
[30] Ricles LM, et al. Function of mesenchymal stem cells following loading of gold nanotracers. Int J Nanomedicine 2011;6:407−16.
[31] Nam SY, et al. In vivo ultrasound and photoacoustic monitoring of mesenchymal stem cells labeled with gold nanotracers. PLoS One 2012;7(5):e37267.

[32] Choi CK, et al. A gold@polydopamine core-shell nanoprobe for long-term intracellular detection of microRNAs in differentiating stem cells. J Am Chem Soc 2015;137(23):7337–46.
[33] Ricles LM, et al. A dual gold nanoparticle system for mesenchymal stem cell tracking. J Mater Chem B Mater Biol Med 2014;2(46):8220–30.
[34] Accomasso L, et al. Fluorescent silica nanoparticles improve optical imaging of stem cells allowing direct discrimination between live and early-stage apoptotic cells. Small 2012;8(20):3192–200.
[35] Gallina C, et al. Human mesenchymal stem cells labelled with dye-loaded amorphous silica nanoparticles: long-term biosafety, stemness preservation and traceability in the beating heart. J Nanobiotechnology 2015;13:77.
[36] Jokerst JV, Khademi C, Gambhir SS. Intracellular aggregation of multimodal silica nanoparticles for ultrasound-guided stem cell implantation. Sci Transl Med 2013;5(177):177ra35.
[37] Novotna B, et al. The impact of silica encapsulated cobalt zinc ferrite nanoparticles on DNA, lipids and proteins of rat bone marrow mesenchymal stem cells. Nanotoxicology 2016;10(6):662–70.
[38] Lee JK, et al. Specific labeling of neurogenic, endothelial, and myogenic differentiated cells derived from human amniotic fluid stem cells with silica-coated magnetic nanoparticles. J Vet Med Sci 2012;74(8):969–75.
[39] Sniadecki NJ, et al. Nanotechnology for cell-substrate interactions. Ann Biomed Eng 2006;34(1):59–74.
[40] Adams GB, et al. Stem cell engraftment at the endosteal niche is specified by the calcium-sensing receptor. Nature 2006;439(7076):599–603.
[41] Dolatshahi-Pirouz A, et al. Micro- and nanoengineering approaches to control stem cell-biomaterial interactions. J Funct Biomater 2011;2(3):88–106.
[42] Dolatshahi-Pirouz A, et al. A combinatorial cell-laden gel microarray for inducing osteogenic differentiation of human mesenchymal stem cells. Sci Rep 2014;4:3896.
[43] Zhou Y, et al. Self-assembly of hyperbranched polymers and its biomedical applications. Adv Mater 2010;22(41):4567–90.
[44] Wang D, et al. Self-assembly of supramolecularly engineered polymers and their biomedical applications. Chem Commun 2014;50(81):11994–2017.
[45] Gelain F, et al. Designer self-assembling peptide nanofiber scaffolds for adult mouse neural stem cell 3-dimensional cultures. PLoS One 2006;1:e119.
[46] Koutsopoulos S, Zhang S. Long-term three-dimensional neural tissue cultures in functionalized self-assembling peptide hydrogels, matrigel and collagen I. Acta Biomater 2013;9(2):5162–9.
[47] Giri S, et al. Telomerase activity and hepatic functions of rat embryonic liver progenitor cell in nanoscaffold-coated model bioreactor. Mol Cell Biochem 2010;336(1–2):137–49.
[48] Castells-Sala C, et al. Influence of electrical stimulation on 3D-cultures of adipose tissue derived progenitor cells (ATDPCs) behavior. Conf Proc IEEE Eng Med Biol Soc 2012;2012:5658–61.
[49] Tam K, et al. A nanoscaffold impregnated with human Wharton's jelly stem cells or its secretions improves healing of wounds. J Cell Biochem 2014;115(4):794–803.
[50] Elkhenany H, et al. Graphene supports in vitro proliferation and osteogenic differentiation of goat adult mesenchymal stem cells: potential for bone tissue engineering. J Appl Toxicol 2015;35(4):367–74.
[51] Mousavi SH, et al. Expansion of human cord blood hematopoietic stem/progenitor cells in three-dimensional nanoscaffold coated with fibronectin. Int J Hematol Oncol Stem Cell Res 2015;9(2):72–9.
[52] Aligholi H, et al. Preparing neural stem/progenitor cells in PuraMatrix hydrogel for transplantation after brain injury in rats: a comparative methodological study. Brain Res 2016;1642:197–208.
[53] Mashhadikhan M, et al. ADSCs on PLLA/PCL hybrid nanoscaffold and gelatin modification: cytocompatibility and mechanical properties. Avicenna J Med Biotechnol 2015;7(1):32–8.
[54] Gorjikhah F, et al. Improving "lab-on-a-chip" techniques using biomedical nanotechnology: a review. Artif Cells Nanomed Biotechnol 2016:1–6.
[55] Sciancalepore AG, et al. A bioartificial renal tubule device embedding human renal stem/progenitor cells. PLoS One 2014;9(1):e87496.

[56] Zhang YS, et al. From cardiac tissue engineering to heart-on-a-chip: beating challenges. Biomed Mater 2015;10(3):034006.
[57] Jastrzebska E, Tomecka E, Jesion I. Heart-on-a-chip based on stem cell biology. Biosens Bioelectron 2016;75:67—81.
[58] Li S, et al. Application of an acoustofluidic perfusion bioreactor for cartilage tissue engineering. Lab Chip 2014;14(23):4475—85.
[59] Mooney E, et al. Carbon nanotubes and mesenchymal stem cells: biocompatibility, proliferation and differentiation. Nano Lett 2008;8(8):2137—43.
[60] Zhu K, et al. Reprogramming fibroblasts to pluripotency using arginine-terminated polyamidoamine nanoparticles based non-viral gene delivery system. Int J Nanomedicine 2014;9:5837—47.
[61] Sohn YD, et al. Induction of pluripotency in bone marrow mononuclear cells via polyketal nanoparticle-mediated delivery of mature microRNAs. Biomaterials 2013;34(17):4235—41.
[62] Chen W, et al. Nonviral cell labeling and differentiation agent for induced pluripotent stem cells based on mesoporous silica nanoparticles. ACS Nano 2013;7(10):8423—40.
[63] Basu S, Haase G, Ben-Ze'ev A. Wnt signaling in cancer stem cells and colon cancer metastasis. F1000Res 2016;5.
[64] Bandhavkar S. Cancer stem cells: a metastasizing menace! Cancer Med 2016;5(4):649—55.
[65] Yang M, Liu P, Huang P. Cancer stem cells, metabolism, and therapeutic significance. Tumour Biol 2016;37(5):5735—42.
[66] Papi A, Orlandi M. Role of nuclear receptors in breast cancer stem cells. World J Stem Cells 2016;8(3): 62—72.
[67] Rinkenbaugh AL, Baldwin AS. The NF-κB pathway and cancer stem cells. Cells 2016;5(2).
[68] Sun JH, et al. Liver cancer stem cell markers: progression and therapeutic implications. World J Gastroenterol 2016;22(13):3547—57.
[69] Mutlu M, et al. miR-200c: a versatile watchdog in cancer progression, EMT, and drug resistance. J Mol Med 2016;94(6):629—44.
[70] Liu Q, et al. Targeted delivery of miR-200c/DOC to inhibit cancer stem cells and cancer cells by the gelatinases-stimuli nanoparticles. Biomaterials 2013;34(29):7191—203.
[71] Wei Q, Lei R, Hu G. Roles of miR-182 in sensory organ development and cancer. Thorac Cancer 2015;6(1):2—9.
[72] Kouri FM, et al. miR-182 integrates apoptosis, growth, and differentiation programs in glioblastoma. Genes Dev 2015;29(7):732—45.
[73] Gul-Uludag H, et al. Polymeric nanoparticle-mediated silencing of CD44 receptor in CD34[+] acute myeloid leukemia cells. Leuk Res 2014;38(11):1299—308.
[74] Ganesh S, et al. Hyaluronic acid based self-assembling nanosystems for CD44 target mediated siRNA delivery to solid tumors. Biomaterials 2013;34(13):3489—502.
[75] Tangudu NK, et al. RNA interference using c-Myc-conjugated nanoparticles suppresses breast and colorectal cancer models. Mol Cancer Ther 2015;14(5):1259—69.
[76] Kim SS, et al. A nanoparticle carrying the p53 gene targets tumors including cancer stem cells, sensitizes glioblastoma to chemotherapy and improves survival. ACS Nano 2014;8(6):5494—514.
[77] Gomez-Cabrero A, Wrasidlo W, Reisfeld RA. IMD-0354 targets breast cancer stem cells: a novel approach for an adjuvant to chemotherapy to prevent multidrug resistance in a murine model. PLoS One 2013;8(8):e73607.

CHAPTER 6

Nanoparticulate Systems for Therapeutic and Diagnostic Applications

Rajashekar Kammari, Nandita G. Das, Sudip K. Das
Butler University, Indianapolis, IN, United States

Contents

1. Introduction	105
2. Why Nanotechnology and Nanomedicine?	106
3. Types of Nanoparticles in Drug Delivery	108
3.1 Nonrigid Nanoparticles	108
3.1.1 Liposomes	*108*
3.1.2 Solid Lipid Nanoparticles	*114*
3.2 Rigid Nanoparticles	119
3.2.1 Biodegradable Polymeric Nanoparticles	*120*
3.2.2 Carbon Nanotubes and Nanohorns	*126*
3.2.3 Iron Nanoparticles	*127*
4. Conclusion	138
References	138

1. INTRODUCTION

The multidisciplinary science of nanotechnology is an emerging field where groupings of atoms and molecules are manipulated at the nanometer levels. The concept of nanotechnology was suggested by Richard Feynman in 1959. The term nanotechnology was first introduced by Taniguchi in 1974 and the strategies of nanotechnology were later described by E. Drexler in 1986. The invention of computer imaging systems and high-power microscopes in the late 1980s revolutionized nanotechnology. Nanotechnology has extensive potential in the fields of pharmacy, physics, biology, and materials science which could combine to contribute toward healthcare. Although the concept of nanotechnology has been explored in healthcare research for the past three decades, it is still considered to be in the early developmental stages as expected therapeutic benefits have not been fully realized [1,2]. Both the academic and industrial communities are investing time and money into the development of nanotherapeutics in order to overcome the perceived challenges and translate the theoretically proven benefits of nanoparticulate systems into clinical advantages. This review mainly focuses on the applications of nanotechnology in drug delivery and diagnosis.

2. WHY NANOTECHNOLOGY AND NANOMEDICINE?

The application of nanotechnology to treat diseases is known as nanomedicine. The US Food and Drug Administration has approved some nanoparticulate formulations and numerous others are under development in various clinical stages. Table 6.1 summarizes some of these nanoparticle formulations [3–6]. Nanoparticulate systems could play a vital role in drug delivery, imaging, and even in surgery as they have a size range similar to that of biological molecules such as proteins, receptors, DNA, and RNA [7]. Nanoparticulate systems are relatively small in size compared to cells but are bigger than most "small molecule"–type drugs, which could improve their retention time in circulation without the risk of clogging the blood vessels, which in turn can improve the bioavailability and pharmacokinetic profile of various drugs. Nanoparticles can utilize a natural process called endocytosis to penetrate cells, which presents a particular advantage in situations where normal entry into cells would be challenging for a given molecule [8]. This feature is also helpful in targeting specific organelles inside the cells such as nuclei in case of gene knockdown using small interfering RNAs (siRNAs) [9–12]. Another interesting feature of nanoparticulate systems is their high surface area-to-volume ratio, which provides a large substrate for attachment of specific moieties for active targeting [13]. Nanoparticles can be surface modified with specific antibodies or peptides to achieve tissue targeting, which reduces the likelihood of nonspecific off-target toxicity [14,15]. The surface properties of nanotherapeutics can be modified according to therapeutic and diagnostic needs, including imparting stealth properties to evade elimination by the reticuloendothelial system, which improves the circulation time and increases drug concentration at the site of action [5,16].

Nanoparticulate technology has opened up potential new avenues in the early detection and treatment of various cancers, biodetection of pathogens, and in the preparation of fluorescent biological labels as they encompass both imaging and therapeutic capabilities. Nanoparticulate technology is also helpful in addressing solubility and stability issues of poorly soluble drugs and in altering their pharmacokinetic profiles to achieve prolonged plasma half-life. Since 1980s, the healthcare community has encountered clinical challenges where resistance has developed against antibiotics and select other traditional therapeutics. It is possible that these issues can be addressed by using nanoparticulate drug delivery systems [4,17]. However, despite the projected therapeutic benefits, there are limitations and challenges with nanotechnology that need to be addressed to improve the odds for success, including the development of better characterization techniques, achieving batch-to-batch consistency, reducing developmental costs and the clinical translation of theoretical design to clinical/therapeutic efficacy [18–20]. Several experimental nanoparticulate systems are known to cause nonspecific inflammatory responses and to possess immunomodulatory properties [21,22]. Other challenges include the detachment of the active targeting moieties before reaching the site of action

Table 6.1 Examples of FDA-approved nanoparticulate formulations

Drug product	Active ingredient	Manufacturer	Indications	FDA approval date
Abraxane	Albumin-bound paclitaxel	Abraxis Bioscience, Astra Zeneca, Celgene	Metastatic adenocarcinoma	2013
			Non–small cell lung cancer	2012
Ferumoxytol	Iron oxide nanoparticles		Breast cancer	2005
			Iron deficiency	2009
Marqibo	Vincristine	Talon Therapeutics	Philadelphia chromosome-negative lymphoblastic leukemia	2012
Oncaspar	PEGasparaginase injectable solution	Enzon	Acute lymphoblastic leukemia	2006
Rapamune	Nanocrystals			2002
Myocet	Liposome-encapsulated doxorubicin	Elan/Sopherion therapeutics	Breast cancer	2000, approved in Europe and Canada
DepoCyt	Liposomal cytarabine	Skye Pharma, Enzon	Lymphomatous meningitis	1999
Ontak	Diphtheria toxin	Seragen	Cutaneous T-cell	1999
AmBisome	Liposomal amphotericin B	Astellas	Fungal infections	1997
Feridex	Iron oxide nanoparticles, injectable solution	AMAG Pharma	Contrast agent for MRI	1996
DaunoXome	Daunorubicin citrate liposomes	Gilead Sciences	HIV-related Kaposi sarcoma	1996
Doxil	PEGylated liposome of doxorubicin hydrochloride	Ortho Biotech	Ovarian cancer	1995
ThermoDox	Heat-activated liposomal doxorubicin	Celsion	Breast cancer, primary liver cancer	2013
Resovist	Iron oxide nanoparticles coated with carboxydextran	Bayer Schering Pharma AG	Liver/spleen lesion imaging	2001, approved in Europe
Endorem	Iron oxide nanoparticles coated with dextran	Guerbet	Liver/spleen lesion imaging	2001, approved in Europe
Genexal-PM	Paclitaxel-loaded polymeric micelle	Samyang	Breast cancer/small cell lung cancer	Marketed in Europe, Korea

FDA, US Food and Drug Administration; *HIV*, human immunodeficiency virus; *MRI*, magnetic resonance imaging; *PEG*, polyethylene glycol.

(pretarget release), which could lead to exaggerated toxicity, and concerns about safety and manufacturability. Moreover, it is acknowledged that nanoparticulate systems are not mainstream in crossing the barrier of regulatory approval [20].

3. TYPES OF NANOPARTICLES IN DRUG DELIVERY

Nanoparticulate systems can be classified into two broad categories based on the integrity of the particles, such as nonrigid nanoparticles, which encompass liposomes and solid lipid nanoparticles, and rigid nanoparticles, which encompass polymeric nanoparticles and inorganic nanoparticles (Fig. 6.1).

3.1 Nonrigid Nanoparticles

Unlike rigid nanoparticles, the nonrigid nanoparticles are known to consist of relatively soft structures that can be easily disrupted by external force. The lipid-based nanoparticles such as liposomes and solid lipid nanoparticles are generally categorized as nonrigid nanoparticles.

3.1.1 Liposomes

The term liposome is derived from two Greek words "lipo" and "soma," which translates to "fat" and "body," respectively. The concept of liposomes was first described by Dr. Alec Bangham in 1964. The breakthrough in research involving liposomes resulted in the approval of some formulations such as Doxil, DaunoXome, ThermoDox, and Marqibo since mid-1990s [4,6,23]. The liposomes can be effectively used to deliver water-soluble drugs (hydrophilic), water-insoluble drugs (hydrophobic), peptides, and nucleic acids.

Liposomes are considered to be biologically inert and biocompatible as they are simplified models of biological membranes and contain amphiphilic phospholipid layers (either natural or synthetic). The phospholipid molecules contain a hydrophilic "head" and a hydrophobic "tail" (hydrocarbon chain). Liposomes are spontaneously formed when a phospholipid layer is disrupted by external force such as sonication or stirring or when it comes in contact with an aqueous phase. The formation of liposomes involves the self-association of phospholipid layers, which makes it spontaneous [24]. The core of

Nanoparticles

Non-rigid nanoparticles
* Liposomes
* Solid-lipid nanoparticles

Rigid nanoparticles
* Bio degradable polymeric nanoparticles
* Carbon nanotubes/nano horns
* Iron nanoparticles

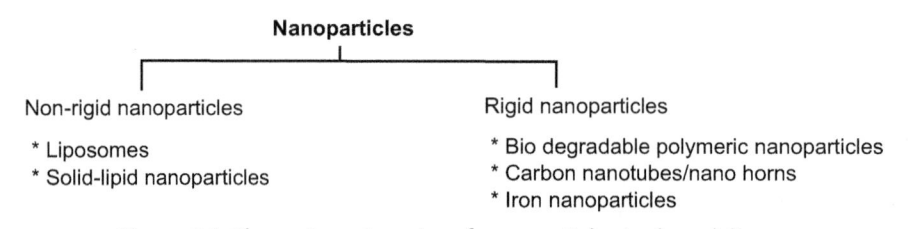

Figure 6.1 The major categories of nanoparticles in drug delivery.

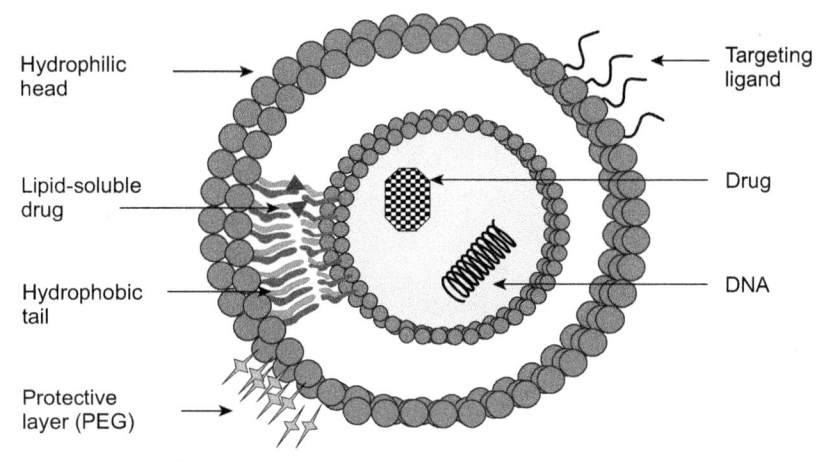

Figure 6.2 Typical bilamellar liposome structure.

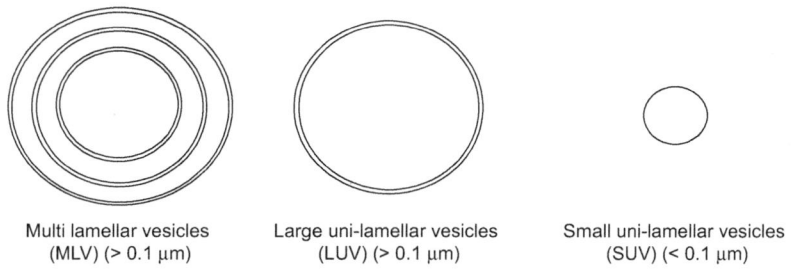

Figure 6.3 Types of liposomes based on the size and number of layers.

the liposome is hydrophilic and the space between the two layers is hydrophobic. This unique feature enables us to load either hydrophilic drugs within the core or hydrophobic drugs between the two phospholipid layers (Fig. 6.2).

Liposomes can be either unilamellar or multilamellar with varying size. The unilamellar vesicles can be further classified as small unilamellar vesicles (SUVs) and large unilamellar vesicles (LUVs) based on their size [25] (Fig. 6.3). Liposomes with a size range of ≤400 nm are known to preferentially accumulate in the tumor tissue by a phenomenon called enhanced permeability and retention effect where the nanosized particles escape through the leaky vasculature [26,27]. However, these conventional liposomes are rapidly eliminated by the mononuclear phagocyte system (MPS), formerly known as the reticuloendothelial system [13]. A popular modification of traditional liposomes, called stealth liposomes, is surface coated with a hydrophilic polymer such as polyethylene glycol and possesses the ability to evade uptake and elimination by the MPS [13,28].

3.1.1.1 Lipid Film Hydration Method for Preparation of Liposomes

The general method of liposome preparation involves four basic steps [29,30]. First, the lipids (either natural or synthetic) are dissolved in appropriate organic solvents. The

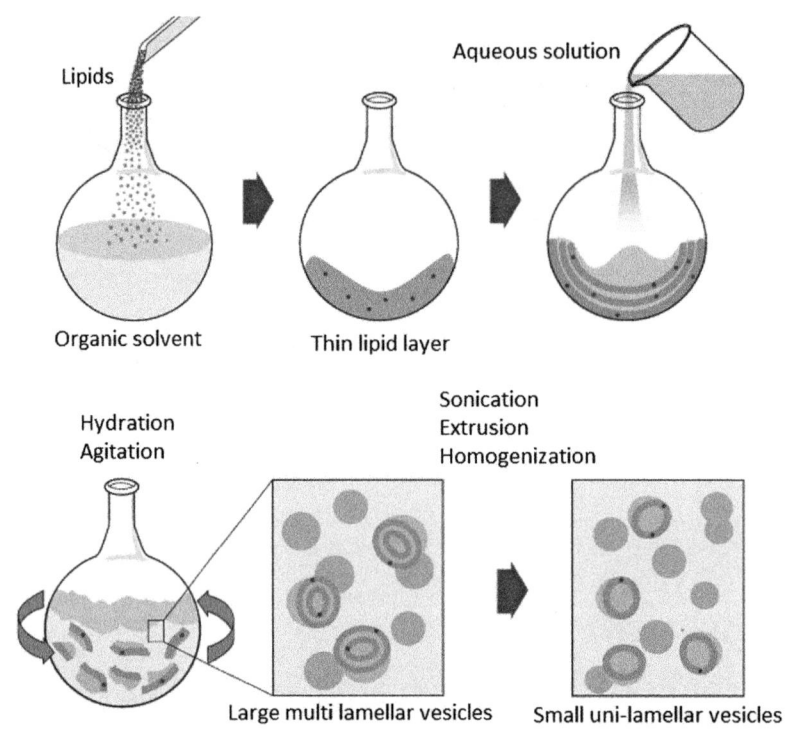

Figure 6.4 Schematic representation of liposome preparation by the lipid film hydration method.

solution is placed against a suitable surface with agitation/rotation and the organic solvent from the lipid solution is evaporated to generate a thin layer of spread-out lipids. The evaporation of organic solvent is facilitated either by increased temperature or by vacuum. Later, the dried thin lipid layer is hydrated with an aqueous phase (usually at or slightly above the transition temperature for the lipids), typically accompanied by agitation. Due to the hydrophobic nature of the tail regions of phospholipids, the liposomes are formed by the process of self-assembly as small sections of the lipids become hydrated in contact with the aqueous medium. Finally, the liposomes are purified using appropriate methods such as ultracentrifugation, gel permeation chromatography, cross-flow microfiltration, or liposome extruder purification [31−33]. The drug loading in liposomes can be done by either passive or active loading methods, as described in the next section (Fig. 6.4).

3.1.1.2 Drug Loading Liposomes by the Passive Loading Method
In the passive loading method, the hydrophobic or hydrophilic drugs are directly added to the thin film of lipids during the formation of vesicles (hydrophilic drug in aqueous phase or hydrophobic drug in organic phase along with lipids) [29,30,34,35]. The trapping efficiency of hydrophobic drugs will depend on the interaction of drug and

hydrophobic lipid bilayer space; however, 100% trapping efficiency is achievable for hydrophobic drugs. On the other hand, the trapping efficiency of hydrophilic drugs is relatively low (30%) due to the limited volume of the encapsulated aqueous component in the liposome core. The trapping efficiency of hydrophilic drugs in liposomes can be increased significantly by using active loading methods such as the pH gradient entrapment method [36].

There are several passive loading techniques for liposome preparation including mechanical dispersion, solvent dispersion, and detergent removal methods.

3.1.1.2.1 Passive Drug Loading by Mechanical Dispersion—Sonication Method
Sonication is one of the simplest and most extensively used methods for the preparation of SUVs. In this method either a probe tip sonicator or a bath-type sonicator is used to disrupt multilamellar vesicles into SUVs. The probe tip sonicator is relatively more powerful than the bath-type sonicator but the former generates more heat, which may pose a higher risk for the degradation of the lipids and the loaded drugs as well. The control of heat generation is relatively easier in the bath-type sonicator than the probe tip sonicator and the overall encapsulation is higher when using the bath-type sonicator compared with the probe tip sonicator.

3.1.1.2.2 Passive Drug Loading by Mechanical Dispersion—Extrusion Method
This technique is also known as the French-press extrusion cell technique. In this method the multilamellar vesicles are passed through a small orifice, which results in pressure-based disruption of the larger vesicles and leads to the formation of SUVs [37]. The size of the liposomes formed by this method is usually larger than that of liposomes formed by sonication. However, the liposomes formed by this method possess the ability of prolonged release of entrapped drugs [38,39].

3.1.1.2.3 Passive Drug Loading by Mechanical Dispersion—Freeze-Thaw Technique
This method is employed in the preparation of LUVs. Initially, the SUVs are frozen rapidly and thawed gradually, during which process the SUVs aggregate. Gentle sonication results in the breakup of the aggregates and the formation of LUVs [40–42]. The encapsulation efficiency of liposomes formed by this method is approximately 30% compared with the sonication method.

3.1.1.2.4 Passive Loading by Solvent Dispersion—Ether Injection Method
This method is also known as the solvent vaporization method. In this method the lipids are dissolved in either diethyl ether or in an ether–methanol mixture. The lipid solution is then rapidly injected into the aqueous phase at 55–65°C, which results in the formation of liposomes. The excess ether is removed by vacuum evaporation. The disadvantage of this method is the production of heterogeneous liposomes with a size range of 70–200 nm [43,44].

3.1.1.2.5 Passive Drug Loading by Solvent Dispersion—Ethanol Injection Method
This method is similar to the ether injection method. In this method, the lipids are dissolved in ethanol and the resultant lipid solution is rapidly injected into the aqueous phase. This results in the formation of multilamellar vesicles. The disadvantages of this method include heterogeneous liposomes with a size range 20—120 nm and the formation of very dilute liposomes. Another concern is the removal of excess ethanol, which forms an azeotropic mixture in aqueous medium [45].

3.1.1.2.6 Passive Drug Loading by Solvent Dispersion—Reverse Phase Evaporation Method
The liposomes produced by this method generally consist of high aqueous volume-to-lipid ratio compared with the liposomes produced by other methods. In this method, the lipids are first dissolved in an organic solvent such as ether or chloroform to form a lipid solution. This solution is then added to the aqueous phase, followed by brief sonication, which results in the formation of inverted micelles. The evaporation of the organic phase from the above solution leads to the formation of a viscous layer of lipids. After reaching a critical point, the layer collapses and the excess phospholipids in the solution form a bilayer around the micelles to generate the liposomes. The main disadvantages of this method include the exposure of drugs to the organic solvents and the brief sonication period, which could potentially adversely affect the formulation components.

3.1.1.3 Purification of Liposomes—Detergent Removal Methods
Detergents or surfactants are normally used to facilitate the dilution of lipids in organic solvents. After the formation of liposomes, the excess phospholipids and detergents should be removed. There are several methods to remove the detergents from liposomal solutions, as described below:

Dialysis: This is the most common method for removing detergents, and can be accomplished by using conventional dialysis bags, which work on the basis of equilibrium dialysis [46,47]. Currently, some commercial dialysis devices such as Slide-A-Lyzer Dialysis Cassettes are also available.

Absorption: In this method the mixed micelles or the liposome solutions are treated with organic polystyrene beads such as the XAD-2 beads or Bio-beads SM2. This method is efficient in removing the detergents with low critical micellar concentration values.

Gel permeation chromatography: In this method the separation column contains pretreated beads that adsorb amphiphilic lipids. However, the intact liposomes percolate through the interbead spaces.

3.1.1.4 In Vitro and In Vivo Studies Involving Liposomes
In 2005 Hao et al. [48] studied the efficiency of liposomes in delivering an anticancer drug topotecan (TPT) to the tumors. They compared the efficiency of S-liposomes and H-liposomes, which comprised soybean phosphatidylcholine and hydrogenated

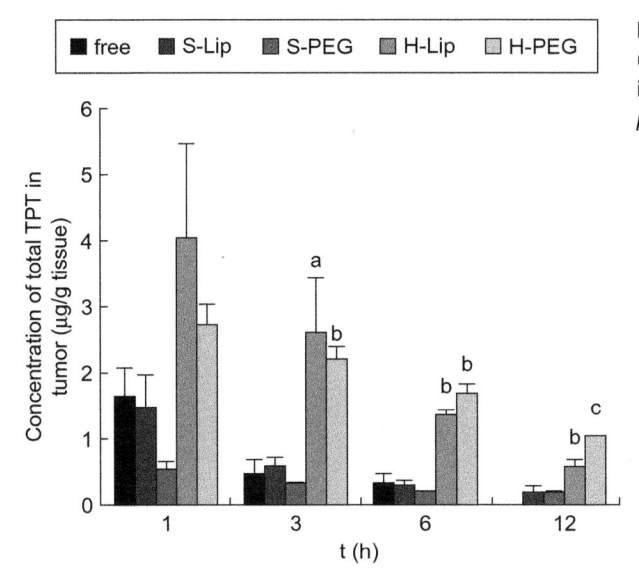

Figure 6.5 Distribution of topotecan (TPT) in tumor tissue following a single intravenous dose [48]. *(Reprinted with permission.)*

soybean phosphatidylcholine, respectively. Fig. 6.5 shows the results obtained by Hao et al., which clearly indicate the high tumor concentration of TPT delivered using the H-liposomes compared with the free drug and S-liposomes.

In another study, Wei et al. [49] studied the biodistribution of gadolinium–diethylene triamine penta-acetate (DTPA) [a magnetic resonance imaging (MRI) contrast agent] encapsulated in paramagnetic liposomes in A549 tumor-bearing mice (Fig. 6.6).

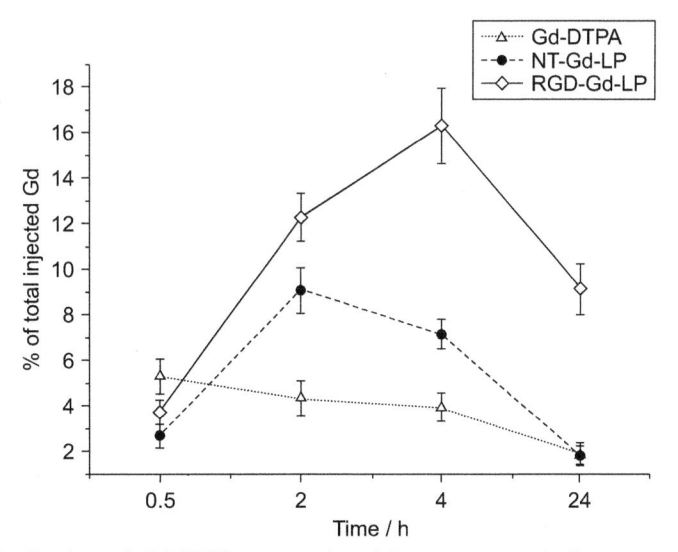

Figure 6.6 Biodistribution of Gd-DTPA encapsulated in paramagnetic liposomes in A549 tumor-bearing mice [49]. *Gd-DTPA*, gadolinium-diethylene triamine penta-acetate; *N-Gd-LP*, nontargeted paramagnetic liposomes; *RGD-Gd-LP*, arginine-glycine-aspartic coupled paramagnetic liposomes. *(Reprinted with permission.)*

They compared the biodistribution of pure Gd-DTPA (Gd-DTPA), nontargeted (N-Gd-Lp), and arginine-glycine-aspartic acid (RGD) coupled (RGD-Gd-LP) paramagnetic liposomes. As expected, the liposomal formulations led to significant improvements in the biodistribution of Gd-DTPA.

3.1.1.5 Challenges Associated With Liposomes

The major problems faced by liposomal formulations include limited long-term stability, difficulties with large-scale production, and rapid elimination by the MPS system as described earlier in this chapter. The stability issues can usually be addressed by freeze-drying the liposomes at low pressure using cryoprotectants such as trehalose. The rapid elimination from the circulation can be thwarted by coating the liposomes with polymers such as polyethylene glycol and chitin derivatives [50]. Such liposomes are commonly referred to as stealth liposomes and they display high retention time in circulation, which ultimately helps in increasing the drug concentration at the site of action [51]. Other problems with liposomal formulations include low encapsulation efficiency, rapid leakage of water-soluble drugs, and other formulation design and manufacturing problems.

3.1.2 Solid Lipid Nanoparticles

Solid lipid nanoparticles are a new generation of colloidal drug carrier systems and consist of surfactant-stabilized lipids that are solid both at room and body temperatures [52]. They combine the advantages of liposomes, polymeric nanoparticles, and emulsions while minimizing some of their individual disadvantages [53,54]. They typically contain a hydrophobic solid matrix core with a phospholipid coating. The hydrophobic tail regions of the phospholipid are embedded into the core matrix and that is why the core exclusively possesses a hydrophobic nature. So it is to be expected that the solid lipid nanoparticles have a higher entrapment efficiency for hydrophobic drugs in the core compared with conventional liposomes [53] (Fig. 6.7).

The solid lipid nanoparticles are suitable for intravenous administration and can be successfully dispersed in aqueous or aqueous-surfactant solutions. Other advantages of solid lipid nanoparticles include easy scale-up and low cost of production, relative

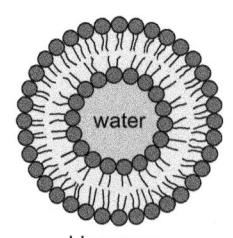

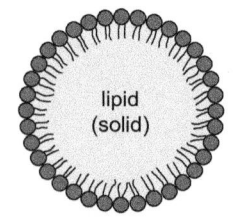

Liposome
(Lipid bilayer enclosing an aqueous core)

Solid lipid nanoparticle (SLN)
Lipid monolayer enclosing a solid lipid core

Figure 6.7 Schematic representation of the structures of liposome and solid lipid nanoparticles.

Table 6.2 Examples of lipids and surfactants used in solid lipid nanoparticle preparations [53]

Lipids	
Triglycerides	Tricaprin, trilaurin, trimyristin, tripalmitin, tristearin
Hard fats	Witepsol W 35, Witepsol H 35, Witepsol H 42, Witepsol E 85
Others	Glyceryl monostearate (Imwitor 900), glyceryl behenate (Compritol 888 ATO), glyceryl palmitostearate (Precirol ATO 5), cetyl palmitate, stearic acid, palmitic acid, decanoic acid, behenic acid

Surfactants (emulsifiers and coemulsifiers)

Soy lecithin, egg lecithin (Lipoid E 80), phosphatidylcholine, poloxamer 188, 182, and 407, poloxamine 908, Tyloxapol, polysorbate 20, 60, and 80, sodium cholate, sodium glycocholate, taurocholic acid sodium salt, taurodeoxycholic acid sodium salt, butanol, butyric acid, dioctyl sodium sulfosuccinate, monooctylphosphoric acid sodium

nontoxic nature, biodegradable composition, and stability against aggregation or coalescence. Other crucial features include the protection offered to the entrapped drugs and prolonged drug release from the matrix [53].

Solid lipid nanoparticles are prepared by using solid lipids (e.g., purified triglycerides, fatty acids, steroids, or waxes), emulsifiers, and water [52]. Table 6.2 summarizes the lipids and emulsifiers currently prevalent in research for solid lipid nanoparticle preparation.

3.1.2.1 Methods to Prepare Solid Lipid Nanoparticles

3.1.2.1.1 Hot Homogenization This is one of the most common methods for the preparation of solid lipid nanoparticles [53,55—58]. In this method, the solid lipids are melted by heating to 5—10°C above its melting temperature. The drug is dissolved, dispersed, or solubilized in the hot melted lipid, followed by the dispersion of the drug lipid melt into an aqueous surfactant solution (heated to the same temperature) to form an oil-in-water preemulsion. The preemulsion is homogenized to obtain a nanoemulsion. In case of laboratory-scale production, a piston-gap homogenizer such as the Avestin B3 homogenizer, M-110L, high-pressure pneumatic lab homogenizer or the Micron lab 40 homogenizer is preferred [59]. In case of large-scale production, there are multiple homogenizers commercially available such as M-110EH or M-700 series microfluidizers. After homogenization, the resultant nanoemulsion is cooled to room temperature to initiate the recrystallization of the lipids to obtain the solid lipid nanoparticles. The recrystallization process can also be induced by techniques such as lyophilization. This technique may not be suitable for hydrophilic drugs as the drug may partition between the lipid and aqueous phases.

In case of temperature-sensitive drugs, it is advised that techniques such as cold homogenization be used even though the exposure time to high temperatures is relatively short.

3.1.2.1.2 Cold Homogenization In this method, the solid lipids are melted by heating to 5–10°C above the melting temperature [53,55–57]. The drug is dissolved, dispersed, or solubilized in the hot melted lipid followed by cooling to room temperature. The resultant substance is then ground to obtain lipid microparticles (50–100 μm). The lipid microparticles are then suspended in a cold aqueous surfactant solution to obtain a presuspension. Finally, the lipid microparticle suspension is homogenized below room temperature to obtain the solid lipid nanoparticles. To minimize the loss of hydrophilic drugs, the aqueous phase can be replaced with liquids in which the dispersed drugs have low solubility, such as select oils or PEG 600.

3.1.2.1.3 Microemulsification In this method, the surfactants/cosurfactants such as lecithin, bile salts, or butanol are dissolved in water to form an aqueous phase [53,60,61]. This aqueous phase is heated to the same temperature as that of molten lipids, following which it is added to the molten lipids under stirring to obtain a thermodynamically stable microemulsion. This mixture is transferred to a cold aqueous medium (2–3°C) under gentle stirring to obtain the solid lipid nanoparticles via the process of precipitation.

3.1.2.2 Solvent Emulsification—Evaporation Method
This method is suitable for the heat-sensitive compounds. First, the lipids are dissolved in an organic solvent that is immiscible in water such as toluene or chloroform [52,62]. Then the lipid solution is transferred to an aqueous phase to form the primary emulsion followed by the evaporation of organic solvent under reduced pressure or vacuum. After the evaporation, the lipids precipitates to form solid lipid nanoparticles [52,53].

3.1.2.2.1 Solvent Emulsification—Diffusion In this method the organic solvents are usually partially miscible with water [52,63,64]. First, the organic solvent such as benzyl alcohol or ethyl formate is saturated with water and then the lipids are dissolved in it. This solution of surfactant is added to a lipid solution in organic solvent at elevated temperatures. Finally, the addition of excess water leads to the diffusion of the organic phase from the emulsion droplets to the continuous phase and leads to the precipitation of the solid lipid nanoparticles.

3.1.2.3 Drug Incorporation in Solid Lipid Nanoparticles
The active drug may incorporate into the solid lipid nanoparticles in three major ways based on the properties of the drug and excipients and their interaction(s) with each other [58]. The three models proposed include the homogenous matrix model, the drug-enriched shell model, and the drug-enriched core model. Homogenous matrix entrapment results when using cold homogenization or hot homogenization with highly

lipophilic drugs. In this model, the drug is dispersed at the molecular level in the solid lipid nanoparticle matrix, which is responsible for the prolonged release of drug over a period of time. Drug-enriched shell entrapment results when phase separation occurs between lipids and the aqueous phase during the formation of solid lipid nanoparticles from liquid drops. Drug release from this type of nanoparticles is very fast and is desirable when the formulation is intended for external application such as topical application for the skin. Drug-enriched core type of entrapment results when the drug precipitates first during the process of nanoparticle formation. The drug release process from these solid lipid nanoparticles is membrane controlled and follows the Fick's law of diffusion. Fig. 6.8 schematically represents the above-stated models:

Several research groups have studied various drugs incorporated in solid lipid nanoparticles. Table 6.3 summarizes some examples [54].

Solid lipid nanoparticles have generated significant interest as a specialty formulation category for various anticancer drugs, for various reasons. For example, Mosallaei et al. have demonstrated the superiority of docetaxel-loaded solid lipid nanoparticles compared with Taxotere, the commercial docetaxel formulation that is injected intravenously. As shown in Fig. 6.9, the docetaxel-loaded solid lipid nanoparticles demonstrate higher cytotoxicity than Taxotere in both colorectal (C 26) and malignant melanoma cells (A375) [74].

In another study, Martins et al. studied the in vitro and in vivo efficacy of camptothecin-loaded solid lipid nanoparticles. The in vitro studies have shown prolonged release of drug for up to 8 h. The in vitro cell viability studies in porcine brain capillary endothelial cells with three types of camptothecin-loaded solid lipid nanoparticles prepared using three different lipids have shown similar cytotoxicity when compared with each other. All camptothecin-loaded solid lipid nanoparticle formulations show superior cytotoxicity compared with the free drug solution and blank (drug-free) nanoparticles (Fig. 6.10) [75].

In 2008, Yaping Li et al. demonstrated that the tumor growth inhibition by targeted docetaxel solid lipid nanoparticles is higher than that by nontargeted solid lipid nanoparticles and free docetaxel solution (Taxotere) in hepatocellular carcinoma-bearing nude mice. A single-dose administration of solid lipid nanoparticles has shown significant

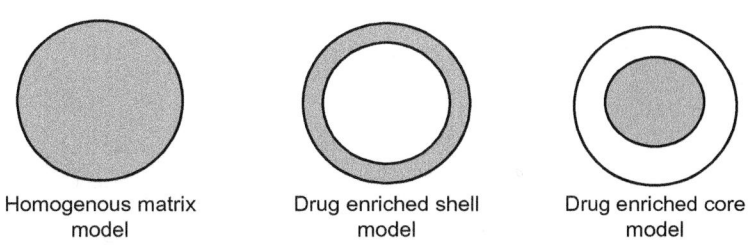

Figure 6.8 Schematic representation of models of drug entrapment in solid lipid nanoparticles.

Table 6.3 Examples of drugs studied in solid lipid nanoparticle formulations

Drug	Research group
Timolol	Cavalli et al. [65]
Deoxycorticosterone	Gasco et al. [66]
Tetracaine	Zur Muhlen et al. [57]
Betamethasone valerate	Westesesn et al. [67]
Piribedil	Demirel et al. [68]
Hydrocortisone	Cavalli et al. [69]
Paclitaxel	Cavalli et al. [70]
Acyclovir	Lukowski et al. [71]
Diazepam	Gasco et al. [72]
Camptothecin	Yang et al. [73]

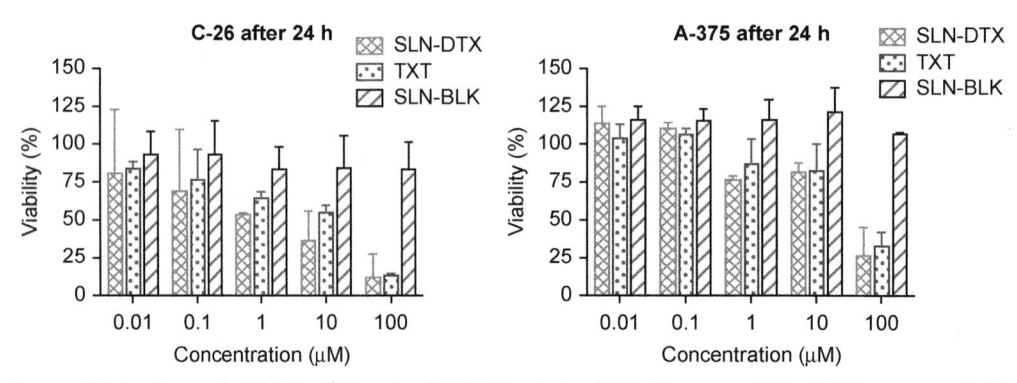

Figure 6.9 In vitro cell viability of docetaxel (DTX)-loaded solid lipid nanoparticles (SLN) compared with the commercially available docetaxel injection Taxotere (TXT) in colorectal C-26 cells and malignant melanoma A 375 cells [74]. *(Reprinted with permission.)*

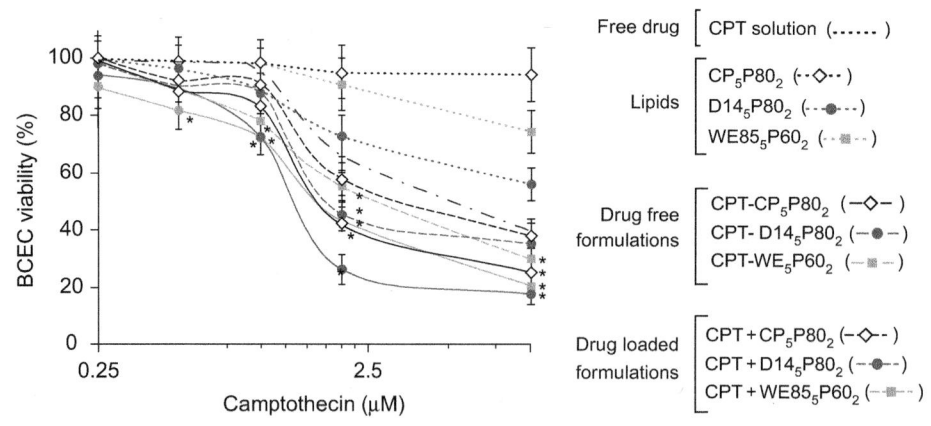

Figure 6.10 In vitro viability of brain capillary endothelial cells (BCECs) exposed for 24 h to camptothecin (CPT) solution, free lipids (CP5P802, D145P802, and WE855P602), drug (CPT)-free formulations, and drug (CPT)-loaded formulations at the CPT concentrations between 0.25 and 10 μM [75]. *(Reprinted with permission.)*

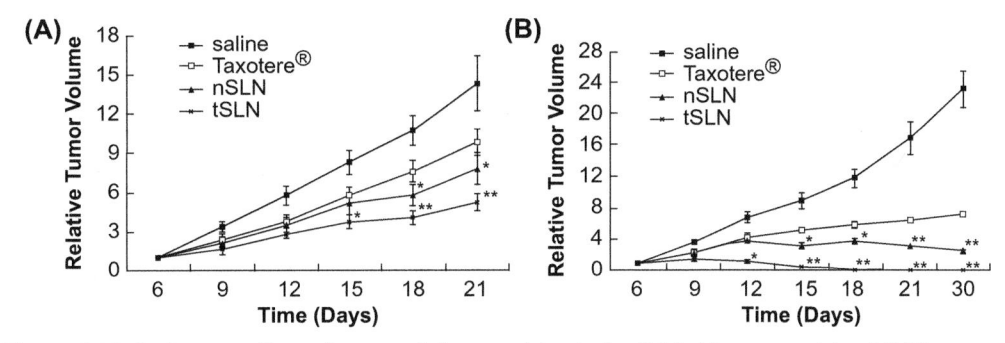

Figure 6.11 Antitumor effect of targeted docetaxel-loaded solid lipid nanoparticles (tSLN), nontargeted docetaxel-loaded solid lipid nanoparticles (nSLN), Taxotere or saline in nude mice bearing hepatoma after a single dose (A) or a schedule of multiple doses (B). *(Reprinted with permission.)*

tumor volume inhibition compared with saline-treated and Taxotere-treated mice (Fig. 6.11A). Moreover, multiple-dose administration showed complete inhibition of tumors in case of targeted docetaxel solid lipid nanoparticle compared with nontargeted docetaxel solid lipid nanoparticle and Taxotere-treated mice (Fig. 6.11B) [76].

3.1.2.4 Challenges Associated With Solid Lipid Nanoparticles

Solid lipid nanoparticles have several advantages over other types of nanoparticulate systems as discussed earlier in this section. However, there are some limitations too, the most challenging being the degradation of active components during the production process. This may be attributed to the stress and strain associated with the homogenization process, whereas fragile molecules such as DNA, siRNA, and peptides need gentle handling. The production of heat during processing may cause drug degradation so the selection of a proper production method is vital. Other problems include particle size and shape variation, coexistence of several different colloidal forms, and drug expulsion from lipid matrix [53].

3.1.2.5 Stability of Solid Lipid Nanoparticles

Solid lipid nanoparticles in general possess adequate stability for periods more than a year (Westesen et al. [67]). Muller et al. found that glyceryl palmitostearate—containing solid lipid nanoparticles are stable for more than 3 years [77]. They also found that the particle size increases when the nanoparticles are exposed to light. Solid lipid nanoparticles can be freeze-dried to aid in long-term storage [77,78].

3.2 Rigid Nanoparticles

Rigid nanoparticles are known to possess significant mechanical strength compared with the lipid-based nonrigid nanoparticles described thus far. Rigid nanoparticles can be divided into three major subcategories including biodegradable polymeric nanoparticles, carbon nanotubes, and iron nanoparticles.

3.2.1 Biodegradable Polymeric Nanoparticles

Polymeric nanoparticles have been used or are under development for various drugs for the treatment of a wide range of diseases such as cancer, diabetes, malaria, and tuberculosis [79–83]. Polymeric nanoparticles generally supersede other nanoparticulate systems with distinct advantages including better targeting abilities, better long-term storage capabilities and high encapsulation efficiency compared with other carriers. These nanoparticles also control drug release properties, improve intracellular penetration, and increase specificity and therapeutic efficacy of encapsulated drugs [84–89]. Fig. 6.12 schematically represents the types of polymeric nanoparticles based on the drug loading.

3.2.1.1 Preparation of Polymeric Nanoparticles

The preparation method and selection of components for the polymeric nanoparticles depends on various parameters such as the desired physicochemical properties, nature of drug, and intended duration of therapy [90].

3.2.1.2 Laboratory-Scale Preparation of Polymeric Nanoparticles

The laboratory-scale nanoparticle preparation methods can be classified into two broad categories: (1) dispersion of preformed polymers or (2) polymerization of monomers. The dispersion of preformed polymers methods include:

1. Solvent evaporation method
2. Spontaneous emulsification method

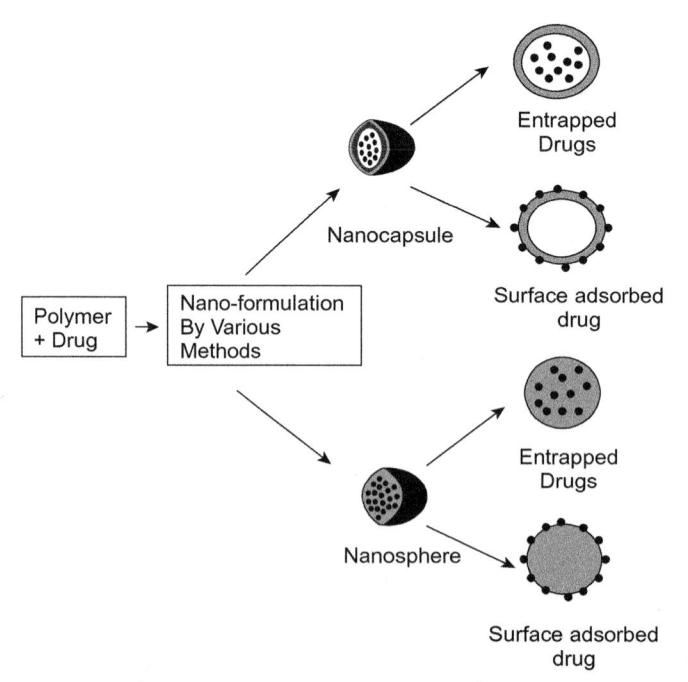

Figure 6.12 Types of polymeric nanoparticles categorized based on drug loading.

3. Salting out/emulsion diffusion method
4. Nonaqueous phase separation method

3.2.1.2.1 Solvent Evaporation Method In this method the preformed polymers such as polylactic acid or poly(D,L-lactic co-glycolic acid) are dissolved in an organic solvent such as chloroform, acetone, or ethyl acetate. The payload drug is generally dissolved in the polymer solution, which is transferred to an aqueous phase that contains a surfactant such as polyvinyl alcohol to form an oil-in-water emulsion [84,90]. The evaporation of organic solvent can be aided by continuing the homogenization process for a sufficient period of time. At the end of the homogenization period, the nanoparticles are collected by ultracentrifugation. A schematic of this method is presented in Fig. 6.13. Process variables such as polymer-to-organic solvent ratio, type of organic solvent, and homogenization speed and time can be modified to achieve the desired particle size and other properties [91].

3.2.1.2.2 Spontaneous Emulsification/Solvent Diffusion Method This is a modification of the solvent evaporation technique [92,93]. In this method, water-miscible solvents such as acetone or methanol are used as the organic phase I and water immiscible solvents such as dichloromethane or chloroform are used as the organic phase II. The interfacial turbulence that is created when these two phases are mixed leads to the formation of nanoparticles. Even though this method produces significantly smaller sized particles, there are some disadvantages such as the presence of residual organic solvent.

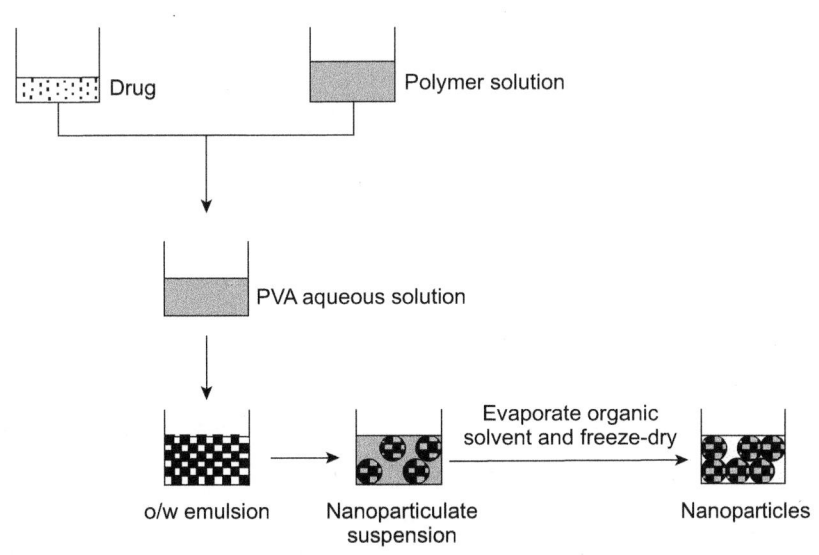

Figure 6.13 Nanoparticle preparation by emulsion solvent evaporation method. *o/w*, oil in water; *PVA*, polyvinyl alcohol.

3.2.1.2.3 Salting Out/Emulsion Diffusion Method

In this method, water-soluble polymers are dissolved in a highly concentrated solution of electrolytes or nonelectrolytes to obtain a viscous gel (aqueous phase) [90,94,95]. This aqueous gel is added to an organic phase such as acetone to obtain an oil-in-water emulsion under vigorous stirring. The formation of nanoparticles is facilitated by adding an excess amount of water, which diffuses the acetone out. The residual organic solvent is removed by continuous stirring or high-speed homogenization. A schematic of this method is presented in Fig. 6.14.

3.2.1.2.4 Nonaqueous Phase Separation Method

This method is suitable for both hydrophilic and lipophilic drugs [90]. Generally, the hydrophilic drugs are dissolved in water and then added to the organic phase. On the other hand, the lipophilic drugs are dissolved in a polymer solution. Once the aqueous phase and organic phase are mixed to form an emulsion, a second organic nonsolvent such as silicone oil (which is miscible with the first organic phase but does not dissolve the drug) is added under vigorous stirring. This results in the extraction of the first organic solvent, which causes the decrease in the solubility of polymer followed by phase separation and formation of a polymer coacervate. This polymer coacervate adsorbs onto the drug molecules to form drug-loaded nanoparticles.

3.2.1.2.5 Nanoparticle Preparation by the Emulsion Polymerization Method

In this method, monomers such as polyalkylcyanoacrylates are mechanically polymerized in the presence of drug to obtain drug-loaded nanoparticles [84,90]. Initially the monomers are dispersed in an aqueous acidic medium in the presence of a surfactant

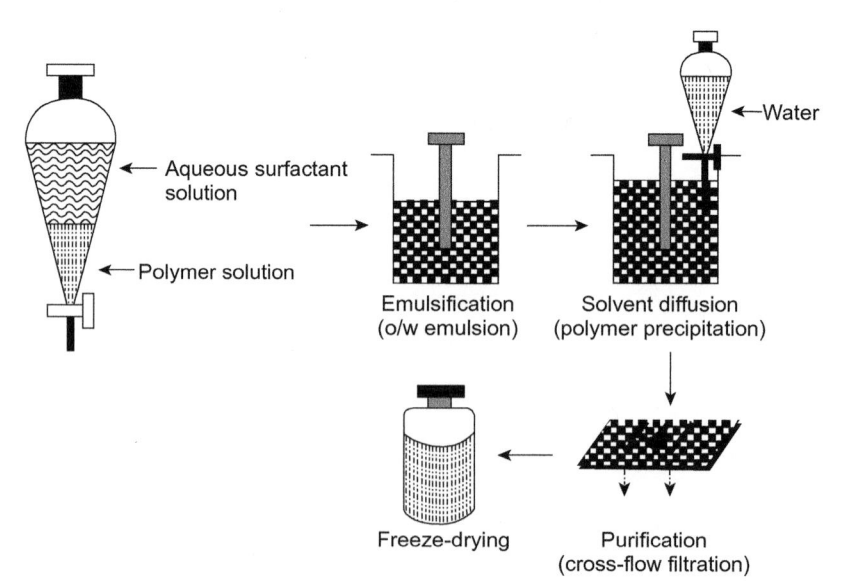

Figure 6.14 Nanoparticle preparation by salting out/emulsion diffusion method.

and stabilizing agent such as polysorbate 20. The drug can be added to the surfactant solution before or at the end of the polymerization process. The mechanism of polymerization has been explained schematically in Fig. 6.15.

Initially, the nonpolar tail ends of surfactant micelles dissolve monomers when they are added to the aqueous acidic medium in the presence of the surfactant and stabilizer solution. Anions such as OH-, CH$_3$O-, and CH$_3$COO- initiate the polymerization process. The monomer molecules enter the core of the surfactant micelles to continue the polymerization process. The polymerization process is favorable between pH 1.5–3. This ensures the stability of the nanoparticles as well. The process of nanoparticle

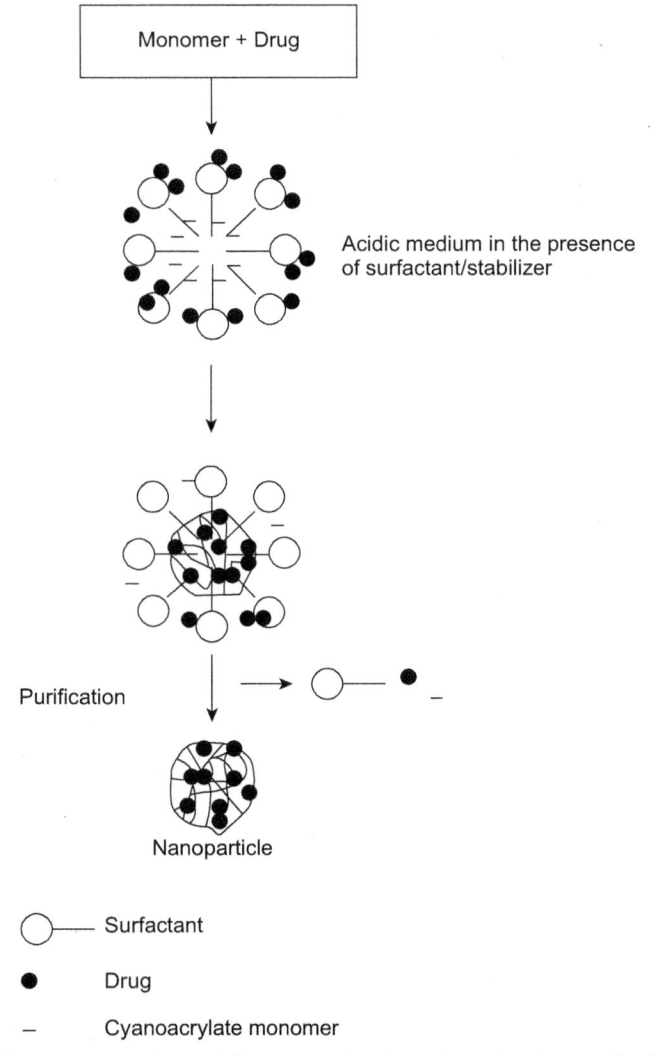

Figure 6.15 Nanoparticle preparation by polymerization method.

formation is facilitated by mechanical stirring. The resultant nanoparticles are collected by ultracentrifugation and finally dispersed in a surfactant-free medium.

3.2.1.3 Large-Scale Production of Nanoparticles

3.2.1.3.1 Supercritical Fluid Technology—Rapid Expansion of Supercritical Solution Unlike the methods discussed earlier in this chapter, supercritical fluid technology does not use organic solvents for the production of nanoparticles [96,97]. This technique is capable of producing nanoparticles of high purity with uniform drug distribution. In this method, the polymer and the drug are dissolved in a supercritical fluid and the solution is allowed to expand as it exits through a tiny nozzle. This results in the decrease in solvent power and the solute precipitates to form solvent-free nanoparticles. This method is suitable for low-molecular-weight polymers only. Most polymers are not soluble in supercritical fluids, which makes it difficult to apply the technique toward the production of a wide variety of nanoparticles.

3.2.1.3.2 Spray Drying Spray drying technology produces nanoparticles of relatively low and uniform size, and it is easy to scale up [90,98]. In this method, the polymer and drugs are dissolved in an organic solvent and sprayed through a nozzle, whereby the droplets are dried simultaneously to obtain the nanoparticles. The size of the nanoparticles can be controlled by modifying the process variables such as spray flow and inlet and outlet temperatures. Spray drying technology can also be combined with freeze-drying (Fig. 6.16). In this modified method, the drug and polymer solution is sprayed through a nozzle into a chamber containing liquid nitrogen and ethanol. The droplets from the nozzle precipitate and collect in the ethanol. The liquid nitrogen evaporates and the organic solvent is extracted by the ethanol, which hardens the nanoparticles. Finally, the nanoparticles are filtered and dried under vacuum.

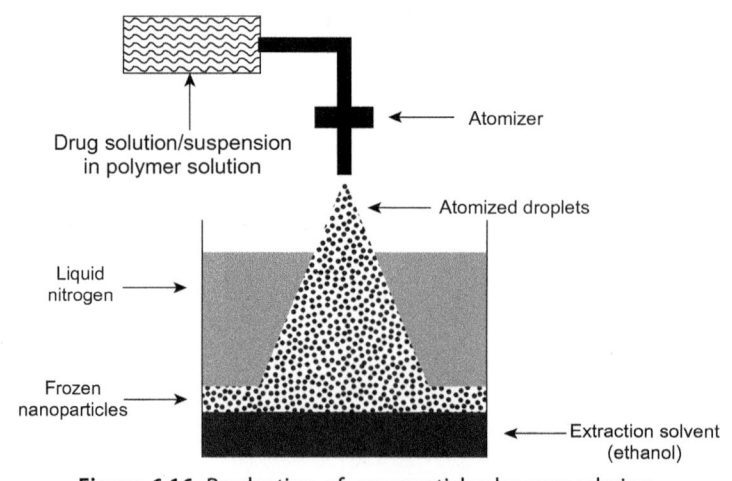

Figure 6.16 Production of nanoparticles by spray drying.

3.2.1.4 In Vitro and In Vivo Studies Involving Nanoparticles

Polymeric nanoparticles have been used for the effective delivery of various anticancer agents and RNA interference—inducing agents such as siRNAs. Dalhman et al. [99] have successfully delivered siRNA to endothelial cells and Susana et al. [100] have used polymeric nanoparticles to deliver GSE24.2 peptide to treat telomerase disorders. Win et al. [101] successfully demonstrated the ability of polymeric nanoparticles to be internalized by Caco-2 cells.

According to Win et al. (Fig. 6.17), nanoparticle uptake by the Caco-2 cells was consistently higher compared with the control (coumarin-6). Fig. 6.18 demonstrates

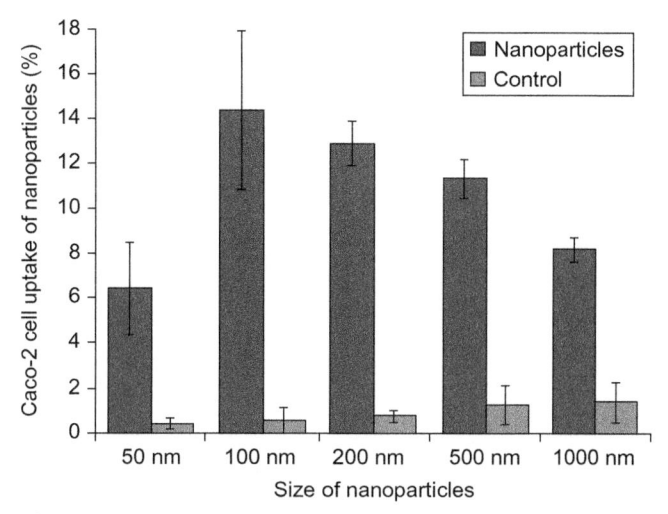

Figure 6.17 Effect of particle size on cellular uptake by Caco-2 cells of polystyrene nanoparticles [101]. *(Reprinted with permission.)*

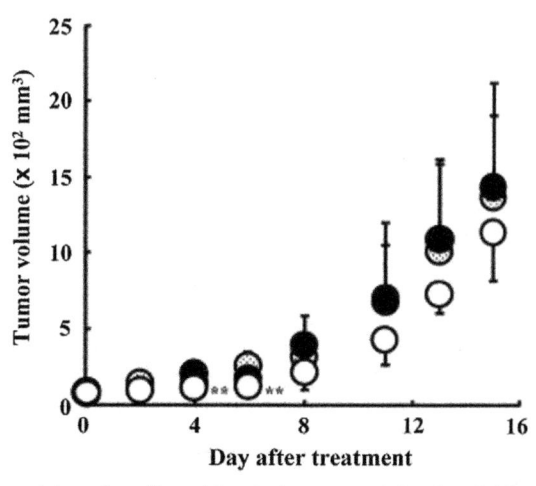

Figure 6.18 In vivo cytotoxicity of paclitaxel-loaded nanoparticles [102]. (*Open circle*, paclitaxel nanoparticles; *closed circle*, saline; *gray circle*, paclitaxel solution.) *(Reprinted with permission.)*

the cytotoxic effect of paclitaxel nanoparticles in C26 tumor-bearing mice studied by the Araki et al. [102].

3.2.1.5 Challenges Associated With Polymeric Nanoparticles

Despite being hailed as the most promising potential carriers for macromolecules such as siRNA and small molecules needing specialized delivery, polymeric nanoparticles face challenges such as nonspecific drug delivery, nonpredictable endosomal release behavior for siRNAs, protein binding, opsonization by macrophages in circulation with subsequent elimination, and undesirable accumulation in liver, spleen, etc.

3.2.2 Carbon Nanotubes and Nanohorns

Carbon nanotubes have gained interest in drug delivery as they have been found capable of delivering vaccines, proteins, peptides, nucleic acids, and other therapeutic agents [103—105]. Carbon nanotubes are formed by the natural folding behavior of graphene sheets. They are commercially available in varying degrees of purity and consist of different structures. Generally, there are two categories of carbon nanotubes depending on the number of graphene sheet layers involved; the first type is the single-walled nanotube (SWNT; diameter 1—2 nm and length 50 nm—1 cm) and the second type is the multiwalled nanotube (length 10—100 nm) [105—109]. The commercially available nanotubes possess a positive charge and hydrophobic nature that make them unsuitable for most drug delivery applications. However, functionalization or modification of these nanotubes makes them dispersible in water and they can serve as potential carriers for a wide variety of compounds. The nanotubes can be modified by various methods [104,105]. Nanotube modification by oxidation involves treatment with strong acids, which results in carboxylic group functionalized nanotubes that are shorter in length. The other commonly used method involves the chemical addition of functional groups to the external walls of the nanotubes (Fig. 6.19).

The modified/functionalized carbon nanotubes are highly soluble in water and can be used as carriers for small and large molecules [110]. The functional groups on modified carbon nanotubes are capable of forming conjugates with drug moieties that would produce a pharmacological effect in the body. The SWNTs have considerably high theoretical surface area (1300 m^2/g), which imparts them with the capability of carrying more than one active moiety, some of which may possess targeting abilities so that the nanotube complex can be useful to deliver drug molecules to the targeted site of action [108]. On the other hand, the multiwalled nanotubes are larger in size so they are capable of delivering large molecules such as DNA and plasmids to the cells [108]. Carbon nanotubes have been used in the development of novel sensors for detecting biological molecules such as proteins and DNA, and in contrasting agents for biological imaging [111—115]. Carbon nanotubes have also been researched for their ability to deliver

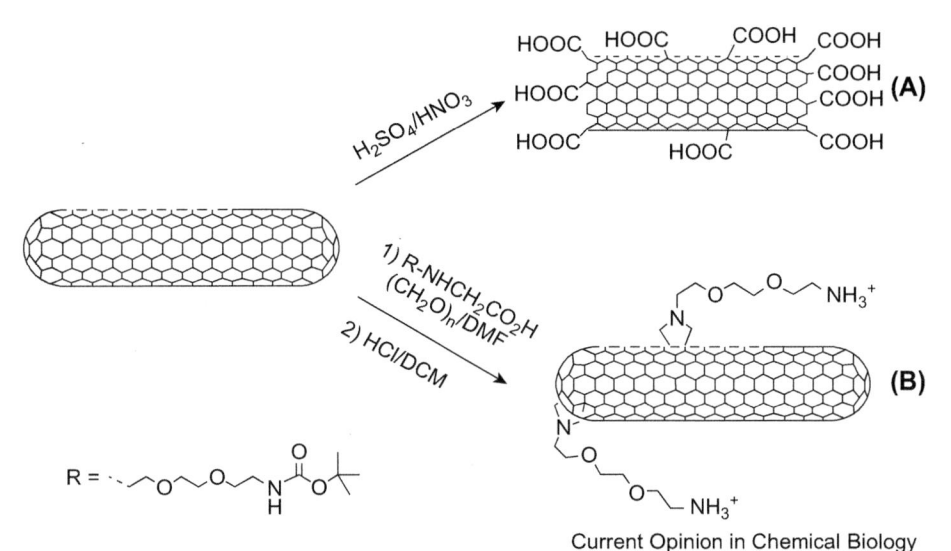

Figure 6.19 Organic functionalization of carbon nanotubes. (A) Treatment with acid to produce carboxylic acid groups, and (B) treatment with amino acids and aldehydes to add desired functional groups on the surface of the nanotube [105]. *(Reprinted with permission.)*

anticancer drugs in in vivo mouse models [116]. Table 6.4 summarizes some molecules conjugated with carbon nanotubes that have been researched for various applications [117].

SWNTs have been studied for the delivery of siRNA. Zhuang et al. conjugated the CXCR4 cell-surface receptor siRNA to SWNTs using a cleavable disulfide bond and determined the in vitro gene knockdown efficiency by fluorescence-activated cell sorting [128]. They also compared the efficacy of the SWNT-associated siRNA with liposomal siRNA (Fig. 6.20) and found higher gene knockdown efficiency with the former.

In another study, Rusling et. al. [116] studied the in vivo efficacy of SWNT-cisplatin-epidermal growth factor (EGF) bioconjugates. The two formulations (control and positive) were injected intravenously and the tumor progression over a period of 10 days was observed. As shown in Fig. 6.21, the positive (the targeted nanotube bioconjugate) has shown significant level of tumor inhibition over a period of 10 days compared to the control (unguided nanotube bioconjugate).

In other studies, carbon nanotubes have been used to successfully deliver various molecules such as vaccines, genes, and drugs for a broad range of diseases including infectious diseases and cancer [117]. However, there continue to be challenges associated with the development of carbon nanotubes for therapeutic purposes such as the toxicity of nonfunctionalized carbon nanotubes, suboptimal stability in physiological conditions, aggregation in vivo, and difficulties in achieving precise drug delivery. Nonfunctionalized multiwalled nanotubes have also been found to be carcinogenic in mouse models [129].

3.2.3 Iron Nanoparticles
Iron oxide nanoparticles/magnetic nanoparticles have the potential to revolutionize current imaging, diagnostic, and therapeutic applications. Magnetic nanoparticles are

Table 6.4 Molecular structures of the carbon nanotube conjugated with different therapeutic agents [117]

Compounds	Application
1	Cell internalization [118–120] Intracellular trafficking [118,119] Cell viability [120] Plasmid DNA delivery [120,121]
3	Cell internalization [118,122,123] Intracellular trafficking [118,122,123] Cell viability [118,122,123]

Cell internalization [118]

Cell internalization [118,124]
Cell viability [124]

Continued

Table 6.4 Molecular structures of the carbon nanotube conjugated with different therapeutic agents [117]—cont'd

Compounds	Application
	Antibiotic delivery [124]
	Cell internalization [125] Cell viability [125] Anticancer delivery [125]

Immunogenic activity [126,127]

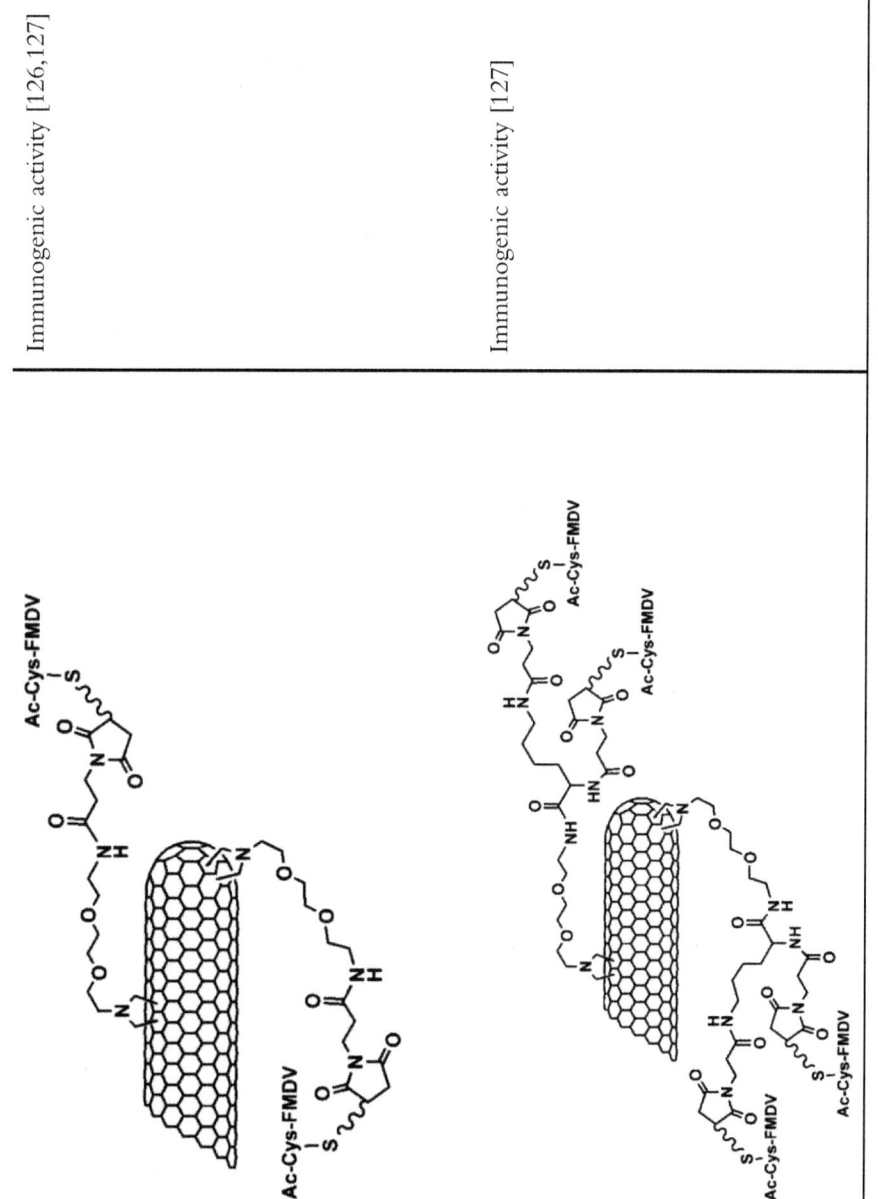

Immunogenic activity [127]

Reprinted with permission.

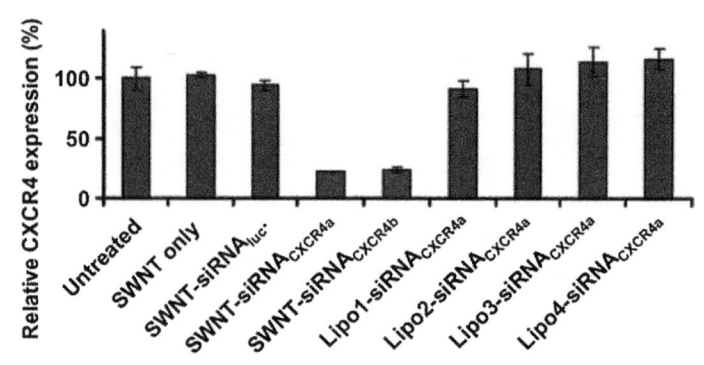

Figure 6.20 CXR4 expression levels after treating with single-walled carbon nanotube (SWNT)—small interference RNA (siRNA) and liposomal siRNA with appropriate controls [128]. *(Reprinted with permission.)*

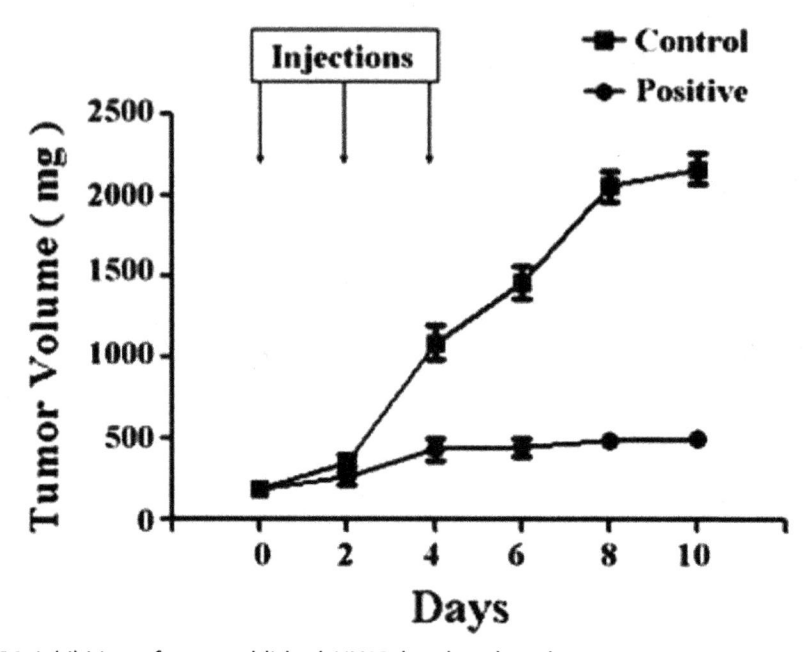

Figure 6.21 Inhibition of pre-established HN12 head and neck squamous carcinoma cells tumor growth by single walled nanotube-cisplatin-epidermal growth factor bioconjugates. The unguided nanotube bioconjugate was labelled as "control" and the targeted nanotube bioconjugate was labelled as "positive" [116]. *(Reprinted with permission.)*

composed of a magnetic core (iron oxide or magnetite) and a biocompatible polymeric shell (dextran or starch) (Fig. 6.22). These nanoparticles have superior targeting abilities compared with other nanoparticle systems due to their responsive properties to magnetic waves. Magnetic nanoparticles are assumed to possess benefits beyond the enhanced permeability and retention effect, which is a common passive targeting technique in case of tumor-targeted nanoparticles. Magnetic nanoparticles have applications in

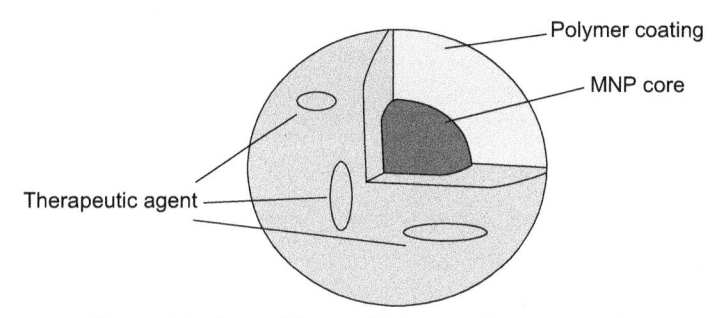

Figure 6.22 Typical iron oxide/magnetic nanoparticle.

immune assays, cancer, cardiovascular diseases, neurological disorders, and as MRI contrasting agents.

The iron oxide core in the magnetic nanoparticle contains magnetite (Fe_3O_4) or maghemite (γFe_2O_3) or a nonstoichiometric composition of both. Magnetic nanoparticles are synthesized by different methods including traditional solution-based wet chemistry, laser pyrolysis, aqueous coprecipitation, and high-temperature decomposition of organometallic precursors.

3.2.3.1 Methods of Preparation
1. Coprecipitation
2. Thermal decomposition
3. Microemulsion
4. Hydrothermal synthesis
5. Sonochemical synthesis

3.2.3.1.1 Coprecipitation In this method, Fe_3O_4 or γFe_2O_3 is synthesized by mixing ferrous ions and ferric ions (usually in a 2:1 molar ratio) in basic solutions either at room temperature or at elevated temperatures. The size and shape of the nanoparticles produced by this method depend on the type of ferrous or ferric salt that has been used, the ratio of ferrous/ferric ions, temperature, etc. This method produces nanoparticles with a wide size distribution. As the process requires high-pH solutions, the by-products of this process require further purification [130].

3.2.3.1.2 Thermal Decomposition This process involves the thermal decomposition of organic compounds such as $Fe(CO)_5$, $Fe(N\text{-nitrosophenylhydroxylamine})_3$, or $Fe(acetylacetonate)_3$. The decomposition is followed by oxidation, which produces high-quality monodispersed iron oxide nanoparticles. The disadvantages of this method include high-temperature requirements and the production of nanoparticles that disperse and dissolve only in nonpolar solvents [130].

3.2.3.1.3 Microemulsion
In this method, first the microemulsion in aqueous phase is prepared with ferric and/or ferrous ions in the presence of 0.1 M HCl to avoid oxidation of the ions. The microemulsion is then precipitated by injecting organic precipitating agents such as cyclohexylamine or oleylamine. The disadvantages of this method include aggregation and stability issues with the nanoparticles [130,131].

3.2.3.1.4 Hydrothermal Synthesis
This method involves the production of nanoparticles by crystallization from an aqueous solution of ions at a high temperature under high vapor pressure. The crystallization can be facilitated by using various wet chemical technologies and this method produces nanoparticles with good monodispersity [130].

3.2.3.1.5 Sonochemical Synthesis
This method involves the usage of sonochemical techniques such as sonication of an aqueous solution of ions to produce nanoparticles. For example, magnetite nanoparticles can be obtained by sonicating an iron (II) acetate aqueous solution [130].

Other methods of iron oxide nanoparticle preparation include electrochemical synthesis, laser pyrolysis technique, and microorganism or bacterial synthesis. Magnetic responsive properties vary based on the method of preparation and surface properties. Table 6.5 summarizes the characteristics of iron oxide nanoparticles prepared by the various methods described.

Iron oxide or magnetic nanoparticles have the tendency to aggregate without surface treatment; therefore the polymer coating over the magnetic core is an integral part of the development of magnetic nanoparticles for biomedical applications. The polymeric coating may also help to escape the MPS and achieve long circulation time. Depending on the type and nature of the polymer coating, magnetic nanoparticles can be categorized into several types. Fig. 6.23 shows three different structures that are possible based on the polymer coating. Table 6.6 presents a literature summary of some polymers that have been used to coat magnetic nanoparticles.

3.2.3.2 Applications of Magnetic Nanoparticles in Drug Delivery
Table 6.7 summarizes some of the therapeutic molecules that have been studied in magnetic nanoparticle formulations. Fig. 6.24 presents the results obtained by Kohler et al., where iron oxide nanoparticles were surface modified with (3-aminopropyl) trimethoxysilane followed by conjugation with an anticancer drug, methotrexate, by the formation of an amide bond between the carboxylic acid of methotrexate and the amine groups on the nanoparticle surface. In vitro cell survival studies with the modified nanoparticles have shown consistent decrease in cell viability compared with free methotrexate in both HeLa and MCF-7 cells [135].

In a similar study, Jain et al. have successfully demonstrated the superior cytotoxic effect of doxorubicin—iron oxide nanoparticles compared with free doxorubicin in MCF7 and PC3 cell lines (Fig. 6.25).

Table 6.5 Comparison of different iron oxide nanoparticles prepared by using different methods [132]

Characteristics of iron oxide nanoparticles	Aerosol/vapor (pyrolysis) method	Gas deposition method	Bulk solution method	Sol–gel method	Microemulsion method
Size and size distribution	About 5–60 nm with broad size distribution	About 5–50 nm with narrow size distribution	About 10–50 nm with broad size distribution	About 20–200 nm with broad size distribution	About 4–15 nm with very narrow size distribution
Morphology	Spherical	Spherical	Spherical (large aggregates)	Spherical with high porosity	Cubic or spherical (no aggregation)
Magnetization values	10–50 emu/g with desired magnetic property	>20 emu/g	20–50 emu/g with superparamagnetic behavior	10–40 emu/g with paramagnetic behavior	430 emu/g with superparamagnetic behavior
Advantages	Fast production rate	Useful for protective coatings and thin film deposition	Large quantities can be synthesized	Particles of desired shape and length can be synthesized, useful for making hybrid nanoparticles	Uniform properties, size of the nanoparticles can be modulated
Disadvantages	Large aggregates are formed	Require very high temperature	Uncontrolled oxidation of magnetite to maghemite, diamagnetic contribution	Products usually contain sol–gel matrix components at their surfaces	Surfactants are difficult to remove; only small quantities of iron oxide can be synthesized

Reprinted with permission.

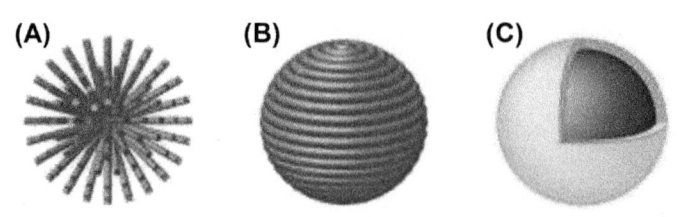

Figure 6.23 Magnetic nanoparticle (MNP) structures and coating schemes. (A) End-grafted polymeric coated MNP; (B) MNP fully encapsulated in polymer coating; (C) Core shell MNP [133]. *(Reprinted with permission.)*

Table 6.6 Synthetic and natural polymers and other materials used to coat magnetic nanoparticles [132,134]

Coating material	Advantages
Polyethylene glycol	Improves blood circulation time, decreases elimination by mononuclear phagocyte system, increases internalization efficiency
Poly(D,L-lactic acid)	Biodegradable, biocompatible
Dextran	Stabilizes colloidal solution. Enhances blood circulation time
Polyvinylpyrrolidone	Stabilizes colloidal solution. Enhances blood circulation time
Polyvinyl alcohol	Prevents coagulation
Polyacrylic acid	Helps in bioadhesion. Improves colloidal stability
Polypeptides	Imparts targeting abilities
Phosphorylcholine	Stabilizes colloidal solution
Polyethyleneimine	Efficient and fast delivery of genetic material, exhibits proton sponge effect
Chitosan	Natural and biocompatible
Gelatin	Natural and biocompatible
Silica	Large surface area, does not require utilization of organic solvent
Silane	Enhances dispersion in biological matrix, significantly improves protein immobilization
Glycerol Monooleate	Does not affect magnetic properties of Fe_2O_3, high entrapment efficiency, can reduce burst release of drugs
Albumin	Does not affect cell proliferation
Gold	Particles exhibit strong magnetic response, uniform coating, protects iron oxide core from oxidation, superior optical properties
Erythrocytes	Easily available, biocompatible, does not exert immunogenic side effects because of autologous nature
Polymethyl methacrylate	Simple, easy to carry out, process can easily be automated
Ethylcellulose	Maintenance of drug concentration at desired site for prolonged period, retains sufficient magnetic responsiveness
Pullulan	Easily prepared, high uptake efficiency
Starch	Natural polymer, can be modified with other polymers such as polyethylene glycol

Table 6.7 Various therapeutic agents used in magnetic nanoparticle systems

Therapeutic molecule	Reference
Chemotherapeutic agents	
Methotrexate	[135,136]
Doxorubicin	[137]
Cisplatin	[138]
Gemcitabine	[138]
Proteins and peptides	
Herceptin (trastuzumab)	[139,140]
Chlorotoxin	[141,142]
DNA and siRNA	
Oligodesoxynucleotides (ODN)	[143]
Antisense survivin ODN	[144]
DNA, siRNA	[145–147]

siRNA, small interfering RNA.

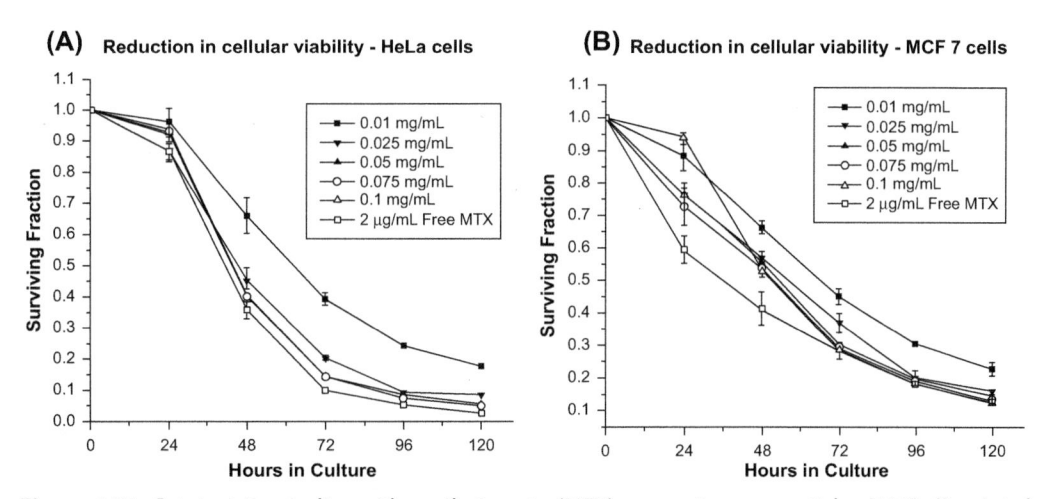

Figure 6.24 Cytotoxicity studies with methotrexate (MTX)-magnetic nanoparticles [135]. *(Reprinted with permission.)*

The challenges associated with iron/magnetic nanoparticles include their inability to cross the blood–brain barrier and the vascular endothelium, tendency to aggregate, unpredictable in vivo behavior, and rapid clearance by the MPS depending on the surface properties, size, and morphology of nanoparticles.

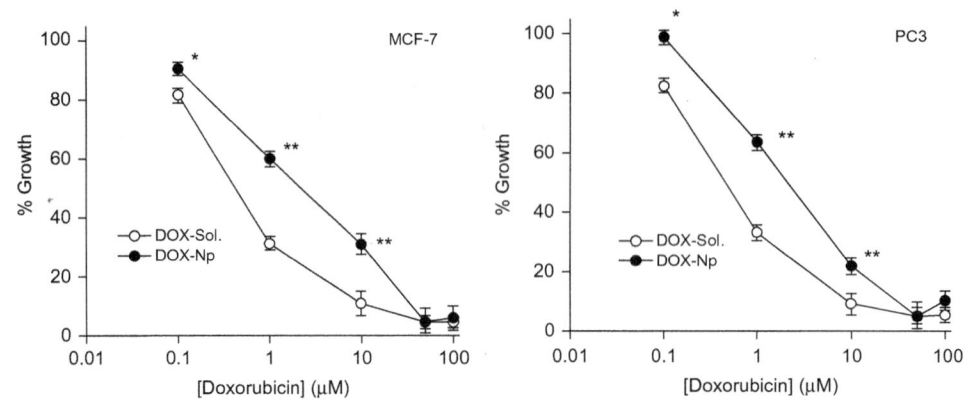

Figure 6.25 Antiproliferative activity of free doxorubicin solution and doxorubicin nanoparticles [137]. *(Reprinted with permission.)*

4. CONCLUSION

Drug delivery using nanoparticulate systems has been steadily gaining intense research attention over the past three decades. Although many small and large molecular drugs have been encapsulated in nanoparticles and successfully tested and found effective in in vitro and in vivo studies, not many drugs are currently approved and available in the market in nanoparticle formulations. The reasons for this include failure to translate the in vivo results into the human clinical trials, premature drug release, rapid elimination by the MPS system, and immunogenic responses. However, multiple studies are underway to understand these challenges and various potential solutions are under serious consideration to remedy the problems to further the efforts being made to achieve ideal nanoparticulate systems for drug delivery. With the rate and extent of research in progress, there is reason to be optimistic that nanoparticulate systems have the potential to revolutionize current treatment strategies in the near future despite all of their present challenges.

REFERENCES

[1] Miyazaki K, Islam N. Nanotechnology systems of innovation—an analysis of industry and academia research activities. Technovation 2007;27(11):661—75.
[2] Sandhiya S, Dkhar SA, Surendiran A. Emerging trends of nanomedicine—an overview. Fundam Clin Pharmacol 2009;23(3):263—9.
[3] Pillai G. Nanomedicines for cancer therapy: an update of FDA approved and those under various stages of development. SOJ Pharm Pharm Sci 2014;1(2):13.
[4] Wang R, Billone PS, Mullett WM. Nanomedicine in action: an overview of cancer nanomedicine on the market and in clinical trials. J Nanomater 2013;2013:12.
[5] Wang M, Thanou M. Targeting nanoparticles to cancer. Pharmacol Res 2010;62(2):90—9.
[6] Torchilin VP. Recent advances with liposomes as pharmaceutical carriers. Nat Rev Drug Discov 2005;4(2):145—60.

[7] Gendelman HE, et al. Nanoneuromedicines for degenerative, inflammatory, and infectious nervous system diseases. Nanomed: Nanotechnol Biol Med 2015;11(3):751−67.
[8] Liu S, Guo Y, Huang R, Li J, Huang S, Kuang Y, Han L, Jiang C. Gene and doxorubicin co-delivery system for targeting therapy of glioma. Biomaterials 2012;33(19):4907−16.
[9] Torchilin V. Tumor delivery of macromolecular drugs based on the EPR effect. Adv Drug Deliv Rev 2011;63(3):131−5.
[10] Huang S, Li J, Han L, Liu S, Ma H, Huang R, Jiang C. Dual targeting effect of Angiopep-2-modified, DNA-loaded nanoparticles for glioma. Biomaterials 2011;32(28):6832−8.
[11] Huang R, Ke W, Han L, Li J, Liu S, Jiang C. Targeted delivery of chlorotoxin-modified DNA-loaded nanoparticles to glioma via intravenous administration. Biomaterials 2011;32(9):2399−406.
[12] Vander Heiden MG. Targeting cancer metabolism: a therapeutic window opens. Nat Rev Drug Discov 2011;10(9):671−84.
[13] Moghimi SM, Hunter AC, Murray JC. Nanomedicine: current status and future prospects. FASEB J 2005;19(3):311−30.
[14] Yokoyama M. Drug targeting with nano-sized carrier systems. J Artif Organs 2005;8:77−84.
[15] Bae YH, Park K. Targeted drug delivery to tumors: myths, reality and possibility. J Control Release 2011;153(3):198−205.
[16] Gamucci O, et al. Biomedical nanoparticles: overview of their surface immune-compatibility. Coatings 2014;4(1):139.
[17] Salata O. Applications of nanoparticles in biology and medicine. J Nanobiotechnol 2004;2(3).
[18] Kumar Khanna V. Targeted delivery of nanomedicines. ISRN Pharmacol 2012;2012:9.
[19] De Jong WH, Borm PJA. Drug delivery and nanoparticles: applications and hazards. Int J Nanomed 2008;3(2):133−49.
[20] Desai N. Challenges in development of nanoparticle-based therapeutics. AAPS J 2012;14(2):282−95.
[21] Luo Y-H, Chang LW, Lin P. Metal-based nanoparticles and the immune system: activation, inflammation, and potential applications. BioMed Res Int 2015;2015:143720.
[22] Zolnik BS, et al. Nanoparticles and the immune system. Endocrinology 2010;151(2):458−65.
[23] Torchilin VP. Targeted pharmaceutical nanocarriers for cancer therapy and imaging. AAPS J 2007;9(2):E128−47.
[24] Malam Y, Loizidou M, Seifalian AM. Liposomes and nanoparticles: nanosized vehicles for drug delivery in cancer. Trends Pharmacol Sci 2009;30(11):592−9.
[25] Sharma A, Sharma US. Liposomes in drug delivery: progress and limitations. Int J Pharm 1997;154(2):123−40.
[26] Greish K, et al. SMA−doxorubicin, a new polymeric micellar drug for effective targeting to solid tumours. J Control Release 2004;97(2):219−30.
[27] Maeda H. The enhanced permeability and retention (EPR) effect in tumor vasculature: the key role of tumor-selective macromolecular drug targeting. Adv Enzyme Regul 2001;41(1):189−207.
[28] Fanciullino R, et al. Development of stealth liposome formulation of 2′-deoxyinosine as 5-fluorouracil modulator: in vitro and in vivo study. Pharm Res 2005;22(12):2051−7.
[29] Wagner A, Vorauer-Uhl K. Liposome technology for industrial purposes. J Drug Deliv 2011:2011.
[30] Akbarzadeh A, et al. Liposome: classification, preparation, and applications. Nanoscale Res Lett 2013;8(1):102.
[31] Alves NJ, et al. Functionalized liposome purification via liposome extruder purification (LEP). Analyst 2013;138(17):4746−51.
[32] Güven A, et al. Rapid and efficient method for the size separation of homogeneous fluorescein-encapsulating liposomes. J Liposome Res 2009;19(2):148−54.
[33] Hwang KJ, Chang YC. The use of cross-flow microfiltration in purification of liposomes. Sep Sci Technol 2004;39(11):2557−76.
[34] Wagner A, et al. GMP production of liposomes—a new industrial approach. J Liposome Res 2006;16(3):311−9.
[35] Patil YP, Jadhav S. Novel methods for liposome preparation. Chem Phys Lipids 2014;177:8−18.
[36] Chonn A, Cullis PR. Recent advances in liposomal drug-delivery systems. Curr Opin Biotechnol 1995;6(6):698−708.

[37] Riaz M. Liposomes preparation methods. Pak J Pharm Sci 1996;9(1):65—77.
[38] Song H, et al. Development of Polysorbate 80/Phospholipid mixed micellar formation for docetaxel and assessment of its in vivo distribution in animal models. Nanoscale Res Lett 2011;6(1):354.
[39] Mozafari MR. Liposomes: an overview of manufacturing techniques. Cell Mol Biol Lett 2005;10(4): 711—9.
[40] Ohsawa T, Miura H, Harada K. Improvement of encapsulation efficiency of water-soluble drugs in liposomes formed by the freeze-thawing method. Chem Pharm Bull 1985;33(9):3945—52.
[41] Llu L, Yonetani T. Preparation and characterization of liposome-encapsulated haemoglobin by a freeze-thaw method. J Microencapsul 1994;11(4):409—21.
[42] Pick U. Liposomes with a large trapping capacity prepared by freezing and thawing of sonicated phospholipid mixtures. Arch Biochem Biophys 1981;212(1):186—94.
[43] Deamer D, Bangham AD. Large volume liposomes by an ether vaporization method. Biochim Biophys Acta (BBA) - Biomembr 1976;443(3):629—34.
[44] Schieren H, et al. Comparison of large unilamellar vesicles prepared by a petroleum ether vaporization method with multilamellar vesicles: ESR, diffusion and entrapment analyses. Biochim Biophys Acta (BBA) - Gen Subj 1978;542(1):137—53.
[45] Batzri S, Korn ED. Single bilayer liposomes prepared without sonication. Biochim Biophys Acta (BBA) - Biomembr 1973;298(4):1015—9.
[46] Alpes H, et al. Formation of large unilamellar vesicles using alkyl maltoside detergents. Biochim Biophys Acta (BBA) - Biomembr 1986;862(2):294—302.
[47] Møller H, Jørgensen N, Forman D. Trends in incidence of testicular cancer in boys and adolescent men. Int J Cancer 1995;61(6):761—4.
[48] Hao YL, et al. In vitro and in vivo studies of different liposomes containing topotecan. Arch Pharm Res 2005;28(5):626—35.
[49] Li W, et al. RGD-targeted paramagnetic liposomes for early detection of tumor: in vitro and in vivo studies. Eur J Radiol 2011;80(2):598—606.
[50] Romberg B, Hennink W, Storm G. Sheddable coatings for long-circulating nanoparticles. Pharm Res 2008;25(1):55—71.
[51] Gabizon AA. Stealth liposomes and tumor targeting: one step further in the quest for the magic bullet. Clin Cancer Res 2001;7(2):223—5.
[52] Wissing SA, Kayser O, Müller RH. Solid lipid nanoparticles for parenteral drug delivery. Adv Drug Deliv Rev 2004;56(9):1257—72.
[53] Mehnert W, Mäder K. Solid lipid nanoparticles: production, characterization and applications. Adv Drug Deliv Rev 2001;47(2—3):165—96.
[54] Müller RH, Mäder K, Gohla S. Solid lipid nanoparticles (SLN) for controlled drug delivery — a review of the state of the art. Eur J Pharm Biopharm 2000;50(1):161—77.
[55] Muller RH, et al. Solid lipid nanoparticles (SLN) - an alternative colloidal carrier system for controlled drug delivery. Eur J Pharm Biopharm 1995;41(1):62—9.
[56] Zur Mühlen A, Mehnert W. Drug release and release mechanism of prednisolone loaded solid lipid nanoparticles. Pharmazie 1998;53(8):552—5.
[57] Zur Mühlen A, Schwarz C, Mehnert W. Solid lipid nanoparticles (SLN) for controlled drug delivery - drug release and release mechanism. Eur J Pharm Biopharm 1998;45(2):149—55.
[58] Müller RH, Radtke M, Wissing SA. Solid lipid nanoparticles (SLN) and nanostructured lipid carriers (NLC) in cosmetic and dermatological preparations. Adv Drug Deliv Rev 2002; 54(Suppl.):S131—55.
[59] Hildebrand GE, et al. Medium scale production of solid lipid nanoparticles (SLN). Proc Control Release Soc 1998;(25):968—9.
[60] Moulik SP, Paul BK. Structure, dynamics and transport properties of micro emulsions. Adv Colloid Interface Sci 1998;78(2):99—195.
[61] Boltri L, et al. Lipid nanoparticles: evaluation of some critical formulation parameters. 1 Proc Control Release Soc 1993;(20):346—7.
[62] Sjostrom B, et al. Structures of nanoparticles prepared from oil-in-water emulsions. Pharm Res 1995; 12(1):39—48.

[63] Trotta M, Debernardi F, Caputo O. Preparation of solid lipid nanoparticles by a solvent emulsification-diffusion technique. Int J Pharm 2003;257(1−2):153−60.
[64] Hu FQ, et al. Preparation of solid lipid nanoparticles with clobetasol propionate by a novel solvent diffusion method in aqueous system and physicochemical characterization. Int J Pharm 2002; 239(1−2):121−8.
[65] Cavalli R, Gasco MR, Morel S. Behaviour of timolol incorporated in liposheres in the presence of a series of phosphate esters. STP Pharma Sci 1992;2(6):514−8.
[66] Gasco MR, Morel S, Carpignano R. Optimization of the incorporation of deoxycorticosterone acetate in liposheres. Eur J Pharm Biopharm 1992;38(1):7−10.
[67] Westesen K, Bunjes H, Koch MHJ. Physicochemical characterization of lipid nanoparticles and evaluation of their drug loading capacity and sustained release potential. J Control Release 1997;48(2−3): 223−36.
[68] Demirel M, et al. Formulation and in vitro-in vivo evaluation of piribedil solid lipid micro- and nanoparticles. J Microencapsul 2001;18(3):359−71.
[69] Cavalli R, et al. Solid lipid nanoparticles as carriers of hydrocortisone and progesterone complexes with β-cyclodextrins. Int J Pharm 1999;182(1):59−69.
[70] Cavalli R, Caputo O, Gasco MR. Preparation and characterization of solid lipid nanospheres containing paclitaxel. Eur J Pharm Sci 2000;10(4):305−9.
[71] Lukowski G, Werner U. Investigation of surface and drug release of solid lipid nanoparticles loaded with acyclovir. Proc Control Release Soc 1998;(25):425−6.
[72] Cavalli R, et al. Sterilization and freeze-drying of drug-free and drug-loaded solid lipid nanoparticles. Int J Pharm 1997;148(1):47−54.
[73] Yang SC, et al. Body distribution in mice of intravenously injected camptothecin solid lipid nanoparticles and targeting effect on brain. J Control Release 1999;59(3):299−307.
[74] Mosallaei N, et al. Docetaxel-loaded solid lipid nanoparticles: preparation, characterization, in vitro, and in vivo evaluations. J Pharm Sci 2013;102(6):1994−2004.
[75] Martins S, et al. Brain delivery of camptothecin by means of solid lipid nanoparticles: formulation design, in vitro and in vivo studies. Int J Pharm 2012;439(1−2):49−62.
[76] Xu Z, et al. The performance of docetaxel-loaded solid lipid nanoparticles targeted to hepatocellular carcinoma. Biomaterials 2009;30(2):226−32.
[77] Muller RH, et al. Solid lipid nanoparticles - a novel carrier system for cosmetics and pharmaceutics. 3rd communication: long-term stability, lyophilisation, spray drying, toxicity, use in cosmetics and pharmaceutics. Pharm Ind 1997;59(7):614−9.
[78] Zimmermann E, Müller RH, Mäder K. Influence of different parameters on reconstitution of lyophilized SLN. Int J Pharm 2000;196(2):211−3.
[79] Kumari A, Yadav SK, Yadav SC. Biodegradable polymeric nanoparticles based drug delivery systems. Colloids Surf B Biointerfaces 2010;75(1):1−18.
[80] Mu L, Feng SS. A novel controlled release formulation for the anticancer drug paclitaxel (Taxol®): PLGA nanoparticles containing vitamin E TPGS. J Control Release 2003;86(1):33−48.
[81] Damgé C, Maincent P, Ubrich N. Oral delivery of insulin associated to polymeric nanoparticles in diabetic rats. J Control Release 2007;117(2):163−70.
[82] Date AA, Joshi MD, Patravale VB. Parasitic diseases: liposomes and polymeric nanoparticles versus lipid nanoparticles. Adv Drug Deliv Rev 2007;59(6):505−21.
[83] Ahmad Z, et al. Alginate nanoparticles as antituberculosis drug carriers: formulation development, pharmacokinetics and therapeutic potential. Indian J Chest Dis Allied Sci 2006;48(3):171.
[84] Soppimath KS, et al. Biodegradable polymeric nanoparticles as drug delivery devices. J Control Release 2001;70(1−2):1−20.
[85] Shenoy DB, Amiji MM. Poly(ethylene oxide)-modified poly(ε-caprolactone) nanoparticles for targeted delivery of tamoxifen in breast cancer. Int J Pharm 2005;293(1−2):261−70.
[86] Schroeder U, et al. Nanoparticle technology for delivery of drugs across the blood−brain barrier. J Pharm Sci 1998;87(11):1305−7.
[87] Raghuvanshi RS, et al. Improved immune response from biodegradable polymer particles entrapping tetanus toxoid by use of different immunization protocol and adjuvants. Int J Pharm 2002;245(1−2): 109−21.

[88] Leroux J-C, et al. Biodegradable nanoparticles—from sustained release formulations to improved site specific drug delivery. J Control Release 1996;39(2—3):339—50.
[89] Alexis F, et al. Factors affecting the clearance and biodistribution of polymeric nanoparticles. Mol Pharm 2008;5(4):505—15.
[90] D'Mello SR, Das SK, Das NG. Polymeric nanoparticles for small-molecule drugs: biodegradation of polymers and fabrication of nanoparticles. Drug Deliv Nanopart Formul Charact 2009:16.
[91] Zambaux MF, et al. Influence of experimental parameters on the characteristics of poly(lactic acid) nanoparticles prepared by a double emulsion method. J Control Release 1998;50(1—3):31—40.
[92] Niwa T, et al. Preparations of biodegradable nanospheres of water-soluble and insoluble drugs with D,L-lactide/glycolide copolymer by a novel spontaneous emulsification solvent diffusion method, and the drug release behavior. J Control Release 1993;25(1—2):89—98.
[93] Murakami H, et al. Preparation of poly (DL-lactide-co-glycolide) nanoparticles by modified spontaneous emulsification solvent diffusion method. Int J Pharm 1999;187(2):143—52.
[94] Allémann E, Gurny R, Doelker E. Preparation of aqueous polymeric nanodispersions by a reversible salting-out process: influence of process parameters on particle size. Int J Pharm 1992;87(1—3): 247—53.
[95] Allémann E, et al. In vitro extended-release properties of drug-loaded poly(DL-lactic acid) nanoparticles produced by a salting-out procedure. Pharm Res 1993;10(12):1732—7.
[96] Tom JW, Debenedetti PG, Jerome R. Precipitation of poly(l-lactic acid) and composite poly(l-lactic acid)-pyrene particles by rapid expansion of supercritical solutions. J Supercrit Fluids 1994;7(1):9—29.
[97] Mishima K, et al. Microencapsulation of proteins by rapid expansion of supercritical solution with a nonsolvent. AIChE J 2000;46(4):857—65.
[98] Johnson O, et al. The stabilization and encapsulation of human growth hormone into biodegradable microspheres. Pharm Res 1997;14(6):730—5.
[99] Dahlman JE, et al. In vivo endothelial siRNA delivery using polymeric nanoparticles with low molecular weight. Nat Nanotechnol 2014;9(8):648—55.
[100] Egusquiaguirre SP, et al. Development of surface modified biodegradable polymeric nanoparticles to deliver GSE24.2 peptide to cells: a promising approach for the treatment of defective telomerase disorders. Eur J Pharm Biopharm 2015;91:91—102.
[101] Yin Win K, Feng S-S. Effects of particle size and surface coating on cellular uptake of polymeric nanoparticles for oral delivery of anticancer drugs. Biomaterials 2005;26(15):2713—22.
[102] Araki T, et al. Formulation and evaluation of paclitaxel-loaded polymeric nanoparticles composed of polyethylene glycol and polylactic acid block copolymer. Biol Pharm Bull 2012;35(8):1306—13.
[103] Martin CR, Kohli P. The emerging field of nanotube biotechnology. Nat Rev Drug Discov 2003; 2(1):29—37.
[104] Bianco A, Prato M. Can carbon nanotubes be considered useful tools for biological applications? Adv Mater 2003;15(20):1765—8.
[105] Bianco A, Kostarelos K, Prato M. Applications of carbon nanotubes in drug delivery. Curr Opin Chem Biol 2005;9(6):674—9.
[106] Bethune DS, et al. Cobalt-catalysed growth of carbon nanotubes with single-atomic-layer walls. Nature 1993;363(6430):605—7.
[107] Iijima S, Ichihashi T. Single-shell carbon nanotubes of 1-nm diameter. Nature 1993;363(6430): 603—5.
[108] Liu Z, et al. Carbon nanotubes in biology and medicine: in vitro and in vivo detection, imaging and drug delivery. Nano Res 2009;2(2):85—120.
[109] Iijima S. Helical microtubules of graphitic carbon. Nature 1991;354(6348):56—8.
[110] Koshino M, et al. Imaging of single organic molecules in motion. Science 2007;316(5826):853.
[111] Chen RJ, et al. Noncovalent functionalization of carbon nanotubes for highly specific electronic biosensors. Proc Natl Acad Sci 2003;100(9):4984—9.
[112] Chen Z, et al. Protein microarrays with carbon nanotubes as multicolor Raman labels. Nat Biotechnol 2008;26(11):1285—92.
[113] Cherukuri P, et al. Near-infrared fluorescence microscopy of single-walled carbon nanotubes in phagocytic cells. J Am Chem Soc 2004;126(48):15638—9.

[114] Welsher K, et al. Selective probing and imaging of cells with single walled carbon nanotubes as near-infrared fluorescent molecules. Nano Lett 2008;8(2):586—90.
[115] Heller DA, et al. Single-walled carbon nanotube spectroscopy in live cells: towards long-term labels and optical sensors. Adv Mater 2005;17(23):2793—9.
[116] Bhirde AA, et al. Targeted killing of cancer cells in vivo and in vitro with EGF-directed carbon nanotube-based drug delivery. ACS Nano 2009;3(2):307—16.
[117] Prato M, Kostarelos K, Bianco A. Functionalized carbon nanotubes in drug design and discovery. Acc Chem Res 2008;41(1):60—8.
[118] Kostarelos K, et al. Cellular uptake of functionalized carbon nanotubes is independent of functional group and cell type. Nat Nanotechnol 2007;2(2):108—13.
[119] Lacerda L, et al. Intracellular trafficking of carbon nanotubes by confocal laser scanning microscopy. Adv Mater 2007;19(11):1480—4.
[120] Pantarotto D, et al. Functionalized carbon nanotubes for plasmid DNA gene delivery. Angew Chem Int Ed 2004;43(39):5242—6.
[121] Singh R, et al. Binding and condensation of plasmid DNA onto functionalized carbon nanotubes: toward the construction of nanotube-based gene delivery vectors. J Am Chem Soc 2005;127(12): 4388—96.
[122] Pantarotto D, et al. Translocation of bioactive peptides across cell membranes by carbon nanotubes. Chem Commun (Camb) 2004;(1):16—7.
[123] Dumortier H, et al. Functionalized carbon nanotubes are non-cytotoxic and preserve the functionality of primary immune cells. Nano Lett 2006;6(7):1522—8.
[124] Wu W, et al. Targeted delivery of amphotericin B to cells by using functionalized carbon nanotubes. Angew Chem Int Ed Engl 2005;44(39):6358—62.
[125] Pastorin G, et al. Double functionalisation of carbon nanotubes for multimodal drug delivery. Chem Commun 2006;(11):1182—4.
[126] Pantarotto D, et al. Synthesis, structural characterization, and immunological properties of carbon nanotubes functionalized with peptides. J Am Chem Soc 2003;125(20):6160—4.
[127] Pantarotto D, et al. Immunization with peptide-functionalized carbon nanotubes enhances virus-specific neutralizing antibody responses. Chem Biol 2003;10(10):961—6.
[128] Liu Z, et al. siRNA delivery into human T cells and primary cells with carbon-nanotube transporters. Angew Chem Int Ed 2007;46(12):2023—7.
[129] Poland CA, et al. Carbon nanotubes introduced into the abdominal cavity of mice show asbestos-like pathogenicity in a pilot study. Nat Nanotechnol 2008;3(7):423—8.
[130] Wu W, He Q, Jiang C. Magnetic iron oxide nanoparticles: synthesis and surface functionalization strategies. Nanoscale Res Lett 2008;3(11):397—415.
[131] Vidal-Vidal J, Rivas J, López-Quintela MA. Synthesis of monodisperse maghemite nanoparticles by the microemulsion method. Colloids Surf A Physicochem Eng Aspects 2006;288(1—3):44—51.
[132] Gupta AK, Gupta M. Synthesis and surface engineering of iron oxide nanoparticles for biomedical applications. Biomaterials 2005;26(18):3995—4021.
[133] Sun C, Lee JSH, Zhang M. Magnetic nanoparticles in MR imaging and drug delivery. Adv Drug Deliv Rev 2008;60(11):1252—65.
[134] Wahajuddin, Arora S. Superparamagnetic iron oxide nanoparticles: magnetic nanoplatforms as drug carriers. Int J Nanomed 2012;7:3445—71.
[135] Kohler N, et al. Methotrexate-modified superparamagnetic nanoparticles and their intracellular uptake into human cancer cells. Langmuir 2005;21(19):8858—64.
[136] Kohler N, et al. Methotrexate-immobilized poly(ethylene glycol) magnetic nanoparticles for MR imaging and drug delivery. Small 2006;2(6):785—92.
[137] Jain TK, et al. Iron oxide nanoparticles for sustained delivery of anticancer agents. Mol Pharm 2005;2(3):194—205.
[138] Yang J, et al. Magnetic PECA nanoparticles as drug carriers for targeted delivery: synthesis and release characteristics. J Microencapsul 2006;23(2):203—12.
[139] Huh Y-M, et al. In vivo magnetic resonance detection of cancer by using multifunctional magnetic nanocrystals. J Am Chem Soc 2005;127(35):12387—91.

[140] Ito A, et al. Magnetite nanoparticle-loaded anti-HER2 immunoliposomes for combination of antibody therapy with hyperthermia. Cancer Lett 2004;212(2):167–75.
[141] Deshane J, Garner CC, Sontheimer H. Chlorotoxin inhibits glioma cell invasion via matrix metalloproteinase-2. J Biol Chem 2003;278(6):4135–44.
[142] Veiseh O, et al. Optical and MRI multifunctional nanoprobe for targeting gliomas. Nano Lett 2005;5(6):1003–8.
[143] Krötz F, et al. Magnetofection—a highly efficient tool for antisense oligonucleotide delivery in vitro and in vivo. Mol Ther 2003;7(5 I):700–10.
[144] Pan B, et al. Dendrimer-modified magnetic nanoparticles enhance efficiency of gene delivery system. Cancer Res 2007;67(17):8156–63.
[145] Schillinger U, et al. Advances in magnetofection—magnetically guided nucleic acid delivery. J Magn Magn Mater 2005;293(1):501–8.
[146] Mykhaylyk O, et al. Magnetic nanoparticle formulations for DNA and siRNA delivery. J Magn Magn Mater 2007;311(1):275–81.
[147] Medarova Z, et al. In vivo imaging of siRNA delivery and silencing in tumors. Nat Med 2007;13(3):372–7.

CHAPTER 7

Peptide and Protein-Based Therapeutic Agents*

Mary Joseph, Hoang M. Trinh, Ashim K. Mitra
University of Missouri—Kansas City, Kansas City, MO, United States

Contents

1. Introduction	146
2. Challenges With Peptide and Protein Therapeutics	147
3. Chemical Modifications	147
3.1 PEGylation	147
3.2 Glycosylation	148
3.3 Mannosylation	149
4. Micro- and Nanotechnology for Biologics in Drug Delivery	150
4.1 Microparticles or Microspheres	150
4.2 Nanoparticles	151
4.3 Solid Lipid NP	152
4.4 Carbon Nanotube	152
4.5 Liposomes	153
4.6 Aquasomes	154
4.7 Micelles	154
5. Protein- and Peptide-Based Therapeutics	155
5.1 Therapeutic Applications	155
5.1.1 Cancer	*155*
5.1.2 Ocular Diseases	*156*
5.1.3 Other Diseases	*157*
5.2 Diagnostic Applications	157
5.2.1 Magnetic Nanoparticles	*157*
5.2.2 Carbon Nanotubes and Gold Nanoparticles	*159*
5.2.3 Other Protein/Peptide Diagnostics	*160*
6. Conclusion	161
References	161

Chapter Objectives

- To outline fundamental concepts of peptide and protein drugs for various therapeutic use.
- To provide an insight on challenges of peptide and protein drug delivery.

*All authors equally contributed to the article.

- To examine effects of glycosylation, PEGylation, and mannosylation in peptide and protein drug delivery.
- To delineate various colloidal systems employed in delivery of peptide and proteins.

1. INTRODUCTION

Peptides and proteins are naturally occurring large molecules with secondary and tertiary structures. These molecules perform a cascade of functions to ensure proper functioning of the body's biological events. Improvements in biotechnology have resulted in a rapid development of peptide and protein therapeutics (PPTs). PPTs can avidly bind to their targets. As a result these compounds are highly potent and specific with possible low toxicity. Several macromolecular drugs are currently available in the market for treatment of a variety of diseases (Table 7.1).

Table 7.1 Peptide and protein therapeutics currently in the market

Drug name	Protein/peptide	Company	Use/disease
Bivalirudin	Peptide	The Medicines Company	Anticoagulant
Cyclosporine	Peptide	Novartis Pharmaceuticals	Immunosuppressant
Jetrea	Protein/enzyme	ThromboGenics Inc.	Vitreomacular adhesion
Elelyso	Protein/enzyme	Pfizer Inc., Protalix BioTherapeutics, Inc.	Type 1 Gaucher diseases
Voraxaze	Protein/enzyme	BTG International Inc.	Toxic methotrexate levels
Surfaxin	Peptide	Discovery Labs	Respiratory distress syndrome
Basaglar	Peptide	Eli Lilly and Company	Type 1 and 2 diabetes mellitus
Naglazyme	Protein/enzyme	Biomarin Pharmaceutical Inc.	Mucopolysaccharidosis
Liraglutide	Peptide	Novo Nordisk	Type 2 diabetes mellitus
Tysabri	Protein	Elan Pharmaceuticals	Multiple sclerosis
Perjeta	Protein	Genentech	Breast cancer
Linzess	Peptide	Ironwood Pharmaceuticals	Irritable bowel syndrome with constipation
Anthrax	Protein	GlaxoSmithKline	Anthrax
Entyvio	Protein	Millennium Pharmaceuticals	Ulcerative colitis/Crohn diseases
Herceptin	Protein	Genentech	Breast cancer
Nucala	Protein	GlaxoSmithKline	Asthma

2. CHALLENGES WITH PEPTIDE AND PROTEIN THERAPEUTICS

Although protein and peptide therapeutics possess high impact in health care, delivery of these agents is limited due to numerous factors. Large molecular size and hydrophilic nature of peptides and proteins prevent these molecules from traversing biological membranes such as gastrointestinal mucosa [1,2]. Such physicochemical properties may cause poor absorption and bioavailability for orally administered protein or peptide drugs. Moreover, these molecules are digested by proteolytic enzymes that are expressed highly in gastrointestinal tract [1]. First-pass metabolism by the liver following oral administration eliminates significant amounts of absorbed drugs [2,3]. Furthermore, low gastric acid pH in the stomach can cause chemical degradation of protein/peptide drugs [3]. Therefore oral delivery is the least favorable route for protein or peptide drugs. Slight modifications of the native confirmation may result in aggregations leading to partial or complete loss of activity [2,4]. The short half-lives of peptide and protein drugs require repeated administration to maintain therapeutic levels [2,3,5]. Nonetheless, frequent intravitreal injections are not patient compliant and may precipitate other complications such as retinal hemorrhage and detachment as is the case with bevacizumab [3,5]. Alternative routes such as nasal and pulmonary routes have been considered for peptide and protein delivery. Despite large surface area and highly vascularized tissue, pulmonary administration has shown limited bioavailability of protein drugs due to degradation by macrophage enzymes and rapid clearance by nasal and respiratory tracts [1].

3. CHEMICAL MODIFICATIONS

Chemical modifications of peptide and protein drugs along with encapsulation in nano/microparticles may stabilize the molecules from hydrolysis and enzymatic effects.

3.1 PEGylation

PEGylation is a chemical modification that involves conjugation of active polyethylene glycol (PEG) to a therapeutic protein/peptide or to a delivery system (nanoparticle). PEGylation offers several advantages such as favorable pharmacokinetics, more stability, and enhanced therapeutic activity [1]. PEGylation of a molecule can cause changes in physicochemical properties such as increase in hydrophilicity, size, and molecular weight, changes in conformation, and steric hindrance of intermolecular interaction [6]. Studies have shown that PEGylation of targeted drug delivery may decrease clearance and enhance delivery of peptide and protein molecules [6,7].

PEGylated poly(lactone-*co*-β-amino ester) nanoparticles for gene delivery were investigated [8]. Results indicate that diblock copolymer containing PEG—poly with 15% ω-pentadecalactone (PDL) (PEG—PPM-15% PDL) micelle particles caused cellular uptake, superior gene transfection efficacy, DNA binding ability, and effective endosomal escape [8]. In vitro antitumor activity was investigated by PEGylating small interference RNA (siRNA) lipoplexes for silencing B-lymphocyte induced maturation protein (BLIMP-1) in lymphoma cells [9]. PEGylation generated stable siRNA lipoplexes of size 300 nm and 80% complexation efficiency [9]. BLIMP-1 protein levels were lower leading to reduction of viability and activation of apoptosis by PEGylated lipoplexes [9]. PEGylated poly(lactic-co-glycolic acid) (PLGA) nanoparticles encapsulated bovine serum albumin (BSA), 200 nm in size and with 48.6% entrapment efficiency, were investigated by Li et al. These nanoconstructs extended the half-life of BSA from 13.6 min to 4.5 h relative to non-PEGylated nanoparticles [10]. PEGylated micelles for protein delivery have also been explored. Jiang et al. studied PEGylated albumin-based polyion complex micelles for protein delivery. PEGylated albumin complex micelles were 15−25 nm in size and inhibited growth of MCF-7 [11]. These micelles may be applied in cancer treatment.

PEGylation of microparticles to improve therapeutic applications such as bioassay, degradation, and release kinetics have been studied by several groups. PEGylated microparticles with neuregulin (NRG) growth factor for myocardial infracted hearts were examined by Pascual-Gil et al. [12]. PEGylated PLGA microparticles encapsulating NRG resulted in the reduction of phagocytosis relative to non-PEGylated microparticles [12]. Controlled release of NRG over 12 weeks was studied. Cardiomyocyte receptors for NRG were activated in animals treated with microparticles loaded with NRG [12]. PEGylated microparticles for microfluidic assay have been also evaluated. PEGylation of magnetic poly (glycidyl methacrylate) microparticles encapsulating BSA was investigated for nonspecific adsorption [13]. Microparticles with 30 kDa PEG produced 45% reduction in nonspecific adsorption of proteins [13]. Moreover, aggregation and adhesion of PEGylated microparticles in microfluidic devices were lower relative to non-PEGylated microparticles [13].

3.2 Glycosylation

Glycosylation is a commonly conserved process in the posttranslational protein modifications of eukaryotes and bacteria [14−16]. However, glycosylation can be introduced by chemical modification in which carbohydrate molecule is conjugated to a protein, peptide, lipid, or nanocarrier in the laboratory. Thirteen monosaccharides and eight different amino acids have been described to be involved in 37 different carbohydrate−protein linkages. In this way, a large variety of glycan structures is created. Carbohydrate moieties are introduced not only to facilitate properties of a protein but also to improve physicochemical, cellular localization, turnover, protein quality control, and ligand interaction [16,17]. It can be either a co- or a postenzymatic translational modification. Glycosylation can be categorized into two groups, N-linked and O-linked. In N-linked glycosylation, the carbohydrate molecule is attached to a nitrogen molecule of arginine or asparagine side chain

[1,6]. On the other hand, in O-linked glycosylation, the oxygen on hydroxyl of tyrosine, threonine, and serine is utilized for conjugation [1,6].

Glycosylated cytochrome c (Cyt c) was immobilized in mesoporous silica nanoparticles (MSNs) for inducing apoptosis in HeLa cells by [18]. Cyt c was modified by glycosylation of lactose to increase stability and reduce proteolytic degradation. Caspase-3 assay demonstrated a 47% activation by Cyt c-SPDP (sulfosuccinimidyl 6-(3′-[2-pyridyldithio]-propionamido)hexanoate) relative to 87% activation observed with Cyt c-lactose bioconjugate [18]. Furthermore, MSN-SPDP-Cyt c did not induce apoptosis, whereas MSN-Cyt c-lactose induced apoptosis in HeLa cells after 72 h [18]. In addition, MSN-Cyt c-lactose demonstrated endosomal escape [18]. These findings indicate that glycosylation can stabilize and reduce enzyme degradation of Cyt c.

3.3 Mannosylation

Mannosylation is another chemical modification that can be incorporated in peptide or protein therapeutics. Mannosylation can be achieved by conjugating mannose with a peptide or protein [1]. Mannosylation can be represented at C-mannosylation [19] or O-mannosylation [20]. Mannosylation on PPTs has been explored in previous years. Mannosylation is feasible since mannose can be conjugated to a carrier system. Either C- or O- mannosylation is recommended depending on the functional group present on a particular carrier system. Conjugation of mannose on delivery system, protein or peptide therapeutic can take the advantage of mannose receptors highly expressed on macrophages, Kupffer, and other cells. Hence mannosylation may assist targeted delivery of therapeutic molecules [1,21].

Mannosylated zwitterionic-based cationic liposomes (Man-ZCL) for human immunodeficiency virus (HIV) DNA vaccines were developed by Qiao et al. Man-ZCL has the ability to conjugate DNA antigen and can offer protection from enzymatic degradation [22]. Man-ZCL exhibits lower toxicity, improved anti-HIV immune responses, and activation of Th1/Th2 mixed immunity as reported in vitro and in vivo studies [22]. Such a delivery system increased the immunogenicity of HIV vaccines. Xiao et al. examined mannosylated bioreducible nanoparticles for inflammatory bowel diseases (IBDs) [23]. A mannosylated bioreducible cationic polymer (PPM) was developed to prepare nanoparticles using sodium triphosphate (TPP) and siRNA (TPP-PPM/siRNA nanoparticles) [23]. TPP-PPM/siRNA nanoparticles showed low cytotoxicity and caused higher cellular uptake [23]. In addition, TPP-PPM/tumor necrosis factor (TNF)-α siRNA nanoparticles demonstrated inhibition of expression and secretion of TNF-α. It also expressed therapeutic response on colitis [23]. Results suggest that such an effective formulation can be utilized in IBD therapy. In vitro and in vivo evaluations of a novel mannosylated dendrimer for delivery of antigen were reported [24]. In vitro studies demonstrated an induced ovalbumin (OVA)-specific T cell response and enhanced antigen presentation when treated with mannosylated dendrimer ovalbumin (MDO). These studies also generated OVA-specific $CD4^+/CD8^+$ T cells and antibody response [24]. Mice tumors treated with MDO either did not grow or produced late onset [24]. These findings confirm that mannosylated dendrimer can serve as a potential carrier not only for vaccine but also for other chemotherapeutics in cancer.

4. MICRO- AND NANOTECHNOLOGY FOR BIOLOGICS IN DRUG DELIVERY

4.1 Microparticles or Microspheres

Microparticles can be referred to as microspheres, which represent small spherical particles, with size ranging from 1 to 1000 μm [25]. Microparticles can be prepared from either natural or synthetic materials. Currently available microparticles are constituted from polymers, ceramic, and glass [26]. Polymeric microparticles as drug delivery vehicle offer several advantages such as ability to encapsulate a wide range of hydrophilic or hydrophobic drugs [27]. In addition, microparticles are more stable in the biological environment relative to liposomes [27]. Microparticles can be designed with a surface-linked targeting moiety. Therefore this system can be exploited for targeted drug delivery [28]. Microparticle encapsulating macromolecule can serve as a shield protecting biologics from degradation [28,29]. Controlled and long-term release is another advantage of the microparticles [28]. Polymeric microparticles made from poly lactic acid (PLA), PLGA, polyethylene, and polystyrene polymers are the most common types of polymer microparticles [25,26]. Polymeric microparticles are composed of biodegradable and biocompatible polymers [25].

Microparticles have been employed to encapsulate several macromolecules for the treatment of many diseases. Vaishya et al. investigated the reversible hydrophobic ion pairing complex strategy to minimize acylation of octreotide during long-term delivery from PLGA microparticles. Higher entrapment efficiency (74—81%) was observed. A large fraction of the peptide was released in the native form. Only less than 7% of peptide was acylated [30]. A microsphere hydrogel drug delivery system was studied by Osswald and Kang-Mieler for controlled and extended in vitro release of bioactive antivascular endothelial growth factor (VEGF) agents (ranibizumab or aflibercept) [31]. Ranibizumab or aflibercept was released from microsphere hydrogel system for 196 days [31]. In addition, released samples were safe, bioactive throughout the release period, and produced significant inhibition of human umbilical vein endothelial cells proliferation relative to free drug [31]. Insulin-loaded double-walled PLGA microsphere exhibited nonporous and spherical structures relative to single polymer microsphere [32]. In addition, double-walled microspheres demonstrated a significantly reduced initial burst release [32]. Moreover, a higher molecular weight protein (BSA) incorporated in double-walled microspheres demonstrated similar results as observed with insulin [33]. A few examples of microparticles encapsulating therapeutic macromolecules are available in the literature. Some of these formulations have shown higher drug entrapment [30] and prolonged release [31]. Microparticles can encapsulate therapeutic macromolecules to treat different pathologies such as ocular diseases, cancer, cardiac disturbances, and inflammation.

4.2 Nanoparticles

In previous years nanotechnology has become the state-of-the-art technology in the field of drug delivery. According to Bawa et al. nanotechnology is "The design, characterization, production, and application of structures, devices, and systems by controlled manipulation of size and shape at the nanometer scale (atomic, molecular, and macromolecular scale) that produces structures, devices, and systems with at least one novel/superior characteristic or property" [34]. Nanoparticles are a colloidal drug delivery system with particle size ranging from 10 to 1000 nm [35]. Just like most other delivery systems, nanoparticles can be prepared from either natural materials such as albumin and gelatin or synthetic materials such as PLGA, PLA, and poly caprolactone. Nanoparticles can be suitable for many applications such as gene and drug delivery systems [36–38], biodetection of pathogens [39,40], fluorescent biological materials [41,42], tumor destruction through heating [43], and tissue engineering [44]. Surface and size can be modified to optimize therapeutic efficacy. Active targeting can be achieved by decorating the ligand on the surface of nanoparticles [45,46]. Nanoparticles can also generate enhanced permeability and retention effect [47]. Because of the small size nanoparticles can not only exhibit longer systemic circulation but also enhance cell penetration [48]. Several methods such as dialysis, solvent evaporation, emulsions, supercritical fluid technology, and solvent displacement/precipitation can be applied in the preparation of nanoparticles [49].

Nanoparticles can encapsulate a wide array of therapeutic molecules, small and large, both hydrophobic and hydrophilic. Nanoparticles can deliver protein or peptide therapeutics for several diseases. Hepatitis B virus (HBV) cytosine phosphate guanosine (HBV-CpG) nanoparticles can induce therapeutic immunity against HBV infection. This delivery system produced strong immunostimulatory effect on lymphocytes, efficient clearance of HBV, and induced anti-hepatitis B surface antigen response in HBV mice models [50]. Surface-enhanced resonance Raman spectroscopy (SERRS) nanoparticles were applied for the detection of lymph node metastases by Spaliviero [51]. SERRS nanoparticles were intravenously injected into mice with prostate cancer. Analysis with fluorescence and Raman imaging indicated that SERRS NPs were localized at higher concentration in the lymph nodes of normal mice relative to metastasized lymph nodes [51]. This technology can serve as a tool to differentiate between normal and metastasized lymph nodes. Theranostic approach utilizing PLGA nanoparticles coated with pH-responsive material was also applied to deliver doxorubicin and indocyanine green [52]. In vivo and ex vivo studies demonstrated accumulation of nanoparticles in solid tumor, where some of the particles permeated into tumor tissues in mice model [52].

4.3 Solid Lipid NP

Solid lipid nanoparticles (SLN) have been developed as an alternative to nanoparticles, liposomes, and microparticles particularly to deliver therapeutic peptides and proteins. These are a new group of lipid emulsion carriers, where solid lipid is being utilized instead of liquid lipid. Several solid lipids such as stearic acid, triglycerides, carnauba wax, beeswax, cetyl alcohol, emulsifying wax, cholesterol butyrate, and cholesterol may be suitable for SLN preparation [53]. The size of SLN ranges between 50 and 1000 nm, similar to other nanocarriers. SLNs can be formulated by several methods such as high-pressure homogenization (hot and cold homogenization) [54–56], solvent injection [57], water in oil in water double emulsion (W/O/W) [58,59], high-shear homogenizer [60,61], solvent emulsification evaporation [62,63], and membrane contactor [64]. One of the advantages of SLNs over other nanocarriers is scale up during production and sterilization, which is otherwise challenging with traditional NPs [65]. The stability of SLN is excellent because the lipid used during preparation does not hydrolyze in aqueous solution relative to other polymers (e.g., PLGA) in nanoparticle preparations. These polymers hydrolyze in aqueous solution; hence lyophilization is essential for NP manufacturing [53]. SLNs display outstanding biocompatibility due to the biodegradable nature of the lipids particularly with hydrophobic drugs [65]. Furthermore, SLNs exhibit high drug loading capacity, are easier to validate, and may be approved by regulatory agencies [65,66]. Controlled release and targeted drug delivery can also be achieved with SLN [65,66]. Several routes of administrations such as oral, rectal, parenteral, ocular, nasal, respiratory, and topical have been selected for SLN delivery [55,65,66]. Several studies have been performed which show SLN may be suitable to deliver protein/peptide therapeutics for various indications [67–70].

4.4 Carbon Nanotube

Carbon nanotube (CNT) is a tubular cylindrical nanostructure of carbon atoms suitable as a drug delivery system. The CNT has a diameter ranging from 1 to 50 nm. These nanotubes can be classified as single-walled CNTs (SWCNTs) or multiwalled CNTs (MWCNTs) [1]. CNT can be considered as a delivery system for macromolecules. Efficacy of indolicidin for immune activation was enhanced by conjugation with gold nanoparticles [71]. Furthermore, CNT-indolicidin protected host cells against bacterial contamination relative to free indolicidin [71]. Similarly, CNT was exploited on intercalated disc assembly in cardiac myocytes [72]. SWCNT with collagen substrate enhanced cardiomyocyte adhesion and maturation as growth supports for neonatal cardiomyocyte [72]. In addition, protein expression, inhibitor of DNA binding assembly, and its functionality were augmented in intercalated disc [72]. CNT may be applied in lung inflammation [73]. SWCNTs are hydrophobic in nature; hence they prevent therapeutic molecules from dispersion in aqueous medium. Adding peptide surfactants to SWCNT (SWCNT/peptide complex) may accelerate the delivery of macromolecules [74]. The peptide sequence is eight amino acids long (Trp—Val—Trp—Val—Trp—Val—Lys—Lys), varied according to the number of tryptophans in the chain [74]. Results indicated that the peptide with the most tryptophans (three) in the chain formed a more stable SWCNT/peptide complex relative to peptide (Trp—Val—Val—Val—Val—Val—Lys—Lys) with fewer tryptophans (one) [74]. Weng et al. have investigated MWCNTs for the delivery of recombined ricin A (RTA). Confocal studies revealed higher cell death for MCF-7, HeLa, HL7702, COS-7, and L-929 cells by MWCNT-RTA conjugates relative to RTA alone [75]. In addition, selective destruction of cancer cells was observed by MWCNT-RTA-HER2 due to recognition of human epidermal growth factor receptor (HER2) receptor on breast cancer cells [75]. These findings clearly demonstrate that CNTs may be exploited to deliver therapeutic macromolecules. Furthermore, various modifications can also be performed on CNTs to enhance solubility and bioavailability of the therapeutic macromolecules.

4.5 Liposomes

Liposome is a spherical vesicle with one or more lipid bilayers. These lipid vesicles can be classified according to lamellarity, i.e., single lamellar/unilamellar with a size ranging between 50 and 250 nm to multilamellar with size 1—5 μm. Liposomes mainly consist of phospholipids and cholesterol. The lipid bilayer structure of liposomes is similar to the cell membrane bilayer. Therefore liposome-mediated drug delivery may be an attractive strategy. Liposomes can encapsulate hydrophilic or lipophilic drugs depending on the core of the vesicle [76]. As a drug delivery system, liposomes have extensively been explored in the pharmaceutical arena due to biodegradable and biocompatible nature, low toxicity, and ability to accommodate hydrophilic and hydrophobic drugs [9,22,77,78]. Flexibility of liposomes can result in passive targeting, which may lead to accumulation in tumor site when a site-specific ligand is attached to the surface [79—81]. Despite all the advantages of using liposomes, there are some shortcomings to this delivery system. High production cost, low solubility due to phospholipid nature, and short half-life are some of the negative factors. Moreover, oxidation and hydrolysis of phospholipids may cause degradation of the vesicle, causing leakage of the encapsulated therapeutic molecules [77].

Several methods can be utilized to prepare liposomes. These methods include dehydration—rehydration method, reverse phase evaporation, vesicle extrusion technique, frozen and thawed multilamellar vesicle (MLV), stable plurilamellar vesicle, and MLVs reverse phase evaporation [76,82,83]. Apart from protection of a drug against enzymatic degradation and targeting delivery, they can be utilized for delivery of antiviral agents [82,84]. In addition to gene delivery, liposomes can be applied for topical delivery of therapeutics and have proved to be effective [85,86]. Delivery of ocular and cancer therapeutic molecules utilizing liposomes has also been explored and found to be feasible [87–92].

4.6 Aquasomes

Aquasomes encompass simple polymers and complex lipid mixture. These vesicles show triple-layered structures comprising core, coating, and drug formed by self-assembly through various bond formations [93]. The method of preparation for aquasomes involves three stages such as formulation of inorganic core, followed by coating the core with polyhydroxyl oligomer, and lastly loading of the drug [93]. Several applications of aquasomes including protein/peptide cargo can provide a vital therapy such as antigen delivery. Aquasomes were prepared by self-assembly of hydroxyapatite and coated with polyhydroxyl oligomers. Consequently these constructs can adsorb BSA as a model antigen [94]. The size of aquasome was from 200 to 220 nm with 30% BSA loading efficiency [94]. The immunological activity of aquasome encapsulating BSA was higher relative to free BSA [94]. In addition, aquasome formulation could stimulate T helper 1 and 2 (Th1 and Th2) immune response [94].

Aquasomes have also been applied in cancer therapy. Kaur et al. developed aquasomes bearing recombinant human interferon α-2b (rhINF-α-2b) for prolonged release and enhanced cytotoxicity in ovarian cancer cells [95]. Results pointed out that rhINF-α-2b-Py-5-P-Aq.somes (with pyridoxal-5-phosphate) exhibited high protein loading, retaining the structural conformation of rhINF-α-2b relative to other aquasomes containing trehalose (Tre), ceramic core, $CaHPO_4$, and cellobiose (Cellob) [95]. Furthermore, aquasomes PEGylated with phospholipid-PEG 2000, rhINF-α-2b released rhINF-α-2b-$CaHPO_4$, rhINF-α-2b-Tre, rhINF-α-2b-Cellob, and rhINF-α-2b-Py-5-P-Aq.somes over 1, 4, 6, and 8 h, respectively [95]. Aquasomes have also been investigated for other diseases such as allergen immunotherapy, which appeared to be effective in mice model [96].

4.7 Micelles

Micelles have attracted attention for the delivery of poorly water-soluble drugs. Micelles are formed by self-assembly of amphiphilic molecules. The structures contain hydrophilic/polar region (head) and hydrophobic/nonpolar region (tail) [1]. Micelles are formed in aqueous solution whereby the polar region faces the outside surface of the micelle and the nonpolar region forms the core. Micelles can deliver both hydrophilic and hydrophobic agents. Such structures can deliver macromolecules because these molecules can provide sustained and controlled release of macromolecules, provide chemical and physical stability of the encapsulated molecules, improve drug pharmacokinetics and favorable tissue distribution, and improve drug bioavailability [1,97]. Formulation of micelle is achieved at above critical micelle concentration [97]. Micelles are usually spherical ranging in size from 2 to 20 nm depending on composition. The most common methods for micelle preparation include oil in water emulsion [98,99], solvent evaporation [100,101], solid dispersion, and dialysis methods [97,102].

Micelles encapsulating therapeutic macromolecules have been explored for a wide range of diseases. Li et al. studied bovine serum albumin (FA-BSA) functionalized polymeric micelles with folate and loaded with superparamagnetic iron oxide (SPION) for tumor targeting and imaging. In vitro imaging results indicated that folate-functionalized micelles can produce higher cellular uptake in hepatoma cells than unmodified micelles [103]. Tumor targeting and imaging capabilities were observed in mice model 24 h after intravenous injection [103]. These outcomes demonstrate that micelles can be applied for tumor targeting and imaging. A novel pancreatic polypeptide (PP) was encapsulated in sterically stabilized micelles (SSMs) and injected into rats for the treatment of pancreatogenic diabetes (PD) [104]. PD rats receiving PP-SSM significantly improved insulin sensitivity, glucose tolerance, and hepatic glycogen relative to controls [104].

5. PROTEIN- AND PEPTIDE-BASED THERAPEUTICS
5.1 Therapeutic Applications
5.1.1 Cancer

In previous years, PPTs have attracted considerable attention in cancer therapeutics, because these are highly potent and selective. This can result in targeted drug delivery with reduced toxicity [2]. PPTs offer high efficacy, safety, and tolerability, which are unique features relative to conventional drugs [2].

A high-affinity peptide ligand LXY30 targeting $\alpha 3$ integrin expressed in human tumors was investigated [105]. LXY30, a cyclic peptide, was stable in human plasma and effective in tumor targeting relative to other peptides screened [105]. In vitro studies indicated that LXY30 was able to bind $\alpha 3\beta 3$ integrin expressing in lung, glioblastoma, and breast cancer [105]. A novel cell-penetrating peptide for the inhibition of β-catenin/LEF-1 signaling was developed for cancer therapy by Hsieh et al. In vivo results revealed that this peptide interacted with β-catenin and inhibited breast cancer cell growth, migration, invasion, colony formation, and suppression of tumor growth in mouse and zebrafish models [106]. Pathway analysis indicated that the peptide downstream target genes were associated with HER2 and interleukin (IL)-9 signaling pathways [106]. These results indicate potential therapeutic applications of the peptide in inhibition of β-catenin/LEF-1. Tumor targeting peptides for non—small cell lung cancer (NSCLC) was studied by McGuire et al. [107]. Several novel peptides indicating individual binding profiles were tested with numerous NSCLC cell lines. These peptides, however, did not bind normal bronchial epithelial cell lines [107]. The binding affinities were between 0.0071 and 40 nM [107].

Monoclonal antibodies, aptamers, and other proteins for the treatment of cancer have been explored extensively. Heo et al. developed an aptamer—antibody complex (oligobody) for targeted cancer cells. In vivo studies with cotinine conjugated t44-OMe aptamer, which is the specific sequence of pegaptanib, were performed. The antibody part resulted in extended pharmacokinetics of the aptamer (t44-Ome) without compromising its binding affinity [108]. Besides, the aptamer of the oligobody was able to penetrate tumor tissues relative to the antibody itself and reduced the tumor in animal model [108]. A monoclonal antibody for the treatment of relapsed chronic lymphocytic leukemia (CLL) was investigated in a phase 1-2 clinical trial. Acalabrutinib (ACP-196), a selective, irreversible inhibitor of Bruton tyrosine kinase was administered to patients with CLL to evaluate safety, efficacy, pharmacokinetics, and pharmacodynamics [109]. No dose limiting toxicity with 95% response rate, 85% partial response, and 10% partial response with lymphocytosis were reported [109].

5.1.2 Ocular Diseases

Diseases associated with the posterior segment of the eye such as age-related macular degeneration (AMD), diabetic macular edema, diabetic retinopathy, macular edema, and retinal vein occlusion may be treated with protein therapeutics. Topical administration of macromolecules for treatment of back of the eye diseases is challenging due to large molecular weight of the proteins in addition to physical and chemical barriers of the eye [110]. As a result, most of PPTs are administered through intravitreal route, which provides specific and targeted treatment for retinal diseases [111]. Over the past few years anti-VEGFs such as bevacizumab and ranibizumab, VEGF trap aflibercept, and aptamer pegaptanib have been indicated for the treatment of ocular neovascular diseases [112—115].

Apart from anti-VEGF drugs, which have shown promising results, new peptide and protein drugs for ocular diseases are emerging. Antisense oligonucleotides for the treatment of ocular diseases are in horizon. Antisense oligonucleotide (ODN17) delivered by cationic nanoemulsion directed at VEGF-R2 for the treatment of corneal neovascularization was investigated by Haqiqit et al. Inhibition of corneal neovascularization was observed in animal models treated with ODN17 nanoemulsion after topical or subconjunctival administration [116]. In retinopathy of prematurity mouse model, a 64% of vitreal neovascularization inhibition was observed after being treated with ODN17 nanoemulsion [116]. These results suggest that antisense oligonucleotides can provide therapeutic effect in ocular diseases. siRNA can be used to inhibit specific gene expression. siRNA can be beneficial to silence genes that are associated with ocular diseases. A phase 1 dose escalation study was performed with siRNA targeting RTP801 gene in patients with AMD [117]. Results indicated that the siRNA (PF-045237655) was well tolerated over a 24-month period after single intravitreal injection. Also, no dose limiting toxicities were observed [117]. These reports confirm that siRNA is safe and well tolerated in patients with AMD. Gene delivery for ocular diseases has gained attention in recent years. Local distribution, transgene duration, and safety of adenovirus carrying luciferase gene were evaluated by Liu et al. Luciferase expression was induced for 64 days following subconjunctival injection [118]. Moreover, adenovirus was dispersed across anterior and posterior eye [118]. Therefore gene delivery may be a promising therapeutic strategy for ocular diseases.

5.1.3 Other Diseases

Cancer and ocular diseases are not the only diseases that can be treated with PPTs. This section will provide a few examples to demonstrate that these agents can be applied to other diseases. A combined delivery of recombinant high mobility group box-1 box A (HMGB1A) peptide and S1Plyase siRNA (siS1Plyase) were investigated in animal models of acute lung injury (ALI) [119]. The siS1Plyase/HMGB1A/R3V6 complex reduced the levels of IL-6 and TNF-α in macrophages. In vivo studies revealed reduction in S1PLyase levels, inflammatory response, and apoptosis in ALI model. Therapeutic cell penetrating peptides (CPPs) for treatment of chronic hepatitis B virus was investigated by Ndeboko et al. Peptide nucleic acids (PNAs) conjugated to CPP (PNA-CPP) was observed in the liver. This construct inhibited duck hepatitis B virus (DHBV) replication [120]. In addition, modified CPP in the absence of PNA was able to inhibit late stages of DHBV replication [120]. Several studies have shown that peptide- and protein-based therapeutics may have potential application in periodontal regeneration. Some of these studies are in clinical trials. Positive results suggest the therapy can speed up repair and regeneration relative to other strategies [121]. Other diseases such as kidney diseases [122,123], Alzheimer [122,124], and bacterial infections [125] have been explored. Table 7.2 summarizes current clinical trials with peptide and protein.

5.2 Diagnostic Applications
5.2.1 Magnetic Nanoparticles

Magnetic nanoparticles (MNPs) have been explored as therapeutic and/or diagnostic tool in medicine. In diagnosis MNPs can serve as contrast agents in magnetic resonance imaging (MRI) [126], cell separation [127,128], purification [129,130], and gene transfer [131,132]. MNPs can be applied as a delivery system for targeted therapy [132] and hyperthermia treatment [133,134]. Detection and immobilization of biomolecules can also be performed by MNPs [135–137]. Numerous diseases may be diagnosed with MNPs such Alzheimer disease [138], gliomas [139], cardiovascular diseases [140], cancer [141,142], and central nervous system autoimmune diseases [143].

Table 7.2 Peptide and protein drugs currently in clinical trials

Molecule	Protein/peptide	Company	Stage/phase	Disease
Epoetin alpha	Protein erythropoietin	University Iowa	II	Neonatal anemia
Daclizumab	Monoclonal antibody	Biogen	III	Relapsing-remitting multiple sclerosis
Human recombinant CC10	Recombinant human protein	Clarassance, Inc.	I	Respiratory distress syndrome in infant
RBX2660	Protein	Rebiotix Inc.	II	*Clostridium difficile* infection
Sikirumab	Human anti–interleukin-6 monoclonal antibody	GlaxoSmithKline	III	Giant cell arteritis
ABT-494	Protein	Abbvie	III	Rheumatoid arthritis
FP-1039		Five Prime Therapeutics, Inc.	I	Cancer
Ibalizumab	Monoclonal antibody	TaiMed Biologics Inc.	III	Human immunodeficiency virus
GW572016	Tyrosine kinase inhibitor	University of New Mexico	I/II	Breast cancer
TTI-621	Fusion protein	Trillium Therapeutics	1	Hematologic malignancies
Ixekizumab/LY2439821	Monoclonal antibody	Eli Lilly	III	Psoriatic arthritis
Nilotinib/AMN107	Kinase inhibitor	Novartis Pharmaceuticals	I/II	Leukemia

https://clinicaltrials.gov/.

MNP has been developed and designed to detect targets such as proteins, peptides, DNA, RNA, pathogens, and tumors. In cardiac diseases, MNP has been utilized to detect plaque. Profilin-1 targeted MNPs were applied to investigate atherosclerosis characteristics in mice model [144]. MNP conjugated with polyclonal profilin-1 antibody and fluorescence dye (PC-NPs) was intravenously administered to atherosclerosis mice model [144]. Immunofluorescence assay discovered high levels of profilin-1 protein inside plaque of diseased mice. Imaging studies showed accumulation of PC-NP in atherosclerotic plaque of carotid artery [144]. This dual-imaging probe may also be applied in diagnosis of plaque in cardiac patients. Another dual molecular probe was explored in ovarian cancer cells. The transfection efficiency of SPION and short hairpin RNA dual-function molecular probe was explored at different iron concentrations (5, 15, 30, 45, 75, and 100 mg/L) [145]. Cell survival rate was above 90% for the first three concentrations and was below 75% for the last three concentrations [145]. When the concentration of the probe was greater than or equal to 45 mg/L, the inhibition of the protein expression level of epidermal growth factor receptor was elevated [145]. MRI analysis displayed lower signal strength with increase in iron concentration in the probe with SKOV3 cell line [145]. These results provide an insight on the role of iron in SPION for diagnosis and treatment. A DNA point mutation can be detected by single based coded (CdS) MNP probes [146]. Adenosine, cytidine, guanosine, and thymidine (A-CdS, C-CdS, G-CdS, and T-CdS) base probes were applied in identifying mutations in DNA [146]. Resonance frequency analysis revealed a change on DNA strand when a mutation was identified. These results were also confirmed with fluorescence analysis [146]. It appears that this technology can be valuable to detect point mutation in DNA strand and can be developed to diagnose genetic cause of diseases.

5.2.2 Carbon Nanotubes and Gold Nanoparticles

Gold nanoparticles have a wide array of applications including molecular diagnosis, imaging, bioinformatics, and targeting therapy [147]. Early and accurate detection of cancer is very important so that proper or personalized medication can be administered. Gold nanoparticle—based calorimetric assay has been developed by Medley et al. for the detection of cancer cells [148]. The assay involves aptamer-conjugated gold nanoparticles. When gold NPs bind to targeted cancer cells, a distinct color change will appear, whereas control noncancerous cells remain unchanged [148]. Aptamer-based biobarcode assays for the detection of Cyt c released from apoptotic cells have been investigated [149]. Sensitivity and specificity of the assay enabled differentiation between cancer and noncancer cells depending on the aptamer used [148]. Kah et al. applied gold nanoparticles with surface modification for early detection of oral cancer [150]. The nanoparticles conjugated to antiepidermal growth factor receptor produced an optical contrast that could differentiate between cancer and normal cells [150]. Furthermore, spectrum analysis from self-enhanced Raman scattering of gold nanoparticles showed a distinct difference between normal saliva and saliva obtained from patient with cancer [150]. These results demonstrate the feasibility of early diagnosis of oral cancer.

Graphene CNT aptasensor was adapted for cardiac myoglobin biomarker by Kumal et al. The aptamer-functionalized nanotube revealed a substantial increase in signal response with a detection limit of around 0.3 ng/mL [151]. This assay can be utilized for the diagnosis of myoglobin screening in patients [151]. SWCNT-based transparent immunosensor has been developed as the biomarker osteopontin (OPN) for the detection of prostate cancer [152]. Monoclonal antibodies specific for OPN were covalently immobilized on the SWCNT with various channel lengths (2, 5, and 10 μm) [152]. Studies indicate that immunosensors were specific for OPN in phosphate buffer saline. Human serum from 1 pg/mL to 1 μg/mL as well as BSA protein with a detection limit of 0.3 pg/mL were detected [152].

5.2.3 Other Protein/Peptide Diagnostics

Several other devices or nanocarriers have been developed in conjunction with peptides/proteins for diagnosis. Silver-gold nanorods generated narrow surface-enhanced Raman scattering (SERS). Photothermal contrast was developed for circulating tumor cell identification [153]. These nanorods consisting of Raman active molecules are antibodies specific to breast cancer and leukocyte-specific CD45 markers [153]. High specific detection provided by antibodies resulted in enhanced SERS signal on these nanorods relative to only gold nanorods [153]. This technology may improve detection and imaging of tumor cells. Similarly, adenosine triphosphate (ATP) was detected through polymerization-induced aggregation of actin-conjugated gold/silver nanorods (G-actin-Au/Ag NRs) [154]. Superior sensitivity, with detection limit of 25 nM for ATP, was observed in comparison with other adenosine nucleotides [154].

Protein microarray technology has significant possibilities in diagnostic applications. A novel multiplex beads-based assay comprising nine tumor-associated antigens was developed for colorectal cancer (CRC) diagnosis [155]. The essay demonstrated 90% specificity, 66% selectivity on CRC patient samples [155]. Protein chips as cancer biomarkers for the detection and diagnosis have also been evaluated for man and woman by Luo et al. Protein chips exhibited pronounced specificity and sensitivity and was free of common interference. Excelled correlation in detection of biomarkers relative with traditional methods were obtained [156]. In addition, male protein chip offered significant diagnostic value on neuron-specific enolase, whereas female protein chip offered diagnosis capability on pro-gastrin-releasing peptide biomarkers [156]. These protein chips may be useful as biomarkers for the diagnosis of various cancers and other diseases.

Lee et al. have studied peptide displaying phage as a diagnostic probe for human lung adenocarcinoma. A novel Pep-1 (CAKATCPAC) demonstrated accurate detection of adenocarcinoma. It also projected highly enhanced targeting ability after ionizing radiation in both cell-derived and patient-derived lung adenocarcinoma xenografts [157]. These results indicate the diagnostic and targeting abilities of Pep-1 in human lung adenocarcinoma.

6. CONCLUSION

PPTs have gained interest in recent years for treatment of diseases. The specificity, tolerability, and highly potent nature of these peptides and proteins have rendered these highly valuable and favorable drugs for further development. A large number of peptide and protein drugs are currently being approved and also in clinical trials. However, peptide and protein drug delivery to the target site still remains a prime concern. Various delivery systems have been developed and investigated to overcome some of the challenges. More advancements are needed to improve therapeutic approaches over existing delivery systems to ensure effective delivery of these compounds.

REFERENCES

[1] Patel A, Cholkar K, Mitra AK. Recent developments in protein and peptide parenteral delivery approaches. Ther Deliv 2014;5(3):337—65.
[2] Fosgerau K, Hoffmann T. Peptide therapeutics: current status and future directions. Drug Discov Today 2015;20(1):122—8.
[3] Vaishya R, et al. Long-term delivery of protein therapeutics. Expert Opin Drug Deliv 2015;12(3): 415—40.
[4] Otvos Jr L, Wade JD. Current challenges in peptide-based drug discovery. Front Chem 2014;2:62.
[5] Patel SP, et al. Novel thermosensitive pentablock copolymers for sustained delivery of proteins in the treatment of posterior segment diseases. Protein Pept Lett 2014;21(11):1185—200.
[6] Pisal DS, Kosloski MP, Balu-Iyer SV. Delivery of therapeutic proteins. J Pharm Sci 2010;99(6): 2557—75.
[7] Caliceti P, Veronese FM. Pharmacokinetic and biodistribution properties of poly(ethylene glycol)-protein conjugates. Adv Drug Deliv Rev 2003;55(10):1261—77.
[8] Chen Y, et al. Enzymatic PEGylated poly(lactone-co-beta-amino ester) nanoparticles as biodegradable, biocompatible and stable vectors for gene delivery. ACS Appl Mater Interfaces 2016;8(1): 490—501.
[9] Belletti D, et al. PEGylated siRNA lipoplexes for silencing of BLIMP-1 in primary effusion lymphoma: in vitro evidences of antitumoral activity. Eur J Pharm Biopharm 2016;99:7—17.
[10] Li Y, et al. PEGylated PLGA nanoparticles as protein carriers: synthesis, preparation and biodistribution in rats. J Control Release 2001;71(2):203—11.
[11] Jiang Y, et al. PEGylated albumin-based polyion complex micelles for protein delivery. Biomacromolecules 2016;17(3):808—17.
[12] Pascual-Gil S, et al. Tracking the in vivo release of bioactive NRG from PLGA and PEG-PLGA microparticles in infarcted hearts. J Control Release 2015;220(Pt A):388—96.
[13] Kucerova J, et al. PEGylation of magnetic poly(glycidyl methacrylate) microparticles for microfluidic bioassays. Mater Sci Eng C Mater Biol Appl 2014;40:308—15.
[14] Abu-Qarn M, Eichler J, Sharon N. Not just for Eukarya anymore: protein glycosylation in Bacteria and Archaea. Curr Opin Struct Biol 2008;18(5):544—50.
[15] Yurist-Doutsch S, et al. Sweet to the extreme: protein glycosylation in Archaea. Mol Microbiol 2008;68(5):1079—84.

[16] Lehle L, Strahl S, Tanner W. Protein glycosylation, conserved from yeast to man: a model organism helps elucidate congenital human diseases. Angew Chem Int Ed Engl 2006;45(41):6802—18.
[17] Marth JD, Grewal PK. Mammalian glycosylation in immunity. Nat Rev Immunol 2008;8(11):874—87.
[18] Mendez J, et al. Delivery of chemically glycosylated cytochrome c immobilized in mesoporous silica nanoparticles induces apoptosis in HeLa cancer cells. Mol Pharm 2014;11(1):102—11.
[19] Doucey MA, et al. Protein C-mannosylation is enzyme-catalysed and uses dolichyl-phosphate-mannose as a precursor. Mol Biol Cell 1998;9(2):291—300.
[20] Loibl M, Strahl S. Protein O-mannosylation: what we have learned from baker's yeast. Biochim Biophys Acta 2013;1833(11):2438—46.
[21] Opanasopit P, et al. In vivo recognition of mannosylated proteins by hepatic mannose receptors and mannan-binding protein. Am J Physiol Gastrointest Liver Physiol 2001;280(5):G879—89.
[22] Qiao C, et al. Enhanced non-inflammasome mediated immune responses by mannosylated zwitterionic-based cationic liposomes for HIV DNA vaccines. Biomaterials 2016;85:1—17.
[23] Xiao B, et al. Mannosylated bioreducible nanoparticle-mediated macrophage-specific TNF-alpha RNA interference for IBD therapy. Biomaterials 2013;34(30):7471—82.
[24] Sheng KC, et al. Delivery of antigen using a novel mannosylated dendrimer potentiates immunogenicity in vitro and in vivo. Eur J Immunol 2008;38(2):424—36.
[25] Ranjan Parida K, Kumar Panda S, Ravana P, Roy H, Manickam M, Talwar P. Microparticles based drug delivery systems: preparation and application in cancer therapeutics. Int Arch Appl Sci Technol 2013;4(3).
[26] Beyatricks KJ, Kavimani S, mohan Maruga Raja MK, Kumar KS. Recent trends in microsphere drug delivery system and its therapeutic applications-a review. Crit Rev Pharm Sci 2013;2(1):1—14.
[27] Vilos C, Velasquez LA. Therapeutic strategies based on polymeric microparticles. J Biomed Biotechnol 2012;2012, 672760.
[28] Nidhi RM, Kaur V, Hallan SS, Sharma S, Mishra N. Microparticles as controlled delivery carrier for the treatment of ulcerative colitis: a brief review. Saudi Pharm J July 2016;24(4):458—72.
[29] Singh MN, et al. Microencapsulation: a promising technique for controlled drug delivery. Res Pharm Sci 2010;5(2):65—77.
[30] Vaishya RD, et al. Reversible hydrophobic ion-paring complex strategy to minimize acylation of octreotide during long-term delivery from PLGA microparticles. Int J Pharm 2015;489(1—2):237—45.
[31] Osswald CR, Kang-Mieler JJ. Controlled and extended in vitro release of bioactive anti-vascular endothelial growth factors from a microsphere-hydrogel drug delivery system. Curr Eye Res 2016:1—7.
[32] Ansary RH, et al. Preparation, characterization, and in vitro release studies of insulin-loaded double-walled poly(lactide-co-glycolide) microspheres. Drug Deliv Transl Res 2016;6(3):308—18.
[33] Ansary RH, et al. Preparation, characterization and in vitro release study of BSA-loaded double-walled glucose-poly(lactide-co-glycolide) microspheres. Arch Pharm Res September 2016;39(9):1242—56.
[34] Bawa R, et al. Protecting new ideas and inventions in nanomedicine with patents. Nanomedicine 2005;1(2):150—8.
[35] Kreuter J. Nanoparticles—a historical perspective. Int J Pharm 2007;331(1):1—10.
[36] Ramezanpour M, et al. Computational and experimental approaches for investigating nanoparticle-based drug delivery systems. Biochim Biophys Acta 2016;1858(7 Pt B):1688—709.
[37] Petrushev B, et al. Gold nanoparticles enhance the effect of tyrosine kinase inhibitors in acute myeloid leukemia therapy. Int J Nanomedicine 2016;11:641—60.
[38] Wang M, et al. Efficient delivery of genome-editing proteins using bioreducible lipid nanoparticles. Proc Natl Acad Sci USA March 15, 2016;113(11):2868—73.
[39] Seo SH, et al. Highly sensitive detection of a bio-threat pathogen by gold nanoparticle-based oligonucleotide-linked immunosorbent assay. Biosens Bioelectron 2015;64:69—73.
[40] Inci F, et al. Nanoplasmonic quantitative detection of intact viruses from unprocessed whole blood. ACS Nano 2013;7(6):4733—45.
[41] Moser F, et al. Cellular uptake of gold nanoparticles and their behavior as labels for localization microscopy. Biophys J 2016;110(4):947—53.

[42] Qi P, et al. Biosynthesis of CdS nanoparticles: a fluorescent sensor for sulfate-reducing bacteria detection. Talanta 2016;147:142–6.
[43] Mahmood M, et al. Engineered nanostructural materials for application in cancer biology and medicine. J Appl Toxicol 2012;32(1):10–9.
[44] Jang H, et al. Observation of a flowing duct in the abdominal wall by using nanoparticles. PLoS One 2016;11(3):e0150423.
[45] Choi CH, et al. Mechanism of active targeting in solid tumors with transferrin-containing gold nanoparticles. Proc Natl Acad Sci USA 2010;107(3):1235–40.
[46] Hatzfeld J. Fluctuations of diphenylamine-DNA in yeast. J Cell Physiol 1974;83(1):159–62.
[47] Bazak R, et al. Passive targeting of nanoparticles to cancer: a comprehensive review of the literature. Mol Clin Oncol 2014;2(6):904–8.
[48] Wilczewska AZ, et al. Nanoparticles as drug delivery systems. Pharmacol Rep 2012;64(5):1020–37.
[49] Pal SL, Jana U, Manna PK, Mohanta GP, Manavalan R. Nanoparticles: an overview of preparation and characterization. J Appl Pharm Sci 2011;1(6):228–34.
[50] Lv S, et al. Nanoparticles encapsulating hepatitis B virus cytosine-phosphate-guanosine induce therapeutic immunity against HBV infection. Hepatology 2014;59(2):385–94.
[51] Spaliviero M, et al. Detection of lymph node metastases with SERRS nanoparticles. Mol Imaging Biol October 2016;18(5):677–85.
[52] Hung CC, et al. Active tumor permeation and uptake of surface charge-switchable theranostic nanoparticles for imaging-guided photothermal/chemo combinatorial therapy. Theranostics 2016;6(3):302–17.
[53] Loxley A. Solid lipid nanoparticles for the delivery of pharmaceutical actives. Drug Deliv Technol 2009;9(8).
[54] Jores K, et al. Investigations on the structure of solid lipid nanoparticles (SLN) and oil-loaded solid lipid nanoparticles by photon correlation spectroscopy, field-flow fractionation and transmission electron microscopy. J Control Release 2004;95(2):217–27.
[55] Muller RH, Mader K, Gohla S. Solid lipid nanoparticles (SLN) for controlled drug delivery – a review of the state of the art. Eur J Pharm Biopharm 2000;50(1):161–77.
[56] Uner M, Yener G. Importance of solid lipid nanoparticles (SLN) in various administration routes and future perspectives. Int J Nanomedicine 2007;2(3):289–300.
[57] Schubert MA, Muller-Goymann CC. Solvent injection as a new approach for manufacturing lipid nanoparticles–evaluation of the method and process parameters. Eur J Pharm Biopharm 2003;55(1):125–31.
[58] Ravanfar R, et al. Preservation of anthocyanins in solid lipid nanoparticles: optimization of a microemulsion dilution method using the Placket-Burman and Box-Behnken designs. Food Chem 2016;199:573–80.
[59] Jo YJ, Choi MJ, Kwon YJ. Effect of palm or coconut solid lipid nanoparticles (SLNs) on growth of *Lactobacillus plantarum* in milk. Korean J Food Sci Anim Resour 2015;35(2):197–204.
[60] Videira MA, Arranja AG, Gouveia LF. Experimental design towards an optimal lipid nanosystem: a new opportunity for paclitaxel-based therapeutics. Eur J Pharm Sci 2013;49(2):302–10.
[61] Trotta M, Debernardi F, Caputo O. Preparation of solid lipid nanoparticles by a solvent emulsification-diffusion technique. Int J Pharm 2003;257(1–2):153–60.
[62] Pooja D, et al. Optimization of solid lipid nanoparticles prepared by a single emulsification-solvent evaporation method. Data Brief 2016;6:15–9.
[63] Jain V, et al. Chitosan-assisted immunotherapy for intervention of experimental leishmaniasis via amphotericin B-loaded solid lipid nanoparticles. Appl Biochem Biotechnol 2014;174(4):1309–30.
[64] Charcosset C, El-Harati A, Fessi H. Preparation of solid lipid nanoparticles using a membrane contactor. J Control Release 2005;108(1):112–20.
[65] Mukherjee S, Ray S, Thakur RS. Solid lipid nanoparticles: a modern formulation approach in drug delivery system. Indian J Pharm Sci 2009;71(4):349–58.
[66] Gross R, et al. Diabetes and impaired response of glucagon cells and vascular bed to adenosine in rat pancreas. Diabetes 1989;38(10):1291–5.
[67] Ma Y, et al. STAT3 decoy oligodeoxynucleotides-loaded solid lipid nanoparticles induce cell death and inhibit invasion in ovarian cancer cells. PLoS One 2015;10(4):e0124924.

[68] Gallarate M, et al. Solid lipid nanoparticles loaded with fluorescent-labelled cyclosporine A: anti-inflammatory activity in vitro. Protein Pept Lett 2014;21(11):1157–62.
[69] Yang R, et al. Preparation of gel-core-solid lipid nanoparticle: a novel way to improve the encapsulation of protein and peptide. Chem Pharm Bull 2010;58(9):1195–202.
[70] Yang R, et al. The influence of lipid characteristics on the formation, in vitro release, and in vivo absorption of protein-loaded SLN prepared by the double emulsion process. Drug Dev Ind Pharm 2011;37(2):139–48.
[71] Sur A, et al. Immune activation efficacy of indolicidin is enhanced upon conjugation with carbon nanotubes and gold nanoparticles. PLoS One 2015;10(4):e0123905.
[72] Sun H, et al. Carbon nanotubes enhance intercalated disc assembly in cardiac myocytes via the beta1-integrin-mediated signaling pathway. Biomaterials 2015;55:84–95.
[73] Frank EA, Birch ME, Yadav JS. MyD88 mediates in vivo effector functions of alveolar macrophages in acute lung inflammatory responses to carbon nanotube exposure. Toxicol Appl Pharmacol 2015;288(3):322–9.
[74] Barzegar A, Mansouri A, Azamat J. Molecular dynamics simulation of non-covalent single-walled carbon nanotube functionalization with surfactant peptides. J Mol Graph Model 2016;64:75–84.
[75] Weng X, et al. Carbon nanotubes as a protein toxin transporter for selective HER2-positive breast cancer cell destruction. Mol Biosyst 2009;5(10):1224–31.
[76] Immordino ML, Dosio F, Cattel L. Stealth liposomes: review of the basic science, rationale, and clinical applications, existing and potential. Int J Nanomedicine 2006;1(3):297–315.
[77] Akbarzadeh A, et al. Liposome: classification, preparation, and applications. Nanoscale Res Lett 2013;8(1):102.
[78] Duehrkop C, et al. Development and characterization of an innovative heparin coating to stabilize and protect liposomes against adverse immune reactions. Colloids Surf B Biointerfaces 2016;141:576–83.
[79] Resnier P, et al. Efficient in vitro gene therapy with PEG siRNA lipid nanocapsules for passive targeting strategy in melanoma. Biotechnol J 2014;9(11):1389–401.
[80] Rauscher A, et al. Influence of pegylation and hapten location at the surface of radiolabelled liposomes on tumour immunotargeting using bispecific antibody. Nucl Med Biol 2014;(41 Suppl.):e66–74.
[81] Gray BP, McGuire MJ, Brown KC. A liposomal drug platform overrides peptide ligand targeting to a cancer biomarker, irrespective of ligand affinity or density. PLoS One 2013;8(8):e72938.
[82] Patil YP, Jadhav S. Novel methods for liposome preparation. Chem Phys Lipids 2014;177:8–18.
[83] Kishimoto T, et al. A case of malignant mesothelioma caused by exposure to asbestos. Nihon Kyobu Shikkan Gakkai Zasshi 1987;25(1):125–9.
[84] Duzgunes N, et al. Delivery of antiviral agents in liposomes. Methods Enzymol 2005;391:351–73.
[85] Kajimoto K, et al. Noninvasive and persistent transfollicular drug delivery system using a combination of liposomes and iontophoresis. Int J Pharm 2011;403(1–2):57–65.
[86] Li J, et al. Gene therapy for psoriasis in the K14-VEGF transgenic mouse model by topical transdermal delivery of interleukin-4 using ultradeformable cationic liposome. J Gene Med 2010;12(6):481–90.
[87] Han W, et al. Efficacy of RNA interference mediated by cationic liposomes. Sheng Wu Gong Cheng Xue Bao 2015;31(8):1239–46.
[88] Shin DH, et al. Synergistic effect of immunoliposomal gemcitabine and bevacizumab in glioblastoma stem cell-targeted therapy. J Biomed Nanotechnol 2015;11(11):1989–2002.
[89] Liguori L, et al. Anti-tumor effects of Bak-proteoliposomes against glioblastoma. Molecules 2015;20(9):15893–909.
[90] Camelo S, et al. Protective effect of intravitreal injection of vasoactive intestinal peptide-loaded liposomes on experimental autoimmune uveoretinitis. J Ocul Pharmacol Ther 2009;25(1):9–21.
[91] Camelo S, et al. Ocular and systemic bio-distribution of rhodamine-conjugated liposomes loaded with VIP injected into the vitreous of Lewis rats. Mol Vis 2007;13:2263–74.
[92] Lajavardi L, et al. Downregulation of endotoxin-induced uveitis by intravitreal injection of vasoactive intestinal peptide encapsulated in liposomes. Invest Ophthalmol Vis Sci 2007;48(7):3230–8.
[93] Umashankar MS, Sachdeva RK, Gulati M. Aquasomes: a promising carrier for peptides and protein delivery. Nanomedicine 2010;6(3):419–26.

[94] Goyal AK, et al. Aquasomes—a nanoparticulate approach for the delivery of antigen. Drug Dev Ind Pharm 2008;34(12):1297—305.
[95] Kaur K, et al. Stealth lipid coated aquasomes bearing recombinant human interferon-alpha-2b offered prolonged release and enhanced cytotoxicity in ovarian cancer cells. Biomed Pharmacother 2015;69:267—76.
[96] Pandey RS, et al. Carbohydrate modified ultrafine ceramic nanoparticles for allergen immunotherapy. Int Immunopharmacol 2011;11(8):925—31.
[97] Xu W, Ling P, Zhang T. Polymeric micelles, a promising drug delivery system to enhance bioavailability of poorly water-soluble drugs. J Drug Deliv 2013:340315.
[98] Penfold J, et al. Adsorption at air-water and oil-water interfaces and self-assembly in aqueous solution of ethoxylated polysorbate nonionic surfactants. Langmuir 2015;31(10):3003—11.
[99] Das K, Maiti S, Das PK. Probing enzyme location in water-in-oil microemulsion using enzyme-carbon dot conjugates. Langmuir 2014;30(9):2448—59.
[100] Mu C, et al. Solubilization of flurbiprofen into aptamer-modified PEG-PLA micelles for targeted delivery to brain-derived endothelial cells in vitro. J Microencapsul 2013;30(7):701—8.
[101] Binkhathlan Z, et al. Encapsulation of P-glycoprotein inhibitors by polymeric micelles can reduce their pharmacokinetic interactions with doxorubicin. Eur J Pharm Biopharm 2012;81(1):142—8.
[102] Kedar U, et al. Advances in polymeric micelles for drug delivery and tumor targeting. Nanomedicine 2010;6(6):714—29.
[103] Li H, et al. Folate-bovine serum albumin functionalized polymeric micelles loaded with superparamagnetic iron oxide nanoparticles for tumor targeting and magnetic resonance imaging. Acta Biomater 2015;15:117—26.
[104] Banerjee A, Onyuksel H. A novel peptide nanomedicine for treatment of pancreatogenic diabetes. Nanomedicine 2013;9(6):722—8.
[105] Xiao W, et al. Discovery and characterization of a high-affinity and high-specificity peptide ligand LXY30 for in vivo targeting of alpha3 integrin-expressing human tumors. EJNMMI Res 2016;6(1):18.
[106] Hsieh TH, et al. A novel cell-penetrating peptide suppresses breast tumorigenesis by inhibiting beta-catenin/LEF-1 signaling. Sci Rep 2016;6:19156.
[107] McGuire MJ, et al. Identification and characterization of a suite of tumor targeting peptides for non-small cell lung cancer. Sci Rep 2014;4:4480.
[108] Heo K, et al. An aptamer-antibody complex (oligobody) as a novel delivery platform for targeted cancer therapies. J Control Release 2016;229:1—9.
[109] Byrd JC, et al. Acalabrutinib (ACP-196) in relapsed chronic lymphocytic leukemia. N Engl J Med 2016;374(4):323—32.
[110] Gaudana R, et al. Ocular drug delivery. AAPS J 2010;12(3):348—60.
[111] El Sanharawi M, et al. Protein delivery for retinal diseases: from basic considerations to clinical applications. Prog Retin Eye Res 2010;29(6):443—65.
[112] Brown DM, et al. Intravitreal aflibercept for diabetic macular edema: 100-week results from the VISTA and VIVID studies. Ophthalmology 2015;122(10):2044—52.
[113] Brown DM, et al. Long-term outcomes of ranibizumab therapy for diabetic macular edema: the 36-month results from two phase III trials: RISE and RIDE. Ophthalmology 2013;120(10):2013—22.
[114] Tolentino M. Systemic and ocular safety of intravitreal anti-VEGF therapies for ocular neovascular disease. Surv Ophthalmol 2011;56(2):95—113.
[115] Ng EW, Adamis AP. Anti-VEGF aptamer (pegaptanib) therapy for ocular vascular diseases. Ann NY Acad Sci 2006;1082:151—71.
[116] Hagigit T, et al. Ocular antisense oligonucleotide delivery by cationic nanoemulsion for improved treatment of ocular neovascularization: an in-vivo study in rats and mice. J Control Release 2012;160(2):225—31.
[117] Nguyen QD, et al. Phase 1 dose-escalation study of a siRNA targeting the RTP801 gene in age-related macular degeneration patients. Eye 2012;26(8):1099—105.

[118] Liu GS, et al. Gene delivery by subconjunctival injection of adenovirus in rats: a study of local distribution, transgene duration and safety. PLoS One 2015;10(12):e0143956.
[119] Oh B, Lee M. Combined delivery of HMGB-1 box A peptide and S1PLyase siRNA in animal models of acute lung injury. J Control Release 2014;175:25—35.
[120] Ndeboko B, et al. Therapeutic potential of cell penetrating peptides (CPPs) and cationic polymers for chronic hepatitis B. Int J Mol Sci 2015;16(12):28230—41.
[121] Reynolds MA, Aichelmann-Reidy ME. Protein and peptide-based therapeutics in periodontal regeneration. J Evid Based Dent Pract 2012;12(3 Suppl.):118—26.
[122] Klein J, et al. The role of urinary peptidomics in kidney disease research. Kidney Int 2016;89(3): 539—45.
[123] Vincenti F, et al. Belatacept and long-term outcomes in kidney transplantation. N Engl J Med 2016; 374(4):333—43.
[124] Di Fede G, et al. Tackling amyloidogenesis in Alzheimer's disease with A2V variants of Amyloid-beta. Sci Rep 2016;6:20949.
[125] Ruhanen H, et al. Potential of known and short prokaryotic protein motifs as a basis for novel peptide-based antibacterial therapeutics: a computational survey. Front Microbiol 2014;5:4.
[126] Egawa EY, et al. A DNA hybridization system for labeling of neural stem cells with SPIO nanoparticles for MRI monitoring post-transplantation. Biomaterials 2015;54:158—67.
[127] Kim YT, et al. Synergistic effect of detection and separation for pathogen using magnetic clusters. Bioconjug Chem 2016;27(1):59—65.
[128] Pivetal J, et al. Development and applications of a DNA labeling method with magnetic nanoparticles to study the role of horizontal gene transfer events between bacteria in soil pollutant bioremediation processes. Environ Sci Pollut Res Int 2015;22(24):20322—7.
[129] Gao Y, et al. A selective and purification-free strategy for labeling adherent cells with inorganic nanoparticles. ACS Appl Mater Interfaces 2016;8(10):6336—43.
[130] Mirahmadi-Zare SZ, et al. Super magnetic nanoparticles NiFe$_2$O$_4$, coated with aluminum-nickel oxide sol-gel lattices to safe, sensitive and selective purification of his-tagged proteins. Protein Expr Purif 2016;121:52—60.
[131] Yuan C, et al. Magnetic nanoparticles for targeted therapeutic gene delivery and magnetic-inducing heating on hepatoma. Nanotechnology 2014;25(34):345101.
[132] Li C, Li L, Keates AC. Targeting cancer gene therapy with magnetic nanoparticles. Oncotarget 2012; 3(4):365—70.
[133] Torres-Lugo M, Rinaldi C. Thermal potentiation of chemotherapy by magnetic nanoparticles. Nanomedicine 2013;8(10):1689—707.
[134] Bellizzi G, Bucci OM. On the optimal choice of the exposure conditions and the nanoparticle features in magnetic nanoparticle hyperthermia. Int J Hyperth 2010;26(4):389—403.
[135] Dzudzevic Cancar H, et al. A novel acetylcholinesterase biosensor: core-shell magnetic nanoparticles incorporating a conjugated polymer for the detection of organophosphorus pesticides. ACS Appl Mater Interfaces 2016;8(12):8058—67.
[136] Hardiansyah A, et al. Core-shell of FePt@SiO2-Au magnetic nanoparticles for rapid SERS detection. Nanoscale Res Lett 2015;10(1):412.
[137] Sun AL, Qi QA, Dong ZL. Label-free electrochemical immunosensor for the determination of feto-protein based on core-shell-shell nanocomposite particles. Protein Pept Lett 2008;15(8):782—8.
[138] Mirsadeghi S, et al. Effect of PEGylated superparamagnetic iron oxide nanoparticles (SPIONs) under magnetic field on amyloid beta fibrillation process. Mater Sci Eng C Mater Biol Appl 2016;59: 390—7.
[139] Chen L, et al. Neuropilin-1 (NRP-1) and magnetic nanoparticles, a potential combination for diagnosis and therapy of gliomas. Curr Pharm Des 2015;21(37):5434—49.
[140] Sharma PA, et al. Nanomaterial based approaches for the diagnosis and therapy of cardiovascular diseases. Curr Pharm Des 2015;21(30):4465—78.
[141] Xue S, et al. 99mTc-labeled iron oxide nanoparticles for dual-contrast (T_1/T_2) magnetic resonance and dual-modality imaging of tumor angiogenesis. J Biomed Nanotechnol 2015;11(6):1027—37.

[142] Vannucci L, et al. In vivo targeting of cutaneous melanoma using an melanoma stimulating hormone-engineered human protein cage with fluorophore and magnetic resonance imaging tracers. J Biomed Nanotechnol 2015;11(1):81−92.
[143] Eitan E, et al. Combination therapy with lenalidomide and nanoceria ameliorates CNS autoimmunity. Exp Neurol 2015;273:151−60.
[144] Wang Y, et al. In vivo MR and fluorescence dual-modality imaging of atherosclerosis characteristics in mice using profilin-1 targeted magnetic nanoparticles. Theranostics 2016;6(2):272−86.
[145] Ge XD, et al. Optimal concentration of superparamagnetic iron oxide-short hairpin RNA dual functional molecular probe transfected into ovarian cancer cells in vitro. Beijing Da Xue Xue Bao 2015;47(5):754−60.
[146] Ye M, et al. A novel method for the detection of point mutation in DNA using single-base-coded CdS nanoprobes. Biosens Bioelectron 2009;24(8):2339−45.
[147] Cai W, et al. Applications of gold nanoparticles in cancer nanotechnology. Nanotechnol Sci Appl 2008;2008(1).
[148] Medley CD, et al. Gold nanoparticle-based colorimetric assay for the direct detection of cancerous cells. Anal Chem 2008;80(4):1067−72.
[149] Lau IP, et al. Aptamer-based bio-barcode assay for the detection of cytochrome-c released from apoptotic cells. Biochem Biophys Res Commun 2010;395(4):560−4.
[150] Kah JC, et al. Early diagnosis of oral cancer based on the surface plasmon resonance of gold nanoparticles. Int J Nanomedicine 2007;2(4):785−98.
[151] Kumar V, et al. Graphene-CNT nanohybrid aptasensor for label free detection of cardiac biomarker myoglobin. Biosens Bioelectron 2015;72:56−60.
[152] Sharma A, et al. Single-walled carbon nanotube based transparent immunosensor for detection of a prostate cancer biomarker osteopontin. Anal Chim Acta 2015;869:68−73.
[153] Nima ZA, et al. Circulating tumor cell identification by functionalized silver-gold nanorods with multicolor, super-enhanced SERS and photothermal resonances. Sci Rep 2014;4:4752.
[154] Liao YJ, et al. Detection of adenosine triphosphate through polymerization-induced aggregation of actin-conjugated gold/silver nanorods. Nanotechnology 2013;24(44):444003.
[155] Villar-Vazquez R, et al. Development of a novel multiplex beads-based assay for autoantibody detection for colorectal cancer diagnosis. Proteomics 2016;16(8):1280−90.
[156] Luo Y, et al. The clinical performance evaluation of novel protein chips for eleven biomarkers detection and the diagnostic model study. Int J Clin Exp Med 2015;8(11):20413−23.
[157] Lee KJ, et al. Application of peptide displaying phage as a novel diagnostic probe for human lung adenocarcinoma. Amino Acids 2016;48(4):1079−86.

CHAPTER 8

Nanotechnology in Intracellular Trafficking, Imaging, and Delivery of Therapeutic Agents

Animikh Ray, Ashim K. Mitra
University of Missouri—Kansas City, Kansas City, MO, United States

Contents

1. Introduction	169
1.1 Nanotechnology in Intracellular Trafficking	171
2. Mechanisms	171
2.1 Clathrin-Mediated Endocytosis	171
2.2 Caveolae-Mediated Endocytosis	172
2.3 Clathrin and Caveolae-Independent Mechanisms	172
2.4 RhoA-Mediated Uptake	173
2.5 Clathrin-Independent Carriers/Glycosylphosphotidylinositol-Anchored Protein Enriched Early Endosomal Compartments Pathway	173
2.6 Flotillin-Mediated Endocytosis	173
3. Macropinocytosis	173
3.1 Phagocytosis	174
3.2 Different Phases in Intracellular Trafficking of Nanomaterials	174
3.3 Early Endocytic Vesicles	174
3.4 Late Endosomes—Multivesicular Bodies	174
3.5 Lysosomes	177
3.6 Intracellular Trafficking of Nanomaterials	178
3.7 Mechanisms of Particle Uptake Into Cell Nucleus	179
3.8 Imaging Technology for Intracellular Trafficking of Nanostructures	180
3.8.1 Confocal Microscopy	*180*
3.8.2 Quantum Dots and Gold Nanoparticles	*181*
3.8.3 Gold Nanoparticles	*183*
4. Conclusion	185
References	185

1. INTRODUCTION

Drug delivery across the cell membrane has been widely investigated by scientists. However, not much work has been done on the fate of therapeutics in the intracellular environment. This review deals with advances in the field of nanotechnology investigating localization of agents in the intracellular environment particularly their role in imaging and diagnosis. It can be stated that subcellular organelle-specific targeting of therapeutic and diagnostic agents has become the new frontier in drug delivery. A variety of pharmaceutical platforms in the nanometer size range, such as liposomes, carbon nanotubes, quantum dots, nanomicelles, and dendrimers, have been investigated for their ability to target subcellular components. Significant improvement has been achieved in the area of organelle-targeted nanocarrier. There is a need to understand the effects of size and shape of nanocarriers on intracellular trafficking and distribution. It is also of paramount importance to determine whether release of therapeutics can be controlled in the intracellular environment. If successful, nanocarriers can be directed toward intracellular organelle where the therapeutics can exert pharmacological effect. Answers to these and similar other questions will lead to a better understanding of targeted intracellular drug delivery.

To answer these questions, the fate of nanocarriers needs to be tracked real time. A rapid enhancement in imaging technologies will allow scientists to explore this area of research. Some of the exciting technological advancements this chapter will review include state-of-the-art confocal microscopes, quantum dots, and gold nanoparticles. Such technologies will allow us to determine disposition of nanocarriers in the intracellular environment with respect to space and time. Rapid improvement in confocal and fluorescent microscopic techniques has given the scientific community an effective tool to image the entry and trafficking of drug-loaded nanocarriers in the intracellular environment. Time-lapsed and z-stacked images provide detailed information about the intracellular environment and delivery of nanoparticles and other nanocarriers. Quantum dots, also referred to as nanocrystals, are made of semiconductor materials. Gradually it has acquired an important position in nanotechnological research. A detailed discussion on quantum dots is beyond the scope if this chapter. However, their role in intracellular imaging and delivery will be examined. Similar to quantum dots, gold nanoparticle is another important imaging and delivery tool.

Pharmaceutical nanocarriers offer an ideal platform to modify disposition of a drug without modifying the molecule itself. Different chemical modifications can be carried out on the components making up the nanocarrier system, which can be loaded with therapeutics. This will lead to targeted therapy without any structural modification of the drug molecule itself. A majority of pharmaceutical nanocarriers are surface modified, which leads to targeted delivery. Another type of targeted delivery that does not involve any modification of nanocarriers is size-dependent targeting. Nanocarriers such as long circulating liposomes and nanoparticles may be able to passively target tissues and cells with leaky vasculature. This is possible due to the enhanced permeability and retention effect. These two different targeting strategies can be classified into active and passive targeting, respectively, and will be discussed in this chapter.

The internal environment of a cell varies vastly from an aqueous buffer solution. In a buffered environment therapeutic molecules have considerable freedom to diffuse and freely interact. The intracellular environment contains cytoskeletal network and numerous organelles. The cytoplasm expresses a large quantity of macromolecules such as proteins and carbohydrates. Hence the diffusion or transport of a therapeutic molecule in such a viscous and crowded environment will be different from that in a buffered solution. Usually diffusion of drug molecules in the intracellular environment is considered to be hindered diffusion reflecting the high degree of molecular crowding. Also, the viscous nature of the cytoplasmic environment and binding of drug molecules to intracellular components may affect diffusion of drugs inside a cell. Another important parameter that needs to be kept in mind while designing nanocarriers is the physicochemical properties of the therapeutic molecule. It plays an important role in the determination of the subcellular fate of drug molecule.

Another important role of nanocarriers that will be reviewed in this chapter will be targeted drug delivery of nanocarriers to different organelles. Special focus will be on nucleus as it is the site of action for many important anticancer drugs such as doxorubicin. How nanocarriers can be effectively sequestered to its targeted site of action inside the cell is an important concept that is discussed in this review. Different targeting moieties are used to specifically target nanocarriers into the organelle. These include peptides, antibodies, DNA, RNA, and other molecules. A detailed knowledge of these targeting moieties is essential to understand how nanotechnology can effectively lead to targeted intracellular delivery. Fig. 8.1 depicts the different parameters affecting intracellular trafficking of different nanoformulations.

1.1 Nanotechnology in Intracellular Trafficking

Nanocarriers such as nanoparticles, nanomicelles, and liposomes have been investigated widely for their ability to deliver therapeutics to intracellular compartments. It is necessary to understand the mechanism of entry of these nanocarriers into the subcellular space crossing the barrier of plasma membrane. This section provides an in-depth account of these mechanisms.

2. MECHANISMS

2.1 Clathrin-Mediated Endocytosis

Cargoes such as nanoparticles usually undertake the clathrin-mediated pathway for translocation across plasma membrane (PM) [1]. Clathrin-mediated endocytosis (CME) begins with accumulation of clathrin from cytoplasm [2]. These clathrins are sequestered at regions of PM referred as clathrin-coated pits (CCPs). This is followed by invagination of CCPs forming separate vesicles that are then detached from the PM to form clathrin-coated vesicles. There are adapter proteins that are responsible for molecular signals that lead to the formation of clathrin-coated vehicles. These adapter proteins interact with numerous regulatory proteins such as AP180 and epsin that control formation of clathrin-coated pits, detachment of vesicles from PM, and the different interactions of these vesicles with cytoskeleton [3].

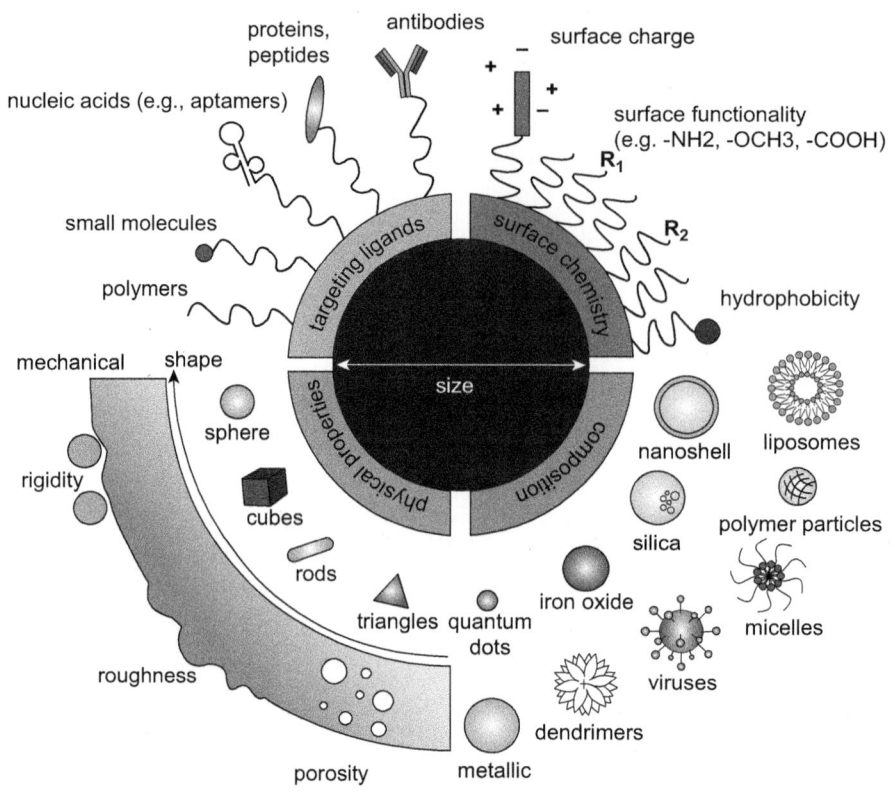

Figure 8.1 Targeting ligands, surface charge, shape, and other parameters critical for nanoformulations such as dendrimers, micelles, and nanoparticles to be delivered to their intracellular compartments. *(Published with permission from the Royal Society of Chemistry.)*

2.2 Caveolae-Mediated Endocytosis

Caveolae are protrusion in PM with a size range of 50–80 nm [4]. These are responsible for uptake of nanocarriers in a clathrin-independent pathway. Structurally caveolae consists of cholesterol, sphingolipids, Glycosylphosphatidylinositol-anchored proteins, and integral membrane proteins caveolin-1 and caveolin-2 [5,6]. Particles having size of ≤100 nm have been observed to utilize pathway mediated by caveolae to gain entry into the intracellular compartment. Finally, uptake of these nanocarriers is completed by detachment of the vesicles from PM, such as CME [7,8].

2.3 Clathrin and Caveolae-Independent Mechanisms

Pathways that are independent of clathrin and caveolae is an active field of research. There is no consensus regarding which pathways are dependent and independent of clathrin and caveolae. However, a majority of scientists agree that broadly they can be classified into three pathways. The commonly accepted clathrin-, caveolae-, and macropinocytosis-independent pathways are RhoA-mediated uptake, clathrin-independent carriers

(CLIC)/glycosylphosphotidylinositol-anchored protein enriched early endosomal compartments (GEEC) pathways, and flotillin-mediated endocytosis [9].

2.4 RhoA-Mediated Uptake

This pathway is regulated by GTPase RhoA. This pathway was initially observed while internalization of β-chain of interleukin-2 receptor (IL-2Rβ) was being investigated. This pathway is independent of clathrin as supported by the fact that IL-2Rβ uptake was influenced by Rac1, p21 (RAC1) activated kinase 1 (PAK1), and PAK2 [10]. These factors are not involved in CME.

2.5 Clathrin-Independent Carriers/Glycosylphosphotidylinositol-Anchored Protein Enriched Early Endosomal Compartments Pathway

Another clathrin- and caveolae-independent mechanism is the CLIC/GEEC pathway. Structurally CLIC/GEEC pathway consists of a ∼40-nm-wide tube-shaped protrusion along with GTPase regulator. It is associated with focal adhesion kinase-1 (GRAF1) and phosphatidylinositol-4,5-bisphosphate 3-kinase [11]. These membrane carriers are attenuated by cdc42 and ARF1.

2.6 Flotillin-Mediated Endocytosis

Flotillins are proteins similar to caveolin-1 embedded in the PM. These proteins appear as a cluster of organized domains within the PM. It has been observed that domains consisting of flotillin get detached from PM in a clathrin-independent manner. Following entry of the vesicles in the cytoplasmic environment, flotillins are found inside multivesicular structures that exhibit close relationship with endosomal processes [12,13].

It has been suggested that flotillin-mediated endocytosis plays a crucial role in nanoparticle uptake. Several studies have shown that flotillin is involved in the uptake of polyplexes and silica nanoparticles. These studies provide evidence of flotillin in endocytic processes that are responsible for nanoparticle entry and trafficking [14,15].

3. MACROPINOCYTOSIS

Classical macropinocytosis is a clathrin- and caveolae-independent mechanism. It involves uptake of high volume of liquid and extracellular substances that are taken up via formation of macropinosomes [16,17]. Structurally macropinocytosis is created by ruffle formation as well as uptake of classical fluid phase markers such as horseradish peroxidase and dextran [18]. The mechanism of uptake is facilitated by a group of small GTPases such as Ras, Cdc42, and Rac1 [19,20]. Macropinocytosis may either take place spontaneously or may be triggered by the influence of growth factors that activate receptor tyrosine kinases. The GTPases and kinases are responsible for signal transduction pathways that induce actin modulation [21]. This in turn induces development of the macropinocytic cup. It has been reported that several cationic nanoparticles are taken up by micropinocytosis. The surface charge of nanocarriers influences their mechanism of uptake [22].

3.1 Phagocytosis

The mechanism of phagocytosis is similar to that of macropinocytosis involving polymerization of actin, which causes membrane ruffling. It takes place when phagocytic cells such as dendritic cells and macrophage engulf particles larger than 0.5 μm [23]. Various types of nanoparticles such as gold and silver use this pathway to enter the intracellular environment [23]. Fig. 8.2 depicts these pathways.

3.2 Different Phases in Intracellular Trafficking of Nanomaterials

As discussed in the previous section, nanoparticles utilize several endocytic pathways to gain entry into the intracellular compartments. Following uptake, nanoparticles are carried along a particular route of endocytosis. The mechanism of nanoparticle uptake into intracellular compartments is a dynamic process with respect to protein content inside endocytic vesicles. During the process of uptake several adapters as well as effector proteins are conjugated or exchanged from surface of vesicular structures containing the nanocarriers [24]. The fusion of endocytic vesicles and process of vesicular maturation may change the nature of protein content on a nanoparticle-containing vesicle. This process begins in early phases of intracellular trafficking. Early endosomes and macropinosomes fuse to form new vesicle [25]. Fig. 8.3 depicts the different events that occur during fusion of endocytic vesicles containing nanoparticles.

3.3 Early Endocytic Vesicles

Endocytic vesicles in the initial stages are a diverse group of structures in the early phase of intracellular trafficking. Early-stage endosomes are characterized by specific marker proteins such as EEA1 or Rab5 and coexist in different subpopulations [26,27]. It has been observed that endosomes that mature in a slow pace exhibit reduced motility. On the other hand, vesicles exhibiting rapid maturation are highly mobile [28].

3.4 Late Endosomes—Multivesicular Bodies

Late endosomes are also referred to as multivesicular bodies (MVBs) [29]. In most cases these vesicles are created from early endosomes. These are physiologically significant events and possibly regulate many important processes such as cell signaling or exocytosis. Structurally, MVBs are 400–1000 nm large cytoplasmic organelles made of small intraluminal vesicles (ILVs) with an average size of approximately 50 nm [30]. As MVBs

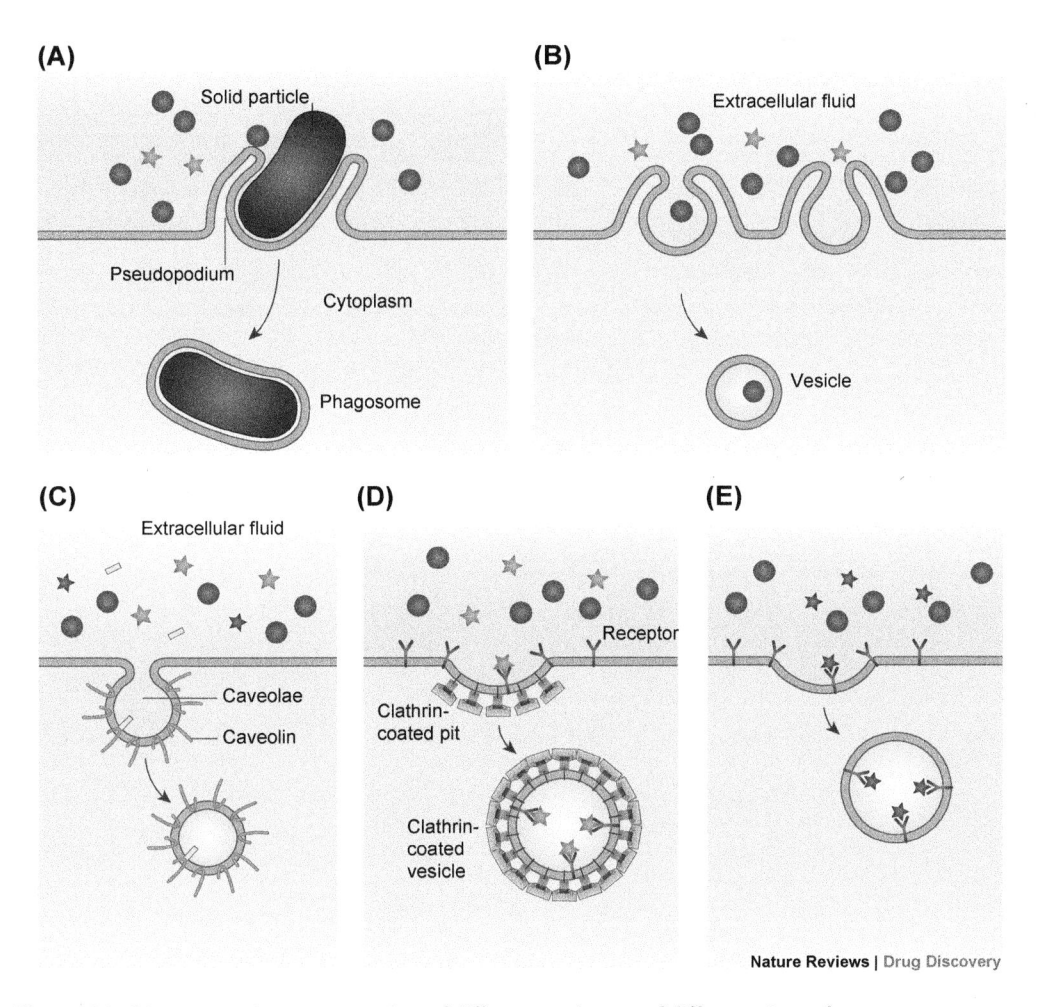

Figure 8.2 Diagrammatic representation of different pathways of different sizes of nanostructure entry into the subcellular space. (A) Phagocytosis; (B) macropinocytosis (>1 µm); (C) clathrin-mediated endocytosis (~60 µm); (D) caveolae-mediated endocytosis (~120 µm); and (E) clathrin-independent and caveolae-independent endocytosis (~90 µm). *(Published with permission from Nature Publishing Group.)*

coalesce with the PM, ILVs are extruded out as exosomes in a process influenced by Rab27b protein [31,32]. It has been observed that cells that are devoid of NPC1 retain nanotransporters within the endosomal system for a longer period compared with healthy cells [33]. This result indicates a significant role of NPC1-dependent cholesterol homeostasis in intracellular trafficking pathways of nanoparticles [34]. Both early and late endosomes play significant roles in intracellular drug delivery strategies [35]. Drugs targeted to mitochondria and nucleus exploit this pathway [36]. Fig. 8.4 depicts utilization of nanostructures within different endocytic vesicles for intracellular drug delivery.

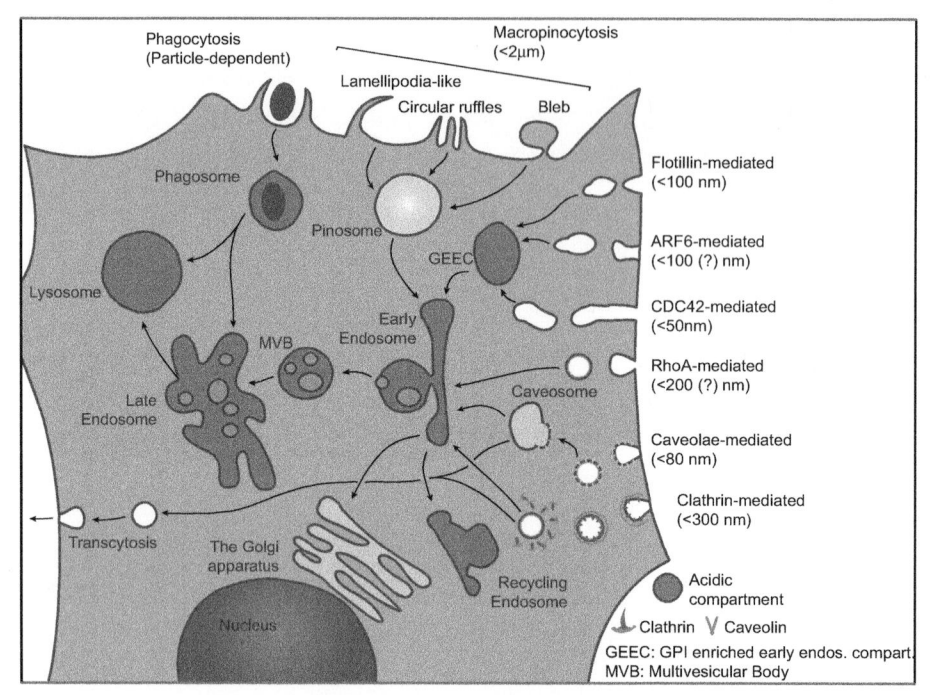

Figure 8.3 Various stages and proteins involved in different stages of endocytic vesicles formation. *(Published with permission from the Royal Society of Chemistry.)*

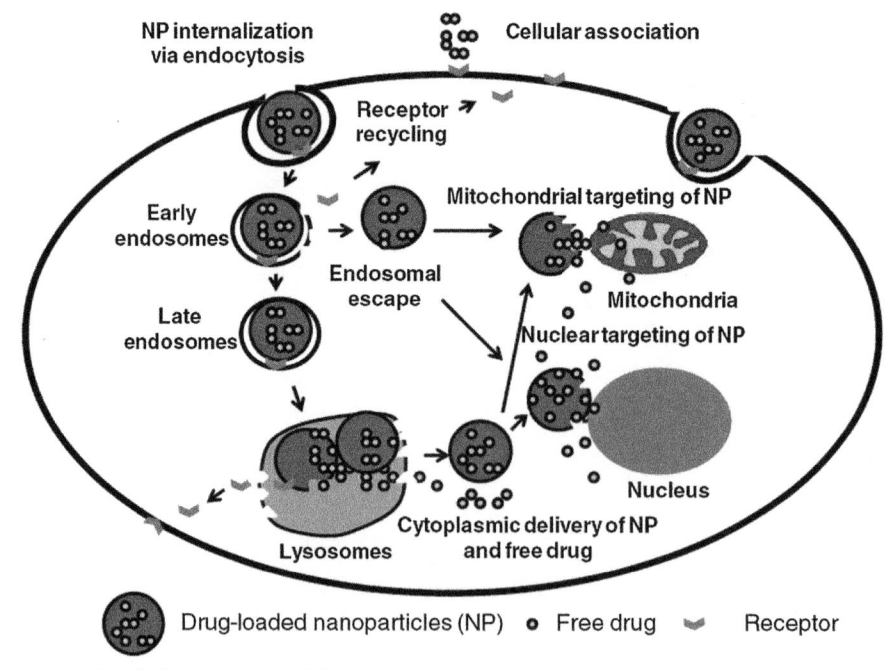

Figure 8.4 Subcellular targeting of functionalized nanoconstructs via the endocytic pathway [37].

3.5 Lysosomes

Lysosomes are considered to be final organelles in endocytic as well as autophagocytic pathways. These vesicles are the final destination for numerous components [38]. Lysosomes can influence biochemical events such as expression of surface receptors and inhibition of microbial infections [39,40]. Microscopic examinations demonstrate that the structure and volume of lysosomes are nonuniform. The internal environment of lysosomes is acidic in nature with a pH of 4.6—5 [41]. This acidity is created and maintained by numerous H+ ATPases. The lysosomal membrane is degraded following treatment of cells with pH-sensitive chitosan nanoparticles encapsulating methotrexate (MTX). Fig. 8.5 depicts the effect of MTX-loaded nanoparticle on lysosomal membrane. This process has been investigated with acridine orange (AO) relocation technique [42]. While designing nanoformulations, investigators need to be careful that the target of the drug delivery system is not the lysosome. These particles need to undergo endosomal escape before formation of lysosome. Once the nanostructures are engulfed by lysosome the particles are degraded and are unable to deliver their payload if the target is nucleus, mitochondria, or some other organelle.

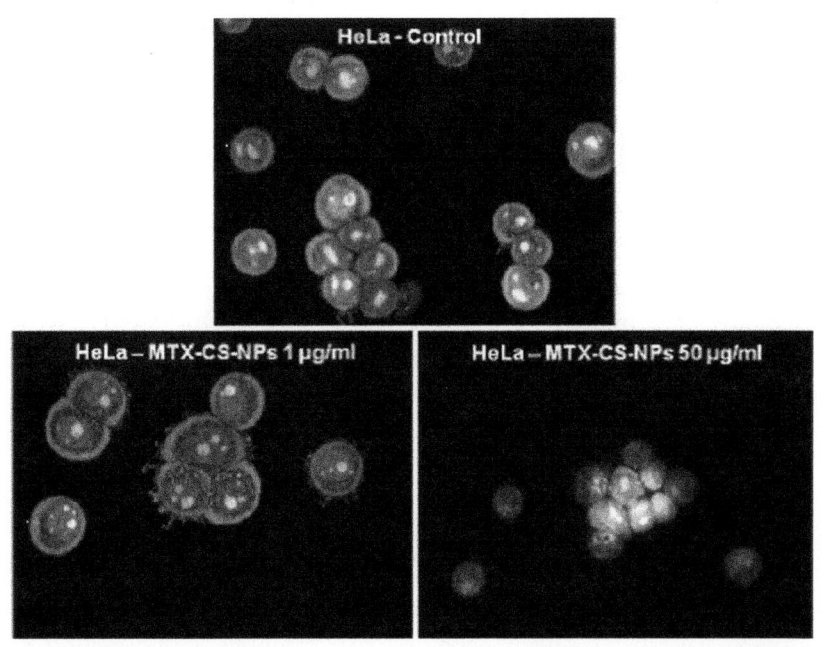

Figure 8.5 Assessment of the effects of chitosan nanoparticles (NPs) encapsulating methotrexate (MTX) (MTX-CS-NPs) on lysosomal membrane permeabilization in HeLa cells as visualized via AO staining. In untreated control cells, lysosomes can be seen as red—orange granules and cytoplasm shows a diffuse green fluorescence. In cells with lysosomal membrane damage (HeLa cells treated with 50 mg/mL MTX-CS-NPs) is evident [42].

3.6 Intracellular Trafficking of Nanomaterials

Studies using polyplexes have revealed active movement of these nanostructures inside endolysosomal vesicles [14]. Several approaches have been adopted to deliver drug-loaded nanocarrier into the subcellular organelles. Nanocarriers by virtue of their particulate nature are believed to be subject to endocytic cellular entry mechanisms and subsequent endolysosomal processing [43]. Nanoconstructs are hypothesized to be ideal for delivery of therapeutics to the endolysosomal system. Significant research is being carried out regarding nanomedicine uptake by the endolysosomal system. This endolysosomal system may act as a target for drug-loaded nanoparticles as many diseases are associated with endosomes and lysosomes. It may potentially act as vehicle for delivery of therapeutics to intracellular sites of action such as mitochondria or nucleus [44]. Drug-loaded nanoconstructs that are endocytosed into clathrin-dependent receptor-mediated endocytosis are prone to degradation by lysosome. Nanoconstructs that undergo uptake by clathrin-independent endocytosis may lead to endosomal accumulation [45]. Hence design of nanoconstruct must consider this aspect while creating a drug delivery platform. The nature of ligand conjugated to nanoconstruct influences whether the drug delivery system successfully deposits its cargo to endosomes or ends up degraded in lysosomes [46].

Biomolecules formed in cytoplasm often include short peptide chains [47]. These short peptide sequences are also referred to as "molecular zip codes." These molecules influence specific uptake of biomolecules into subcellular organelles [48,49]. Such short peptides are usually identified by an import mechanism located in the specific organelle. These molecular zip codes may be exploited to deliver nanoconstructs into different subcellular compartments. Mitochondria and nucleus are the two most widely targeted organelles currently being investigated. The reason is that these two organelles are probably critical to the pathology of numerous diseases. Hence these organelles are attractive targets for drug-loaded nanoconstructs [50]. Numerous liposomal formulation modified surface conjugated with mitochondriotropic ligands have enhanced efficacy of anticancer drugs. Gold nanoparticles have been widely selected to deliver into the nucleus with ligands such as adenoviral nuclear localization signal (NLS) and fragments of domain that bind to integrin [40]. To enhance uptake of therapeutic DNA into nucleus, a capped 3.3-kilobase pair cytomegalovirus luciferase-NLS gene containing a NLS peptide (PKKKRKVEDPYC) was created [51]. Transfection was enhanced a thousandfold due to presence of the peptide chain. Nanoconstructs may be conjugated to ligands that carry them toward the target organelle or these particles may be prepared with inherent predisposition toward a particular organelle. Some examples of the targeted ligand approach have been already included. An example of the second approach is the use of mitochondriotropic amphiphilic dequalinium chloride [52–54]. This molecule can undergo self-assembly to form vesicles referred to as DQAsomes or

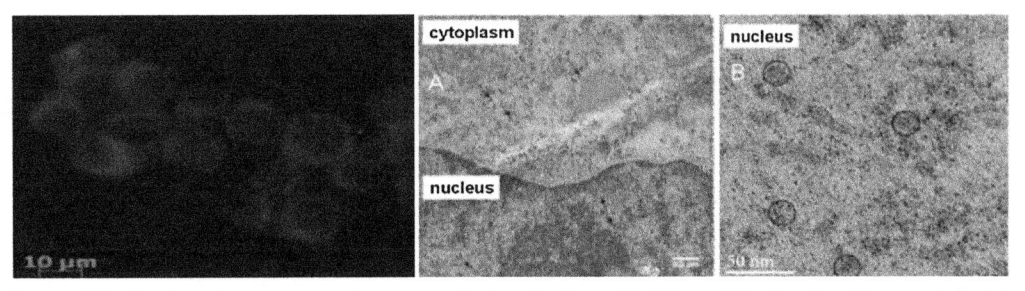

Figure 8.6 Confocal images showing separate localization of differentially localized layered double hydroxide nanoparticles. (A) Hexagonal sheets; (B) nanorods. *(Published with permission from the Royal Society of Chemistry.)*

dequalinium (DQA)-based liposome-like vesicles. DQAsomes are composed of mitochondriotropic molecules and are considered to be ideal for mitochondria-specific delivery of therapeutic macromolecules. These vesicles can also be an excellent vehicle for delivery of small molecule drugs, especially anticancer therapeutics, which cause apoptosis by their pharmacological action in the mitochondria. Another mitochondria-specific nanoformulation is referred to as mitochondria-porter liposomes [55]. These vesicles fuse to the membrane of mitochondria and release their content in the inner mitochondrial environment. Hence these constructs are able to specifically deliver their cargo to the mitochondria.

The shape and surface architecture of nanoconstructs also play a vital role in subcellular disposition of drug-loaded nanoconstructs [56]. A change in surface architecture may lead to a change in predisposition of nanoconstructs toward a particular subcellular organelle. As an example, fluorescein isothiocyanate—tagged layered double hydroxide (LDH) nanoparticle can be fabricated into hexagonal sheets with average diameter range of 50—150 nm and thickness of 10—20 nm [57]. These nanoparticles can also be formed into nanorods with a diameter of 30—60 nm and length of 100—200 nm. The nanorods are preferentially deposited into nucleus, whereas the hexagonal sheets remain trapped in the cytoplasm. It has been hypothesized that a microtubule-controlled transport phenomenon is responsible for rapid uptake of nanorods in the nucleus. Fig. 8.6 shows particle uptake with different localization profiles of differentially fabricated LDH nanoparticles.

3.7 Mechanisms of Particle Uptake Into Cell Nucleus

The cell nucleus is perhaps the most significant organelle in terms of drug delivery. It is the site of action where many critical anticancer drugs such as doxorubicin exert their pharmacological action [58]. It is the ultimate site of action for gene expression. The exact mechanism of plasmid DNA delivery by lipoplexes following endosomal escape is not clearly delineated. The nucleopore complex (NPC), which controls nucleocytoplasmic transport, plays a crucial role in human and other eukaryotic cells [59]. The NPC influences both active and passive transport across the nuclear membrane. Passive transport is a nonspecific mechanism for transport of particles not bigger than 10 nm diameter and with molecular weight not more than 25 kDa [60]. Passive diffusion does not involve expenditure of any energy as it never takes place against concentration gradient. Facilitated or active transport on the other hand involves expenditure of energy. In case of active nuclear transport that energy is presented in the form of GTP. Active transport may be for or against the concentration gradient. Active transport may work against concentration gradients where the cutoff diameter of particles is approximately 50 nm with molecular weight ranging from 25–75 kDa. Thachenko et al. [61] have predicted a cutoff size ideal for targeted nuclear delivery of nanoparticles. This work suggests particles should ideally have diameters less than 100 nm to cross cell membrane and less than 30 nm to be imported into nucleus through the NPC.

Active transport across the NPC often needs the conjugation of nanoparticles or plasmid DNA to a nuclear localization signal. This peptide causes the specific uptake of particles through the NPC. This peptide forms a conjugate with nuclear membrane importers such as karyopherin alpha and beta [62]. Another similar peptide known as cell-penetrating peptide (CPP) allows particles to cross the cell membrane and escape the endosomal vesicles [63]. If the drug-loaded particles or plasmid DNA cannot escape the endosomal vesicles, these constructs may have a high probability of being degraded in lysosomes. Hence CPP and NLS should be considered while designing a drug-loaded nanoformulation targeted at the nucleus.

3.8 Imaging Technology for Intracellular Trafficking of Nanostructures
3.8.1 Confocal Microscopy
Confocal microscopy, most frequently confocal laser scanning microscopy, is a powerful technique that allows enhanced optical resolution and contrasted images. It uses a spatial pinhole added to the confocal plane of lens. This mechanism removes light rays that are out of focus. As a result, 3-D reconstruction becomes a possibility. The set of images that are captured at varying depths via optical sectioning can be reconstructed into a 3-D image that provides enhanced structural information [64]. Advances in confocal microscopy have expanded the horizon of investigation into intracellular trafficking of nanoconstructs. To better evaluate this phenomenon confocal microscopes utilize a strategy referred to as Z-stacking (also called as focus stacking). It is a digital image processing method. It combines several images captured at several focal distances. This process gives rise to a composite image with a bigger depth of field than any of the individual images from which the composite image is created. It can be very useful to capture in-focus images of objects that are under high magnification as depth of field is lowered with

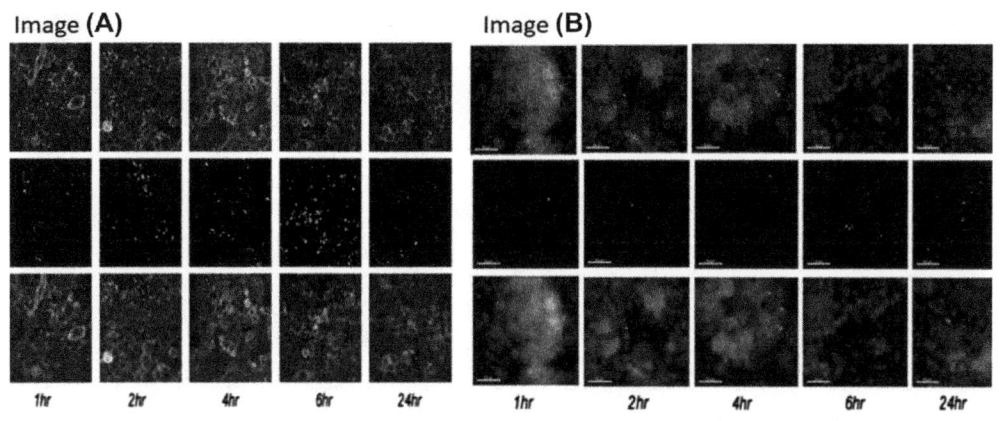

Figure 8.7 (A) Nanoparticle (NP) uptake in OK cells. Z-stack images for 1-, 2-, 4-, 6-, and 24-h time points are shown. Green channel *(row 1)*, red channel *(row 2)*, and color overlay *(row 3)* images are provided. Green denotes the cell perimeter (α5 label for Na$^+$/K$^+$ pump), whereas red indicates rhodamine NPs. Scale bar represents 50 μm. (B) NP uptake in human bronchial epithelial cells. Z-stack images for 1-, 2-, 4-, 6-, and 24-h time points are shown. Green channel *(row 1)*, red channel *(row 2)*, and color overlay *(row 3)* images are provided. Green denotes the cell perimeter (α5 label for Na$^+$/K$^+$ pump), whereas red indicates rhodamine NPs. Scale bar represents 50 μm. *(Published with permission from Elsevier.)*

magnification. Confocal laser scanning microscopy coupled with Z-stacking is a powerful tool for tracking intracellular localization of nanoconstructs [65].

Poly(lactic-co-glycolic acid) (PLGA) nanoparticles encapsulating fluorescent rhodamine has been investigated for disposition in the subcellular organelle with the help of confocal microscopy using the Z-stacking method. This imaging technique can provide images of the nanoparticles localized in Golgi bodies and early endosomes of human bronchial epithelial cells and to a much lesser extent in lysosomes [66]. Fig. 8.7 shows PLGA nanoparticle encapsulating rhodamine imaged by confocal laser scanning microscopy using Z-stacking.

3.8.2 Quantum Dots and Gold Nanoparticles

A quantum dot is a microcrystalline semiconductor nanostructure [67]. It is able to restrict movement of conduction band electrons, valence band holes, or excitons in all three spatial directions. It has been applied extensively to track and image the intracellular fate of nanoparticles. A significant advantage of quantum dot over traditional fluorescent techniques is that it does not photobleach significantly, which allows investigators freedom to design experiments [68]. However, quantum dots do possess fluorescent properties (albeit without significant photobleaching), which render them an attractive system for diagnostic and therapeutic tool. In one study quantum dots were observed in endosomal and lysosomal vesicles (Fig. 8.8). This trafficking mimics the pathway traversed by drug-loaded nanoparticles. Quantum dots coupled with transmission electron

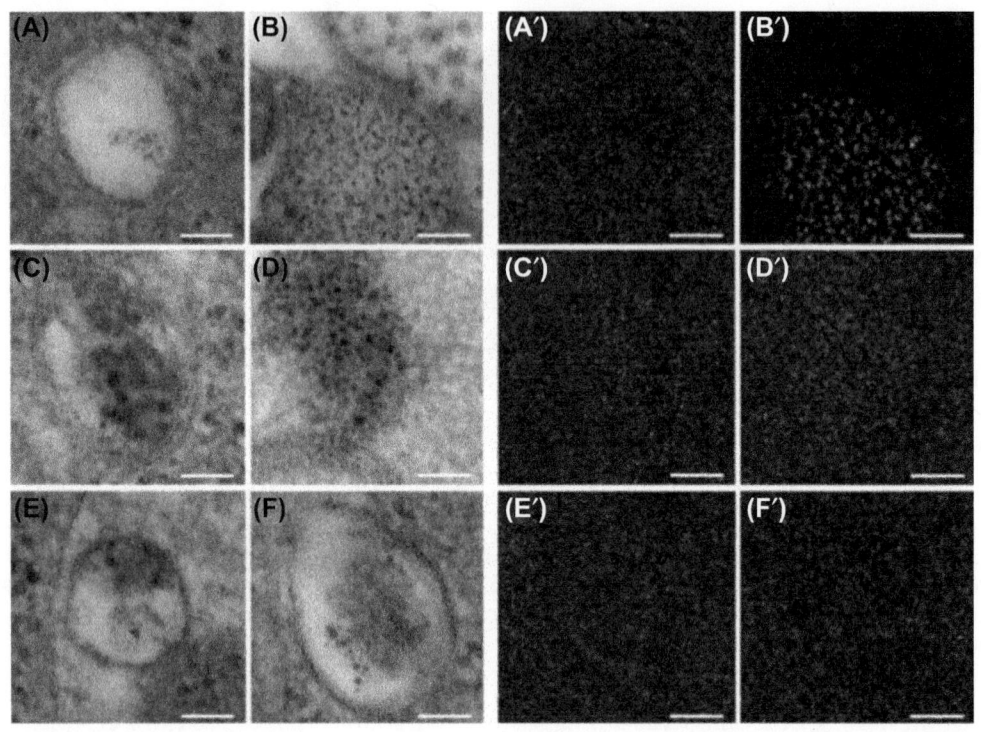

Figure 8.8 Different intracellular areas were scanned for S and Cd. Parts A–F represent the areas selected in this figure and parts A′–F′ show the corresponding S/Cd electron spectroscopic images. Images B and B′ show a homogenous distribution of quantum dots within an intracellular vesicle with a specific signal for S/Cd, whereas other images are only related to noisy unspecific S/Cd background. No further analysis on these structural origins was performed, but it is assumed that the structures present in A, D, and F are contaminants of transmission electron microscopy embedding and staining with heavy metals, whereas the structures in C and E possibly represent protein or lipid aggregates. All scale bars equate to 50 nm [69].

microscopy and confocal microscopy are being explored as powerful tools to investigate intracellular trafficking of nanosized structures.

Apart from endosomal and lysosomal compartments, quantum dots may also be targeted to other organelles such as mitochondria and nucleus [70]. Conjugation of 23 amino acid nuclear and 28 amino acid mitochondrial localization signals leads to localization of quantum dots into nucleus and mitochondria, respectively. Quantum dots are localized in their respective compartments within 30 min of beginning of cellular uptake [70]. Conjugation of signaling peptides to quantum dots provides an idea of mechanisms and pathways responsible for uptake by specific organelles. This process allows us to develop drug-loaded nanoconstructs that can be specifically targeted to particular organelles. Peptide-conjugated quantum dots also allow us to determine the localization kinetics of nanostructures in different targeted organelles (Fig. 8.9).

3.8.3 Gold Nanoparticles

Gold nanoparticles are considered to be an important platform for pharmaceutical and biomedical applications. This is due to their physicochemical properties. The inert core does not produce any cytotoxicity. Gold nanoparticles absorb and scatter under

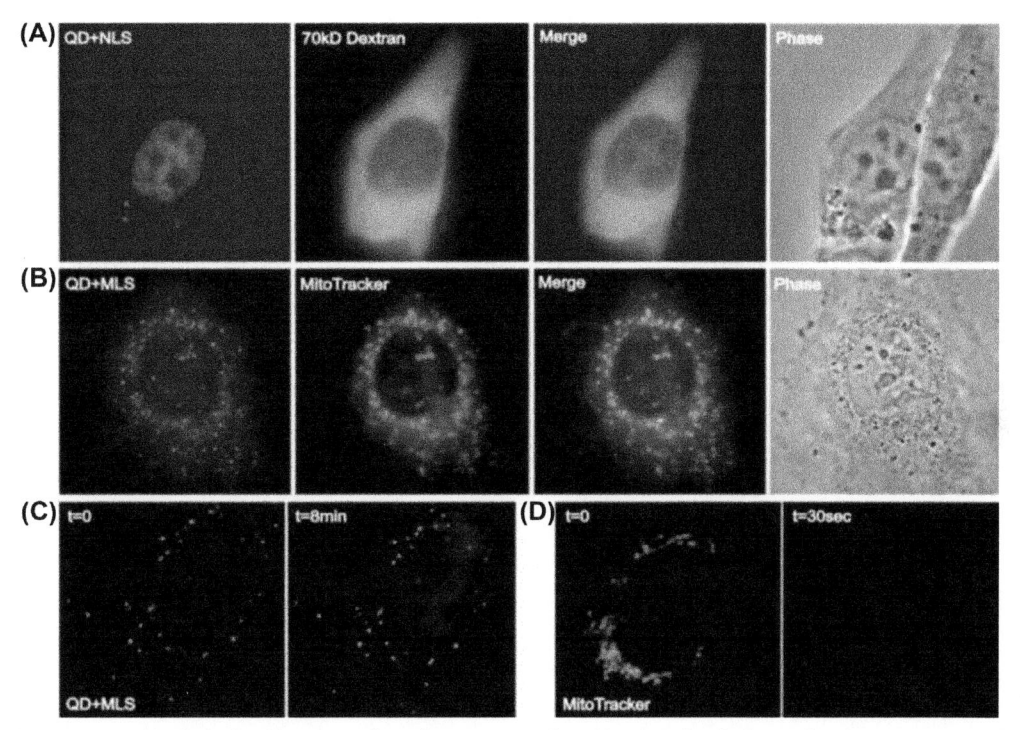

Figure 8.9 Subcellular localization of single quantum dots (QDs). Polyethylene glycol—QDs were conjugated to localization peptides, which allow active targeting to nucleus (A) and mitochondria (B). These nanoconstructs were delivered to 3T3 fibroblast cells via microinjection. (C) Quantum dots remain fluorescent even after 8 min of mercury lamp exposure. (D) Conventional mitotracker dye photo bleaches at similar exposure. *(Published with permission from John Wiley and Sons.)*

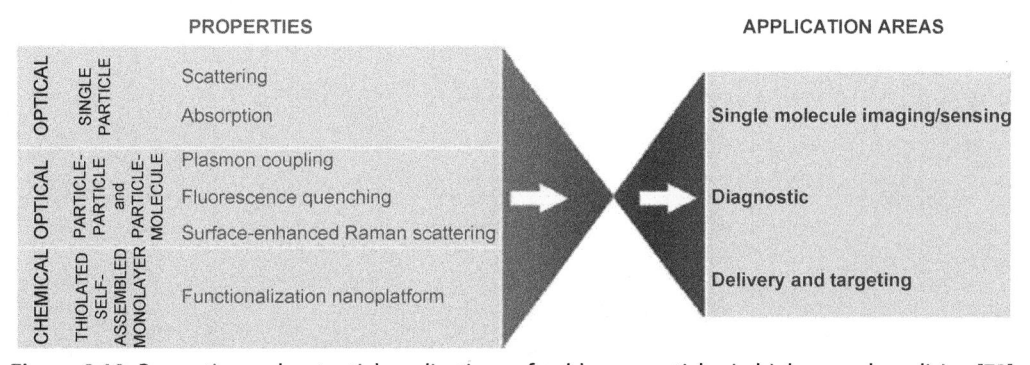

Figure 8.10 Properties and potential applications of gold nanoparticles in biology and medicine [73].

Table 8.1 Comparison of gold nanoparticles subcellular localization using different methods of cellular delivery [73]

Method	Gold core size (nm)	Capping	Subcellular localization	Toxicity	References
CPP	16	94% PEG, 2% Tat, 2% NLS, 2% penetratin	Cytoplasmic and nuclear	Not reported	[14]
CPP	~20	Nuclear localization sequence and receptor-mediated endocytosis peptides	Nucleus	~5% death	[74]
CPP	12	Sweet arrow peptide	Endosomal	Not reported	[71]
CPP	2.8	Tat peptide	Cytosolic around the mitochondria and in nucleus	Low cytotoxicity below 10 µM	[67,70]
CPP	20	BiotinylatedTat-HA2, PEG-SH, antiactin antibodies	Cytoskeleton (cytoplasm)	Not reported	[75]
PEI	4	PEI	Mainly endosomal and some nuclear localization	20–30% death	[76]
SLO toxin	5 and 10	90% CALNN–10% CALNN–PEG	Endosomal and cytosolic	Toxicity controlled by protocol optimization	Shaheen et al., unpublished data
Liposomes	1.4	Phospholipid	Lysosomes near the nuclear membrane	Not reported	[77]
Transferrin	14–100	Transferrin	Endosomal	Nontoxic	[56,78]
Ultrasound	100	DDPE	Endosomal	Nontoxic	[79]
Microinjection	11–32	Nucleoplasms	Nuclear and cytoplasmic	Not reported	[80]

CPP, cell-penetrating peptide; *NLS*, nuclear localization signal; *PEG*, polyethylene glycol.

resonance light both at the visible and near-infrared spectrum [71]. The plasmon resonance of these bands can be optimized over a wide spectral range. It is done by modification of parameters such as component of the particles, size, and shape [72]. Light scattering property of gold nanoparticle is strong enough to be easily detected. The signal is stronger than most fluorophores and like quantum dots does not undergo photobleaching [73]. For nanoparticles below 30 nm, light absorption is more than its scattering. This phenomenon can be utilized for imaging by photothermal microscopy. It can also be easily imaged by transmission as well as scanning electron microscopy. Hence gold nanoparticles are better suited to study mechanism and kinetics of particle movement across the nucleopore complex [73].

The potential applications of gold nanoparticles include but are not limited to bioimaging, single molecule tracking, biosensing, drug delivery, transfection, and diagnosis. Bioconjugation of relevant ligands to gold nanoparticle leads to specific targeting of tumor cells with minimal uptake into normal cells. It has the potential to provide efficient diagnostic and therapeutic strategies in neoplastic disorders. Fig. 8.10 depicts the different significant applications of gold nanoparticles. Table 8.1 depicts different subcellular localization of gold nanoparticles when conjugated with various ligands.

4. CONCLUSION

This review provides a synopsis of the research being carried out in the field of intracellular drug delivery. It also outlines some of the critical parameters that need to be factored in while designing nanostructures with site of action inside the cell. As mentioned previously this exciting field of research is still in early stages. A lot of work needs to be done to answer many important questions.

REFERENCES

[1] Smith PJ, et al. Cellular entry of nanoparticles via serum sensitive clathrin-mediated endocytosis, and plasma membrane permeabilization. Int J Nanomed 2012;7:2045—55.
[2] Ferreira F, et al. Endocytosis of G protein-coupled receptors is regulated by clathrin light chain phosphorylation. Curr Biol 2012;22(15):1361—70.
[3] Ford MG, et al. Curvature of clathrin-coated pits driven by epsin. Nature 2002;419(6905):361—6.
[4] Mayor S, Pagano RE. Pathways of clathrin-independent endocytosis. Nat Rev Mol Cell Biol 2007; 8(8):603—12.
[5] Thomsen P, Roepstorff K, Stahlhut M, van Deurs B. Caveolae are highly immobile plasma membrane microdomains, which are not involved in constitutive endocytic trafficking. Mol Biol Cell 2002;13(1): 238—50.
[6] Simons K, Ikonen E. Functional rafts in cell membranes. Nature 1997;387(6633):569—72.
[7] Hao X, et al. Caveolae mediated endocytosis of biocompatible gold nanoparticles in living Hela cells. J Phys Condens Matter 2012;24(16):164207.
[8] Wang Z, Tiruppathi C, Minshall RD, Malik AB. Size and dynamics of caveolae studied using nanoparticles in living endothelial cells. ACS Nano 2009;3(12):4110—6.
[9] Doherty GJ, McMahon HT. Mechanisms of endocytosis. Annu Rev Biochem 2009;78:857—902.

[10] Grassart A, Dujeancourt A, Lazarow PB, Dautry-Varsat A, Sauvonnet N. Clathrin-independent endocytosis used by the IL-2 receptor is regulated by Rac1, Pak1 and Pak2. EMBO Rep 2008;9(4): 356–62.
[11] Lundmark R, et al. The GTPase-activating protein GRAF1 regulates the CLIC/GEEC endocytic pathway. Curr Biol 2008;18(22):1802–8.
[12] Ge L, et al. Flotillins play an essential role in Niemann-Pick C1-like 1-mediated cholesterol uptake. Proc Natl Acad Sci USA 2011;108(2):551–6.
[13] Strauss K, et al. Exosome secretion ameliorates lysosomal storage of cholesterol in Niemann-Pick type C disease. J Biol Chem 2010;285(34):26279–88.
[14] Vercauteren D, et al. Dynamic colocalization microscopy to characterize intracellular trafficking of nanomedicines. ACS Nano 2011;5(10):7874–84.
[15] Kasper J, et al. Flotillin involved uptake of silica nanoparticles and responses of an alveolar-capillary barrier in vitro. Eur J Pharm Biopharm 2013;84(2):275–87.
[16] Liberali P, et al. The closure of Pak1-dependent macropinosomes requires the phosphorylation of CtBP1/BARS. EMBO J 2008;27(7):970–81.
[17] Dharmawardhane S, et al. Regulation of macropinocytosis by p21-activated kinase-1. Mol Biol Cell 2000;11(10):3341–52.
[18] Fujii M, Kawai K, Egami Y, Araki N. Dissecting the roles of Rac1 activation and deactivation in macropinocytosis using microscopic photo-manipulation. Sci Rep 2013;3:2385.
[19] Grimmer S, van Deurs B, Sandvig K. Membrane ruffling and macropinocytosis in A431 cells require cholesterol. J Cell Sci 2002;115(Pt. 14):2953–62.
[20] Mercer J, Helenius A. Vaccinia virus uses macropinocytosis and apoptotic mimicry to enter host cells. Science 2008;320(5875):531–5.
[21] Hoon JL, et al. Functions and regulation of circular dorsal ruffles. Mol Cell Biol November 2012; 32(21):4246–57.
[22] Harush-Frenkel O, et al. Surface charge of nanoparticles determines their endocytic and transcytotic pathway in polarized MDCK cells. Biomacromolecules 2008;9:435–43.
[23] Kim S, et al. Phagocytosis and endocytosis of silver nanoparticles induce interleukin-8 production in human macrophages. Yonsei Med J 2012;53(3):654–7.
[24] Rink J, Ghigo E, Kalaidzidis Y, Zerial M. Rab conversion as a mechanism of progression from early to late endosomes. Cell 2005;122(5):735–49.
[25] Mercer J, Helenius A. Gulping rather than sipping: macropinocytosis as a way of virus entry. Curr Opin Microbiol 2012;15(4):490–9.
[26] Spang A. On the fate of early endosomes. Biol Chem 2009;390(8):753–9.
[27] Mu FT, et al. EEA1, an early endosome-associated protein. EEA1 is a conserved alpha-helical peripheral membrane protein flanked by cysteine "fingers" and contains a calmodulin-binding IQ motif. J Biol Chem 1995;270(22):13503–11.
[28] Lakadamyali M, Rust MJ, Zhuang X. Ligands for clathrin-mediated endocytosis are differentially sorted into distinct populations of early endosomes. Cell 2006;124(5):997–1009.
[29] Hanson PI, Cashikar A. Multivesicular body morphogenesis. Annu Rev Cell Dev Biol 2012;28: 337–62.
[30] Murk JL, et al. Influence of aldehyde fixation on the morphology of endosomes and lysosomes: quantitative analysis and electron tomography. J Microsc 2003;212(Pt. 1):81–90.
[31] Ostrowski M, et al. Rab27a and Rab27b control different steps of the exosome secretion pathway. Nat Cell Biol 2010;12(1):19–30. sup pp. 11–13.
[32] Denzer K, Kleijmeer MJ, Heijnen HF, Stoorvogel W, Geuze HJ. Exosome: from internal vesicle of the multivesicular body to intercellular signaling device. J Cell Sci 2000;113(Pt. 19):3365–74.
[33] Sahay G, et al. Efficiency of siRNA delivery by lipid nanoparticles is limited by endocytic recycling. Nat Biotechnol 2013;31(7):653–8.
[34] Cruz JC, Sugii S, Yu C, Chang TY. Role of Niemann-Pick type C1 protein in intracellular trafficking of low density lipoprotein-derived cholesterol. J Biol Chem 2000;275(6):4013–21.
[35] Rajendran L, et al. Subcellular targeting strategies for drug design and delivery. Nat Rev Drug Discov 2010;9:29–42.

[36] Sakhrani NM, Harish P. Organelle targeting: third level of drug targeting. Drug Des Devel Ther 2013; 7:585—99.
[37] Çağdas M, Sezer AD, Bucak S. Liposomes as potential drug carrier systems for drug delivery. In: Sezer AD, editor. Application of nanotechnology in drug delivery. InTech; 2014. http://dx.doi.org/10.5772/58459.
[38] Galvez T, Gilleron J, Zerial M, O'Sullivan GA. SnapShot: mammalian Rab proteins in endocytic trafficking. Cell 2012;151(1):234.
[39] Sandin P, Fitzpatrick LW, Simpson JC, Dawson KA. High-speed imaging of Rab family small GTPases reveals rare events in nanoparticle trafficking in living cells. ACS Nano 2012;6(2):1513—21.
[40] Schroder BA, Wrocklage C, Hasilik A, Saftig P. The proteome of lysosomes. Proteomics 2010;10(22): 4053—76.
[41] Mellman I, Fuchs R, Helenius A. Acidification of the endocytic and exocytic pathways. Annu Rev Biochem 1986;55:663—700.
[42] Noguiera DR, et al. Mechanisms underlying cytotoxicity induced by engineered nanomaterials: a review of in vitro studies. Nanomaterials 2014;4:454—84.
[43] Sahay G, et al. Endocytosis of nanomedicines. J Control Release August 3, 2010;145(3):182—95.
[44] Prokop A, Davidson JM. Nanovehicular intracellular delivery systems. J Pharm Sci September 2008; 97(9):3518—90.
[45] Herd H, et al. Nanoparticle geometry and surface orientation influences mode of cellular uptake. ACS Nano March 26, 2013;7(3). http://dx.doi.org/10.1021/nn304439f.
[46] Ulbrich K, et al. Targeted drug delivery with polymers and magnetic nanoparticles: covalent and non-covalent approaches, release control, and clinical studies. Chem Rev 2016;116(9).
[47] Walter P, et al. The protein translocation machinery of the endoplasmic reticulum. Philos Trans R Soc Lond B Biol Sci 1982;300(1099):225—8.
[48] Allen TD, et al. The nuclear pore complex: mediator of translocation between nucleus and cytoplasm. J Cell Sci 2000;113(Pt. 10):1651—9.
[49] Stoffler D, Fahrenkrog B, Aebi U. The nuclear pore complex: from molecular architecture to functional dynamics. Curr Opin Cell Biol 1999;11(3):391—401.
[50] Intracellular delivery: Fundamentals and applications. In: Prokop A, editor. Fundamental Biomedical Technologies; 2011.
[51] Zanta MA, Belguise-Valladier P, Behr JP. Gene delivery: a single nuclear localization signal peptide is sufficient to carry DNA to the cell nucleus. Proc Natl Acad Sci USA 1999;96(1):91—6.
[52] D'Souza GG, et al. DQAsome-mediated delivery of plasmid DNA toward mitochondria in living cells. J Control Release 2003;92(1—2):189—97.
[53] D'Souza GG, Boddapati SV, Weissig V. Mitochondrial leader sequence—plasmid DNA conjugates delivered into mammalian cells by DQAsomes co-localize with mitochondria. Mitochondrion 2005;5(5):352—8.
[54] D'Souza GG, et al. Nanocarrier-assisted sub-cellular targeting to the site of mitochondria improves the pro-apoptotic activity of paclitaxel. J Drug Target 2008;16(7):578—85.
[55] Yamada Y, et al. MITO-Porter: A liposome-based carrier system for delivery of macromolecules into mitochondria via membrane fusion. Biochim Biophys Acta 2008;1778(2):423—32.
[56] Murugan K, et al. Parameters and characteristics governing cellular internalization and trans-barrier trafficking of nanostructures. Int J Nanomedicine 2015;2015(10):2191—206.
[57] Oh JM, et al. Intracellular drug delivery of layered double hydroxide nanoparticles. J Nanosci Nanotechnol 2011;11:1632—5.
[58] Deepthi A, et al. Targeted drug delivery to the nucleus and its potential role in cancer chemotherapy. J Pharm Sci Res 2013;5(2):48—56.
[59] Wente SR, Rout PM. The nuclear pore complex and nuclear transport. Cold Spring Harb Perspect Biol 2010;2(10):a000562.
[60] Sykes EA, et al. Investigating the impact of nanoparticle size on active and passive tumor targeting efficiency. ACS Nano 2014;8(6):5696—706.
[61] Tkachenko, et al. Multifunctional gold nanoparticle—peptide complexes for nuclear targeting. J Am Chem Soc 2003;125(16):4700—1.

[62] Moroianu J, Blobel G, Radu A. The binding site of karyopherin alpha for karyopherin beta overlaps with a nuclear localization sequence. Proc Natl Acad Sci USA 1996;93(13):6572—6.
[63] Erazo-Oliveras A, Muthukrishnan N, Baker R, Wang T-Y, Pellois J-P. Improving the endosomal escape of cell-penetrating peptides and their cargos: strategies and challenges. Pharmaceuticals (Basel, Switz) 2012;5(11). http://dx.doi.org/10.3390/ph5111177.
[64] Zhou X, et al. Double-exposure optical sectioning structured illumination microscopy based on Hilbert transform reconstruction. PLoS One 2015;10(3):e0120892.
[65] Smith IO, Ren F, Baumann MJ, Case ED. Confocal laser scanning microscopy as a tool for imaging cancellous bone. J Biomed Mater Res 2006;79B:185—92.
[66] Cartiera MS, Johnson KM, Rajendran V, Caplan MJ, Saltzman WM. The uptake and intracellular fate of PLGA nanoparticles in epithelial cells. Biomaterials 2009;30(14):2790—8.
[67] Kramer IJ, Sargent EH. The architecture of colloidal quantum dot solar cells: materials to devices. Chem Rev 2014;114:863—82.
[68] Walling MA, Novak JA, Shepard JRE. Quantum dots for live cell and in vivo imaging. Int J Mol Sci 2009;10(2):441—91.
[69] Brendenberger C, et al. Intracellular imaging of nanoparticles: is it an elemental mistake to believe what you see? Part Fibre Toxicol 2010;7:15.
[70] Derfus AM, et al. Intracellular delivery of quantum dots for live cell labelling and organelle tracking. Adv Mater June 17, 2004;16(12).
[71] Huang X, El-Sayed M. Gold nanoparticles: optical properties and implementations in cancer diagnosis and photothermal therapy 2010;1(1):13—28.
[72] Sonnichsen C, Franzl T, Wilk T, von Plessen G, Feldmann J, Wilson O, et al. Drastic reduction of plasmon damping in gold nanorods. Phys Rev Lett 2002;88:077402.
[73] Yguerabide J, Yguerabide EE. Light-scattering submicroscopic particles as highly fluorescent analogs and their use as tracer labels in clinical and biological applications I. theory. Anal Biochem 1998;262:137—56.
[74] Tkachenko AG, Xie H, Coleman D, Glomm W, Ryan J, Anderson MF, et al. Multifunctional gold nanoparticle peptide complexes for nuclear targeting. J Am Chem Soc 2003;125:47001.
[75] Kumar S, Harrison N, Richards-Kortum R, Sokolov K. Plasmonic nanosensors for imaging intracellular biomarkers in live cells. Nano Lett 2007;7:133843.
[76] Thomas M, Klibanov AM. Non-viral gene therapy: polycation-mediated DNA delivery. Appl Microbiol Biotechnol 2003;62:2734.
[77] Chithrani DB, Dunne M, Stewart J, Allen C, Jaffray DA. Cellular uptake and transport of gold nanoparticles incorporated in a liposomal carrier. Nanomedicine 2009;6:1619.
[78] Yang PH, Sun XS, Chiu JF, Sun HZ, He QY. Transferrin-mediated gold nanoparticle cellular uptake. Bioconj Chem 2005;16:4946.
[79] Soman NR, Marsh JN, Lanza GM, Wickline SA. New mechanisms for non-porative ultrasound stimulation of cargo delivery to cell cytosol with targeted perfluorocarbon nanoparticles. Nanotechnology 2008;19:185102.
[80] Feldherr CM, Lanford RE, Akin D. Signal-mediated nuclear transport in Simian-virus 40-transformed cells is regulated by large tumor-antigen. Proc Natl Acad Sci USA 1992;89:110025.

CHAPTER 9

Electrospun Nanofibers in Drug Delivery: Fabrication, Advances, and Biomedical Applications

Vibhuti Agrahari[a], Vivek Agrahari[a], Jianing Meng[a], Ashim K. Mitra
University of Missouri—Kansas City, Kansas City, MO, United States

Contents

1. Introduction	190
1.1 Process of Electrospinning	190
1.2 Parameters Influencing the Electrospinning Process and Fiber Characteristics	191
1.2.1 Concentration	192
1.2.2 Polymer Molecular Weight	192
1.2.3 Conductivity	192
1.2.4 Viscosity	194
1.2.5 Flow Rate	194
1.2.6 Applied Voltage	194
1.2.7 Distance Between the Needle Tip and Collector	194
1.2.8 Environmental Factors (Humidity and Temperature)	194
1.2.9 Collector Types	195
2. Stimuli-Responsive Nanofibers in Drug Delivery Applications	195
2.1 pH-Responsive Systems	195
2.2 Light-Activated Systems	195
2.3 Thermoresponsive Systems	199
2.4 Ultrasound-Responsive Systems	200
2.5 Enzyme-Responsive Systems	200
2.6 Oxidative Stress—Responsive Systems	200
2.7 Carbohydrate-Responsive Systems	200
2.8 Multiresponsive Systems	201
2.9 Challenges in Stimuli-Responsive Drug Delivery Applications of Nanofibers	201
3. Applications of Electrospun Nanofibers	201
3.1 Electrospun Nanofibers in Tissue Engineering	201
3.1.1 Skin Tissue Engineering	202
3.1.2 Bone Tissue Engineering	203
3.1.3 Cardiac Tissue Engineering	204
3.1.4 Nerve Tissue Engineering	205
3.2 Electrospun Nanofibers Applications in Dentistry	205
3.3 Electrospun Nanofibers Application in Ocular Injuries	206

[a] Authors contributed equally.

3.4 Electrospun Nanofibers in Drug Delivery	207
3.4.1 Transdermal Drug Delivery System	*208*
3.4.2 Cancer Therapy	*208*
3.5 Electrospun Nanofibers in Biomedical Application	209
3.6 Biosensor and Immunoassay	209
4. Conclusion	210
References	211

1. INTRODUCTION

Nanomedicine approaches play an important role in drug delivery [1,2]. Currently, electrospun nanofibers (NFs) are extensively applied in drug delivery systems. NF formulations offer various advantages in drug delivery such as high drug loading efficiency, flexibility to be formulated in various shapes, high surface-to-volume ratio, and high porosity [1]. These benefits render drug-loaded NFs an attractive candidate in formulations development. Furthermore, the encapsulation of labile molecules in NFs can enhance the drug stability in a harsh biological environment.

NFs are defined as fibers with a diameter less than 1000 nm (1 μm) [3]. These structures can be manufactured using the electrospinning process. Electrospinning is a simple and highly versatile technique that allows the generation of ultrathin fibers from a variety of polymeric and composite materials [4]. The simplicity of the procedure, high surface-to-volume ratio of the NF mesh, wide variety in usable polymers, and the possibility of large-scale production make electrospinning technology attractive for tissue engineering, drug delivery, and other biomedical applications (Fig. 9.1).

1.1 Process of Electrospinning

Electrospinning utilizes electrostatic forces as a driving force to generate polymeric fibers [5]. A typical electrospinning system is described in Fig. 9.2. This system consists of four major components: (1) a glass syringe containing a polymer spinneret, which is connected to a high voltage supply and can be a needle or a coaxial that can generate core–shell NFs; (2) a high-voltage power supply, which injects finite polarity charge (typically positive) into the polymer solution; (3) a syringe pump that forces the polymer solution through the spinneret; and (4) a grounded collector, which can be a sheet of aluminum or a rotating drum collector [6].

As the pump plunger pushes the syringe, a polymer solution droplet is formed at the tip of the spinneret. Subsequently electric charges can cause the power supply extended into the polymer solution via the metallic needle. When a sufficiently high electrical potential is applied to the droplet, it assumes electrical charges. The reciprocal of charges repulsion creates a force that is opposite to the surface tension of the polymer droplet. At a critical voltage, the electrical force of the charges overcomes the force due to surface tension. This energy causes the spherical droplet to elongate and assume a conical shape

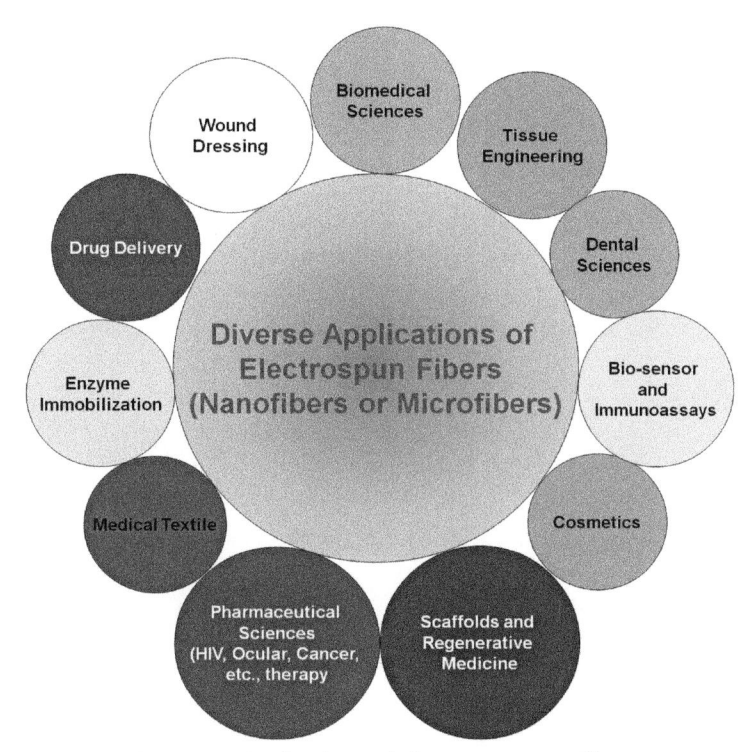

Figure 9.1 Applications of electrospun nanofibers.

known as Taylor cone. It is followed by the eruption of a jet from the tip of the Taylor cone. The jet of the polymer solution flows in the direction of the electric field toward the grounded collector. During this process, charges migrate to the surface of the jet. Electrostatic repulsive force leads to the whipping of the jet, which allows the polymer chains to stretch in the solutions. As a result, the jet is elongated and the diameter is further reduced. The solvent of the polymer is evaporated, so that the fiber is deposited on the grounded collector [7−9].

1.2 Parameters Influencing the Electrospinning Process and Fiber Characteristics

The electrospinning process can be governed by several factors, such as polymer solution, process, and ambient parameters. The polymer solution parameters include concentration viscosity, conductivity, molecular weight, and surface tension. The process parameters include applied electric field (voltage), tip to collector distance, and flow rate. All of these parameters lead to fibers with various properties. These factors are classified as the composition of the polymer solutions and processing parameters [10]. The compositions

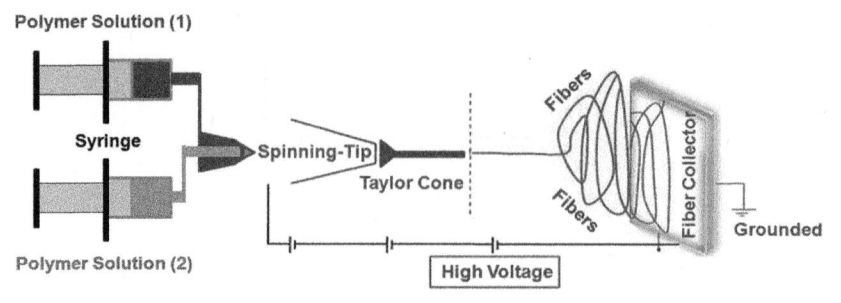

Figure 9.2 Schematic representation of the electrospinning process.

of the polymer solutions include concentration, molecular weight, surface tension, viscosity, and conductivity, whereas process parameters include applied voltage, tip to collector distance, and flow rate. Ambient parameters encompass the humidity and temperature of the environment. Each of these parameters significantly controls the fiber morphology, diameter, and quality. By proper optimization and selection of these parameters, the desired morphology and diameter of fibers can be obtained as discussed further in the following subsection and summarized in Table 9.1.

1.2.1 Concentration

The concentration of polymer solution plays an important role in the fiber formation process. Every polymer has an optimal concentration range. Within this window, the diameter of the NF increases with the polymer concentration. If the solution is diluted, electrospray process takes place instead of electrospinning, as the liquid jet is broken up into droplets by the surface tension of the solution. It leads to the formation of beaded fibers or a mixture of beads and fibers [11].

1.2.2 Polymer Molecular Weight

Another important factor in electrospinning is molecular weight of the polymer. In solution, molecular weight reflects the entanglement of polymer chains, which causes the liquid jet to overcome the surface tension and ultimately form smooth NFs [12]. Molecular weight of the polymer has a performed effect on electrical/rheological properties. Similar to the concentration, high molecular weight favors the formation of microribbons. A high-molecular-weight solution generates fibers with larger diameters, whereas low-molecular-weight polymers tend to form beads.

1.2.3 Conductivity

The conductivity of the solution can control the fiber diameter distribution. A solution with very low conductivity cannot be electrospun, as the surface of the droplet does not

Table 9.1 Effects of processing variables on nanofiber morphology and properties

Electrospinning parameters	Value	Effects on Fiber diameter	Effects on Fiber morphology
Process parameters			
Flow rate	↑	↑	Beaded and thick fiber. High flow rates produced fibers that are not completely dried
Needle-to-collector distance	↓	↓	Beaded fiber if the distance is too short or long. Formation of thick fibers
Applied voltage	↑	↓	Beaded fibers
Needle inner diameter	↑	↑	Beaded fibers
Solution parameters			
Polymer molecular weight	↑	↕ such as viscosity, type of the polymer, concentration	Less bead formation. Smooth fiber
Polymer concentration	↑	↑ (within a range)	Bead formation after a certain concentration
Polymer solubility	↑		
Solution viscosity	↑	↑ (within a range)	Lower bead formation
Solution conductivity	↑	↓ but broad distribution in diameter	Bead-free fibers
Solvent dielectric constant	↑	↓	Lower bead formation
Solvent volatility	↑	↑	Pore formation
Surface tension	↑	↓	Jet is more likely to break up into droplets generating beaded fibers
Other parameters			
Humidity	↑	↓	Beaded fibers and pores formation
Temperature	↑	↓	
Collector type		• Smoother fibers resulted from metal collectors; more porous fiber structure was obtained using porous collectors • Aligned fibers were obtained using a conductive frame, rotating drum, or a wheel-like bobbin collector	

↑, Increase; ↓, decrease; ↕, depends on other variables.

carry any charge to form a Taylor cone. As a result, no electrospinning can take place. An increase in the conductivity of the polymer solution tends to lower the fiber diameter. However, polymer solutions with conductivity beyond a critical value are extremely unstable under the strong electric fields, causing a broad diameter divergence. The solution conductivity is determined by the polymer type, solvent, and salt concentration [13]. High solution conductivity can be achieved by changing the solvent, such as by using organic acids. Adding salts, such as NaCl and KH_2PO_4, can also tune the conductivity [4]. Highly conductive solutions are extremely unstable in the presence of strong electric fields, which result in a broad diameter fiber distribution.

1.2.4 Viscosity

The fiber diameter and morphology are strongly affected by the viscosity of the polymer solution during the electrospinning process. No continuous fiber formation will be possible with very low solution viscosity and with very high viscosity it is difficult to create jet injection from polymer solution. Thus an optimal viscosity of polymer solution is required for an effective electrospinning process [12].

1.2.5 Flow Rate

The flow rate of the polymer solution controls the diameter and morphology of the fibers. With higher flow rates, the diameter of the fibers increases accordingly. If the flow rate is extremely high, the solvent may not evaporate completely during the transfer from the spinneret to the collector. It may lead to beaded morphologies [14]. Several studies were undertaken to establish any relationship between solution flow rate and fiber morphology and diameter. High flow rates may also result in beaded fibers because of the insufficient drying time.

1.2.6 Applied Voltage

The voltage is one of the most important factors among the electrospinning process variables. The charged jets ejected only from the Taylor cone can apply voltage higher than the critical voltage. Higher voltage results in higher electrostatic repulsive force on the liquid jet, which favors the narrowing of fiber diameter [13].

1.2.7 Distance Between the Needle Tip and Collector

The diameter of the fibers increases as the distance between the needle and the collector is lowered. If it is too short, beaded morphologies can occur due to inadequate fiber drying [4].

1.2.8 Environmental Factors (Humidity and Temperature)

Besides the solution and electrospinning parameters, environmental factors such as relative humidity and temperature also affect the morphology and diameter of the fibers through the solidification process. However, this effect is generally rather limited compared with other parameters. The fiber diameter is usually decreased with the increase of temperature causing lower viscosity of the polymer solutions. Small pores on the surface of the fibers in addition to the beaded fibers maybe generated due to the higher humidity.

1.2.9 Collector Types
Type of collector is another important aspect in the electrospinning process. Usually, aluminum collectors are selected in the electrospinning process. However, difficulty in transferring collected fibers coupled with the need for aligned fibers necessitates other collectors such as conductive paper/cloth or rotating wheel. Due to diminished conductive area, beaded fibers are produced due to decreased surface area. The alignment of fiber is determined by the type of the collector and rotation speed [4].

2. STIMULI-RESPONSIVE NANOFIBERS IN DRUG DELIVERY APPLICATIONS

A stimuli-responsive nanocarrier provides a smart system for various therapeutic applications [15]. Generally, stimuli-responsive systems are able to enhance/trigger the release of therapeutic drugs in response to triggering signals (intrinsic or extrinsic). The intrinsic signals include pH, temperature, enzymes, and oxidative stress, whereas external stimuli constitute magnetic field, light, and heat [15,16]. These stimuli are applied as a triggering element in nanocarrier drug delivery systems [17,18]. The release of therapeutic molecules is controlled in a spatial and temporal manner [19]. Here, we have briefly summarized different stimuli that have been applied for triggering the drug release from NFs (Fig. 9.2). The delivery systems, which release active molecules in response to specific stimuli at the target site, are shown in Table 9.2 and Fig. 9.3.

2.1 pH-Responsive Systems
Variations in pH have been exploited to trigger drug release from delivery systems [18]. The use of polymers with ionizable groups (carboxylic, sulfonate, and amino) undergo conformational and/or solubility changes in response to environmental pH variation to release therapeutic molecules. pH-responsive systems are suitable for thermolabile drugs. Several NF systems have been developed with pH-sensitive polymers such as poly (ε-caprolactone) (PCL), poly (lactic acid-co-glycolic acid) (PLGA), and silk. Polymers with ionizable groups are classified into two types: weak polyacids and weak polybases. Poly (acrylic acid) and poly (methacrylic acid) are commonly used as pH-responsive polyacids, whereas poly(N,N-dimethylamino ethylmethacrylate) and poly(N,N-diethylaminoethylmethacrylate) are pH-responsive polymeric bases [20,34,35].

2.2 Light-Activated Systems
Light can be used as an external stimulus since its intensity can be precisely controlled. Light-sensitive materials have been used a lot as drug delivery systems. These delivery systems

Table 9.2 Stimuli-sensitive nanofiber delivery systems in pharmaceutical and biomedical applications

Stimulus	Active moiety	Polymer	Target diseases	Comments	References
pH	Doxorubicin	Silk	Breast cancer	Thixotropic silk hydrogels provide improved injectability to support sustained release, suggesting promising applications for localized chemotherapy	[20]
	Doxorubicin	Poly (ε-caprolactone) (PCL)	Gastric cancer and vaginal delivery of antiviral drugs or antiinflammatory drugs	The pH-responsive drug delivery systems based on PCL nanofibers have the potential in oral delivery of anticancer drugs for treating gastric cancer and vaginal delivery of antiviral drugs or antiinflammatory drugs, to deliver them to the specific target, and minimize their toxic side effects	[21]
	Etravirine and TDF	Cellulose acetate phthalate (CAP)	Human immunodeficiency virus (HIV)	The pH-dependent release properties have been carefully studied and we show that the released antiviral drugs, together with the CAP, which has been reported to have intrinsic antimicrobial activity, efficiently neutralize HIV in vitro	[22]
		Polyurethane (PU) and CAP	HIV	CAP imparts pH responsiveness to the core–shell structure giving the fibers potential for semen sensitive intravaginal drug delivery	[23]
	Paracetamol	Triblock copolymers	Various applications	The local delivery and controllable release profiles make these fibers as potential implantable drug carriers and functional coatings of medical devices	[24]

Temperature	Paclitaxel	PCL	Liver cancer	The approach developed here uses the nanofibers and nanoparticles together for the treatment of cancer	[25]
	Ibuprofen	Poly(N-isopropylacrylamide) and PCL	Various applications	Composite design can provide a novel approach to suppress the burst effect in drug delivery systems for potential pharmaceutical applications	[26]
	Ketoprofen	Poly(N-isopropylacrylamide), ethyl cellulose	Various applications	This study demonstrated that electrospun-blend PNIPAAm/EC fibers comprise effective and biocompatible materials for drug delivery systems and tissue engineering	[27]
Light	Polymethylmethacrylate (PMMA) nanofibers doped with silver nanoparticles (AgNPs) and *meso*-tetraphenylporphyrin (TPP)	PMMA nanofibers doped with AgNPs and TPP	Antibacterial	Results suggest that the proposed material is a promising option for the photodynamic inactivation of bacteria	[28]
	Fluorescein isothiocyanate–bovine serum albumin	poly(N-isopropylacrylamide-co-polyethylene glycol acrylate)		These results suggest that light-responsive fibrous nanocomposites can be utilized in applications such as drug delivery	[29]
Moisture	Maraviroc	Polyvinylpyrrolidone or poly(ethylene oxide)	HIV	Water-soluble electrospun materials can rapidly release maraviroc upon contact with moisture and that drug delivery is faster (less than 6 min under sink conditions) when maraviroc is electrospun in polyvinylpyrrolidone fibers containing an excipient wetting agent	[30]

Continued

Table 9.2 Stimuli-sensitive nanofiber delivery systems in pharmaceutical and biomedical applications—cont'd

Stimulus	Active moiety	Polymer	Target diseases	Comments	References
Hydrogen peroxide	Rhodamine B	Polyvinyl alcohol (PVA)/polyoxalate (PVA/POX NFs) blended	Inflammatory diseases	Nanofibrous PVA/POX can potentially be used to target numerous inflammatory diseases that overproduce hydrogen peroxide and may become a potential candidate for use as a local drug delivery vehicle	[31]
pH + glucose	Lectins	ConA and Jacalin	Removal of toxins from the solution	These functional nanofibers can therefore be easily modified and hence can be used for quick removal of selective proteins or toxins from the solution	[32]
pH + temperature	Nifedipine (NIF)	Poly(N-isopropylacrylamide)-co-poly(acrylic acid) [P(NIPAAm-co-AAc)]		The release amount of NIF from the nanofibers could be controlled effectively by adjusting the temperature or pH value of the aqueous medium and incorporating the hydrophobic PU	[33]

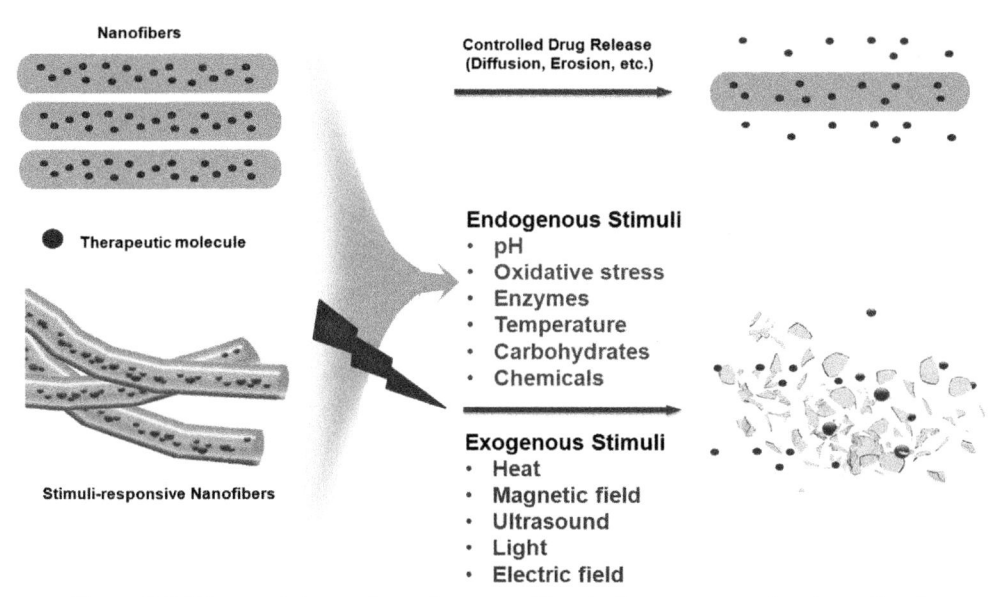

Figure 9.3 Triggered drug release from nanofiber in the presence of various stimuli.

incorporate light-sensitive groups such as azobenzene, stilbene, and triphenylmethane into the formulation, which respond to a specific wavelength. The light-sensitive polymers are hydrophilic, biocompatible, and biodegradable. However, the limitations of light-sensitive polymers include inconsistent response due to leaching of chromophores during swelling or contraction of the system, and a slow response is achieved with stimulus. These polymers can be divided into ultraviolet (UV)- and visible light—sensitive systems on the basis of the wavelength that triggers the phase transition. Visible light-sensitive polymers are preferred over UV-sensitive polymers because of their availability, safety, and ease of use [19,36,37].

2.3 Thermoresponsive Systems

Rise in temperature is associated with several ailments including cancer. In thermoresponsive drug delivery systems, thermosensitive polymers undergo abrupt change in solubility in response to a small change in temperature [38]. Thermosensitive polymers exhibit a phase transition in solution at a temperature at the lower critical solution temperature. This process can cause conformational changes in the polymer material that triggers drug release [39]. The most commonly used thermosensitive polymers include poly(N-isopropyl acrylamide), poly(N,N-diethylacrylamide), poly(N-vinylalkylamide), poly(N-vinyl caprolactam), pluronics, polysaccharide, chitosan, and PLGA/polyethylene glycol (PEG) triblock/pentablock copolymers. The major advantages of thermosensitive polymeric systems are the avoidance of toxic organic solvents, ability to deliver both hydrophilic and lipophilic drugs, and sustained drug release. In spite of these advantages several drawbacks associated with these systems include high-burst drug release, low mechanical strength leading to potential dose dumping, instability of thermolabile drugs, lack of biocompatibility, and gradual pH lowering of the system due to acidic degradation products of the polymers [40–42].

2.4 Ultrasound-Responsive Systems

The intensity of ultrasound energy can be tailored and applied over a small area of the body. The mechanism of ultrasound involves a medium that focuses, reflects, and refracts the ultrasonic waves. Ultrasound-sensitive vehicles have the potential to treat cancers because of their invasive character, ability to penetrate deeply into the human body, and ease of control. However, clinical use of this system may still require repeated use, with many related disadvantages such as patient noncompliance, higher risk of sonication side effects, and the associated cost [43].

2.5 Enzyme-Responsive Systems

Enzymes play a central role in cell regulation. These proteins are not only important targets in therapeutics, but also essential for formulation development. Drug delivery systems, especially nanocarriers can be monitored to deliver or release drugs via enzymatic conversion of the vehicles. For instance, if the enzyme level is higher at a target site or the enzymatic activity is higher in diseased tissue, this imbalance can trigger higher drug release at the target site [17,42,44,52].

2.6 Oxidative Stress–Responsive Systems

Oxidative stress is caused predominantly by the accumulation of hydrogen peroxide (H_2O_2), which may potentially be useful as a stimulus for targeted drug delivery. Oxidation-responsive polymers show great potential in the biomedical field and drug delivery applications. Although oxidative stress–responsive NF systems are slow in development, this stimulus can be targeted in future stimuli-sensitive approaches for diseases associated with oxidative stress such as the posterior eye segment diseases [41,70].

2.7 Carbohydrate-Responsive Systems

Carbohydrate-responsive systems have gained attention in drug delivery. These systems are designed to produce the triggered drug release in response to specific chemicals such as sugars (glucose, fructose, and mannose). These polymers have garnered considerable attention because of their application in both sensing and delivery (insulin) applications. In spite of these advantages, the major limitations are short response duration and biocompatibility issues [45].

2.8 Multiresponsive Systems

Dual- or multiresponsive nanocarrier are exciting developments in the field of stimuli-sensitive drug delivery. These systems in general can orthogonally respond to two or more stimuli. The combination involves pH and ionic strength, pH and thermoresponsiveness, or pH and carbohydrates. These dual-responsive systems are developed by a combination of two monomers having responsiveness to different stimuli. Of the multiresponsive systems, pH and temperature-responsive NFs are the most studied. One potential advantage of dual-responsive systems is the fact that one stimulus can be utilized to load the carrier, whereas a second one can be used to trigger the release. However, the design of multiresponsive NF remains a challenge because these systems are composed of several blocks, each with a different stimulus [19,46].

2.9 Challenges in Stimuli-Responsive Drug Delivery Applications of Nanofibers

Rapid progress has been made in the development of stimuli-responsive polymeric NFs in biomedical applications. However, a majority of these systems have not made it past the preclinical stages due to several limitations and challenges. There are several limitations of NF stimuli-responsive systems that need to be solved before these systems can proceed to clinical trial. The complex formulation steps, scaling up of the synthesis, and use of multiple components need to be simplified. External stimuli sources need improvement to achieve better tissue penetration without causing any damage to other nonspecific tissues. Although the NFs have been successfully fabricated, these systems have not been thoroughly investigated relative to stimuli-responsive potential. Moreover, potential toxicity of polymers involved in the stimuli-sensitive therapeutics including the slow response of NFs needs improvement and further evaluation. In addition to the above-mentioned challenges, the degradation product of any stimuli-sensitive system must be biocompatible and safe before it can be translated. These barriers impede the optimal performance of stimuli-responsive delivery systems. Although there are many challenges, a number of opportunities in the development of smart polymeric drug delivery systems are being contemplated.

3. APPLICATIONS OF ELECTROSPUN NANOFIBERS
3.1 Electrospun Nanofibers in Tissue Engineering

A wide variety of methods have been reported in the literature for the fabrication of tissue engineering scaffolds [47]. Electrospun NF scaffolds have exhibited an excellent cell growing capability. Biocompatible and biodegradable NFs are generally preferred over conventional scaffolds because of their ability to provide a native environment for tissue regeneration. It is initiated by cellular adhesion to the matrix or neighboring cells.

Most tissues and cells are underlain or surrounded by a natural extracellular matrix (ECM). These tissues are able to organize cells into the ECM, facilitate cell migrations, activate signal transduction pathways, and coordinate cellular functions. NFs have a unique ability of mimicking ECM of the target cell and tissues [48,49].

Among the synthetic polymers, PLGA is considered to be the ideal material for tissue regeneration because of its biodegradable nature, easy spinnability, and multiple focal adhesion points. The results revealed that PCL electrospun NF scaffolds could enhance MC3T3-E1 preosteoblast cell adhesion and proliferation as well as assistance in the cell [50]. The limitations of electrospun NF in tissue engineering can be overcome by generating a 3D instead of 2D environment. Three-dimensional scaffolds have more exposed inner surface area and pore size allowing enhanced infiltration of the cell compared with the 2D conventional scaffold. Attempts have been made to fabricate larger intrafiber pore size to allow the scaffolds to be present as 3D instead of a 2D environment. Three dimensional scaffolds may be fabricated by combining multiple polymers, i.e., NFs [51]. Various solubility and stretching properties render the polymers in the flight between the needle and collector. The controlled large intrafiber pore size will result in the infiltration of cells into the electrospun blended NF scaffold. Due to wettability of the polymer blends a unique construct may be prepared, which promotes cell infiltration and adhesion. Electrospun NF is one of the examples of 3D scaffolds offering several applications in tissue engineering such as vascular grafts, nerve regeneration, and bone regeneration.

3.1.1 Skin Tissue Engineering

An electrospun NF has contributed to the development of innovative grafting scaffolds for skin. For instance, high porosity of electrospun NFs could provide larger structural space of accommodation for the grafted cells. It also facilitates migration, cell proliferation, oxygen exchange, and nutrient delivery in wound healing. The small pore size of nanofibrous scaffolds provides dehydration and limits the wound infection. The tunable mechanical properties of electrospun NFs also prevent wound contraction during implantation. Various natural polymers such as collagen, gelatin, silk, chitosan, and fibrinogen have been fabricated into NFs for wound healing. Cell culture suggests that NFs favored the attachment and proliferation of keratinocytes or fibroblasts. Vatankhah et al. developed cellulose acetate/gelatin electrospun NFs to mimic dermis ECM (a complex combination of proteins and polysaccharides). Electrospun cellulose acetate/gelatin 25:75 NFs represent distinct adherence features and high proliferation of human dermal fibroblasts based on data [53]. In another study, animal data suggest that early-state healing in the collagen NF was promoted with the absence of surface tissue debris, and prominent capillary and fibroblast proliferation. However, limitation of natural polymer includes low resistance to enzymatic degradation and weak mechanical properties. In contrast, biodegradable synthetic polymers, such as poly(glycolic acid) (PGA), poly(lactic acid) (PLA), PCL, and their copolymers, are commonly used for skin and other tissue engineering (TE) due to their favorable mechanical properties. To investigate the relationship between the degradation properties of NFs and their efficacy for dermal regeneration, PLA and PLGA with different lactide/glycolide mole fractions (85:15, 75:25, and 50:50) were mixed and electrospun into NFs. In vivo studies showed that poly-L-lactic acid (PLLA) NFs remained stable after 12 months of implantation, whereas NFs of PLGA 85:15, 75:25 lost 50% of their original masses after 4 and 3 months, respectively. PLGA (85:15, 75:25) NFs appears to generate favorable biodegradable scaffolds for dermal replacement supporting the growth of keratinocyte, fibroblast, and endothelial cells [54]. The degradation rate can match the healing rate in defected tissue. Similarly, other degradable composite NFs, such as PLGA/dextran, PCL/gelatin, poly(lactic acid-co-caprolactone) (PLCL)/fibrinogen have been fabricated for skin tissue engineering, and promising results were obtained [55].

Wound dressing protects the wound from microorganisms. It absorbs exudates and accelerates the healing process. In cases of burns, diabetic ulcers, and split-skingraft-donor sites the wound healing process is prolonged. Electrospun NFs can efficiently absorb exudates and adjust the wound moisture [56]. The high porosity of nanofibrous membranes contributes to air permeability required for cell respiration. The relatively small pore size of NFs can preserve the wound from bacterial infections. Several advantages such as enhanced homeostasis, flexibility in dressing, mechanical strength, and functionalization with various bioactive molecules are offered by the NF dressings. A NF also possesses the advantage of scar-free regeneration by conducting the normal skin cell proliferation. Electrospun NFs of polyvinyl alcohol (PVA), poly(vinyl acetate), and a blend loaded with ciprofloxacin hydrochloride were studied as wound dressings. Addition of poly (vinyl acetate) to PVA NFs muted drug release at earlier stages, prolonging drug release [57]. In another study, dynamic interactions of fusidic acid—loaded electrospun PLGA NFs with wound bacteria have been explored [58]. In vitro microbiological tests showed bacterial colonization of fibers forming a thick layer of biofilm. Interestingly, the preexposure of membrane to wound bacteria causes significant improvement in drug release rate, which was the consequence of the changes in fiber morphology as well as the reduction in pH of the incubation medium. However, loading of adequate concentrations of fusidic acid into the NFs can remarkably prohibit bacterial biofilm formation [58]. Epidermal growth factor—loaded silk NFs can also accelerate the healing process by compressing the time of wound closure [59].

3.1.2 Bone Tissue Engineering
Bone is a physically hard, rigid, and strong connective tissue. It microscopically contains relatively small number of cells [60]. This tissue contains abundant ECM in the form of collagen NFs and stiffening inorganic substrate, such as hydroxyapatite (HAp) [61]. Therefore the unique bone ECM is an organic—inorganic nanofibrous composite, in

which osteocytes are able to function. Bone ECM-mimicking scaffolds, electrospun composite NFs of degradable polymers and calcium phosphate are subject of substantial investigations. Polymeric mineralized nanofibrous composites fabricated by soaking electrospun PLLA or PLLA/collagen NFs in calcium chloride solution and disodium phosphate solution [62]. The researchers noticed bone-likenano-HAp can successfully be deposited on both NFs, whereas the formation of nano-HAp on PLLA/collagen NFs is more rapid and uniform relative to PLLA NFs. Moreover, nano-HAp-deposited NFs shows enhanced capture efficacy of human fetal osteoblast cells within 20 min [63]. Later on, novel bone scaffold has been developed by simultaneous electrospraying of nano-HAp on electrospun gelatin NFs, as well as spin/spray gelatin/HA nanofibrous composite. This scaffold displays higher mechanical properties and promoted cell proliferation, alkaline phosphatase activity, and mineralization of osteoblast cells relative to pure gelatin NFs [64].

Stem cell—based therapy for bone regeneration is an active research area of many scientists. Among stem cells, mesenchymal stem cells have been widely applied in bone TE due to easy availability, self-renewing ability, and potential of osteogenic differentiation [65]. Incorporation of nano-HAp into electrospun NFs may promote cell adhesion and proliferation and even enhance osteogenic differentiation of mesenchymal stem cells. Novel nano-hydroxyapatite/PLGA composite scaffolds with high porosity and well-controlled pore architectures is developed. This newly developed composite scaffolds may serve as an excellent 3D substrate for cell attachment and migration in bone tissue engineering [66]. Similarly, Peng et al. suggest that chitosan/HAp nanofibrous scaffolds not only supported better cell attachment and proliferation of mouse mesenchymal stem cells but also promoted the osteogenic differentiation by upregulating osteogenic gene expression, even in the absence of osteogenic supplementation [67]. Various concentrations (0—50%) of nano-HAp are blended into PCL to fabricate electrospun PCL/HAp NFs for bone TE. Results suggest that mesenchymal stem cells on NFs accelerate cell proliferation rate and enhance osteogenic differentiation capability with increasing concentrations of HAp in PCL nanofibers [60,68]. Besides HAp, other calcium salts, including beta-tricalcium phosphate, calcium carbonate, and even calcium phosphate cements, have been incorporated into polymeric nanofibers for bone TE, indicating that polymer/bioceramics nanofibrous composites are promising scaffolds for accelerating bone regeneration [69].

3.1.3 Cardiac Tissue Engineering

Cardiac TE has gained attention as it promises to revolutionize the treatment of patients with end-stage heart failure. Electrospun NFs have been considered promising scaffolds due to tunable mechanical properties. Orientation of fibers can cause myocardial regeneration. Cell alignment in myocardial tissues and aligned ECM play important roles in the expression and function of cardiac cells. To mimic the cell alignment of myocardium and enhance cardiac differentiation, a tissue engineered cardiac graft has been generated by simultaneously electrospinning elastic polyurethane NFs and electrospraying mesenchymal stem cells [71]. By controlling the processing parameters, the tissue constructs are designed to possess the fibrous and anisotropic structure with mechanical response similar to native myocardium. Enhanced cardiac differentiation is detected in the aligned cardiac nanofibrous graft due to higher expression of cardiac markers, such as GATA4, Nkx2.5, and MEF2C. For instance, biodegradable and aligned nonwoven PLGA nanofibrous membranes are electrospun to provide isotropic or anisotropic growth of neonatal rat CMs. Cell orientation and elongation are enhanced in aligned NFs. PLA/carbon nanotube NFs may be electrospun as a conductive platform to direct mesenchymal stem cell differentiation toward a cardiomyocytes lineage under electrical stimulation [64,72].

3.1.4 Nerve Tissue Engineering

Another application of electrospun NFs is in nerve regeneration. The aim is to develop an effective neural network for bridging gaps in damaged peripheral or central neurons. The function of neural scaffolds is to direct axonal sprouting and promotion of neurotrophic factor diffusion. Electrospun NFs are suitable materials for nerve TE as these structures not only provide substrate topographical guidance to direct neural cells growth but also mimic the neural fibrous ECM. Xie et al. reported that the aligned PCL NFs not only enhance the differentiation of embryonic stem cells into neural lineages but also direct neurite outgrowth. The application of electrical stimulation in nerve tissue engineering has become an emerging approach to promote neurite growth and differentiation. Electrically conductive NFs have been developed as a crucial substrate for electrical stimulation. Therefore conductive polymers, such as polypyrrole, polyaniline (PANi), poly (3,4-ethylenedioxythiophene), and even carbon nanotubes, can be incorporated into NFs during electrospinning. Conductive polymer-contained NFs may enhance the proliferation of nerve cells. Rat neural stem cells on PLLA/PANi scaffolds exhibit higher proliferation than PLLA NFs after 8 days in cell culture [73,74].

3.2 Electrospun Nanofibers Applications in Dentistry

Electrospinning is an excellent technique for fabricating tissue engineering scaffolds in dentistry. A variety of materials including natural polymers (silk, collagen, chitosan), synthetic polymers (PVA, polydioxanone), and nanocomposites (HAp blends) have been electrospun for tissue engineering of oral and dental tissues, i.e., pulp dentin complex, guided tissue regeneration for periodontium, caries prevention, modification of resin composites, implant surface modification, and cartilage regeneration. The major advantage of electrospinning is its ability to produce complex geometry of nanofibrous scaffolds that can be used for dentin-pulp complex regeneration. The goal of dentin-pulp complex regeneration is to restore the mechanical and physical attributes of the tooth structure. Electrospun NF has been of interest for the repair of defects in periodontal tissues such as alveolar bone, periodontal ligament, and cementum. Biodegradable polymers such as collagen, PLGA, PLA, and PCL possess the disadvantage of poor porosity, surface alignment, and lack of biological functionality. To overcome these drawbacks, significant research has been conducted on electrospun NF, which provides enhanced porosity, cell attachment, and fiber alignment to use in periodontal regeneration. Although electrospinning has added exciting new prospects in the field of periodontal tissue regeneration, much work is needed to validate the application of electrospun nanofibrous scaffolds in the clinical stage with respect to mechanical and biological properties as well as the underlying mechanisms [75].

3.3 Electrospun Nanofibers Application in Ocular Injuries

Injured or damaged corneal epithelium represents one of the frequent causes of impaired vision or even blindness. Ocular injuries require immediate management that may allow critical function restoration and minimize tissue loss. Such processes may be appropriate for ocular repair dressing, cleansing solutions, and antibiotics. Current treatment for ocular surface injuries includes the suturing of human amniotic membrane over the injury site. However, the membrane is costly and fragile, and the treatment is possible only with the most advanced surgical settings. Another option includes synthetic bandages that are usually available for more severe open globe injuries. However, synthetic bandages lack the flexibility and transparency required to restore the globe integrity in addition to monitoring the wound until permanent treatments can be available.

A biologically inspired ocular repair dressing, known as BIOcular, has been designed to fill the unmet need. BIOcular dressings are composed of biopolymeric hydrogel and NF. The hydrogel provides control release and NF provides the mechanical properties. The dressing is designed to treat corneal abrasions and ulcers on the surface of the eye. This dressing also provides resistance to bacterial penetration. It naturally resorbs over time. The dressing has a refractive index of 1.335 similar to cornea (1.38). It allows visible light transmission of 85% (http://lunainc.com/synthetic-bandages-ocular-injury-treatment/). BIOcular dressings are compatible with primary human corneal epithelial cells. If the corneal damage is extensive, it may also involve the limbal region. Such defect can lead to limbal stem cell (LSC) deficiency. LSCs are essential for the regeneration of the corneal epithelium in normal and diseased states. Absence leads to corneal neovascularization, chronic inflammation, and persistent epithelial defects, all of which may result in a visual disability or often lead to blindness. The effective way to treat LSC deficiency is the transplantation of the intact limbal tissue containing LSCs or the transfer of ex vivo expanded stem cells [76,77]. In recent years, promising scaffolds for the growth and transfer of various types of SCs have been possible due to NF. NFs enables production of the required porosity and a specified basic weight in addition to the large surface area. It can mimic the structure of ECM proteins, which provide support for stem cell growth. Biocompatibility of NFs can be obtained by natural polymers, such as chitosan, gelatin, or collagen, or synthetic polymers, such as PVA, polyamide, and poly (L-lactic acid). During seeding of NFs with SCs, the stability of nanofibrous architecture in aqueous solutions and optimal biocompatibility should be monitored. Various SC types grow on NFs or even better than on plastic surfaces. Under standard conditions, LSCs are cultured for 2–3 weeks on plastic dishes. The cells are then detached and transferred onto NF scaffolds for additional 24 or 48 h to allow cells to adhere. Then, cell-seeded scaffolds are transferred onto the ocular surface with the cell side facing down on the ocular surface and fixed by sutures. In addition to their ability to serve as a SC carrier, NFs can be loaded with various pharmacologically active substances. These agents can promote SC growth and/or attenuate the local inflammatory reaction occurring after stem cell transplantation [78].

3.4 Electrospun Nanofibers in Drug Delivery

The aim of designing an electrospun NFs in drug delivery system is to control drug release over a definite period depending on medical conditions [79]. The rate of drug release can be tailored on the basis of fiber diameter, porosity, and drug-binding mechanisms for various applications. To date, a large number of small and biomolecules, including genes, proteins, and enzymes, have been successfully incorporated into electrospun NFs, mainly by two approaches: blending electrospinning and coaxial electrospinning.

Compared with blended NFs, the coaxial NFs reduce initial burst release with a longer release period. PLCL NFs containing tetracycline hydrochloride (TCH) may be fabricated by two methods, i.e., blending and coaxial electrospinning. TCH from both types of NFs exhibits differences in burst release. For the blended NFs, 60–80% of loaded TCH is released within the first 5 h, whereas in the case of coaxial electrospun NFs, burst release is reduced to only 5–10% followed by stable and sustained release [63,72,80].

In another study, bovine serum albumin (BSA) is selected as a model protein and incorporated into PCL NFs by blending and coaxial electrospinning [81]. Similarly, coaxial NFs have exhibited more sustained release profiles compared with blended nanofibers. Moreover, addition of PEG into PCL NFs can be preserved up to 5% of the initial biological activity of the protein. Another approach of electrospun nanofiber involves the release of multiple drugs without changing the release kinetics of any agent. To study the release of multiple drugs, a composite drug delivery system consisting of NF/particle electrospun is currently indicated. Various particles such as PLGA nanoparticles and alginate and chitosan microspheres have been successfully incorporated into electrospun NFs. This strategy may improvise the combination of both hydrophobic and hydrophilic drugs. For instance, Xu et al. have encapsulated a hydrophilic protein molecule BSA into chitosan microspheres and another hydrophobic model drug benzoin in PLLA solution [82].

Electrospinning may allow the fabrication of PLLA fiber/chitosan microsphere composites to investigate dual release of these two drugs. Chitosan microspheres are dispersed uniformly in the NFs. Additionally, hydrophilic BSA shows a short-term release, whereas hydrophobic benzoin generates relatively longer and sustained release. The mesoporous silica nanoparticles have also been incorporated into electrospun NFs to investigate the dual drug release system. A choice of mesoporous silica nanoparticles is based on large specific surface area, mesoporous structure, and surface fictionalization. This technology is emerging as a promising delivery system. These studies have confirmed that a composite approach of nanofiber/particle enables the sustained and independent release of multiple drugs [63].

3.4.1 Transdermal Drug Delivery System
Electrospun NFs can also be utilized as a transdermal drug delivery system (TDDS). A TDDS is designed to facilitate delivery through the skin. It is an alternative way of delivering sensitive drugs that are greatly affected by first-pass metabolism. Additionally, controlled drug release from a TDDS significantly improves drug efficacy due to reduced fluctuations in the drug level. Low-molecular-weight drugs can be effectively transported through the skin. However, transdermal delivery of large hydrophilic drugs is still limited. Electrospun NFs for transdermal delivery of antiinflammatory agents, vitamins, and antioxidant drugs have been successfully delivered with hydrogel polymers like PVA and cellulose acetate as drug carriers. Yun et al. have fabricated a TDDS by electrospinning of poly (vinyl alcohol)/poly (acrylic acid)/multiwalled carbon nanotube (PVA/PAA/MWCNT) NFs containing ketoprofen. The swelling properties and drug-release behavior of the NFs are significantly altered by modulating the concentration of the MWCNTs [80,83].

3.4.2 Cancer Therapy
Cancer therapy is extremely challenging to medical science. So far, a wide range of therapeutic agents have been developed to treat various types of cancers. These therapeutic agents are associated with several drawbacks, such as poor solubility and instability in the biological environment, low concentration at tumor site, adverse effects on healthy tissues, low efficacy in solid tumors, and high rate of elimination by the reticuloendothelial system. To overcome these challenges, novel delivery systems such as liposomes, nanomicelles, hydrogels, and nanoparticles have been studied [84]. Among these electrospun fabrics loaded with anticancer drugs appear to be promising approach. For instance, extremely hydrophobic antitumor agents, due to poor solubility and instability render it difficult to have sustained release of active drug molecules with suitable concentrations over a sufficient period of time. To solve these problems, hydroxyl camptothecin

(HCPT), an insoluble and unstable anticancer drug, has been loaded in poly (D,L-lactic acid)-PEG electrospun NFs using 2-hydroxypropyl-β-cyclodextrin (HPCD) as a solubilizer. HCPT-loaded electrospun fibers caused much higher inhibitory activity against human mammary gland MCF-7 cancer cells compared with the free drug during the first 72 h of incubation. However, a biphasic release (a significant initial burst release followed by very slow or negligible release during incubation time) is observed. To overcome this problem, emulsion electrospinning of HCPT was investigated in the presence of HPCD to fabricate core—shell NFs. Compared with the blend electrospinning technique, constant release is achieved due to the formation of preferential HCPT/HPCD complexes. Interestingly, the core—shell HCPT-loaded fibers display higher inhibitory activity (>20 times) against human hepatocellular carcinoma cells (Hep G2) than free HCPT over 72 h incubation [80,85].

3.5 Electrospun Nanofibers in Biomedical Application

Electrospun NF scaffolds possess properties of interconnection between pores and cell adhesion, infiltration, migration, and proliferation, while permitting free exchange of cell nutrients and wastes in addition to a high surface-to-volume ratio. Other characteristics of the electrospun NF include surface modification of bioactive molecules, cell recognizable ligands, and the ability of imitating natural ECM in addition to the mechanical strength, biocompatibility, and biodegradability. Electrospun NF shows remarkable application in drug delivery, wound dressing, medical implants, biosensors, and dental surgery (as discussed earlier). Electrospun NF offers a cost-effective method to mimic native ECM composed of an interlocking meshwork of proteins and glycosaminoglycans. Other important raw materials include PCL, PLA, PGA, PLGA, and PLCL. These copolymers are very suitable because of their ease of processing, mechanical properties, and biocompatibility. Natural polymers, such as collagen, gelatin, chitosan, and silk fibroin, have also been electrospun into NF scaffolds for biomedical applications [86].

3.6 Biosensor and Immunoassay

Biosensors have been widely utilized for environmental, food, and clinical applications. These structures are analytical devices for the detection of biological components (analytes) such as detection of gases and biological analytes. These sensors are present in low amounts and concentrations; therefore sensitivity and limit of detection play very important roles. Owing to the high surface area-to-volume ratio electrospun NF has been recognized to enlarge the surface area of the detector substrate. This process increases the sensitivity and limit of detection of biosensors without the need for the large sample size. Additionally, electrospun NFs can easily be functionalized through the incorporation of doping agents through surface modification either during or after spinning [63].

NF biosensor technology has been utilized in glucose detection. High sensitivity and selectivity are required for glucose detection. Glucose oxidase (GOD) has been widely used to fabricate glucose biosensors. It is highly sensitive and selective to glucose. GOD enzyme shows good stability at a wide pH range. GOD has been successfully employed in various electrospun NFs. Ren et al. fabricated PVA/GOD electrospun NFs as glucose biosensor. The measurements suggest that nanofibrous enzymatic electrodes exhibit a rapid response (1 s) and a higher response current (l A level) to glucose at normal and diabetic levels. The linear response is in the range from 1 to 10 mM and the limit of detection (LOD) of 0.05 mM of the biosensor meets the requirements of glucose detection in medical diagnosis. However, the intrinsic nature of the enzyme and insufficient stability limit the application of GOD-based sensors. More attention is needed to develop nonenzymatic glucose sensing. For this purpose, carbon, metals (Au, Pt, Ni, and Cu), and their oxides have been exploited as electrode materials to construct enzyme-free glucose sensors. For instance, CuO NFs have been prepared by electrospinning with subsequent thermal treatment processes for glucose nonenzymatic detection. This biosensor produces high sensitivity (431.3 $\mu A/cm^2/mM$), fast response (about1 s), and long-term stability [63,87].

Enzyme-linked immunosorbent assay (ELISA) is the gold standard immunoassay for research and in the clinical setting because of its sensitivity and simple detection. However, long analysis time and low selectivity limit the use of ELISA. Tsou et al. reported electrospun silica NF membranes for ELISA. LOD of nanofibrous ELISA is only 1.6 pM, 32 times lower than that of conventional ELISA with polystyrene well plates, and the detection time is reduced to only 1 h [63].

4. CONCLUSION

The electrospinning technique provides an inexpensive way to produce NFs from many types of polymers. These NFs have distinctive properties such as low weight, small fiber diameter, high surface area, and porosity. The properties of electrospun NFs such as fiber diameter and mechanical and surface properties can be easily modified by adjusting the electrospinning parameters. This technology is suitable for both natural and synthetic polymers. Moreover, the design of experimental approaches is an important tool in drug delivery applications and can be implemented in NF fabrication approaches for better therapeutic efficacy. The experimental design approaches have been successfully applied in analytical and formulation research [88–90]. Polymer electrospun NFs are important tools in the development of new products such as permeable NF materials, biosensors, and artificial organs in addition to immunobioassays. The tunable properties of NF make it an attractive candidate to use in tissue regeneration. Electrospun NFs in tissue engineering can grow tissues as a replacement. The electrospun NF can play a significant role in tissue regeneration such as skin grafting, nerve, cardiac, and bone. It can be included in wound dressings, dental restoration, ocular injuries, and drug delivery systems. NFs can be indicated in accidents or inherited defects without triggering severe immune responses. The extended application of electrospun NFs has been combined with other materials. Incorporation of NFs into hydrogels and nanoparticles may improve the mechanical properties of the "nanocomposite" system. Furthermore, novel stimuli systems, such as thermoresponsive polymers, pH-sensitive polymers, chemical cross-linked hydrogels, and supramolecular polymers, have been synthesized to fabricate into advanced nanofiber-based delivery systems in many biomedical applications.

Even though electrospun NF offers distinctive advantage, still there are limitations to this technology. A major challenge is difficulty in fabricating 3D scaffolds with macropores. The small pore size of electrospun NFs limits proper cellular infiltration into the fibers. However, other strategies, such as gas-forming, pyrogen-leaching, low-temperature spinning, have been employed to increase the pore size. Another issue remaining is how this promising technology can be transferred from the laboratory to production site. More studies are required for large-scale production of NFs with consistent fiber quality. In addition, environmental issues must be ascertained since this process is associated with solvent/solution in electrospinning. Besides, degradation rate and bioactivity of electrospun NFs need further investigation especially for tissue engineering and biomedical applications. To summarize, electrospun NFs are promising candidates for translation to clinical application.

REFERENCES

[1] Agrahari V, Agrahari V, Mitra AK. Nanocarrier fabrication and macromolecule drug delivery: challenges and opportunities. Ther Deliv 2016;7(4):257–78.
[2] Meng J, Agrahari V, Youm I. Advances in targeted drug delivery approaches for the central nervous system tumors: the inspiration of nanobiotechnology. J Neuroimmune Pharmacol 2016 [Epub ahead of print].
[3] Meng J, Agrahari V, Ezoulin MJ, Zhang C, Purohit SS, Molteni A, Dim D, Oyler NA, Youan BC. Tenofovir containing thiolated chitosan core/shell nanofibers: in vitro and in vivo evaluations. Mol Pharm December 5, 2016;13(12):4129–40.
[4] Bhardwaj N, Kundu SC. Electrospinning: a fascinating fiber fabrication technique. Biotechnol Adv 2010;28(3):325–47.
[5] Yoshimoto H, Shin YM, Terai H, Vacanti JP. A biodegradable nanofiber scaffold by electrospinning and its potential for bone tissue engineering. Biomaterials 2003;24(12):2077–82.
[6] Luo CJ, Stoyanov SD, Stride E, Pelan E, Edirisinghe M. Electrospinning versus fibre production methods: from specifics to technological convergence. Chem Soc Rev 2012;41(13):4708–35.
[7] Liang D, Hsiao BS, Chu B. Functional electrospun nanofibrous scaffolds for biomedical applications. Adv Drug Deliv Rev 2007;59(14):1392–412.
[8] Zeugolis DI, Khew ST, Yew ES, Ekaputra AK, Tong YW, Yung LY, et al. Electro-spinning of pure collagen nano-fibres — just an expensive way to make gelatin? Biomaterials 2008;29(15):2293–305.
[9] Ghasemi-Mobarakeh L, Prabhakaran MP, Morshed M, Nasr-Esfahani MH, Ramakrishna S. Electrospun poly(epsilon-caprolactone)/gelatin nanofibrous scaffolds for nerve tissue engineering. Biomaterials 2008;29(34):4532–9.

[10] Garg K, Bowlin GL. Electrospinning jets and nanofibrous structures. Biomicrofluidics 2011;5(1): 13403.
[11] Sharma R, Singh H, Joshi M, Sharma A, Garg T, Goyal AK, et al. Recent advances in polymeric electrospun nanofibers for drug delivery. Crit Rev Ther drug Carrier Syst 2014;31(3):187−217.
[12] Klossner RR, Queen HA, Coughlin AJ, Krause WE. Correlation of chitosan's rheological properties and its ability to electrospin. Biomacromolecules 2008;9(10):2947−53.
[13] Ding F, Deng H, Du Y, Shi X, Wang Q. Emerging chitin and chitosan nanofibrous materials for biomedical applications. Nanoscale 2014;6(16):9477−93.
[14] Dehghani F, Annabi N. Engineering porous scaffolds using gas-based techniques. Curr Opin Biotechnol 2011;22(5):661−6.
[15] Aghabegi Moghanjoughi A, Khoshnevis D, Zarrabi A. A concise review on smart polymers for controlled drug release. Drug Deliv Transl Res 2016;6(3):333−40.
[16] Stoddard RJ, Steger AL, Blakney AK, Woodrow KA. In pursuit of functional electrospun materials for clinical applications in humans. Ther Deliv 2016;7(6):387−409.
[17] Agrahari V, Zhang C, Zhang T, Li W, Gounev TK, Oyler NA, et al. Hyaluronidase-sensitive nanoparticle templates for triggered release of HIV/AIDS microbicide in vitro. AAPS J 2014;16(2): 181−93.
[18] Zhang T, Zhang C, Agrahari V, Murowchick JB, Oyler NA, Youan BB. Spray drying tenofovir loaded mucoadhesive and pH-sensitive microspheres intended for HIV prevention. Antivir Res 2013;97(3):334−46.
[19] Huang C, Soenen SJ, Rejman J, Lucas B, Braeckmans K, Demeester J, et al. Stimuli-responsiveelectrospun fibers and their applications. Chem Soc Rev 2011;40(5):2417−34.
[20] Wu H, Liu S, Xiao L, Dong X, Lu Q, Kaplan DL. Injectable and pH-responsive silk nanofiber hydrogels for sustained anticancer drug delivery. ACS Appl Mater Interfaces 2016;8(27):17118−26.
[21] Jiang J, Xie J, Ma B, Bartlett DE, Xu A, Wang CH. Mussel-inspiredprotein-mediated surface functionalization of electrospun nanofibers for pH-responsive drug delivery. Acta Biomater 2014;10(3): 1324−32.
[22] Huang C, Soenen SJ, van Gulck E, Vanham G, Rejman J, Van Calenbergh S, et al. Electrospun cellulose acetate phthalate fibers for semen induced anti-HIV vaginal drug delivery. Biomaterials 2012; 33(3):962−9.
[23] Hua D, Liu Z, Wang F, Gao B, Chen F, Zhang Q, et al. pH responsive polyurethane (core) and cellulose acetate phthalate (shell) electrospun fibers for intravaginal drug delivery. Carbohydr Polym 2016;151:1240−4.
[24] Qi M, Li X, Yang Y, Zhou S. Electrospun fibers of acid-labile biodegradable polymers containing ortho ester groups for controlled release of paracetamol. Eur J Pharm Biopharm 2008;70(2):445−52.
[25] Che HL, Lee HJ, Uto K, Ebara M, Kim WJ, Aoyagi T, et al. Simultaneous drug and gene delivery from the biodegradable poly(epsilon-caprolactone) nanofibers for the treatment of liver cancer. J Nanosci Nanotechnol 2015;15(10):7971−5.
[26] Tran T, Hernandez M, Patel D, Wu J. Temperature and pH responsive microfibers for controllable and variable ibuprofen delivery. Adv Mater Sci Eng 2015;2015:6.
[27] Hu J, Li HY, Williams GR, Yang HH, Tao L, Zhu LM. Electrospun poly(N-isopropylacrylamide)/ethyl cellulose nanofibers as thermoresponsive drug delivery systems. J Pharm Sci 2016;105(3): 1104−12.
[28] Elashnikov R, Lyutakov O, Ulbrich P, Svorcik V. Light-activated polymethylmethacrylate nanofibers with antibacterial activity. Mater Sci Eng C Mater Biol Appl 2016;64:229−35.
[29] Ramanan VV, Hribar KC, Katz JS, Burdick JA. Nanofiber−nanorod composites exhibiting light-induced reversible lower critical solution temperature transitions. Nanotechnology 2011;22(49): 494009.
[30] Ball C, Woodrow KA. Electrospun solid dispersions of maraviroc for rapid intravaginal preexposure prophylaxis of HIV. Antimicrob Agents Chemother 2014;58(8):4855−65.
[31] Phromviyo N, Lert-Itthiporn A, Swatsitang E, Chompoosor A. Biodegradable poly(vinyl alcohol)/polyoxalate electrospun nanofibers for hydrogen peroxide-triggered drug release. J Biomater Sci Polym Ed 2015;26(14):975−87.

[32] Wang Y, Kotsuchibashi Y, Uto K, Ebara M, Aoyagi T, Liu Y, et al. pH and glucose responsive nanofibers for the reversible capture and release of lectins. Biomater Sci 2015;3(1):152–62.

[33] Lin X, Tang D, Yu Z, Feng Q. Stimuli-responsive electrospun nanofibers from poly(N-isopropylacrylamide)-co-poly(acrylic acid) copolymer and polyurethane. J Mater Chem B 2014;2(6):651–8.

[34] Kanamala M, Wilson WR, Yang M, Palmer BD, Wu Z. Mechanisms and biomaterials in pH-responsive tumour targeted drug delivery: a review. Biomaterials 2016;85:152–67.

[35] Karimi M, Eslami M, Sahandi-Zangabad P, Mirab F, Farajisafiloo N, Shafaei Z, et al. pH-Sensitivestimulus-responsive nanocarriers for targeted delivery of therapeutic agents. Wiley Interdiscip Rev Nanomed Nanobiotechnol 2016;8(5):696–716.

[36] Qiu Y, Park K. Environment-sensitive hydrogels for drug delivery. Adv Drug Deliv Rev 2001;53(3):321–39.

[37] You J, Shao R, Wei X, Gupta S, Li C. Near-infrared light triggers release of Paclitaxel from biodegradable microspheres: photothermal effect and enhanced antitumor activity. Small 2010;6(9):1022–31.

[38] Mura S, Nicolas J, Couvreur P. Stimuli-responsive nanocarriers for drug delivery. Nat Mater 2013;12(11):991–1003.

[39] Agrahari V, Agrahari V, Hung WT, Christenson LK, Mitra AK. Composite nanoformulation therapeutics for long-term ocular delivery of macromolecules. Mol Pharm 2016;13(9):2912–22.

[40] Schmaljohann D. Thermo- and pH-responsive polymers in drug delivery. Adv Drug Deliv Rev 2006;58(15):1655–70.

[41] Ganta S, Devalapally H, Shahiwala A, Amiji M. A review of stimuli-responsive nanocarriers for drug and gene delivery. J Control Release 2008;126(3):187–204.

[42] Fleige E, Quadir MA, Haag R. Stimuli-responsive polymeric nanocarriers for the controlled transport of active compounds: concepts and applications. Adv Drug Deliv Rev 2012;64(9):866–84.

[43] Zhao YZ, Du LN, Lu CT, Jin YG, Ge SP. Potential and problems in ultrasound-responsive drug delivery systems. Int J Nanomedicine 2013;8:1621–33.

[44] Hu Q, Katti PS, Gu Z. Enzyme-responsive nanomaterials for controlled drug delivery. Nanoscale 2014;6(21):12273–86.

[45] Priya James H, John R, Alex A, Anoop KR. Smart polymers for the controlled delivery of drugs — a concise overview. Acta Pharm Sin B 2014;4(2):120–7.

[46] Guragain S, Bastakoti BP, Malgras V, Nakashima K, Yamauchi Y. Multi-stimuli-responsive polymeric materials. Chemistry 2015;21(38):13164–74.

[47] Hu X, Liu S, Zhou G, Huang Y, Xie Z, Jing X. Electrospinning of polymeric nanofibers for drug delivery applications. J Control Release 2014;185:12–21.

[48] Ingavle GC, Leach JK. Advancements in electrospinning of polymeric nanofibrous scaffolds for tissue engineering. Tissue Eng Part B Rev 2014;20(4):277–93.

[49] Son YJ, Kim WJ, Yoo HS. Therapeutic applications of electrospun nanofibers for drug delivery systems. Arch Pharm Res 2014;37(1):69–78.

[50] Smith IO, McCabe LR, Baumann MJ. MC3T3-E1 osteoblast attachment and proliferation on porous hydroxyapatite scaffolds fabricated with nanophase powder. Int J Nanomedicine 2006;1(2):189–94.

[51] Park YR, Ju HW, Lee JM, Kim DK, Lee OJ, Moon BM, et al. Three-dimensional electrospun silk-fibroin nanofiber for skin tissue engineering. Int J Biol Macromol December 2016;93(Pt B):1567–74.

[52] Agrahari V, Meng J, Ezoulin MJ, Youm I, Dim DC, Molteni A, Hung WT, Christenson LK, Youan BC. Stimuli-sensitive thiolated hyaluronic acid based nanofibers: synthesis, preclinical safety and in vitro anti-HIV activity. Nanomedicine (Lond) November 2016;11(22):2935–58.

[53] Vatankhah E, Prabhakaran MP, Jin G, Mobarakeh LG, Ramakrishna S. Development of nanofibrous cellulose acetate/gelatin skin substitutes for variety wound treatment applications. J Biomater Appl 2014;28(6):909–21.

[54] Blackwood KA, McKean R, Canton I, Freeman CO, Franklin KL, Cole D, et al. Development of biodegradable electrospun scaffolds for dermal replacement. Biomaterials 2008;29(21):3091–104.

[55] Beachley V, Wen X. Polymer nanofibrous structures: fabrication, biofunctionalization, and cell interactions. Prog Polym Sci 2010;35(7):868–92.

[56] Rho KS, Jeong L, Lee G, Seo BM, Park YJ, Hong SD, et al. Electrospinning of collagen nanofibers: effects on the behavior of normal human keratinocytes and early-stage wound healing. Biomaterials 2006;27(8):1452—61.

[57] Jannesari M, Varshosaz J, Morshed M, Zamani M. Composite poly(vinyl alcohol)/poly(vinyl acetate) electrospun nanofibrous mats as a novel wound dressing matrix for controlled release of drugs. Int J Nanomedicine 2011;6:993—1003.

[58] Said SS, Aloufy AK, El-Halfawy OM, Boraei NA, El-Khordagui LK. Antimicrobial PLGA ultrafine fibers: interaction with wound bacteria. Eur J Pharm Biopharm 2011;79(1):108—18.

[59] Erfurt-Berge C, Renner R. Recent developments in topical wound therapy: impact of antimicrobiological changes and rebalancing the wound milieu. Biomed Res Int 2014;2014. 819525.

[60] Holzwarth JM, Ma PX. Biomimetic nanofibrous scaffolds for bone tissue engineering. Biomaterials 2011;32(36):9622—9.

[61] Sheikh FA, Kanjwal MA, Macossay J, Barakat NA, Kim HY. A simple approach for synthesis, characterization and bioactivity of bovine bones to fabricate the polyurethane nanofiber containing hydroxyapatite nanoparticles. Express Polym Lett 2012;6(1).

[62] Shin SH, Purevdorj O, Castano O, Planell JA, Kim HW. A short review: recent advances in electrospinning for bone tissue regeneration. J Tissue Eng 2012;3(1). 2041731412443530.

[63] Kai D, Liow SS, Loh XJ. Biodegradable polymers for electrospinning: towards biomedical applications. Mater Sci Eng C Mater Biol Appl 2014;45:659—70.

[64] Braghirolli DI, Steffens D, Pranke P. Electrospinning for regenerative medicine: a review of the main topics. Drug Discov Today 2014;19(6):743—53.

[65] Shin M, Yoshimoto H, Vacanti JP. In vivo bone tissue engineering using mesenchymal stem cells on a novel electrospun nanofibrous scaffold. Tissue Eng 2004;10(1—2):33—41.

[66] Huang YX, Ren J, Chen C, Ren TB, Zhou XY. Preparation and properties of poly(lactide-co-glycolide) (PLGA)/nano-hydroxyapatite (NHA) scaffolds by thermally induced phase separation and rabbit MSCs culture on scaffolds. J Biomater Appl 2008;22(5):409—32.

[67] Peng H, Yin Z, Liu H, Chen X, Feng B, Yuan H, et al. Electrospun biomimetic scaffold of hydroxyapatite/chitosan supports enhanced osteogenic differentiation of mMSCs. Nanotechnology 2012; 23(48):485102.

[68] Gentile P, Chiono V, Carmagnola I, Hatton PV. An overview of poly(lactic-co-glycolic) acid (PLGA)-based biomaterials for bone tissue engineering. Int J Mol Sci 2014;15(3):3640—59.

[69] Richardson SM, Kalamegam G, Pushparaj PN, Matta C, Memic A, Khademhosseini A, et al. Mesenchymal stem cells in regenerative medicine: focus on articular cartilage and intervertebral disc regeneration. Methods 2016;99:69—80.

[70] Agrahari V, Agrahari V, Mandal A, Pal D, Mitra AK. How are we improving the delivery to back of the eye? Advances and challenges of novel therapeutic approaches. Expert Opin Drug Deliv December 28, 2016:1—17.

[71] Guan J, Wang F, Li Z, Chen J, Guo X, Liao J, et al. The stimulation of the cardiac differentiation of mesenchymal stem cells in tissue constructs that mimic myocardium structure and biomechanics. Biomaterials 2011;32(24):5568—80.

[72] Lu Y, Huang J, Yu G, Cardenas R, Wei S, Wujcik EK, et al. Coaxial electrospun fibers: applications in drug delivery and tissue engineering. Wiley Interdiscip Rev Nanomed Nanobiotechnol 2016;8(5): 654—77.

[73] Xie J, MacEwan MR, Schwartz AG, Xia Y. Electrospun nanofibers for neural tissue engineering. Nanoscale 2010;2(1):35—44.

[74] Ghasemi-Mobarakeh L, Prabhakaran MP, Morshed M, Nasr-Esfahani MH, Baharvand H, Kiani S, et al. Application of conductive polymers, scaffolds and electrical stimulation for nerve tissue engineering. J Tissue Eng Regen Med 2011;5(4):e17—35.

[75] Seo S-J, Kim H-W, Lee J-H. Electrospun nanofibers applications in dentistry. J Nanomater 2016; 2016:7.

[76] Sejpal K, Bakhtiari P, Deng SX. Presentation, diagnosis and management of limbal stem cell deficiency. Middle East Afr J Ophthalmol 2013;20(1):5—10.

[77] Dua HS, Saini JS, Azuara-Blanco A, Gupta P. Limbal stem cell deficiency: concept, aetiology, clinical presentation, diagnosis and management. Indian J Ophthalmol 2000;48(2):83—92.

[78] Holan V, Javorkova E. Mesenchymal stem cells, nanofiber scaffolds and ocular surface reconstruction. Stem Cell Rev 2013;9(5):609–19.

[79] Katti DS, Robinson KW, Ko FK, Laurencin CT. Bioresorbable nanofiber-based systems for wound healing and drug delivery: optimization of fabrication parameters. J Biomed Mater Res B Appl Biomater 2004;70(2):286–96.

[80] Zamani M, Prabhakaran MP, Ramakrishna S. Advances in drug delivery via electrospun and electrosprayed nanomaterials. Int J Nanomedicine 2013;8:2997–3017.

[81] Zhang YZ, Wang X, Feng Y, Li J, Lim CT, Ramakrishna S. Coaxial electrospinning of (fluorescein isothiocyanate-conjugated bovine serum albumin)-encapsulated poly(epsilon-caprolactone) nanofibers for sustained release. Biomacromolecules 2006;7(4):1049–57.

[82] Xu J, Jiao Y, Shao X, Zhou C. Controlled dual release of hydrophobic and hydrophilic drugs from electrospun poly(l-lactic acid) fiber mats loaded with chitosan microspheres. Mater Lett 2011; 65(17–18):2800–3.

[83] Yun J, Im JS, Lee Y-S, Kim H-I. Electro-responsive transdermal drug delivery behavior of PVA/PAA/MWCNT nanofibers. Eur Polym J 2011;47(10):1893–902.

[84] Mitra AK, Agrahari V, Mandal A, Cholkar K, Natarajan C, Shah S, et al. Novel delivery approaches for cancer therapeutics. J Control Release 2015;219:248–68.

[85] Xie C, Li X, Luo X, Yang Y, Cui W, Zou J, et al. Release modulation and cytotoxicity of hydroxycamptothecin-loaded electrospun fibers with 2-hydroxypropyl-beta-cyclodextrin inoculations. Int J Pharm 2010;391(1–2):55–64.

[86] Agarwal S, Wendorff JH, Greiner A. Use of electrospinning technique for biomedical applications. Polymer 2008;49(26):5603–21.

[87] Su X, Wei J, Ren X, Li L, Meng X, Ren J, et al. A new amperometric glucose biosensor based on one-step electrospun poly(vinyl alcohol)/chitosan nanofibers. J Biomed Nanotechnol 2013;9(10): 1776–83.

[88] Youm I, Agrahari V, Murowchick JB, Youan BB. Uptake and cytotoxicity of docetaxel-loaded hyaluronic acid-grafted oily core nanocapsules in MDA-MB 231 cancer cells. Pharm Res 2014;31(9): 2439–52.

[89] Meng J, Zhang T, Agrahari V, Ezoulin MJ, Youan BB. Comparative biophysical properties of tenofovir-loaded, thiolated and nonthiolated chitosan nanoparticles intended for HIV prevention. Nanomedicine (Lond) 2014;9(11):1595–612.

[90] Agrahari V, Meng J, Zhang T, Youan BB. Application of design of experiment and simulation methods to liquid chromatography analysis of topical HIV microbicides stampidine and HI443. J Anal Bioanal Tech 2014;5(1).

CHAPTER 10

Nanosystems for Diagnostic Imaging, Biodetectors, and Biosensors

Gayathri Acharya[1], Ashim K. Mitra[2], Kishore Cholkar[3]
[1]GlaxoSmithKline, Collegeville, PA, United States; [2]University of Missouri—Kansas City, Kansas City, MO, United States; [3]Ingenus Pharmaceuticals/RiconPharma LLC, Denville, NJ, United States

Contents

1. Introduction	217
2. Nanosystems as Platforms for Advanced Diagnostic Imaging	218
2.1 Iron Oxide Nanoparticles	218
2.2 Quantum Dots	220
2.3 Gold Nanoparticles	221
2.4 Carbon Nanotubes	222
2.5 Silica Nanoparticles	222
2.6 Liposomes	223
2.7 Nanomicelles	224
2.8 Dendrimers	225
3. Diagnostic Imaging With Nanosystems	226
3.1 Magnetic Resonance Imaging	227
3.2 Optical Imaging	228
3.3 Nuclear Imaging	230
3.4 Computed Tomography	230
3.5 Ultrasound	231
4. Biological Sensors	232
4.1 Glucose Sensors	233
4.1.1 Immobilized Enzyme Film Glucose Biosensors	*234*
4.1.2 Nanoparticle/Carbon Nanotube—Based Glucose Biosensors	*235*
4.1.3 Mechanism of Nonenzymatic Glucose Biosensors	*238*
4.2 Microcantilever	239
4.2.1 Mechanism of Microcantilever Deflection	*239*
5. Conclusions	244
References	244

1. INTRODUCTION

Nanotechnology has been on the forefront of medical breakthroughs since its advent. The very potential of a nanosystem lies in its ability to act as an individual nanosized unit or device, with numerous physicochemical properties. Nanosystems are extremely valuable in biomedical applications. This technology is taking modern medicine to a whole new level with personalized medicine. An interdisciplinary approach to merge multifunctional nanosystems, high-performance imaging techniques, and computers to develop multimodal tissue targeting, diagnosis, and therapy has become the current state-of-the-art cancer treatment modality. The objective of this chapter is to outline the fundamentals for selecting and designing nanosystems for applications in diagnostic imaging and biodetectors/biosensors. Nanoparticles are designed as a single delivery system for a combined approach of tissue targeting, cellular imaging, molecular diagnosis, drug delivery, and photothermal therapy. The strategy is to develop personalized medicine especially for cancer. Such combinatorial approach of combining therapy with diagnostics represents theranostics. It includes diagnosis, therapy, and image-guided prognosis making personalized medicine a reality.

2. NANOSYSTEMS AS PLATFORMS FOR ADVANCED DIAGNOSTIC IMAGING

Imaging is an essential part of disease prognosis and contrast agents play an important part. Contrast agents enhance the imaging of tissue structure. Contrast agents have become indispensable in the field of medical diagnosis. Despite image-enhancing ability low efficiency of the target tissue requires high concentrations to obtain the desired effect [1]. Although many safer options have been introduced for contrast agents, their ability to passively diffuse into the surrounding area around the target tissue is a major drawback [1]. Nanosystems lower toxicity of the contrast agents, by adding target specificity to the system, which in turn reduces the dose required. Nanosystems offer larger surface area and smaller size compared with traditional contrast agents along with low toxicity. These properties can be streamlined to diagnose the pathological tissue by modifying the charge, size, shape, and target-specific surface moiety [2—4]. Some of the strategies for drug loading and functionalization of nanosystems are depicted in Fig. 10.1.

2.1 Iron Oxide Nanoparticles

Iron oxide nanoparticles are composed of iron oxide particles of size 1—100 mm. The two primary biocompatible forms of iron oxide are magnetite (Fe_3O_4) and the oxide form maghemite (γ-Fe_3O_4). Magnetic fluids, data storage, catalysis, and biomedical applications are some of the key applications. In biomedical research, magnetic nanoparticles are applied in magnetic bioseparation, biological detection, detoxification, immunoassays, hyperthermia, medical diagnosis, tissue repair, tumor therapy, and targeted drug delivery [3]. Advantages of various polymers used in functionalization of iron oxide nanoparticles is shown in Table 10.1. Iron oxide nanoparticles are known to improve imaging contrast in magnetic resonance imaging (MRI) [3,5].

Iron oxide nanoparticles tend to aggregate due to their large surface to volume ratio exhibiting strong supraparamagnetic properties. Physicochemical properties such as the particle size, distribution, and concentration are invaluable for adjusting the optical

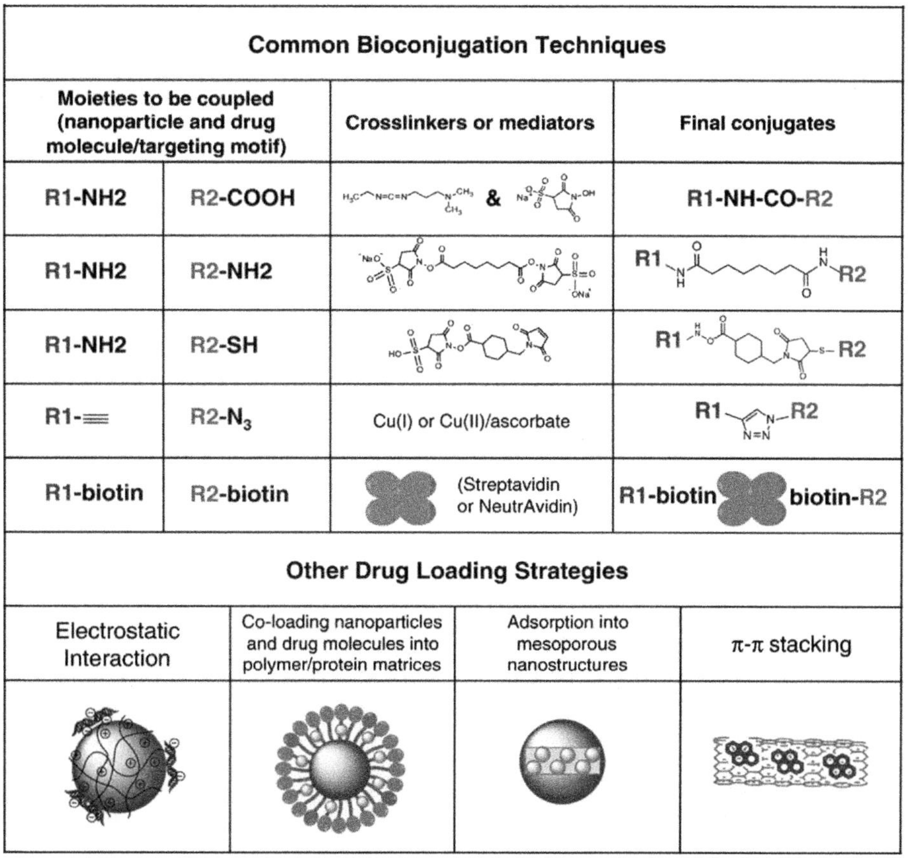

Common Bioconjugation Techniques		
Moieties to be coupled (nanoparticle and drug molecule/targeting motif)	Crosslinkers or mediators	Final conjugates
R1-NH2 / R2-COOH	EDC & Sulfo-NHS	R1-NH-CO-R2
R1-NH2 / R2-NH2	BS3 crosslinker	R1-NH-CO-(CH2)n-CO-NH-R2
R1-NH2 / R2-SH	Sulfo-SMCC	R1-NH-CO-...-S-R2
R1-≡ / R2-N₃	Cu(I) or Cu(II)/ascorbate	R1-triazole-R2
R1-biotin / R2-biotin	(Streptavidin or NeutrAvidin)	R1-biotin···biotin-R2

Other Drug Loading Strategies			
Electrostatic Interaction	Co-loading nanoparticles and drug molecules into polymer/protein matrices	Adsorption into mesoporous nanostructures	π-π stacking

Figure 10.1 Strategies used for drug loading and functionalization of nanosystems [3].

and magnetic properties. Combinatorial therapies assisted by iron oxide nanoparticles are indicated in cancer therapy. Fe$_3$O$_4$ nanoparticles can provide targeted drug delivery and enhance imaging and therapeutics through high localization at the target site under magnetic field. Synergistically these nanoparticles also cause tumor cell death via localized hyperthermia under alternating magnetic fields and/or photon application (with therapeutic agents) that generates heat [6].

Multiple techniques are applied for the synthesis of magnetic nanoparticles. Although coprecipitation of iron salts is the most common method, desired size range and nonuniform distribution of the particle are some of the drawbacks [6]. Sonolysis, electrospray synthesis, flow injection synthesis, polyol method, sol–gel reaction, hydrothermal synthesis, and microemulsions are just a few of these techniques [5]. Naked iron oxide nanoparticles are highly unstable. This material oxidizes in air due to strong chemical activity from the large surface to volume ratio that leads to loss of magnetism and dispersibility. To enhance the stability of the particles, the particles are often surface modified or coated to protect the

Table 10.1 Advantages of various polymers for functionalization of iron oxide nanoparticles [6]

	Polymers	Advantages
Natural polymers	Dextran	Enables optimum polar interactions with iron oxide surfaces, improves the blood circulation time, stability, and biocompatibility
	Starch	Improves the biocompatibility, good for magnetic resonance imaging, and drug target delivery
	Gelatin	Used as a gelling agent, hydrophilic emulsifier, biocompatible
	Chitosan	Nontoxic, alkaline, hydrophilic, widely used as nonviral gene delivery system, biocompatible, and hydrophilic
Synthetic polymers	Poly(ethyleneglycol)	Enhance the hydrophilicity and water solubility, improves the biocompatibility, blood circulation times
	Poly(vinyl alcohol)	Prevents agglomeration, giving rise to monodispersibility
	Poly(lactic acid)	Improves the biocompatibility, biodegradability, and low toxicity in human body
	Alginate	Improves the stability and biocompatibility
	Polymethylmethacrylate	Generally used as thermosensitive drug delivery and cell separation
	Polyacrylic acid	Improves stability and biocompatibility as well as bioconjugation

nanoparticle as well as to introduce advanced functionality. Both organic and inorganic compounds can be conjugated for surface functionalization [6].

2.2 Quantum Dots

Quantum dots are nanosized crystals that act as semiconductors depending on the temperature and purity of the material. The tight size range (2—10 nm) of quantum dots manifests quantum mechanics—like properties [3]. Quantum dots are researched as contrast agents for diagnosis and detection, due to narrow emission spectra, high light stability, and wide and continuous absorption spectra. Additionally, the energy spectrum of these nanosystems can also be tailored by controlling the size, shape, and energy levels. Smaller quantum dots require high energy for electrons to enter an excited state. It results in high-energy frequency and smaller wavelength, emitting light at the blue end of the spectrum. Conversely, large quantum dots emit light at the red end of the spectrum [3]. The structure of quantum dots comprises a semiconductor core made of heavy metals [like cadmium selenide (CdSe), lead selenide (PbSe), or indium arsenide (InAs)] and an outer shell [zinc sulfide (ZnS), cadmium sulfide (CdS)] to prevent toxicity. CdSe/ZnS quantum dots are currently the most commonly available commercial products [7]. Numerous methods have been utilized to synthesize quantum dots, i.e., plasma synthesis, electrochemical assembly, and viral assembly. Colloidal synthesis is still the most common technique [8].

Quantum dots are very stable against photobleaching and can be considered as alternatives for traditional fluorescent indicator dyes and proteins. These materials exhibit tunable luminescence and electrical properties that are employed in various biological applications such as imaging, DNA detection, and cell sorting, labeling, and tracking [8]. Despite their size, quantum dots can be combined with other nanosystems for widening their applications [3].

2.3 Gold Nanoparticles

Gold nanoparticles have been extensively studied over the last decade in numerous therapeutic applications. By definition gold nanoparticles are composed of nanosized colloidal gold particle suspended in water or other liquids that exhibit optical, electronic, and molecular recognition properties [2]. These unique properties of gold nanoparticles can also be fine-tuned to obtain desired effect by adjusting the size, shape, and surface chemistry [9]. These nanoparticles also come in various shapes such as nanorods, nanostars, nanocubes, nanotriangles, nanoclusters, and nanoshells, each with a unique set of properties and applications. Nanoparticles of noble metals like gold display surface plasmon resonance, a property that is responsible for strong electromagnetic fields with high optical absorption and emission properties [10–12]. Contrary to quantum dots are the smaller gold nanoparticles that absorb light in the lower wavelength region reflecting red light. As their size increases these dots emit more clear or translucent color [12].

Gold nanoparticles can be prepared by chemical, physical, and biological methods. Most commonly the process involves reduction of dissolved chloroauric acid (H[AuCl$_4$]) to generate Au$^+$ ions from Au^{3+} ions, followed by disproportionation reaction, three Au$^+$ ions generate one Au^{3+} and two Au^0 ions. The Au^0 ions act as nucleation centers around which Au$^+$ ions are reduced. The resulting unstable surface charge on particles is then stabilized with surfactants to prevent aggregation resulting in dispersion within colloidal suspension [10].

Photodynamic therapy (PDT) is a treatment with a combination of drug and photosensitizer agents, which are exposed to certain wavelength of visible light to trigger photochemical reaction. This generates singlet oxygen molecules that cause tumor cell death. Several confounding factors are involved in this type of therapy with limited application. Gold nanoparticles are biocompatible with low cytotoxicity rendering them one of the safest candidates for biomedical applications like imaging (sensory probes), therapeutic drug delivery, and catalysis [3]. Larger gold nanoparticles (>40 nm) are applied for imaging because of high scattering properties. Smaller particles

(<20 nm), applied for photothermal therapy, are capable of absorbing most of the incident light energy creating sufficient heat to denature proteins leading to tumor cell death [11,12].

2.4 Carbon Nanotubes

Carbon nanotubes (CNTs) are one-dimensional systems made of one-atom-thick sheet of graphite (called graphene) rolled up into a seamless cylinder with diameter in the order of a nanometer. Although the diameter of a nanotube is just a few nanometers (approximately 50,000 times smaller than the width of a human hair) in size, these constructs can be up to several millimeters in length. The length to diameter ratio of these nanosystems exceeds 10,000 times rendering CNTs with novel properties. CNTs have a wide variety of applications including biomedical imaging, electronics, optics, and other fields of materials science. These nanotubes exhibit extraordinary strength and electrical and optical properties and are efficient heat conductors. The optical properties of CNTs include effective absorption, fluorescence, and Raman spectroscopy.

CNTs are generally prepared by simple chemical vapor deposition method [13]. Other techniques include arc discharge, laser ablation, and high-pressure carbon monoxide disproportionation. In the chemical vapor deposition process, hydrocarbon polymer vapors are passed through a catalyst reactor at high temperature [13]. Nanotubes grow on the catalyst and are subsequently cooled and collected [14]. The unique physicochemical properties of carbon nanoparticles enable delivery of a variety of hydrophilic and hydrophobic drugs and even codelivery of two different drug molecules for combinatorial therapy. Functionalization of CNT has expanded the applications as a delivery platform for diverse molecules such as peptides, proteins, plasmid DNA, and synthetic oligodeoxynucleotides [15]. In fact these tubes can be even functionalized for targeted drug delivery in hard-to-reach tumor cells. CNTs are widely studied as potential theranostic agents and they can deliver both diagnostic/contrast and therapeutic agents [3,16].

2.5 Silica Nanoparticles

Silica nanoparticles are mesopores (2- to 50-nm pores) of silica that display unique physicochemical properties [17]. These nanocarriers can be prepared in a variety of sizes and shapes including nanohelices, nanotubes, nanozigzags, and nanoribbons. With tunable optical, electrical, and mechanical properties, these particles are applied in catalysis, PDT, adsorption, separation, diagnostic sensors, and therapeutic drug delivery [18].

Silica nanoparticles are synthesized with surfactants like cetyltrimethylammonium bromide as templates (or structure-directing agents) and tetraethyl orthosilicate or sodium metasilicate (Na_2SiO_3) as the silica precursors. With the deep understanding of the sol—gel techniques, a variety of nanoparticles with precise shapes and sizes were developed to meet the growing need for multifunctional nanosystems [19]. Although by nature silica particles are hydrophilic in nature, this material can be surface modified with silanol groups (~SiOH) to add required functionalization with basic silane chemistry [17].

Organic silica is widely recommended as a supplement and a therapeutic agent in amelioration of bone- and skin-related conditions. Small size and positive surface charge of organic silica-based nanoparticles render them an ideal platform for drug and gene therapy where negatively charged membrane enhances cellular uptake. These materials are also biocompatible with low toxicity. The mesoporous particle surface enables controlled delivery of the therapeutic agent. Fluorophore-doped organic silica nanoparticles are well known as optical sensors [20]. Photoluminescence properties along with the ability to entrap drug (either hydrophilic or hydrophobic) can be tuned by changing the drug/dye type. Although fluorophore-doped organic silica nanoparticles are attractive as theranostic agents, functionalization of the surface for tumor cell targeting has widened their application as biosensors with very low cytotoxicity [3,21].

2.6 Liposomes

Liposomes (also known as phospholipid bilayer vesicles) are spherical lipid bilayer membranes that represent models of cell membranes. Liposomes are composed of two main components: phospholipids and cholesterol. Phospholipids are amphipathic molecules composed of a glycerol backbone, two fatty acid tails, and a polar head group. Liposomes are viewed as aqueous cores with a hydrophobic membrane cap. These vesicles display a unique property to encapsulate both hydrophilic and hydrophobic drugs simultaneously. Depending on the size, surface charge, and lipid blend, drug is released from vesicles via three primary mechanisms such as cell fusion, endocytosis, and diffusion. Due to biocompatibility and biodegradability along with minimal toxicity, several clinically approved liposomal formulations have been developed for diagnostic imaging and biosensing [22].

Breakdown of liposome preparation involves four main steps: (1) drying of lipids from organic solvents, (2) redispersion of the lipids in aqueous media (containing drug/dye), (3) mechanical dispersion of liposomes to obtain the desired size, and (4) purification. Several techniques are applied for mechanical dispersion of liposomes such as sonication, membrane extrusion, French pressure cell extrusion, freeze thawing, and microemulsification.

As discussed earlier, liposomes are carriers of both hydrophilic and lipophilic drugs/dyes, which render these systems ideal candidates for theranostic application. Liposomes of certain size ranges may be engulfed by the macrophage phagocytosis process rendering these vesicles ideal carriers for targeting parasitic and infectious diseases. For imaging purposes, nanobubbles of contrast or diagnostic agent can be entrapped into the liposomal core or embedded into the bilayer membrane [23]. A schematic representation of liposomal modification in drug delivery and imaging is shown in Fig. 10.2.

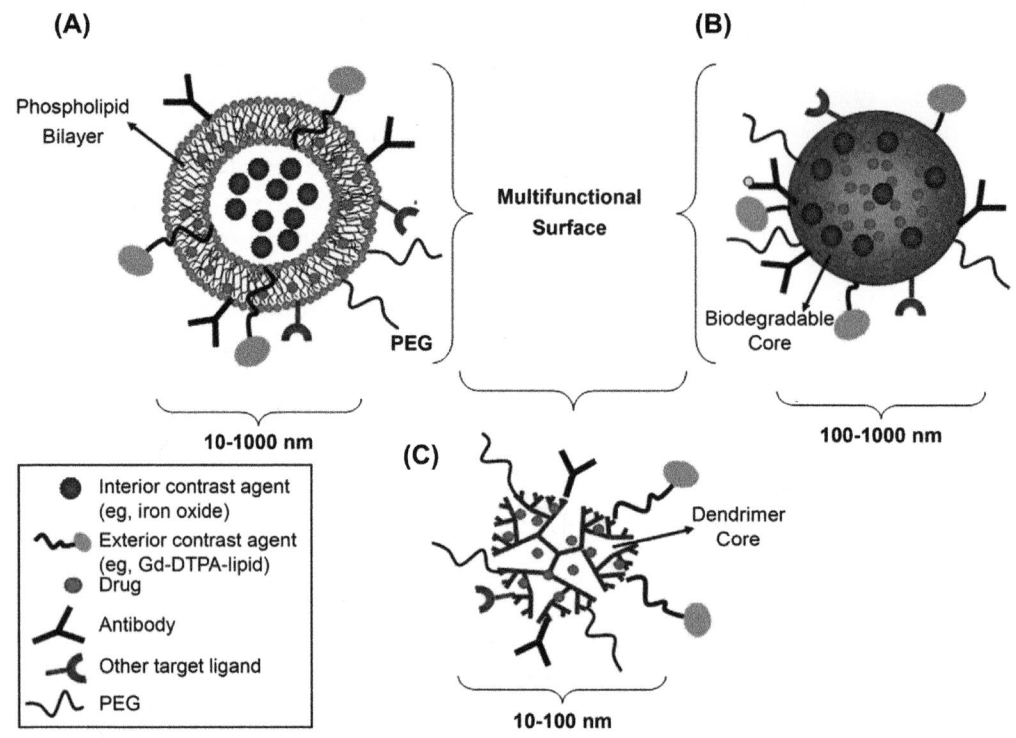

Figure 10.2 Schematic representation of nanosystems functionalized for theranostic properties: (A) liposomal system, (B) solid biodegradable polymer nanoparticles, and (C) dendrimer [32].

2.7 Nanomicelles

Nanomicelles are amphiphilic molecules formed by spherical arrangement of hydrophilic and hydrophobic moieties in aqueous media. The shape and size of micelles depend on the architecture of the surfactant molecules and solution conditions, i.e., pH, temperature, ionic strength, and surfactant concentration. Given the malleable surface and amphiphilic nature, nanomicelles are one of the most widely selected platforms for the development of theranostics. Nanomicelles can be modified to merge imaging and cancer treatment.

pH-responsive nanomicelles are formed by self-assembled two polymers, poly(ethylene glycol)-b-poly(L-lactic acid) [PEG-p(L-LA)] and poly(ethylene glycol)-b-poly(L-histidine) [PEG-p(L-His)] in aqueous solution. The contrast agent [gadolinium (Gd^{3+})] is attached to the hydroxyl group of PEG-p(L-LA) via chelating agent diethylenetriaminopentaaceticacid dianhydride (DTPA) to produce PEG-p(L-LA)-DTPA-Gd [24,25]. These nanomicelles destabilize following passive accumulation in the acidic pH of the tumor; due to charged water-soluble polymeric molecules the contrast agent is released. Additionally, modification of nanomicelles with a positively charged surface augments the accumulation of nanomicelles in the negatively charged tumor cellular membrane [24]. MRI of pH-responsive cancer-targeted micelle enables detection of tumors ~3 mm^3 in size within a few minutes [24].

In recent years, lysosomes have been identified as organelles that regulate numerous cellular processes and maintain cellular homeostasis. Irrespective of the type of cancer or multidrug resistance, acidic lysosomes can be regarded as novel diagnostic and pharmacological targets for cancer therapy [26]. In one study, combining cancer-specific aptamer, pH-sensitive fluorescent probe BDP-688, and R16FP photosensitizer integrated into a nanomicelle resulted in high tumor specificity [27]. Fluorescence triggered active visualization of lysosomal pH and site-specific near-infrared (NIR, 700–1000 nm) PDT in the presence of photosensitizer generates reactive oxygen species. It causes lysosome membrane permeation, which in turn causes cathepsin-activated apoptosis [27].

Nanomicelles as magnetic iron oxide nanoparticle carrier have been extensively studied to enhance drug concentration at target site and to reduce concentration, which ultimately reduces toxicity. The magnetic nanomicelle system triggers four-step action: (1) ligand-based targeted delivery, (2) magnetism-enhanced accumulation and retention, (3) ultrasonication-induced internalization, and (4) pH-responsive drug release. Folic acid (FA) conjugated with carboxymethyl lauryl chitosan (CLC) was developed to form iron oxide nanoparticles carrying hybrid nanomicelles. FA-CLC is a tumor-targeted pH-sensitive molecule that facilitates encapsulation of hydrophobic drugs and releases the cargo in acidic environment [28]. The FA segment in the FA-CLC molecule can target FA receptor overexpressing tumor tissue and negatively charged tumor blood vessels. CLC on the other hand triggers pH-sensitive drug release, as well as generates iron oxide nanoparticles [28].

NIR organic dyes like indocyanine green and cypate delivered in conjugation with targeted theranostic nanoparticles offer many advantages over traditional PDT [29]. Cypate along with Ce6 photosensitizer encapsulated with monomethoxy poly(ethylene glycol) and decylamine-grafter poly(L-aspartic acid) [mPEG-*b*-PAsp (DA)] nanomicelle system provides precise tumor localization and anticancer activity. Such a multifunctional micellar platform activity demonstrated synergistic anticancer effect under photothermal and PDT [25,29].

2.8 Dendrimers

Dendrimers are highly symmetrical polymeric three-dimensional (3D) structures with three structural components. A single core formation called central core/shell is followed by repetitively branched tree-like structure. The shell surrounds the core called the interior dendrimers. The outer shell can be functionalized with surface groups. A dendrimer core contributes to cavity size, absorption, capture, and release of drug. The functionalized exterior contributes to drug targeting, solubility, and chelation [30]. Dendrimers represent multifunctional nanosystems for various theranostic applications especially cancer. The surface chemistry of dendrimers can be modified to obtain desired tissue targeting, solubility, thermal stability, therapy, dendritic sensors, and gene and transdermal drug delivery [25]. These constructs are primarily utilized as contrast agent carriers for magnetic resonance, radionuclide, and fluorescence imaging and also as controlled drug delivery nanosystems [25].

Dendrimers can be synthesized by various methods including divergent and convergent methods and click chemistry. Usually the synthesis of dendrimers progresses outward in a step-by-step manner from a multifunctional core shell that reacts with monomers with one reactive group and two dormant groups [30]. It is followed by activation of the outward functional groups for further reaction with more monomers. Self-assembling dendrimers have also been developed with core shell molecules that self-assemble or recognize ditopic or polytopic core structures forming dendrimers.

Dendrimers have been indicated in various cancer-related therapies and diagnostic modalities. The nanoscale size, large multivalent surface area, well-defined polymer architecture, and quantized building blocks make dendrimers one of the most advanced nanosystems. Dendrimers can be customized to fit any application based on size, polymer type (used in building its structure), and surface modification. MRI contrast agents like Gd^{3+} are docked onto dendrimer surface via magnetic resonance chelates like DTPA and tetraazacyclododecane tetraacetic acid that capture the metal ions onto the surface [31]. Gd^{3+} dendrimers can be utilized as intravascular contrast agents owing to blood pool imaging properties. A schematic of dendrimers functionalization for theranostic application is depicted in Fig. 10.1. PEG-core dendrimer-based iodinated contrast agents display a longer systemic half-life, low immunogenicity, and improved solubility. It is suitable as a multimodal theranostic agent for intravascular diseases. Like other advanced nanosystems dendrimers can also be utilized as dual-modality agents such as G2 poly(amidoamine) (PAMAM) dendrimers with Gd^{3+} and fluorophore [32]. Rhodamine green is applied in MRI and fluorescence dual imaging in peritoneal ovarian cancer. Similarly, G6 PAMAM dendrimers labeled with Cy5.5 and Gd have been developed to combine MRI and optical imaging with enhanced resolution in sentinel lymph nodes draining in breast tissue [33].

3. DIAGNOSTIC IMAGING WITH NANOSYSTEMS

Modern medical imaging has accomplished way more than its intended application with the amalgamation of nanosystems. Typically there are many different types of diagnostic tools each with their own advantages and disadvantages (Table 10.2). All diagnostic imaging techniques have certain intensity threshold requirements for differentiating the tissue of interest from its background. Imaging is dependent on four main processes: (1) pharmacokinetics of the agent, (2) type of imaging technique, (3) period required for image acquisition, and (4) dimensions of the tissue. Some of the current image modalities include nuclear imaging, optical imaging, MRI, computed tomography (CT), and

Table 10.2 Advantages and disadvantages of different imaging modalities [35]

Imaging modality	Advantages	Disadvantages
X-ray computed tomography (CT)	• Best bone structure visualization • High temporal resolution	• Radiation exposure
Magnetic resonance (MR)	• Best soft-tissue visualization • No radiation dose	• Compatibility issues • Trade-off between temporal, spatial resolution, and sensitivity • High cost
Radionuclide imaging (PET, SPECT)	• Whole body, high sensitivity functional imaging • Multilabeling capability	• Radiation exposure • Lack of anatomic information but can be combined with CT or MR
Ultrasound	• Real time imaging • No radiation dose • Low cost	• Image quality is operator dependent • Limited penetration depth (especially in the presence of bony structures) • Limited imageable area
Optical imaging	• Single probe detection • No radiation dose • Subcellular resolution • Multilabeling capability • Low cost	• Limited penetration depth • Semiquantitative

PET, positron emission tomography; *SPECT*, single-photon emission computed tomography.

ultrasound. Research and clinical applications of these imaging modalities are summarized in Fig. 10.3. Aforementioned techniques can be applied with large tissue specimens that do not require precise depiction of the pathological area. These techniques can be enhanced to diagnose small tumors or tissues, with the addition of contrast agents that enhance the signal of the pathological area relative to background tissue. The chemical property of the contrast agent, tissue concentration, and type of imaging technique are crucial to the imaging of finer vasculature. Although contrast agents are extensively used in diagnostic imaging, the concentration injected to obtain desired tissue concentration may cause long-term accumulation and acute toxicity.

3.1 Magnetic Resonance Imaging

MRI constitutes a medical imaging modality that involves pulses of radio waves and powerful magnetic fields [34]. Due to its enhanced sensitivity relative to other imaging modalities, MRI can detect even minute changes in tissue structure caused by trauma, inflammation, or infections in small tumors and blood vessels. In an MRI scan, a strong

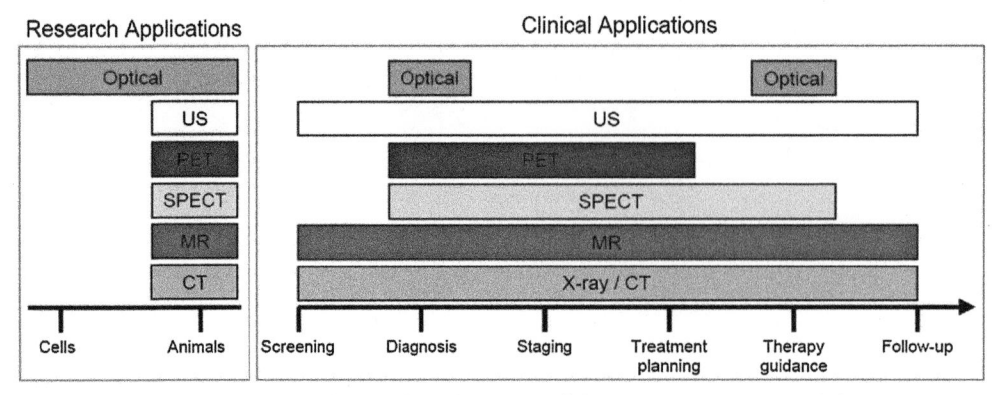

Figure 10.3 Research and clinical applications of diagnostic imaging modalities [35].

magnetic field is created to align the protons of hydrogen atoms, which are then exposed to pulsed radio waves causing the protons to spin [35]. Spinning of protons in the body produces a weak signal that is detected and processed by computers into readable images [36]. Unlike ionizing radiation, radio waves and magnetic fields have no proven adverse effects on the human body, but their impact on overall health or safety during the first trimester of pregnancy is uncertain. MRI is most commonly indicated to assess abnormalities or injuries to bones, joints, blood vessels, spinal cord, tendons, ligaments, pelvis, abdomen, chest, and breast tissue [36]. However, a magnetically active contrast substance adds to the imaging capabilities of MRI for detecting even smaller internal abnormalities [37]. MRI has two proton relaxation parameters, longitudinal and transverse, i.e., T_1 and T_2, respectively. Agents enhancing the T_1 relaxivity spike the signal intensity during imaging, whereas T_2 agents reduce the intensity. Paramagnetic compounds such as transition or lanthanide metal ions are the most commonly selected T_1 contrast agents [38]. Chelated organic gadolinium III (Gd^{3+}) or paramagnetic complexes combined with nanosystems (such as dendrimers, nanomicelles, silica nanoparticles, perfluorocarbon nanoparticles or nanotubes) are introduced intravenously as T_1 contrast agents to enhance longitudinal relaxation times [38]. Unlike Gd^{3+}, superparamagnetic iron oxide nanoparticles can be tuned to enhance T_1 relaxation or shorten T_2 relaxation times depending on the particle size. Despite these advantages contrast agent uses are restricted due to detection limits, low concentrations, and lack of target tissue specificity. Application of combinatorial therapy with magnetism and ultrasound significantly enhances therapeutic efficacy of theranostics thereby reducing dose-dependent toxicities.

3.2 Optical Imaging

Optical imaging requires nonionizing radiation and photon interaction with biological systems to capture high-resolution images of soft tissues. This technique generates images by exciting electrons to capture cellular absorption, emission, reflection, scattering, polarization, coherence, and fluorescence of visible, ultraviolet, and infrared light depending on cell properties [35,36]. Optical imaging techniques are highly efficient due to nonionizing radiation. Hence this technique is applied in diagnosis, treatment monitoring, and also long, repetitive procedures [39]. More than the diagnostic technique, optical imaging is famous for its compact, portable, and cost-effective design flexibility. Types of optical imaging are endoscopy, optical coherence tomography, photoacoustic imaging, diffuse optical tomography, Raman spectroscopy, super-resolution microscopy, and terahertz tomography. Given their unique properties, optical imaging can be utilized for detecting gastrointestinal problems, skin cancer, tumors angiogenesis, neuronal activity, and single cell characterization.

Fluorescence-based optical imaging can be applied to study and understand complex biological alterations in cellular pathways, interactions, structures, functions, sensitivity, and noninvasive properties. However, autofluorescene (natural emission of light) and absorption limit the penetration depth and sensitivity of the process. There are numerous contrast enhancing dyes and labels that can aid in optical fluorescence imaging. A variety of nanosystems, especially the ones with excellent optical properties like gold nanoparticles, quantum dots, and emissive polymerosomes, are often doped with fluorescent dyes to overcome these drawbacks [40]. Organic fluorescent dyes by and large are doped with nanoparticles made of silica, calcium phosphates, lipoproteins, or polymeric nanoparticles [41–43]. The type of nanoparticle can be selected based on several factors including disease, drug type, administration route, and mechanism of particle uptake at the target site [40].

Silica nanoparticles are optically transparent with tunable morphology. The particles are prepared with simple surface fabrication through basic silane chemistry. These constructs are used in fluorescent diagnostic imaging nanoparticles and biosensors. Calcium phosphate nanoparticles on the other hand are fabricated for targeted genes and drug delivery with surface modification. Lipoprotein nanosystems are nonimmunogenic, biodegradable, and biocompatible in nature with controllable both hydrophobic and hydrophilic agents. Moreover, lipoprotein delivery systems can minimize rapid clearance by reticuloendothelial system improving drug circulation time. Polymeric nanoparticles are also widely screened for safety and efficacy in optical imaging and theranostics [44]. Several US Food and Drug Administration (FDA)-approved polymers can be attractive carriers for fluorescent dyes [43]. Both hydrophilic [polyacrylamide, polyurethanes, poly(hydroxyethyl methacrylamide), poly(ethylene glycols) (PEGs), and Pluronic] and hydrophobic [polyacrylonitrile, poly(D,L-lactic-co-glycolic acid) (PLGA), and polystyrene] polymers have been explored for applications in bioimaging and biosensing [42]. Quantum dots and lanthanides are often used as inorganic fluorophores for optical imaging [42]. As discussed earlier, quantum dots are fluorescent inorganic nanoparticles that have size-tunable emission wavelength spectra and resistance to photobleaching [45]. More interestingly, quantum dots have a wide absorption spectrum that allows single excitation source to excite multiple quantum dots of different size. Given their unique narrow and symmetrical emission wavelength, quantum dots allow for easy differentiation and hence particles of different colors can be used simultaneously to obtain complex cellular imaging without overlap. Despite their advantages, quantum dots are limited by their complex surface chemistry and nanotoxicity [46]. Noble metal nanoparticles (like gold and silver) have unique surface plasmon resonance, which is enhanced and tunable radiative and nonradiative properties [47]. Gold nanoparticles make excellent fluorescent particles with dual application in photothermal therapy and optical imaging [12].

3.3 Nuclear Imaging

Nuclear imaging, also known as gamma scintigraphy, is a medical imaging technique that is often combined with CT to assess disease severity and treatment effect. Although the technique by itself is noninvasive, small doses of radiopharmaceuticals (short-lived gamma radioisotope) are administered via oral, intravenous, or inhalation route for emitting gamma rays. The emitted radiation is then scanned using gamma detectors such as single-photon emission CT or the positron emission tomography to obtain 3D computerized images. Nuclear imaging is used in various types of cancers, neurological disorders, and cardiovascular, gastrointestinal, and endocrinal diseases [35]. In addition to the diagnostic applications, nuclear imaging can also be selected to treat certain cancers such as non-Hodgkin lymphoma and thyroid-related tumors by radioimmunotherapy. Radionuclide (tracers) imaging has become the most attractive and powerful modality for molecular imaging in personalized cancer therapy. Nanomaterials radiolabeled with gamma-emitting radionuclides are utilized in this technique. Most of the nanosystems have been radiolabeled to obtain multifunctional systems such as dendrimers, nanomicelles, quantum dots, nanoparticles (polymer, silica, gold, iron oxide), CNTs, and even liposomes [48]. Many radionuclides have been studied for tumor accumulation such as ^{111}In, ^{99m}TC, ^{67}Ga, ^{64}Cu, and ^{18}F, but unfortunately none of them have reached the clinical stage [49]. Liposomes are highly promising multifunctional nanosystems for fluorescent bioimaging, radiotherapy, and delivery of antiangiogenic agents. Vescan is a liposomal-based tracer doped with ^{111}In, which showed tumor-specific accumulation in high concentrations. However, it has not been approved by the FDA for clinical studies [50]. PEGylated liposomes have high circulation half-life compared with liposomes [51].

3.4 Computed Tomography

CT, also known as X-ray-computed tomography, utilizes ionizing radiation through special computer-aided X-ray equipment. CT produces fine cross-sections and 3D images of biological tissue. It is the preferred diagnostic method for tumor detection and measurement of size, shape, and location [26]. This particular imaging modality is primarily applied in scanning soft tissues such as coronary arteries, cardiovascular tissue, and aneurysms of abdomen, chest, brain, lungs, and pelvic areas. Similar to X-rays, CT is noninvasive and painless, but it can also aid in theranostic application [26]. There has been tremendous progress in the last few years and a full-body CT scan has become the norm for annual general checkups.

Iodinated organic CT contrast agents are aromatic water-soluble molecules widely indicated in CT scanning. Iodine presents low contrast efficacy with short circulation half-life and poor vascular permeability. Moreover, high doses of iodine are required to overcome renal clearance to obtain the required concentration at the target site [52]. Nanoparticles tagged with contrast agents can be designed to target drug delivery and prolong circulation requiring relatively low doses of contrast agent [53]. Liposomes, polymeric nanoparticles, nanosuspensions, nanoemulsions, nanocapsules, nanomicelles, and dendrimers can be utilized in the development of contrast agent combined with multifunctional nanosystems [44,52]. Typical nanosystems in the size range of 10–80 nm are large enough to circumvent renal clearance, and also small enough to prevent uptake by macrophage. As a result, these nanoconstructs distribute in the body reducing the risk of potential toxicity [52,54]. Liposomes are extremely valuable as contrast agent carriers but their uptake by reticuloendothelial systems limit their circulation time, which causes leakage of contrast material and subsequent renal toxicity [52]. To overcome these drawbacks, PEGylated stealth liposomes were developed with controlled size ~100 nm that enhance circulation times of iodinated contrast agents (iopamidol, iodixanol, or iohexol) [53].

Self-assembling nanoparticles made of chitosan and folate conjugated poly-γ-glutamic acid are radiolabeled with ^{99m}Tc. This construct can target folate receptor overexpressing tumor cells. These specially designed nanoparticles range between 75 and 200 nm. These particles are large enough to avoid rapid renal clearance, thereby prolonging circulation time, and promote passive tumor accumulation and active tumor cell internalization through folate receptors [55]. MonomethoxyPEG-polyalanine-poly-[ε,N-(2,3,5-triiodobenzoyl)]-L-lysine copolymer self-assembles to form amphiphilic nanomicelles with size range of 10–80 nm, which have all the intended properties for tumor angiogenesis [53]. Unlike polymeric nanoparticles, dendrimers offer a more symmetric structure that can be tailored to fit a wide variety of bioimaging applications.

3.5 Ultrasound

Ultrasound or sonography is a diagnostic imaging technique similar to the technique applied in oceanographic studies. Ultrasound produces higher frequency sound waves that are pulsed into the tissue with a probe. These pulses are reflected or absorbed (echos) at varying degrees depending on the tissue. Such pulses are recorded as electrical impulses and images [36]. Ultrasound is the most common, noninvasive, and safest way of examining internal organs without the use of harmful radiation [56]. It is widely applied in pregnancy to determine the growth and development of a fetus. Other than pregnancy, ultrasound is applied to detect tumors, congenital vascular malformations, and organs like pelvis, abdomen, heart, thyroid, kidneys, liver, uterus, ovaries, and blood vessels [36]. Over the last decade, insoluble gas microbubbles encapsulated in protein/liposomal shell had been clinically indicated as contrast agents [56]. These commercially available microbubbles are in the micrometer range with poor circulation half-lives that limit tumor penetration and targetability [57]. Moreover, these microsized contrast agents are unstable during sonication. These molecules generate low endothelial layer permeability, rendering them unfavorable for tumor permeation and targeting. In case of ultrasound contrast agents, nanoparticles overcome most of the limitations with their physicochemical properties (mainly nanosize) and ease of surface functionalization. Popularity of nanosystems as carriers for ultrasonication contrast agents stems from their enhanced stability, tumor targeting, and application in multiplex imaging modality. However, in this scenario nanosized gas-filled vesicles enhance contrast to noise ratio because of their hollow inner shell echogenicity [44]. Various types of nanosystems have been studied as nanocarriers including liposomes, dendrimers, nanomicelles, quantum dots, emulsions, polymers, and silica nanoparticles.

Mesoporous silica nanoparticles (MSNs) are inorganic, porous solid nanoparticles with high circulation half-life than traditional microbubbles. MSN is amenable to conjugation with tumor overexpressing receptor antibody (such as Herceptin). It allows the conjugate to increase tumor cell accumulation and selectivity for contrast enhancement with real-time imaging [58].

Poly(lactic acid) nanoparticles encapsulating ultrasound contrast agents such as SF_6 gas improves weak echogenicity of dense hydrophobic gases. The particle size in these nanosystems ($\sim$200 nm) is crucial for passive tumor accumulation via enhanced permeability and retention (EPR effect) of tumor cells [59,60]. Advancements in the development of contrast-enhancing nanosystems have also advanced dual imaging system with multimodal contrast agents. Copper oxide nanoparticles are proven to demonstrate magnetic, acoustic, and high thermal conductivity [61]. The multifunctional nanoparticles reduce T_1 relaxation times for MRI and enhance attenuation coefficient for ultrasound imaging. Moreover, simple surface modification of these nanoparticles enables target-specific visualization and simultaneous thermal ablation of tumor cells [44,61].

4. BIOLOGICAL SENSORS

Sensors are devices that measure, amplify, and convert a physical quantity into a measurable unit as a signal. Biosensors are the analytical tools resulting from multidisciplinary research. These devices are powerful analytical tools that find applications in medicine, pharmacy, dentistry, environmental diagnostics, and food processing industries. Classification of sensors is based on the input signal domains or transduction modes. Moreover, it

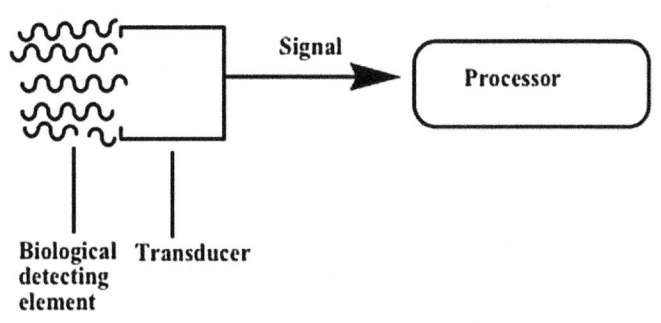

Figure 10.4 Schematic representation of a biosensor.

also depends on the type of molecule. Sensors may be broadly classified as physical and chemical sensors. Mostly, biological sensors belong to class of chemical sensors. Biological sensors consist of three parts: (1) a detecting element (biological), (2) a transducer, and (3) a signal processing unit. Basic biosensor schematic is presented in Fig. 10.4.

At present such sensors are advanced with immobilization of analytes such as, but not limited to, enzymes, antibodies, and chemicals. However, in the following section of this chapter we focused and limited our discussion to glucose biosensors and microcantilevers, which are immobilized with enzymes. Other devices are not discussed because these may be beyond the scope of this chapter.

4.1 Glucose Sensors

Biosensors such as glucose biosensor have been well studied. This device is currently available as self-usable biological device. It is well known that glucose is the source of energy for living organisms and metabolism of glucose generates ATP (source of energy). Insulin, a pancreatic hormone, metabolizes and regulates blood glucose levels by traversing glucose from blood stream into the cells. Low insulin production causes increased blood glucose level, leading to diabetes. Treatment options include insulin administration as subcutaneous injections. Patients suffering from diabetes require continuous glucose monitoring to regulate blood glucose level. In 1962 Leland C Clark developed a biological sensor to monitor blood glucose continuously [62]. Advances in research and technology resulted in the development of novel devices that directly display digital readout of the glucose concentration from microliter blood samples.

In recent years, there has been growing interest in immobilizing biomolecules on a substrate and nanoparticle approach for glucose determination. Also, research is being focused on the development of novel nonenzymatic glucose biosensors. An advanced implantable miniature electrical transducer that monitors glucose continuously was developed [63]. However, implantable devices raised concerns in regards to biocompatibility. In 1996 MiniMed (Northridge, CA, USA) developed a biocompatible commercial glucose monitoring system (CGMS) which received FDA approval. This device monitored the glucose levels in the patients and alerted patients to potential fluctuations in glucose levels by an alarm. However, this device is associated with a major drawback of not producing the real-time glucose measurement [64]. Research advance by MiniMed resulted in development of Real-Time system. The FDA approved the new CGMS, which displayed glucose concentration on the insulin pump [65–67]. However, the CGMS was not user friendly to children and adolescents suffering from type 1 diabetes. It is not due to the device itself rather because of the device adherence. Moreover, it was observed that the CGMS did not find any conclusive benefit in pregnant women.

Glucose oxidase (GOD) [68] is an enzyme that binds to beta-D-glucopyranose and breaks down sugar into its metabolites. It has been utilized as an amperometric biosensor for diagnostic instruments and for controlling blood sugar in diabetic patients. Such glucose biosensors may be broadly classified into three types, namely: (1) immobilized enzyme film glucose biosensors, (2) nanoparticle/CNT-based glucose biosensors, and (3) nonenzymatic glucose biosensors. These biosensors are briefly discussed in the following sections.

4.1.1 Immobilized Enzyme Film Glucose Biosensors

In this type of biosensors, the enzyme GOD is adsorbed or entangled in the fibrous membrane of the polymers such as poly(vinyl alcohol) (PVA), PLGA, polypyrrole, and poly(o-phenylenediamine) with a covalent linkage. Fig. 10.5 represents a schematic representation of such biosensor.

Miao et al. performed electropolymerization of nonconductive polymer for fabrication onto a planer screen printed electrode to prepare a glucose biosensor [69]. In this device ferrocene was utilized as a mediator for the amperometric glucose response. Glucose measurement was carried out with potentiostating at a potential of 0.3 V. The device has a linear range up to 25 mM with a fast response time of 100 s and sensitivity of 16.6 nA/mM. In another study, Guanglei et al. developed a new efficient and superior glucose biosensor by immobilizing GOD [68] with electrospinning into PVA fibrous membrane [70]. Membrane immobilization exhibited a rapid response of 1 s. A higher response current of microampere level to glucose was observed in normal and diabetic levels. The electrospinning technique is superior, convenient, and 100 times more efficient than electropolymerization. Moreover, higher sensitivities and lower detection limits are achieved with enzyme immobilized on gold polypyrrole nanocomposite [71]. This biosensor demonstrates very low detection limit, 2×10^{-6} M, and very high sensitivity, 1.09 mA/M, for glucose with a fast response time less than 10 s. Au-pyrrole biosensors have an excellent operational stability up to 100 assays. Gold-pyrrole biosensors demonstrated higher operational stability relative to electropolymerized and electrospun biosensors.

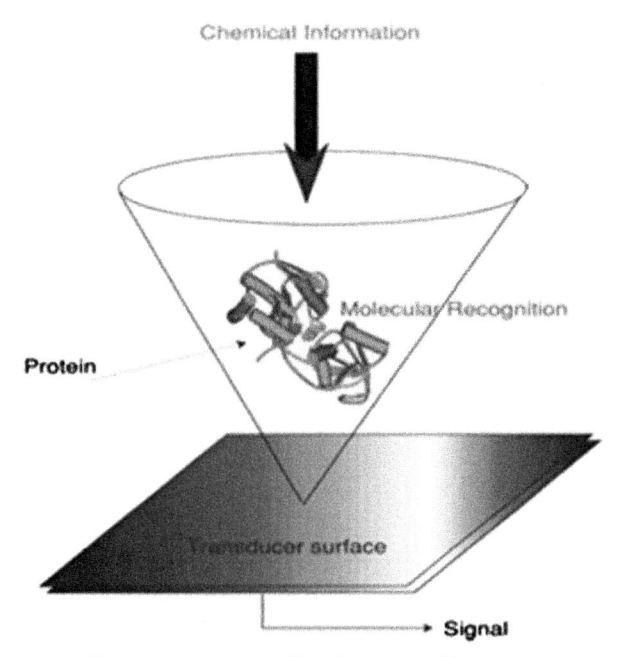

Figure 10.5 Immobilized enzyme biosensor.

4.1.2 Nanoparticle/Carbon Nanotube–Based Glucose Biosensors

Current research interest is focused on nanotechnology. Gold nanoparticles exhibit attractive properties such as small size, high surface area, and good biocompatibility for biosensor application. In most cases, gold nanoparticles are prepared by reduction of $HAuCl_4$ with citrate. Gold nanoparticles self-assemble onto the electrode surface and at the final stage enzymes are immobilized effectively on nanoparticle surface. For example, immobilization of GOD, gold nanoparticle composite, and polyaniline nanofibers are used for the development of novel glucose biosensor (Fig. 10.6) [72].

Nafion (NF) is also prepared for the biosensor development for the elimination of interferences of electroactive compounds such as ascorbic acid, uric acid, glutathione, and L-cysteine, to glucose response. GOD is immobilized with high loading efficiency and activity because of the presence of large surface area and microgaps in nanocomposites. Such nanocomposites can provide excellent conductivity. Advantage of biosensor includes the rapid transmission of electrons and enhanced current response due to the presence of high surface to volume ratio of nanocomposites. Biosensor storage stability demonstrated less than 5% decrease in the response over 2 weeks. Immobilization of GOD on gold nanoparticles electrodeposited on indium tin oxide electrode surface has been fabricated and studied [73]. This biosensor is a disposable amperometric glucose biosensor. Gold nanoparticles provide direct electron transfer between GOD and electrode surface with an effective catalytic activity toward the reduction of

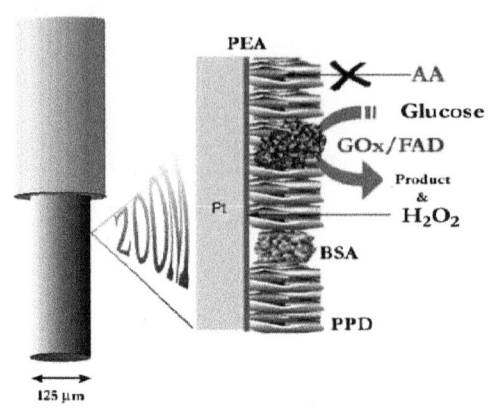

Figure 10.6 Nanoparticle-based glucose biosensor. *AA*, ascorbic acid; *BSA*, bovine serum albumin; *FAD*, flavin adenine dinucleotide; *GOx*, glucose oxidase; *PPD*, poly-phenylenediamines.

glucose. The rate constant for heterogenous electron transfer was evaluated to be $3.7\,s^{-1}$. The biosensor exhibited a linear range from 0.04 to 4.8 mmol/L and a 0.015-mmol/L detection limit.

Other studies were conducted with fabrication of glucose biosensors that includes electrostatic interactions between CNTs and cationic surfactant/polymers. Enzyme, GOD, is bound to CNT through electrostatic interactions. The negative charges in the enzyme and the positive charge in the CNT provided the bonding. Currently, in the fabrication of CNTs, a single-walled, multilayer film was plated on the surface of the working electrode. It is based on the alternate electrostatic adsorption of charged individual components. Multi-wall carbon nanotubes (MWCNTs) with positive surface charge were wrapped with poly (diallyldimethylammonium chloride). The assembly was fabricated by layer-over-layer deposition of GOD. Initially single-walled CNT with electrodeposited enzyme generated an immobilization matrix. This construct serves as an amperometric glucose biosensor [74]. The electrode surface was modified by the single-walled CNT and enzyme [68]. The latter was immobilized with 11-(ferrocenyl)-undercyltrimethyl ammonium bromide. GOD was immobilized onto the single-wall CNT. This single-walled CNT has found its application in direct transfer of electron from GOD. Such direct electron transfer from GOD to CNT is determined with cyclic voltameter. This biosensor can be applied to measure D-glucose concentration. The range of the relation between concentration and steady state current is between 0.04 and 0.38 mM. The biosensor demonstrated a residual activity above 94% after 42 days of preparation indicating the utility of such device in identification and quantification of D-glucose. Moreover, the biosensor demonstrated high mechanical strength and stability.

As previously discussed with NF, electrospinning-based nanofibrous composite electrode has been developed. A nanofibrous composite electrode,

PMMA-MWCNT(PDDA)/GOD-nafion-NFE, for the detection of glucose has been demonstrated [75]. High loading of GOD into electrospun matrix has been achieved due to the fibrous morphology and wrapping of PDDA over MWCNTs. Such MWCNT-based biosensors offer advantages over the immobilized enzyme-based biosensors. These biosensors demonstrate an excellent detection limit (1 μM), linear response range (20 μM—15 mM), response time of ~8 s, and operational stability and are free from electrochemical interferences. Moreover, such biosensors exhibit high selectivity, sensitivity, stability, and good reproducibility relative to others. Superior performance of the biosensor is attributed to the electrocatalytic activity toward hydrogen peroxide (H_2O_2) with a pronounced oxidation current at +100 mV.

A combination approach of the nanoparticle deposition onto the CNTs was implemented. Deposition of Pt nanoparticles on MWCNTs for the development of novel biosensor has been reported [76]. In this type, the enzyme is immobilized with chitosan-SiO_2 solgel. NF coating is applied to minimize or completely eliminate interferences. These biosensors exhibited higher stability and electrocatalytic activity with a better response over the linear range of 1 μM—23 mM with lower limit of detection of 1 μM. The response time for the biosensor was 5 s with a high sensitivity of 58.9 μA/mM/cm². Furthermore, a better and improved biosensor has been reported with Pb nanowires [77]. In another study, a glucose biosensor was prepared by crosslinking and immobilizing GOD with bovine serum albumin matrix on a platinum electrode. This platinum electrode was further modified with gold nanoparticles-decorated Pb nanowires. This novel biosensor demonstrated greater sensitivity, 135.5 μA/mM, and a detection limit of 2 μM. It had a linear response range of 5—2200 μM and the response time was <5 s. This device exhibited good reproducibility, long-term stability, and relatively good antiinterference in comparison with the other developed nanobiosensors.

A novel glucose biosensor based on the combination of enzyme, MWCNT, and neutral red for the determination of glucose was developed [78]. Following the carbodiimide reaction the neutral red was covalently immobilized on the MWCNT. The enzyme, GOD, was covalently bound to neutral red and the NF was bound to GOD resulting in MWNT-NR-GOD-NF nanobiocomposite. This nanobiocomposite was coated on the electrode. Hydrogen peroxide is liberated due to enzymatic reaction with glucose by GOD. The reaction of glucose with neutral dye-functionalized CNT aids in selective detection of glucose. This device shows good stability, antiinterferent ability, and an enormous determination range (1×10^{-8} to 1×10^{-3} M with a detection limit of 3×10^{-9} M) with a response time of 4 s.

4.1.2.1 Mechanism of Implantable Biosensor
The above two types of biosensors work on the same principle, i.e., enzymatic conversion of glucose to pyruvate and hydrogen peroxide by GOD. The by-product produced,

hydrogen peroxide, is further reduced and the potential difference is measured with the help of a signal processor. The signal processor amplifies the signal and the digital reading is observed on the display.

4.1.2.2 Nonenzymatic Glucose Biosensors

For the determination of glucose concentration in biological and chemical samples a biosensor has been developed. However, researchers are working toward the development of novel nonenzymatic biosensor. The most commonly faced problem is the insufficient stability of the biosensor that originated from the enzyme, which is very difficult to overcome. GOD is very stable relative to other enzymes. However, this enzyme may be degraded due to thermal and chemical insults. Moreover, the enzyme may be degraded during fabrication and storage. Moreover, GOD is easily affected by the severe interferences from other oxidizable species in the samples such as ascorbic and uric acids. The electrodes need to be poised at ≥ 7 V vs Ag/AgCl for the electrochemical detection of hydrogen peroxide. Because of all these limitations, researchers have focused on the development of enzymeless glucose biosensors. Enzymeless biosensors have the advantages of stability, simplicity, being oxidation free, and most importantly reproducibility.

Enzymeless biosensors have been developed with disposable pencil graphite electrode. Glucose detection based on overoxidized polypyrrole nanofiber electrode modified with cobalt(II)pthalocyanine tetrasulfonate has been developed [79]. This newly developed enzymeless biosensor displays electrocatalytic activity in alkaline solution for the oxidation of glucose. The performance for glucose determination was significantly improved with a wide linear range, 0.25–20 mM, long-term stability, low percentage of interference, and highly reproducible response. The detection limit is 0.1 mM.

A higher ordered nickel nanowire array electrode for the determination of electrocatalytic oxidation of glucose in alkaline medium has been developed [80]. The linear range for quantification of glucose is 5.0×10^{-7} to 7.0×10^{-3} M with a high sensitivity of 1043 μA/mM. The lower detection limit is 1×10^{-7} M. The biosensor is free of interference from oxidizable species, exhibiting good reproducibility and long-term stability. This novel Ni-nanowire assay provides an improved method for the development of enzymeless biosensor.

4.1.3 Mechanism of Nonenzymatic Glucose Biosensors

The mechanism for the nonenzymatic glucose biosensors is similar to that of the enzymatic glucose biosensors. The difference lies in the absence of enzyme for glucose detection. The mechanism of nonenzymatic glucose biosensor is described as the chemical reaction that occurs on the biosensor surface as follows:

$$NiO + OH^- - e^- \rightarrow NiO(OH)$$

$$Ni + 2OH^- - 2e^- \rightarrow NiO + H_2O$$

$$Ni(II) - e^- \rightarrow Ni(III)$$

The Ni(OH)O produced will oxidize the glucose to glucolactone liberating two protons. This reaction is catalyzed by Ni(III)/(II) redox couple according to the following reactions:

$$Ni(OH)_2 + OH^- \rightarrow NiO(OH) + H_2O + e^-$$

$$NiO(OH) + glucose \rightarrow Ni(OH)_2 + glucolactone$$

Ni(III) rapidly oxidizes glucose at the anode to produce Ni(II). As a result the concentrations of Ni(II) and Ni(III) species are changed. This causes an increase in the anodic peak current with simultaneous diminishing cathode peak current. These potential changes can be taken into account to generate electric signal for the detection of glucose in test samples.

4.2 Microcantilever

Microcantilevers (MCs) are ultrasensitive biosensors for multiple analyte detections. These MCs are suitable for diverse applications such as in screening of diseases, point mutation detection, and blood glucose monitoring. Moreover, MCs can be considered as detectors for chemical and biological warfare agents. Advantages of such biosensors include nonhazardous sample procedure, low sample requirement, high sensitivity, low cost, and rapid response. Moreover, nanoelectromechanical systems have been developed for the nanocantilevers in sensing applications. A novel technology enhanced the sensitivity limit for counting of molecules. High-throughput analysis and ultrasensitive detection with these detectors may improve the availability of highly sensitive miniaturized biological sensors in the near future.

4.2.1 Mechanism of Microcantilever Deflection

Microcantilevers work on the principle of specific analyte adsorption to probe and bend the cantilever causing energy minimization. This binding of molecules to one side of thin material makes the opposite side inert. It generates a differential stress between the two surfaces. This differential surface stress causes the material to deform, which provides a method of detecting molecular adsorption. Fig. 10.7 depicts a schematic for the basic mechanism of a microcantilever.

Mathematically, surface stress (σ) and surface free energy (γ) can be related to Shuttleworth equation [81] as in Eq. (10.1):

$$\sigma = \gamma + (d\gamma/d\varepsilon) \tag{10.1}$$

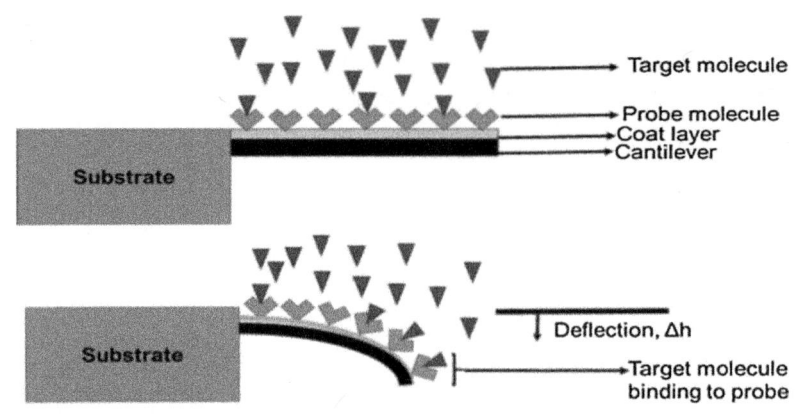

Figure 10.7 Basic mechanism of microcantilever. Specific analyte binds to probe molecule and alters intermolecular interactions within a self-assembled monolayer on one side of cantilever beam. This process produces large surface stress to bend cantilever beam generating motion.

Surface strain ($d\varepsilon$) is defined as the ratio of the change in surface area to the total area ($d\varepsilon = dA/A$).

On the other hand, Sotney's equation [82] relates the difference in surface stress ($\Delta\sigma$) between the chemically modified surface and the other inert surface with the cantilever deflection (Δh) as shown in Eq. (10.2):

$$\Delta h = \frac{4(1-\nu)L^2}{Et^2}(\Delta\sigma_1 - \Delta\sigma_2) \qquad (10.2)$$

where ν the Poisson's ratio of the material, E is the Young's elastic modulus of the cantilever material, t is the thickness, and L is the length of the cantilever.

In the following sections the applications of biosensors, i.e., micro- and nanocantilevers, in disease diagnostics are discussed. Mostly, cantilevers are indicated for detection of coronary heart diseases, nucleotide polymorphisms, and antibody—antigen or DNA hybridization.

4.2.1.1 Microcantilevers as Cancer Detectors

Microcantilever surface coated with antibodies specific to prostate cancer antigen (PSA) has been developed [83]. When PSA-coated microcantilever interacts with positive blood samples of patients with cancer, antigen—antibody interactions caused the bending of the cantilever. The nanometer angle bending of the cantilever was detected optically by a low-power laser beam with a photodetector. Such microcantilever assay is highly sensitive relative to conventional biochemical techniques and enzyme-linked immunosorbent assay. Moreover, microcantilever assay is less expensive than fluorescent tags or radiolabel molecules. In another study, Lee et al. demonstrated the detection of PSA resonance frequency shift of piezoelectric nanomechanical microcantilever [84].

Table 10.3 provides more insights into the applications of microcantilever in cancer detection.

Anti-myoglobin monoclonal antibody was coated on the microcantilever upper surface with sulfosuccinimidyl 6-[3-(2-pyridyldithio)-propionamido] hexanoate (sulfo-LC-SPDP) cross-linker [85]. Human serum myoglobin binding to anti-myoglobin caused a deflection of the microcantilever. A low concentration of myoglobin (85 ng/mL) can be easily detected, which demonstrates high sensitivity of the biosensor.

4.2.1.2 Microcantilevers in Coronary Heart Diseases

Adsorption of low-density lipoproteins and the oxidized form on heparin can be differentiated with biosensing microcantilevers [86]. Such an ability to differentiate these two species is of clinical interest. This differentiation and identification are clinically important parameters because their uptake from plasma favors the oxidized form. It is believed that the oxidized forms of low-density lipoproteins are responsible for accumulation of cholesterol in the aorta. It is associated with the first stage of coronary heart disease. Moreover, this technique is employed to study and identify conformational changes in two plasma proteins such as immunoglobulin G (IgG) and bovine serum albumin.

4.2.1.3 Microcantilevers in Nucleotide Polymorphisms

Polymorphism within the gene sequence and genome, i.e., single nucleotide polymorphisms (SNPs) is a major concern of genomics research. Point mutations may lead to genetic diseases such as thalassemia, Tay—Sachs disease, and Alzheimer disease.

Early detection of SNPs may aid in early diagnosis and treatment. Microcantilevers are helpful in detecting such single base pair mismatches with extreme sensitivity for specific biomolecular recognition interactions, i.e., between the probe and target DNA sequences. Sensitivity of microcantilevers is within the pico- to femtogram range. For example, thiolated DNA probes are immobilized on the gold-coated microcantilever. A net positive deflection of the microcantilever is achieved with hybridization of fully complementary target DNA sequence. A net positive deflection may result because of the reduction in configurational entropy of double-stranded DNA versus single-stranded DNA. Hybridization of the probe DNA with target DNA with base-pair mismatches results in a net negative deflection of the microcantilever. This is because of enhanced repulsive forces applied on the microcantilever surface. The deflection is greater for target DNA with two base pair mismatches relative to single base pair mismatch. The degree of repulsion is directly proportional to the number of base pair mismatches [87]. Moreover, multiple label-free biodetection and quantitative DNA binding assays have been demonstrated with nanomechanical microcantilever [88].

Table 10.3 Microcantilevers in cancer diagnosis

Microcantilever	Disease	Probe molecule	Target molecule/cells	Remarks	References
Silicon substrate	Liver cancer diagnosis	AFP antibody	AFP antigen	Cantilever arrays fabricated with microelectromechanical systems technology have been established to eliminate interference of the adsorption-induced stiffness changes. Sensitivity of the sensor was ~8 pg/mL	[94]
Gold-coated cantilevers	Human adenocarcinoma breast cancer	Peptide sensors such as cRGDfC	Breast cancer cell lines like MCF7 and MDA-MB-231	Noncancerous cell lines such as MCF10A and HUVEC served as control. Cancerous cells demonstrated significantly high binding specificity (280 nm) relative to noncancerous (90 nm)	[95]
Gold-coated self-sensing piezoresistors integrated biosensor	Diabetes	Self-assembled monolayer of 4-mercaptophenylboronic acid	Glucose	The cantilever bending and glucose concentration were demonstrated at glucose concentrations of 5 and 25 mM. Magnitudes of cantilever bending were proportional to glucose concentration	[96]
	Diabetes	Immobilization of glucose oxidase	Glucose	No interferences for glucose detection have shown on the measurement of blood glucose level by this technique	[97]

Piezoresistive microcantilevers fabricated with silicon-on-insulator substrate	Breast cancer	Si$_3$N$_4$ as stress compensating layer	Breast cancer cells	Force sensor may be used as a tool for cancerous and benign breast tissue demarcation. Helpful to characterize histological tissue samples	[98]
Label-free microcantilever array aptasensor	Liver cancer	HepG2 cell-specific aptamers	HepG2 cells	The aptasensor exhibits high specificity over not only human liver normal cells, but also other cancer cells of breast, bladder, and cervix tumors. The linear relation ranges from 1×10^3 to 1×10^5 cells/mL, with a detection limit of 300 cells/mL (S/N = 3). Our work provides a simple method for detection of liver cancer cells with advantages in terms of simplicity and stability	[99]
Gold-coated microcantilever	Pathogens like *Salmonella enterica* strains	anti-S.e. Heidelberg antibody	Liver cancer cells	Successfully detected whole pathogenic organisms. High sensitivity and selectivity, low analyte volume, real-time detection in fluids, air, and possibility to create a portable and implantable device	[100]

4.2.1.4 Biochips in Microcantilevers

Studies have demonstrated that bending of microfabricated cantilevers biochips have advantages over earlier microcantilevers [89,90]. Sensing elements in biochips with mechanical detection systems consist of bimaterial such as Au—Si beams. In general, the Au side is coated with a receptor, which upon binding with a ligand like proteins or biological agents, is tensioned or relieved. Such binding causes microcantilever deflection. Microcantilever deflection is found to be proportional to the analyte concentration. Bindings in biomolecular applications include antibody—antigen bindings or DNA hybridization of a pair of DNA strands with complementary sequences [90]. Advantages of biochip microcantilevers are that they do not require (1) external power, (2) labeling, and (3) external electronics or fluorescent molecules or signal transduction for their operation.

4.2.1.5 Nanocantilevers

Nanocantilevers are 90 nm thick made from silicon nitride. These constructs can detect a single piece of DNA [91] with a mass of about 0.23 attograms (1 attogram = 10^{-18} g). Gold dots of nanometer size were placed at the very end of cantilevers. This acts to capture agents for sulfide-modified double-stranded DNA. Scanning laser beams are employed to measure vibrational frequencies of cantilevers. Another laboratory developed ultrathin (10-nm-thick) resonant nanocantilevers with aluminum-molybdenum composites [92]. Similarly, nanocantilevers with varying length and thickness (30 nm) functionalized with antibodies for virus are under investigation [93].

5. CONCLUSIONS

Challenges with cancer diagnosis, treatment, and emergence of multidrug-resistant phenotypes need novel personalized treatment strategies. Interdisciplinary research has helped to develop several nanotechnology-based imaging systems, sensors, and detectors that can be combined with cancer therapies to provide combinatorial advantage known as theranostics. Current research focus has been on the development of such patient-compliant imagining systems and biodetectors. Gold nanoparticles, quantum dots, iron nanoparticles, liposomes, dendrimers, and nanomicelles are now being pursued as a tool for diagnosis and imaging agent. Microcantilevers are powerful biochemical sensors that are being explored at large. Various applications of microcantilevers in disease diagnosis such as cancer, diabetes, and pathogen detection will be helpful in early detection, prevention, and treatment.

REFERENCES

[1] Ten Dam MA, Wetzels JF. Toxicity of contrast media: an update. Neth J Med 2008;66(10):416—22.
[2] Nune SK, et al. Nanoparticles for biomedical imaging. Expert Opin Drug Deliv 2009;6(11): 1175—94.

[3] Xie J, Lee S, Chen X. Nanoparticle-based theranostic agents. Adv Drug Deliv Rev 2010;62(11): 1064−79.
[4] Casciaro S. Theranostic applications: non-ionizing cellular and molecular imaging through innovative nanosystems for early diagnosis and therapy. World J Radiol 2011;3(10):249−55.
[5] Laurent S, et al. Magnetic iron oxide nanoparticles: synthesis, stabilization, vectorization, physicochemical characterizations, and biological applications. Chem Rev 2008;108(6):2064−110.
[6] Wu W, He Q, Jiang C. Magnetic iron oxide nanoparticles: synthesis and surface functionalization strategies. Nanoscale Res Lett 2008;3(11):397−415.
[7] Valizadeh A, et al. Quantum dots: synthesis, bioapplications, and toxicity. Nanoscale Res Lett 2012; 7(1):480.
[8] Walling MA, Novak JA, Shepard JR. Quantum dots for live cell and in vivo imaging. Int J Mol Sci 2009;10(2):441−91.
[9] Zhou J, et al. Functionalized gold nanoparticles: synthesis, structure and colloid stability. J Colloid Interface Sci 2009;331(2):251−62.
[10] Boisselier E, Astruc D. Gold nanoparticles in nanomedicine: preparations, imaging, diagnostics, therapies and toxicity. Chem Soc Rev 2009;38(6):1759−82.
[11] Jain S, Hirst DG, O'Sullivan JM. Gold nanoparticles as novel agents for cancer therapy. Br J Radiol 2012;85(1010):101−13.
[12] Huanga X, El-Sayed MA. Gold nanoparticles: optical properties and implementations in cancer diagnosis and photothermal therapy. J Adv Res 2010;1(1):13−28.
[13] Dai H. Carbon nanotubes: synthesis, integration, and properties. Acc Chem Res 2002;35(12): 1035−44.
[14] Gao F, et al. Functionalized carbon nanotube theranostic agents for microwave diagnostic imaging and thermal therapy of tumors. In: EuCAP. The Hague: IEEE; 2014. p. 691−3.
[15] Liang H, et al. Functional DNA-containing nanomaterials: cellular applications in biosensing, imaging, and targeted therapy. Acc Chem Res 2014;47(6):1891−901.
[16] Martincic M, Tobias G. Filled carbon nanotubes in biomedical imaging and drug delivery. Expert Opin Drug Deliv 2015;12(4):563−81.
[17] Tang F, Li L, Chen D. Mesoporous silica nanoparticles: synthesis, biocompatibility and drug delivery. Adv Mater 2012;24(12):1504−34.
[18] Schulza A, McDonagh C. Intracellular sensing and cell diagnostics using fluorescent silica nanoparticles. Soft Matter 2012;8(9):2579−85.
[19] García-Calzón JA, Díaz-García EA. Synthesis and analytical potential of silica nanotubes. TrAC 2012; 35:27−38.
[20] Qian J, et al. Bio-molecule-conjugated fluorescent organically modified silica nanoparticles as optical probes for cancer cell imaging. Opt Express 2008;16(24):19568−78.
[21] Slowing II, et al. Mesoporous silica nanoparticles for drug delivery and biosensing applications. Adv Funct Mater 2007;17(8):1225−36.
[22] Akbarzadeh A, et al. Liposome: classification, preparation, and applications. Nanoscale Res Lett 2013; 8(1):102.
[23] Bozzuto G, Molinari A. Liposomes as nanomedical devices. Int J Nanomed 2015;10:975−99.
[24] Kim KS, et al. A cancer-recognizable MRI contrast agents using pH-responsive polymeric micelle. Biomaterials 2014;35(1):337−43.
[25] Torchilin VP. Multifunctional nanocarriers. Adv Drug Deliv Rev 2006;58(14):1532−55.
[26] Brigger I, Dubernet C, Couvreur P. Nanoparticles in cancer therapy and diagnosis. Adv Drug Deliv Rev 2002;54(5):631−51.
[27] Tian J, et al. A multifunctional nanomicelle for real-time targeted imaging and precise near-infrared cancer therapy. Angew Chem Int Ed Engl 2014;53(36):9544−9.
[28] Chen HP, et al. A novel micelle-forming material used for preparing a theranostic vehicle exhibiting enhanced in vivo therapeutic efficacy. J Med Chem 2015;58(9):3704−19.
[29] Guo M, et al. Dual imaging-guided photothermal/photodynamic therapy using micelles. Biomaterials 2014;35(16):4656−66.
[30] Abbasi E, et al. Dendrimers: synthesis, applications, and properties. Nanoscale Res Lett 2014;9(1):247.

[31] Longmire M, Choyke PL, Kobayashi H. Dendrimer-based contrast agents for molecular imaging. Curr Top Med Chem 2008;8(14):1180–6.
[32] Fahmy TM, et al. Nanosystems for simultaneous imaging and drug delivery to T cells. AAPS J 2007;9(2):E171–80.
[33] Tomalia DA, Reyna LA, Svenson S. Dendrimers as multi-purpose nanodevices for oncology drug delivery and diagnostic imaging. Biochem Soc Trans 2007;35(Pt 1):61–7.
[34] Sinha VR, et al. Poly-epsilon-caprolactone microspheres and nanospheres: an overview. Int J Pharm 2004;278(1):1–23.
[35] Zheng J, Jaffray DA, Allen C. Nanosystems for multimodality in vivo imaging. In: Torchilin V, editor. Multifunctional pharmaceutical nanocarriers. New York: Springer; 2008. p. 409–30.
[36] Di Paola M, et al. Echographic imaging of tumoral cells through novel nanosystems for image diagnosis. World J Radiol 2014;6(7):459–70.
[37] Geraldes CF, Laurent S. Classification and basic properties of contrast agents for magnetic resonance imaging. Contrast Media Mol Imaging 2009;4(1):1–23.
[38] Estelrich J, Sanchez-Martin MJ, Busquets MA. Nanoparticles in magnetic resonance imaging: from simple to dual contrast agents. Int J Nanomed 2015;10:1727–41.
[39] Law GL, Wong WT. An introduction to molecular imaging. In: Long N, Wong WT, editors. The chemistry of molecular imaging. Hoboken (NJ): John Wiley & Sons; 2014. p. 408.
[40] Xiao L, Yeung ES. Optical imaging of individual plasmonic nanoparticles in biological samples. Annu Rev Anal Chem (Palo Alto Calif) 2014;7:89–111.
[41] Chen M, et al. Nanoparticles in fluorescence optical imaging. In: Yang X, editor. Nanotechnology in modern medical imaging and interventions. Nova Science Publishers, Inc.; 2013. p. 331.
[42] Coll JL. Cancer optical imaging using fluorescent nanoparticles. Nanomedicine (London) 2011;6(1):7–10.
[43] Pansare VJ, et al. Composite fluorescent nanoparticles for biomedical imaging. Mol Imaging Biol 2014;16(2):180–8.
[44] Abeylath SC, et al. Combinatorial-designed multifunctional polymeric nanosystems for tumor-targeted therapeutic delivery. Acc Chem Res 2011;44(10):1009–17.
[45] Jiang S, Gnanasammandhan MK, Zhang Y. Optical imaging-guided cancer therapy with fluorescent nanoparticles. J R Soc Interface 2010;7(42):3–18.
[46] Tobin EH. Nanotechnology applications for infectious diseases. In: Brenner S, editor. The clinical nanomedicine handbook. CRC Press; 2013. p. 365.
[47] Wolfbeis OS. An overview of nanoparticles commonly used in fluorescent bioimaging. Chem Soc Rev 2015;44(14):4743–68.
[48] Srivatsan A, Chen X. Recent advances in nanoparticle-based nuclear imaging of cancers. Adv Cancer Res 2014;124:83–129.
[49] Abou DS, Pickett JE, Thorek DL. Nuclear molecular imaging with nanoparticles: radiochemistry, applications and translation. Br J Radiol 2015;88(1054):20150185.
[50] Ting G, et al. Nanotargeted radionuclides for cancer nuclear imaging and internal radiotherapy. J Biomed Biotechnol 2010;2010.
[51] Xing Y, et al. Radiolabeled nanoparticles for multimodality tumor imaging. Theranostics 2014;4(3):290–306.
[52] Liu Y, Ai K, Lu L. Nanoparticulate x-ray computed tomography contrast agents: from design validation to in vivo applications. Acc Chem Res 2012;45(10):1817–27.
[53] Lusic H, Grinstaff MW. X-ray-computed tomography contrast agents. Chem Rev 2013;113(3):1641–66.
[54] Walkey CD, et al. Nanoparticle size and surface chemistry determine serum protein adsorption and macrophage uptake. J Am Chem Soc 2012;134(4):2139–47.
[55] Polyak A, et al. (99m)Tc-labelled nanosystem as tumour imaging agent for SPECT and SPECT/CT modalities. Int J Pharm 2013;449(1–2):10–7.
[56] Kothapalli SVVN. Ultrasound contrast agents loaded with magnetic nanoparticles: acoustic and mechanical characterization. Stockholm, Sweden: Department of Medical Engineering, School of Technology and Health, KTH - Royal Institute of Technology; 2013.

[57] Zheng SG, Xu HX, Chen HR. Nano/microparticles and ultrasound contrast agents. World J Radiol 2013;5(12):468–71.
[58] Milgroom A, et al. Mesoporous silica nanoparticles as a breast-cancer targeting ultrasound contrast agent. Colloids Surf B Biointerfaces 2014;116:652–7.
[59] Kwon S, Wheatley MA. Gas-loaded PLA nanoparticles as ultrasound contrast agents. In: Magjarevic R, Nagel JH, editors. World congress on medical physics and biomedical engineering 2006. Springer Berlin Heidelberg; 2006. p. 275–8.
[60] Bae KH, Chung HJ, Park TG. Nanomaterials for cancer therapy and imaging. Mol Cells 2011;31(4): 295–302.
[61] Perlman O, Weitz IS, Azhari H. Copper oxide nanoparticles as contrast agents for MRI and ultrasound dual-modality imaging. Phys Med Biol 2015;60(15):5767–83.
[62] Clark LC. Monitor and control of blood and tissue oxygen tensions. Trans Am Soc Artif Intern Organs 1956;2:41.
[63] Updike SJ, Hicks GP. The enzyme electrode. Nature 1967;214:986–8.
[64] Mastrototaro JJ. The MiniMed continuous glucose monitoring system. Diabetes Technol Ther 2000; 2(Suppl. 1):S13–8.
[65] Diabetes Research in Children Network (DirectNet) Study Group. The accuracy of the CGMS in children with type 1 diabetes: results of the diabetes research in children. Net-work (DirectNet) accuracy study. Diabetes Technol Ther 2003;5:781–9.
[66] Diabetes Research in Children Network (DirectNet) Study Group. The accuracy of the Guardian RT continuous glucose monitor in children with type 1 diabetes. Diabetes Technol Ther 2008; 10:266–72.
[67] Mastrototaro J, Shin J, Marcus A, Sulur G, STAR, Clinical Trial Investigations. The accuracy and efficacy of real time continuous glucose monitoring sensor in patients with type 1 diabetes. Diabetes Technol Ther 2008;10:385–90.
[68] Doijad RC, et al. Formulation and targeting efficiency of Cisplatin engineered solid lipid nanoparticles. Indian J Pharm Sci 2008;70(2):203–7.
[69] Miao Y, Chen J, Wu X. Construction of a glucose biosensor by immobilizing glucose oxidase within a poly(o-phenylenediamine) covered screen printed electrode. Online J Biol Sci 2006;6(1):18–22.
[70] Ren G, Xu X, Liu Q, Cheng J, Yuan X, Wu L, Wan Y. Electrospun poly(vinyl alcohol)/glucose oxidase biocomposite membranes for biosensor applications. React Funct Polym 2006;66:1559–64.
[71] Njagi J, Andreescu S. Stable enzyme biosensors based on chemically synthesized Au-polypyrrole nanocomposites. Biosens Bioelectron 2007;23:168–75.
[72] Xian Y, Hu Y, Liu F, Xian Y, Wang H, Jin L. Glucose biosensor based on Au nanoparticles-conductive polyaniline nanocomposite. Biosens Bioelectron 2006;21:1996–2000.
[73] Wang J, Wang L, Di J, Tu Y. Disposable biosensor based on immobilization of glucose oxidase at gold nanoparticles eletrodeposited on indium tin oxide electrode. Sens Actuators 2008;135:283–8.
[74] Sato N, Okuma H. Development of single-wall carbon nanotubes modified screen-printed electrode using a ferrocene-modified cationic surfactant for amperometric glucose biosensor applications. Sens Actuators 2008;B129:188–94.
[75] Manesh KM, Kim HT, Santosh P, Gopalan AI, Lee K-P. A novel glucose biosensor based on immobilization of glucose oxidase into multiwall carbon nanotubes-polyelectrolyte-loaded electrospun nanofibrous membrane. Biosens Bioelectron 2008;23:771–9.
[76] Zou Y, Xiang C, Sun Li-X, Xu F. Glucose biosensor based on electrodeposition of platinum nanoparticles onto carbon nanotubes and immobilizing enzyme with chitosan-SiO$_2$ sol-gel. Biosens Bioelectron 2008;23:1010–6.
[77] Wang H, Wang X, Zhang X, Qin X, Zhao Z, Miao Z, Huang N, Chen Q. A novel glucose biosensor based on the immobilization of glucose oxidase onto gold nanoparticles-modified Pb nanowires. Biosens Bioelectron 2009;25(1):142–6.
[78] Shoba Jeykumari DR, Sriman Narayanan S. A novel nanobiocomposite based glucose biosensor using neutral red functionalized carbon nanotubes. Biosens Bioelectron 2008;23:1401–11.
[79] Ozcan L, Sahin Y, Turk H. Non-enzymatic glucose based on overoxidized polypyrrole nanofiber electrode modified with cobalt(II)phthalocyanine tetrasulfonate. Biosens Bioelectron 2008;28: 512–7.

[80] Lu L-M, Zhang L, Qu F-L, Lu H-X, Zhang X-B, Wu ZS, Huan S-Y, Wang Q-A, Shen G-L, Yu R-Q. A nano-Ni based ultrasensitive nonenzymatic electrochemical sensor for glucose: enhancing sensitivity through a nanowire array strategy. Biosens Bioelectron 2009;25:218−23.
[81] Shuttleworth R. The surface tension of solids. Proc Phys Soc Lond 1950;63A:444−57.
[82] Stoney GG. The tension of metallic films deposited by electrolysis. Proc R Soc A, Math Phys Eng Sci 1909;82:553.
[83] Wu G, et al. Bioassay of prostate-specific antigen (PSA) using microcantilevers. Nat Biotechnol 2001; 19(9):856−60.
[84] Lee JH, et al. Immunoassay of prostate-specific antigen (PSA) using resonant frequency shift of piezoelectric nanomechanical microcantilever. Biosens Bioelectron 2005;20(10):2157−62.
[85] Arntz Y, Seelig JD, Lang HP, Zhang J, Hunziker P, Ramseyer JP, Meyer E, Hegner M, Gerber C. Label-free protein assay based on a nanomechanical cantilever array. Nanotechnology 2003;14: 86−90.
[86] Battison FM, Ramseyer J-P, Lang HP, Baller MK, Gerber C, Gimzewski JK, Meyer E, Guntherodt H-J. A chemical sensor based on a microfabricated cantilever array with simultaneous resonance-frequency and bending readout. Sens Actuators B 2001;77:122−31.
[87] Hansen KM, et al. Cantilever-based optical deflection assay for discrimination of DNA single-nucleotide mismatches. Anal Chem 2001;73(7):1567−71.
[88] McKendry R, et al. Multiple label-free biodetection and quantitative DNA-binding assays on a nanomechanical cantilever array. Proc Natl Acad Sci USA 2002;99(15):9783−8.
[89] Fodor SP, et al. Multiplexed biochemical assays with biological chips. Nature 1993;364(6437): 555−6.
[90] Rowe CA, et al. Array biosensor for simultaneous identification of bacterial, viral, and protein analytes. Anal Chem 1999;71(17):3846−52.
[91] Ilic B, et al. Enumeration of DNA molecules bound to a nanomechanical oscillator. Nano Lett 2005; 5(5):925−9.
[92] Nelson-Fitzpatrick N, Fischer LM, Evoy S, Ophus C, Wang Y, Mitlin D, Lee Z-H, Radmilovic V, Dahmen U. Fabrication and characterization of ultra thin resonant nanocantilevers in aluminium-molybdenum composites. In: The nanotechnology conference and trade show. CA, Boston: University of Alberta; 2006.
[93] Gupta AK, et al. Anomalous resonance in a nanomechanical biosensor. Proc Natl Acad Sci USA 2006;103(36):13362−7.
[94] Shuaipeng W, Jingjing W, Yinfang Z, Jinling Y, Fuhua Y. Cantilever with immobilized antibody for liver cancer biomarker detection. J Semicond 2014;35(10):104008.
[95] Etayash H, Jiang K, Azmi S, Thundat T, Kaur K. Real-time detection of breast cancer cells using peptide-functionalized microcantilever arrays. Sci Rep 2005;5:13967.
[96] Jianlin Z, Jiancheng Y, Xiaomei Y. A glucose biosensor based on piezoresistive microcantilevers. Solid-State and Integrated Circuit Technology (ICSICT), IEEE; 2012. p. 1−3.
[97] Pei J, Tian F, Thundat T. Glucose biosensor based on the microcantilever. Anal Chem 2004;76(2): 292−7.
[98] Pandya HJ, Roy R, Chen W, Chekmareva MA, Foran DJ, Desai JP. Accurate characterization of benign and cancerous breast tissues: aspecific patient studies using piezoresistive microcantilevers. Biosens Bioelectron 2015;63:414−24.
[99] Chen X, Pan Y, Liu H, Bai X, Wang N, Zhang B. Label-free detection of liver cancer cells by aptamer-based microcantilever biosensor. Biosens Bioelectron 2016;79:353−8.
[100] Weeks B, Camarero J, Noy A, Miller AE, De Yoreo JJ. Development of a microcantilever-based pathogen detector. Scanning 2003;25(6):297−9.

CHAPTER 11

Micro- and Nanotechnology-Based Implantable Devices and Bionics

Rohit Bisht[1], Abhirup Mandal[2], Ashim K. Mitra[2]
[1]University of Auckland, Auckland, New Zealand; [2]University of Missouri—Kansas City, Kansas City, MO, United States

Contents

1. Introduction	249
2. Biocompatibility Issues of Implants	252
3. Microtechnology-Based Implantable Devices and Bionics	258
3.1 Sensing Systems	262
3.2 Drug Delivery Devices	269
4. Nanotechnology-Based Implantable Devices and Bionics	272
4.1 Sensing Systems	274
4.2 Drug Delivery Devices	277
5. Conclusions and Future Perspectives	280
References	281

1. INTRODUCTION

Micro- and nanotechnology-based biomedical implantable devices are collectively known as bionic implants. The term bionic refers to the study of artificial systems that can mimic the biological systems. Implantable devices have demonstrated significant potential for wide applications including biosensing and drug delivery. The market of implantable devices is expected to grow at a cumulative annual growth rate of 7.1% and may be able to reach $17.82 billion by 2017 [1]. Over the past few years, the micro- and nanoelectromechanical systems (MEMS and NEMS) technology-based next generation of implantable biomedical devices has enabled the design of small size biomedical devices. These small size systems can be implanted with minimally invasive procedures intended for drug delivery, diagnosing, monitoring, and treating various diseases. The next-generation biomedical implants (BMIs) are applied in various medical applications, such as (1) central and peripheral neural BMIs, such as neuronal and retinal implants; (2) cardiovascular BMIs, such as stents, vascular grafts, heart valves, and pacemakers; (3) orthopedic, such as bone grafts, fusion, and sensor devices; (4) pressure sensors; (5) immunoisolation devices; and (6) drug delivery systems. These devices also show great potential for the treatment of a number of critical diseases in emergency situations without the support of a physician or medical practitioner [2]. However, the major challenges with implant technologies currently are the better host acceptability and reduced foreign body reactions of the body toward implants. Micro-/nanotechnology has the ability to modify the design and properties of these implantable systems to overcome the present challenges, and result in better diagnosis and management of the diseases. The micro- and nanotechnology have significantly reduced the size of whole device to a minimally invasive implantable form. Surface modification techniques and biocompatible material selection improved the biocompatibility between the implant and the biological medium. Figs. 11.1–11.4 display different polymeric microfabrication techniques, such as microinjection molding, hot embossing, casting, and stereolithography.

Advancement in the field of micro-/nanotechnology-based devices make possible the programmed drug release to achieve specific control over drug release. Table 11.1 displays different forms of implantable devices and working principles. Figs. 11.5–11.7 show a schematic illustration of the different types of implantable devices and mechanisms involved.

Currently, several US Food and Drug Administration (FDA)-approved implantable devices are in use for the management of various diseases. In 1977 Alzet pump (ALZA/Durect Corp., Cupertino, CA, USA), an implantable drug delivery system for animal research, was introduced and remained as a gold standard [31] (Fig. 11.8A). Another implantable pump, iPrecio microinfusion pump (Primetech), consists of integrated electronics for preprograming of a complex drug delivery regimen before implantation [32]. A battery-powered motor to drive a set of pins is provided, which generates a peristaltic actuation for controlled delivery of the dissolved drug from the reservoir (Fig. 11.8B). The Duros micropump technology delivers peptides and proteins at a

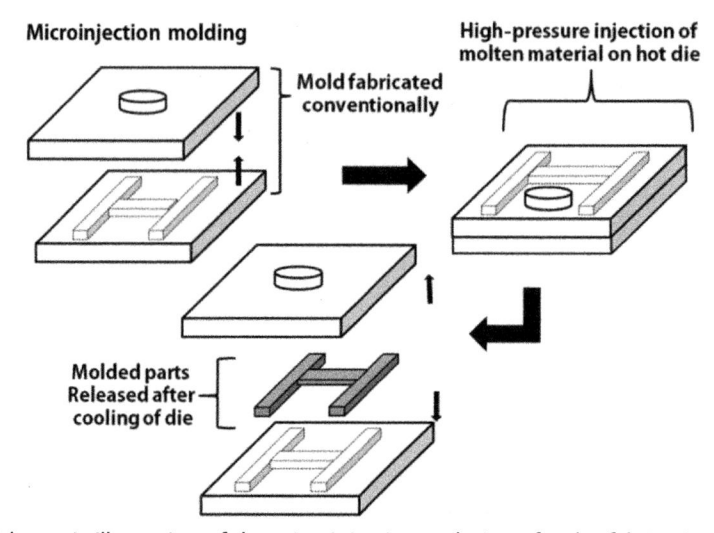

Figure 11.1 Schematic illustration of the microinjection technique for the fabrication of implantable microdevices.

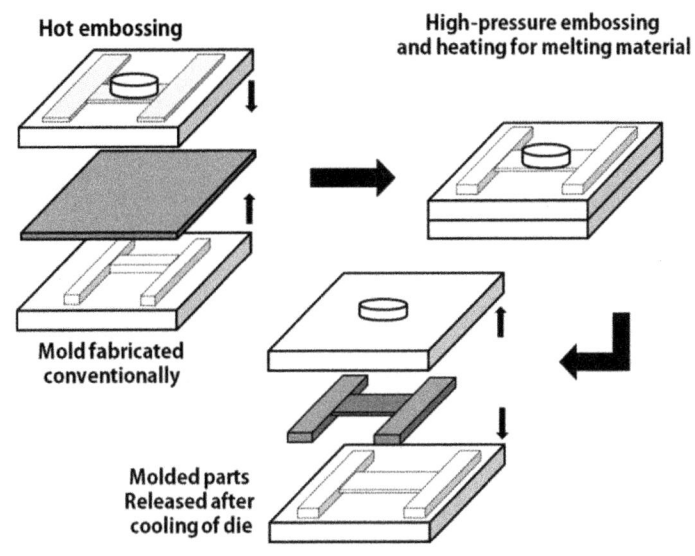

Figure 11.2 Schematic illustration of the hot embossing technique used for the fabrication of implantable microdevices.

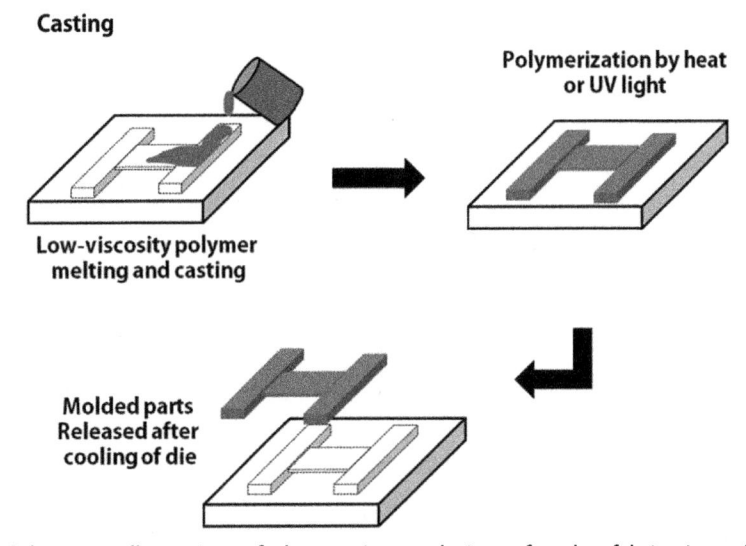

Figure 11.3 Schematic illustration of the casting technique for the fabrication of implantable microdevices.

constant rate over 3–12 months [33] (Fig. 11.9A). Duros was also investigated for the delivery of several therapeutic agents, such as sufentanil for the management of chronic pain in combination with the Chronogesic pain therapy system, exenatide (type 2 diabetes), and ω-interferon (hepatitis C) [34]. Synchromed II (Medtronic, Minneapolis,

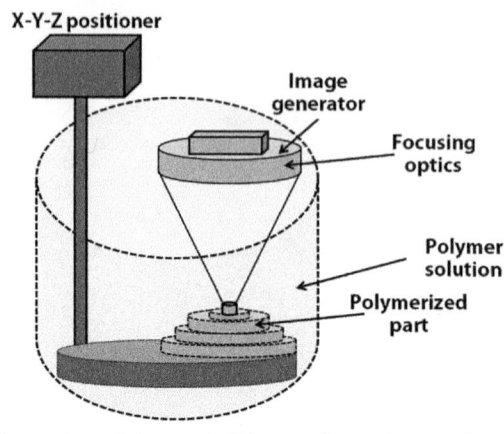

Figure 11.4 Schematic illustration of the stereolithography technique for the fabrication of implantable microdevices.

MN, USA) consists of a programmable drug infusion system for precise drug delivery in chronic therapy (Fig. 11.9B). In addition, this system is also fitted with catheter to deliver specific amounts of baclofen directly to the intrathecal space and cerebrospinal fluid (CSF) [35]. The Codman 3000 (Codman and Shurtleff/Johnson and Johnson, New Brunswick, NJ, USA) is provided with a pressurized gas expansion mechanism to deliver drug into the intraspinal space [36]. Prometra (Flowonix, Medical, Mt. Olive, NJ, USA; FDA approved in 2012) and Medstream (Codman and Shurtleff/Johnson and Johnson; FDA approved in 2011) are based on a similar pressurized gas expansion actuation technique along with battery-facilitated valves to regulate drug flow [37,38]. Table 11.2 depicts some micro- and nanodevices developed to date for biomedical applications.

2. BIOCOMPATIBILITY ISSUES OF IMPLANTS

The success of any implantable device mainly depends upon its in vivo reliability, cytocompatibility, and durability throughout its proposed duration of action. Typically, tissue inflammation and immunological responses can arise within a short time span following implantation [69]. The possible inflammation responses caused by tissue injuries following device implantation is due to natural immunological responses. A series of wound healing mechanisms comes into play after tissue injury resulting from device implantation [70,71]. Fig. 11.10 shows the sequence of events from an immune response against implant leads to the formation of fibrous capsules around the implantable system. The material properties of the implantable devices, such as the shape, size, surface chemistry, roughness, design, porosity, composition, contact duration, and degradation, are mainly responsible for possible immunological responses [72–76].

Table 11.1 Different types of micro- and nanotechnology-based drug delivery devices

Device type	Mechanism	Advantages	Disadvantages	References
Reservoir-based drug-delivery devices	The drug released slowly either through orifices located in the reservoir wall or when an impermeable seal is removed	Simple design with ease of application	Refilling of drug is not possible	
Passive diffusion-based reservoir devices	Delivery of drug through reservoir is regulated by a nanoporous membrane that is biodegradable, electrochemically or electrically removable (metal thin film), or shrunken by application of thermal energy (hydrogel block valve)	Simple design with more control over the drug release	Small dose volumes with slow release rate	[3–8]
Actively directed reservoir devices	Drug released by the electrochemical dissolution of a metal capping film. Thermal energy and prepressurizing the reservoir can also be used to achieve drug release	Rapid drug release under emergency conditions	Small dose volumes and refilling of drug is not possible	[2,9–11]
Drug-infusion micropumps	Require electrical power or other sources of energy (e.g., chemical or mechanical) to supply the pressure differential for drug release	Can be refilled to allow chronic dosing	More complicated than simple reservoirs	

Continued

Table 11.1 Different types of micro- and nanotechnology-based drug delivery devices—cont'd

Device type	Mechanism	Advantages	Disadvantages	References
Passive micropumps	*Osmotic micropumps*: With the development of osmotic gradient, osmotic pumps works continuously with continuous drug release. The pump is for single use	Do not require electrical power alternative sources	Single use	[12–14]
	Spring-powered micropumps: These are spring pressurized dual-reservoir-pump systems having smallest size and low weight	Allows multidrug capability; dose can be accurately delivered with the help of smart, electronically activated microvalves; it can be refilled		[15–17]
Active micropumps	*Electrostatic micropumps*: Drug released due to a mechanical force results from the attraction between closely spaced (at the micron scale) but oppositely charged metallic plates. The fluid can be refilled from a reservoir. Both reciprocating and peristaltic diaphragm-type electrostatic micropumps have been developed	Rapid mechanical response with low power consumption	Work over short distances limits the fluid volume that can be displaced with each stroke. Moreover, high voltages are required for operation	[18–20]

Piezoelectric micropumps: Piezoelectric thin film or sheet attached to a flexible diaphragm and application of appropriate electronic control signal, the diaphragm can pump fluid in a pulsatile manner	Piezoelectric mechanisms provide a high force and a fast mechanical response	Require high voltages	[21–23]
Electrochemical micropumps: A small current or voltage applied for the generation of oxygen and hydrogen gas bubbles, which provide excess pressure used to drive a flexible diaphragm, which displaces drug from the reservoir	Low power consumption with large mechanical displacement		[24–26]
Thermal micropumps: Displacement of drug through diaphragm is induced via thermally induced material expansion or phase change (e.g., liquid to gas)		The long thermal time constant limits the mechanical response time. High power consumption	[27–30]

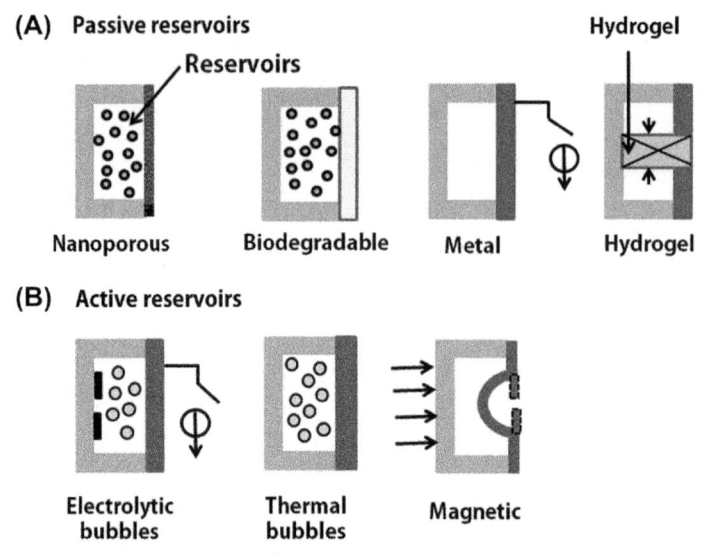

Figure 11.5 (A) Passive reservoir: release of drug is regulated by a membrane that may be modified to be nanoporous, biodegradable, electrochemically or electrically removable (metal thin film), or shrunken by using thermal energy (hydrogel block valve). (B) Active reservoir: drug is actively displaced from the reservoir by electrolytically produced bubbles, thermally generated bubbles, and modulation of membrane through magnetic effect.

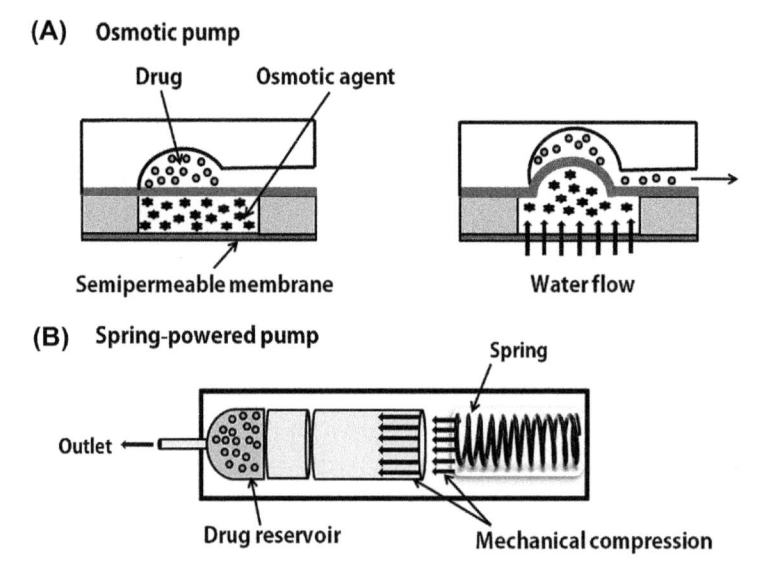

Figure 11.6 (A) Osmotic pumps: osmotic agent regulates water uptake through semipermeable membrane, which deflects flexible diaphragm and displaces drug from the reservoir. (B) Spring-powered pump: spring provides the mechanical compression that displaces the drug from the reservoir and the valve in line with the pump outlet regulates the flow of the drug from the reservoir.

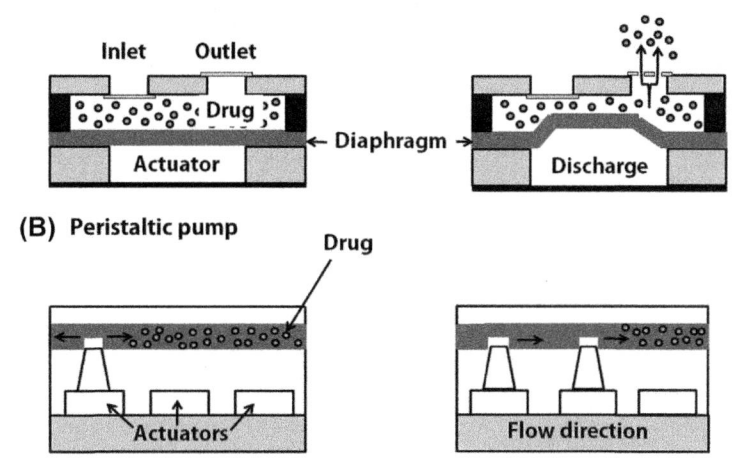

Figure 11.7 (A) Reciprocating pump: reciprocating actuator is responsible for pumping. During the operation, the two opposing one-way regulates the filling and emptying of the drug chamber above the diaphragm. (B) Peristaltic pump: it consists of three pumping actuators. Drug displacement is achieved by the actuator activated in a precise sequence.

Till date, various polymers have been used for the fabrication of implantable devices, such as collagen [77], chitosan [78], alginate [79], hyaluronan [80], dextran [81], poly(lactic acid) [82], poly(lactic-*co*-glycolic acid) (PLGA) [83], poly(ethylene glycol) [84], 2-hydroxy ethyl methacrylate [85], and poly(vinyl alcohol) [86]. These materials are generally considered to be biocompatible [87]. For the safe local and systemic application of the materials used in the fabrication of devices, in-depth in vitro and in vivo biocompatibility investigations are required [87,88]. The International Organization for Standardization (ISO) 10993 provides

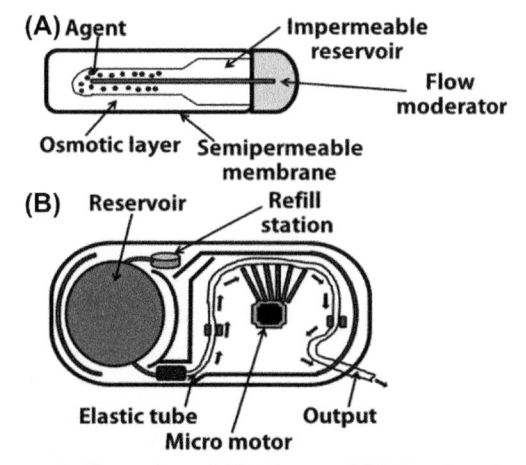

Figure 11.8 Schematic illustration of (A) Alzet and (B) iPrecio microinfusion pumps.

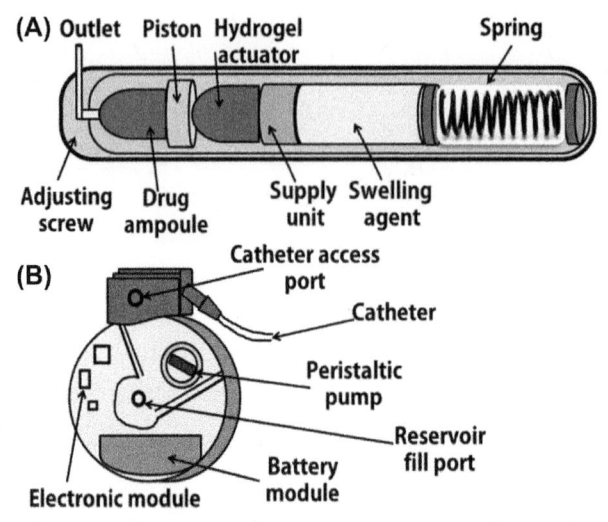

Figure 11.9 Schematic illustration of (A) Duros and (B) Synchromed II micropumps.

a series of standards for evaluating the biocompatibility of a medical device. ISO 10993-5 covers in vitro testing including positive and negative control materials, extraction conditions, choice of cell lines, and cell media. Moreover, important aspects of the test procedures, including tests on extracts and tests on direct and indirect contents, are described in this document [89]. Methods based on the assessment of cytotoxicity, mutagenesis/carcinogenesis, and cell biofunction are used to evaluate biocompatibility and biofunctionality of medical devices [90–93]. While maintaining sensor functionality, the negative responses can be minimized by use of biocompatible outer coatings, such as hydrogel coating over the implants that are able to mimic the body tissue. Antiinflammatory agents incorporated inside the coating, which are released at the local site of implant application, have been very effective in preventing inflammation and fibrosis. Two different strategies have been employed to overcome inflammation responses against implantable devices, such as combination of an implantable device and a drug delivery system where drug will enhance implant biocompatibility or reduce inflammation responses [94,95]. Another strategy may be the modification of preparation procedure and components of implantable devices having high degree of biocompatibility or safety profile. Biocompatibility of the implantable devices needs careful consideration, not only from a chemistry standpoint, but also from a biological perspective for safe and effective clinical application.

3. MICROTECHNOLOGY-BASED IMPLANTABLE DEVICES AND BIONICS

Over the past decades, advancements in microfabrication technologies have enabled the development of microdevices, such as microneedles, micropumps, microvalves, and microbionic systems for drug delivery, diagnostics, neural prosthetics, minimally invasive

Table 11.2 List of some micro- and nanodevices for biomedical applications

Device	Material	Study results	References
Biosensor	Zinc oxide nanowire	Successfully measured K^+ ion concentration	[39]
	Polydimethylsiloxane	Successfully measured glucose concentration	[40]
	Epoxy-polyurethane membrane	Stable for 4—8 months	[41]
	Sulfonic acid functionalized hydroxyl-terminated hyperbranched polyester	Successfully integrated biocompatible and anticoagulation coating on biosensor	[42]
Stents	Stent-316 stainless steel, Ti-Ni-Ta alloy Au-Cr film	Response time 260 ms and output frequency of 2 Hz	[43]
	Poly (D,L-lactic-*co*-glycolic acid) with sirolimus and triflusal	Exhibited significant reduction in restenosis	[44]
	Liquid crystal polymer	Enabled precise and accurate measurements of wireless transmitted data	[45]
	Formula 418 cook medical	Successful reception of wireless data up to a range of 50 cm (FDA approved)	[46]
	Polyethylene stent with magnetoelastic sensor array	Successful reception of wireless signals up to a range of 7.5 cm	[47]
Micro-nano needles	Carbon nanosyringe arrays	Successfully delivered different cargos in cytoplasm of the cell	[48]
	Atomic force microscope silicon tip to nanoneedle	Delivered proteins directly in cell	[49]
	MWCNT nanoneedle attached to tungsten tip	Exhibited detection of glucose, ascorbic acid, cytochrome in volumes <1 pL	[50]
	Silicon-based microneedle array	Successfully delivered protein to dermal layer	[51]
	Ultrasharp silicon microneedle	Force of insertion with single microneedle less than 10 nN	[52]
Micro-nano reservoirs	Gold	Gold corrosion is biocompatible	[53]
	Poly(L-lactic acid)	PLA showed slow degradation relative to PLGA membrane	[8]
	Poly(lactic-*co*-glycolic acid)	Different polymers with varied molecular weights degrades over a span of time and showed pulsatile drug delivery	[8]

Continued

Table 11.2 List of some micro- and nanodevices for biomedical applications—cont'd

Device	Material	Study results	References
Micro-nano pumps	Carbon nanotubes coated with poly(lactide)-poly(ethylene glycol) (CNT-PLA-PEG)	Biocompatible polymer-coated CNTs with low toxicity in vivo and in vitro; increased drug efficiency from 12% to 50%	[54]
	Polyetheretherketone	Achieved 98.5% cell manipulation success rate	[55]
	Poly(methyl methacrylate)	Thick diaphragm (1.3 mm) dispensed volume varying from 500 pL to 250 nL at a flow rate of 250 nL/s	[55]
	SAM-*N*-(triethosilylpropyl)-*O*-polyethylene oxide	Imparts hemocompatibility to silicon-based device	[56]
	Silicone	Minimizes flow resistance and demonstrated optimal delivery to site with one-sided valve in catheter to avoid back flow	[24]
Micro-nano actuators	Polyvinylidene fluoride with silver electrode encapsulated in PMMA	Piezoelectric actuator stimulated bone growth and exhibits bone area increment	[57]
	C2-C12-collagen film integrated with silicon MEMS device	Depict successful locomotive motion	[58]
	Polypyrrole-based electrostatic actuation	Require faster actuation speed to image with a catheter	[59]
Tissue engineering	Core-polyethylene glycol/polyacrylic acid	Successfully demonstrate cell growth with contingency on covalent tethering of collagen	[60]
	Resorbable chitosan	Successful recording of physiological signals for over 12 months	[61]
	Biodegradable polyurethane scaffolds	Completely resorbs scaffold after 3 months with slight inflammatory response	[62]
Coatings	Dexamethasone-loaded nitrocellulose coatings	Sustain drug release for over 16 days	[63]

Table 11.2 List of some micro- and nanodevices for biomedical applications—cont'd

Device	Material	Study results	References
	Micropatterned titanium dioxide	Pattern size-dependent antiinflammatory coating	[64]
	Nanosilver	Reduction in cytokine concentration and lower lymphocyte and mast cell infiltration	[65]
	Perfluorocarboxylate ionomer	Lower mineralization on coating and exhibits better cracking-resistant property	[66]
	Carboxymethyl-PEG-carboxymethyl	Exhibits hemocompatibility	[67]
Self-assembled monolayer	Carboxyl terminal	Successfully deploy PDMS probes	[68]

MEMS, microelectromechanical systems; *MWCNT*, multiwalled carbon nanotube; *PDMS*, polydimethylsiloxane; *PLA*, poly(L-lactic acid); *PLGA*, poly(D,L-lactic-*co*-glycolic acid); *PMMA*, Poly(methyl methacrylate).

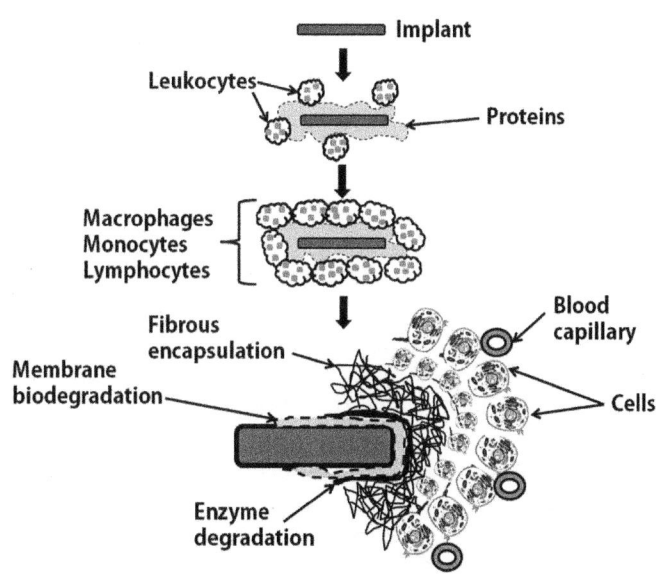

Figure 11.10 Sequence of events that are initiated by the immune system of the body against the implant leading to the formation of fibrous capsules around the implantable system.

surgery, and tissue engineering [96]. Advancement in the field of microfabrication techniques have resulted in the development of MEMS, bioMEMS, lab-on-a-chip (LOC), micro-total analysis systems, and other microdevices. These advancements in microtechnology offer various benefits, such as portability, ease of implantation, excellent performance, low cost, and more control over the release of the therapeutic molecules. In addition, the ease of integration of the system with electronic elements allows straightforward control over the system [97]. As mentioned earlier, the major challenge with the development and application of microfabricated implantable devices is the biocompatibility of the materials used in their fabrication. Materials with low toxicity profile have been used for the development of implantable devices, such as polymers [e.g., liquid crystal polymers, parylene, polydimethylsiloxane (PDMS)], metals (e.g., nitinol, titanium, stainless steel, and platinum), and various inorganics and ceramics (e.g., zirconia and alumina). To date, various microfabricated sensors with the MEMS technology use bioincompatible materials such as Si, poly-Si, SiO_2, Si_3N_4, SiC, and SU-8 epoxy photoresists [89,98]. In the following sections, we describe in detail the characteristics and challenges with various types of microdevices.

3.1 Sensing Systems

Microfabricated implantable sensing devices have been used for analysis of blood and other body fluids. Till date, LOC, microarray systems, and microfluidic devices integrated with sensors have been developed that can detect a specific change in the environment. In case of biosensors, the devices are fabricated in such a way that the integrated sensor can interact and sense a small and specific change in the biological system or its components. Thin membrane film is an easy example of the most common type of pressure sensors. The pressure variation from the surrounding environment results in deflection of the membrane film, which is transduced with the help of piezoresistors on the membranes or conductors present on both sides [99]. Several MEMS (MEMS pressure and acceleration sensor) have been developed for diagnostic analysis including cardiac pacemakers, cardioverter defibrillators, implantable cardiac resynchronization devices, cochlear stimulators, as well as neurological pulse generators for deep brain, spinal, visual cortex, retinal, and sacral nerve stimulations [100−103]. Biomedical applications of MEMS have been discussed in various reviews [100−102,104]. A repeating sequence of photolithography, etching, and deposition steps can be used for the structural configuration of devices, such as traces (thin metal wires), interlayer connections, reservoirs, valves, or membranes, in a layer-by-layer fashion [100,105,106].

Several MEMS systems have been developed as sensing devices for the better diagnosis and management of the diseases. For example, measurement of intraocular pressure (IOP) plays an important role in the effective diagnosis and improvement in the management of glaucoma, which can cause vision loss. Collins et al. [107,108] proposed an implantable small sized pressure sensor intended to fit in an artificial lens to sense the change in IOP. Mokwa et al. [109] introduced an IOP sensor fitted with a coil on flex, flip chip pressure sensor and implantable chip (IC) embedded in a lens. Another biosensor has been developed, which consists of parallel-resonant inductive-capacitive circuit. It is fabricated with electrodeposition of copper on a microfabricated chip with a pressure-sensitive

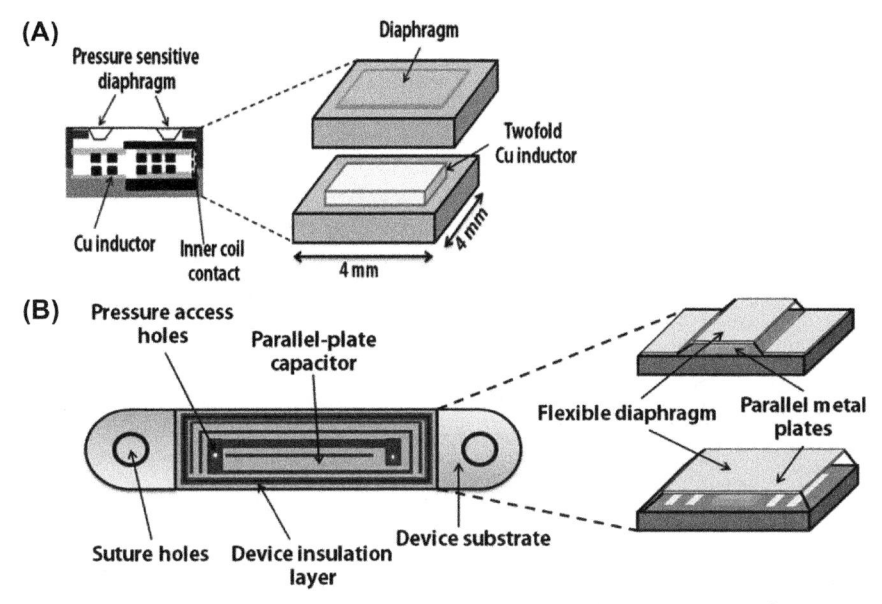

Figure 11.11 Implantable intraocular pressure sensors. (A) The device consists of two silicon chips and the pressure-sensitive diaphragm is present on the top silicon chip. Twofold copper inductors act as sensitive element. (B) Microfabricated implantable parylene-based wireless passive intraocular pressure sensors. A flexible diaphragm chamber can sense an electrical signal in response to pressure change.

diaphragm for IOP measurement [110] (Fig. 11.11A). Chen et al. [111] developed a microfabricated implantable parylene-based wireless passive IOP sensor consisting of an integrated capacitor and an inductor coil to facilitate passive wireless sensing. Parylene is a biocompatible material suitable for the development of minimally invasive intraocular implants (Fig. 11.11B). The effectiveness and stability of the sensor have been evaluated in a live rabbit eye for 6 months. There was no sign of inflammatory response or fibrosis following device implantation, which indicates biocompatibility in the intraocular environment.

Microfabricated implantable devices have also been applied in patients with head injury or having elevated intracranial pressure (ICP), such as chronic hydrocephalus, brain tumors, and abscesses. In terms of mobility, microfabricated wireless implantable devices are more effective over catheter-based systems and allow continuous monitoring of postoperative ICP [112–114]. In 1979 Cosman et al. [115] introduced a pressure sensor integrated with a shunt valve system and a detector stays outside the body for pressure measurement. The same system has also been applied for the measurement of ventricular fluid pressure in relation to change in body positions in normal individuals and patients with implanted shunts [116].

In 1988 Talamonti et al. [117] introduced a microfabricated implanted device integrated with microcoil for the measurement of ICP. An implantable telemetric

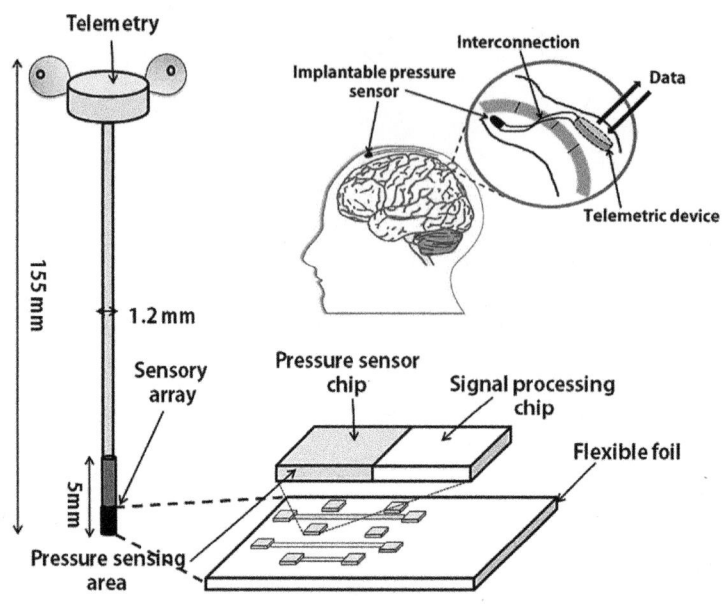

Figure 11.12 Microfabricated telemetric device for intracranial pressure sensing.

endosystem (ITES) has been developed for pressure detection. The device is integrated with surface microfabricated polysilicon membranes, which showed significant results compared with a commercially available sensor when tested in vitro in 0.9% NaCl solution [118] (Fig. 11.12). The possible toxicity of ITES on mouse fibroblast cell line (L 929) indicated its biocompatible nature. Another ITES system has been reported, which consists of surface-microfabricated capacitive-type pressure sensor (0.8 mm × 2 mm × 0.5 mm), and was fabricated in an eight-mask metal oxide semiconductor-like process [119]. The device is integrated with low-power application-specific integrated circuit along with capacitance for telemetry and energy transmission. A biocompatible silicone-based coating over the device ensures long-term implantation. Treatment with standard copper (Cu)-based flex substrates and aluminum (Al)-electroplated microcoils can further enhance the device biocompatibility. The low power consumption of below 100 pA at 3.5 V, which can be powered telemetrically, supports the targeted biomedical application of the device.

In 2000 Flick et al. [120] reported an implantable device consisting of a sensor element combined with a transcutaneous telemetric interface used for measuring the intracorporal pressure and temperature. The device is integrated with a small chip (4 mm × 4 mm × 1 mm) that facilitates a minimally invasive implantation. The device is integrated with complementary metal oxide semiconductor (CMOS)-compatible pressure and temperature sensor with a pulse-width modulated output. This device is very useful for capturing special signals in emergency situations. Microtechnology-based implant devices and bionics have also been developed as a cardiovascular pressure sensor in patients with heart failure. Microtechnology-based devices on catheters are superior over fluid-filled catheters with external transducers and are common in clinic and animal research [121]. Wireless implantable microsystems developed for continuous blood pressure monitoring offer significant opportunities for better management of cardiovascular diseases and improved quality of life. These advanced microdevices overcome the limitations associated with such devices, i.e., catheter whip and limited frequency response. Small size of these devices will enhance the accessibility to small places, which is not possible with earlier conventional devices. Microdevices developed till date are based on piezoresistive material; strain gage pressure sensor and tip pressure catheters utilize an optical technique. Various microdevices developed have been patented and reported in various publications [122–127].

Esashi et al. [128] developed a microfabricated pressure sensor (0.7 mm × 3.5 mm × 0.8 mm) to be placed at the tip of a catheter for the measurement of blood pressure in patients with heart failure. The microfabricated pressure sensor has the pressure sensitivity of 3.45×10^{-5}/mm Hg and the temperature coefficient at zero pressure is 0.17 mm Hg/°C. The IC integrated with the sensor has an output frequency change of about 7 kHz for 1000 mm Hg. Ritzema-Carter et al. [129] studied a percutaneously implanted permanent left atrial pressure monitoring system (HeartPOD Savacor, Inc., USA), which can be admitted into a patient with acute coronary syndrome. This device is useful in detecting left ventricular dysfunction before coronary artery bypass grafting and symptomatic heart failure. Small handheld computers are used to communicate with the implant by radiofrequency digital telemetry. Walton et al. [130] developed a microfabricated implantable device, HeartPOD, for direct measurement of left atrial pressure in patients with congestive heart failure (Fig. 11.13A). Safe monitoring of intracardiac pressures was evaluated in an animal model where the device functioned reliably with accurate pressure measurements. Magalski et al. [131] reported on an implantable hemodynamic monitoring device (IHM) for continuous measurement of heart rate, patient activity levels, and right ventricular systolic and diastolic, and estimated pulmonary artery diastolic pressures in patients with chronic heart failure (CHF). IHM devices were implanted in 32 patients with CHF and were examined with right heart catheterization at implantation and studied for 3, 6, and 12 months. The microfabricated IHM device generated accurate and precise data over time, which indicates its successful clinical application. A permanent implantable device was placed percutaneously in the right pulmonary artery via the internal jugular vein for monitoring pulmonary artery pressure in a clinical setting for heart failure therapy [132] (Fig. 11.13B).

Schnakenberg et al. [133] developed a microfabricated implantable silicone capsule, which can be placed in the arterial system via a guiding catheter for monitoring intravascular pressure. A transponder chip with a monolithically integrated capacitive pressure sensor and a ferrite-based antenna were integrated within silicon capsule (Fig. 11.13C). The integrated chip inside the capsule operates at a nominal power supply voltage of 3 V.

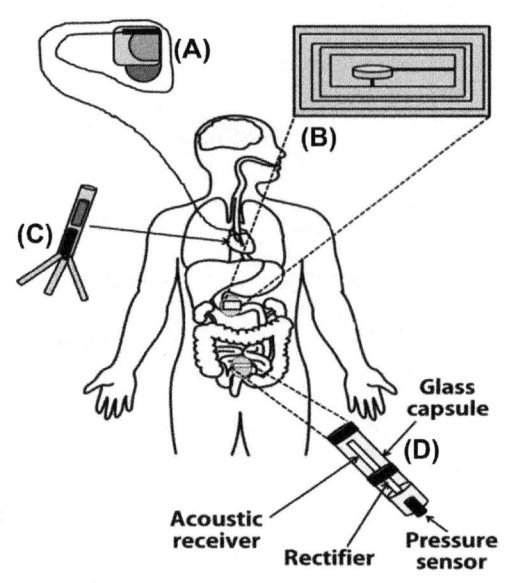

Figure 11.13 Microfabricated implantable devices. (A) HeartPOD system for measuring cardiovascular blood pressure; (B) ENDOCOM implantable wireless pressure sensor for follow-up with abdominal aortic aneurysm stent; (C) Intravascular pressure monitoring system, and (D) implantable bladder pressure sensor.

Till date, various microfabricated devices for monitoring blood pressure and atrial or ventral dysfunction have been developed. These devices have been patented and are currently undergoing clinical trials [134–139]. Currently, microtechnology-based implantable devices are also employed in the diagnosis and management of patients with renal dysfunction [140,141]. In general, catheterization and catheter-based sensors are commonly utilized in the monitoring of urinary bladder volume. However, application of these devices has been associated with invasive nature and risk of infection on prolonged use, and thus are only suitable for short-term use. A bladder pill (40 mm × 5 mm) has been developed for monitoring internal bladder pressure, which is inserted into the bladder through minimally invasive cystoscopy [142]. This small size device consumes on average of 350 μA. This low-cost, flexible system is fitted inside an F20 cystoscope for implantation (Fig. 11.13D). Kim et al. [143] reported an implantable pressure-sensing system (40 mm × 8 mm) fitted with a piezoelectric cantilever, which converts sound vibration harmonics at the resonant frequency into electrical power, which ultimately charges a capacitor. On oscillation of piezoelectric cantilever at its natural resonant frequency, it sends a high-frequency signal that can be detected with an external receiver. This frequency corresponds to the measured pressure. Such device is evaluated in vivo by implanting it inside a pig's bladder. When pressure is changed from 0 to 20 cm H_2O, the corresponding resonant frequency oscillated from 250 to 232 kHz, resulting in a sensitivity of 1 kHz/cm H_2O (20 cm H_2O is the maximum pressure in an anesthetized pig generated with saline injection). A pressure sensitivity of 1 kHz/cm H_2O is achieved with minimal misalignment sensitivity (26% drop at 90-degree misalignment between the implanted device and acoustic source); 60% drop at 90-degree misalignment was noted between the implanted device and radiofrequency receiver coil.

A remotely powered implantable wireless pressure sensor (ENDOCOM) has been reported for monitoring pressure in abdominal aortic aneurysms [144]. Effectiveness of the sensor has been evaluated in vivo using porcine model. Numerical modeling is used to determine the optimal position of the sensor in the aneurysmal sac. A small pill-shaped microfabricated device is reported, which is linked with a remote receiver through wireless radiofrequency. This device is helpful in monitoring the health of a fetus during and after in utero fetal surgery [145]. Langenfeld et al. [146] developed biomechanical endocardial sorin transducer (BEST) sensor to monitor peak endocardial acceleration (PEA, unit g) during the isometric systolic contraction of the heart (dP/dtmax). The BEST sensor is incorporated in the tip of a pacing lead and measures PEA directly near the myocardium. In a clinical study, the device was implanted with a dual-chamber pacemaker Living-1 (Sorin) in 105 patients with physical and mental stress conditions. The sensor functioned properly in short and long duration among 98% of patients for 1–2 months and 1 year after implantation. Kudo et al. [147] reported on a novel biosensor fabricated with functional polymers, such as hydrophobic PDMS and hydrophilic 2-methacryloyloxyethyl phosphorylcholine copolymerized with dodecyl methacrylate, and used for glucose measurement. The sensor was integrated with flexible hydrogen peroxide electrode (Pt working electrode and Ag/AgCl counter/reference electrode) consisting of immobilized glucose oxidase. These flexible hydrogen peroxide electrodes were fabricated by photolithography and ion beam sputtering techniques. The performance of the device was evaluated by measuring glucose level in phosphate buffer saline (pH 7.0). The current output of the glucose sensor was related to the glucose level linearly over a range of 0.06–2.00 mmol/L, with a correlation coefficient of 0.997.

Microdevices have showed their valuable contribution for safe and effective diagnosis and management of ocular disorders. Hornig et al. [148] developed retinal implants consisting of multielectrode arrays to selectively stimulate individual neurons in blind subjects with retinal degeneration. These epiretinally positioned stimulation electrodes were combined with computer model of a retinal segment, which indicate the stimulation focus can be moved laterally, which resulted in activation of differently located neurons. Activation of retinal neuron through microdevices has shown a significant effect in improving vision loss. Humayun et al. [149] reported a retinal prosthetic system for electrical stimulation of the retinal surface in blind individuals with end-stage retinitis pigmentosa or age-related macular degeneration. The device consists of an array of electrodes (5 mm × 5 mm or 3 mm × 3 mm) (Fig. 11.14A). The electrode array consists of fairly

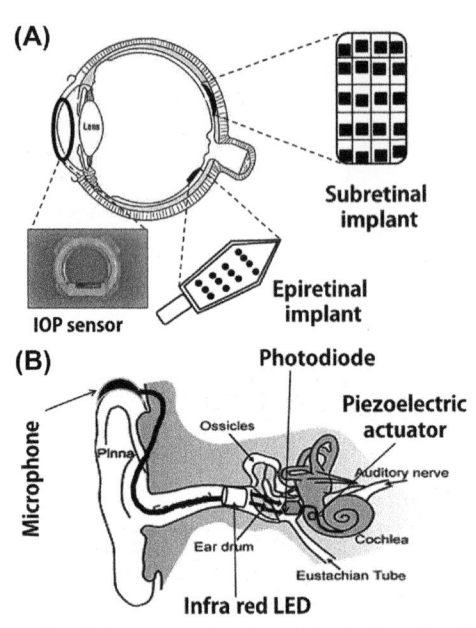

Figure 11.14 Microelectromechanical systems implantable devices for (A) eye and (B) ear. *IOP*, intraocular pressure; *LED*, light-emitting diode.

large electrodes (diameter ∼125 mm) compared with the diameter of a typical retinal neuron ganglion cell (diameter ∼10–20 mm). Large electrodes are helpful in maintaining the current density below safe thresholds for long-duration simulation of neural tissues. The device and the approach of device implantation offer benefits such as less invasion and ease of implantation. Zrenner et al. [150] investigated the long-term stability and biocompatibility of the subretinal microphoto diodes array (MPDAs) implants in rats. After 4 months of MPDA implantation with an area of 0.48–0.8 mm^2 and a thickness of 50 mm, the retina above the implanted MPDA was still intact. The implant showed excellent biocompatibility with retinal cells cultured on the implant material. In another study, an artificial silicon retina (ASR) microchip was developed for the treatment of vision loss from retinitis pigmentosa [151] (Fig. 11.14A). The ASR microchip is of 2 mm diameter integrated in a silicon-based device containing 5000 microelectrode-tipped microphotodiodes powered by incident light. In clinical investigation, ASR microchips were implanted in the right eyes of six patients with retinitis pigmentosa. The results showed no signs of implant rejection, possible infection, inflammation, erosion, neovascularization, and retinal detachment in any patient. The implanted device had improved visual function in all patients.

MEMS-guided electrical stimulation also showed significant effect in restoring "hearing" in patients having irreversible conduction hearing loss like damaged hair cells in the inner ear. Wise et al. [152] reported on a hybrid electrode array as an implantable MEMS-based cochlear prosthesis intended to restore hearing to profoundly deaf patients (Fig. 11.14B). The electrode array fabricated with a 3-μm bulk silicon microfabrication technique provides high-density stimulation, which improves sound perception, minimizes insertion damage, and optimizes implant placement. A commercial AMI 0.5-μm 2P/3M mixed-signal processor is used to fabricate signal processing chip. The position sensors have effective gage factors of 10—20. Young et al. [153] designed, implemented, and characterized an implantable MEMS (2.5 mm × 6.2 mm) with a capacitive accelerometer-based middle ear microphone for a hearing aid. The sensor has a sensing area of 1 mm × 1 mm with an integrated chip area of 2 mm × 2.4 mm and is interfaced with a custom-designed low-noise electronic IC chip over a flexible substrate. The implant system showed a minimal sound detection level of 60-dB sound pressure level (SPL) at 500 Hz and 35-dB SPL at 2 kHz in a 200-Hz bandwidth when attached to the umbo along its desired sensing axis.

Jackson et al. [154] reported MEMS microflex interconnect technology for fabrication of a new generation of Bio-MEMS devices that involve movable microelectrodes implanted in brain tissue. The device is fitted with electrothermal V-beam actuators to move microelectrodes off the edge of the chip and into the brain to monitor neuronal activity. The device is integrated with three highly doped polysilicon microelectrodes (4 μm × 50 μm × 5000 μm) and their movement was controlled by low-voltage square waveforms (8—10 V). On implantation, the device was bonded to the skull of the animal with poly(methyl methacrylate). The extended penetration of the microelectrode into the brain was done through craniotomy. In another study, thermal influence of an integrated 3-D Utah electrode array device was investigated where it is implanted in the brain for cortical neural signal recording by numerical simulation with finite element analysis [155]. In vitro and in vivo studies validated the numerical simulation by noninvasive temperature detection employing an infrared thermal camera. The noninvasive nature of detection avoids bleeding, which is a limitation associated with temperature probe inserted in the tissue. In another study, MEMS-based sensors were developed for direct measurement of bone stress [156]. The device is fabricated with the CMOS-MEMS processes and is permanently implanted within open fractures, or embedded in bone grafts, or placed on implants at the interfaces between bone and prosthetics (Fig. 11.15). The dimension of silicon CMOS chip surface was 60 μm × 60 μm × 60 μm. The stress sensor integrated with an array of piezoresistive pixels, which can detect a stress tensor at the interfacial area between the MEMS chip and bone, with a resolution of 100 Pa, in 1 s averaging. However, an in vivo study is still needed to evaluate its ability to measure and quantify biomechanical properties. This device can be used to gain new knowledge about bone regeneration and remodeling at the microscale, which may be helpful for clinical management of bone diseases and trauma.

3.2 Drug Delivery Devices

Conventional drug delivery systems fail to deliver drug in a more precise manner and in some cases it may reach more than the safe concentration at the site of action and thus

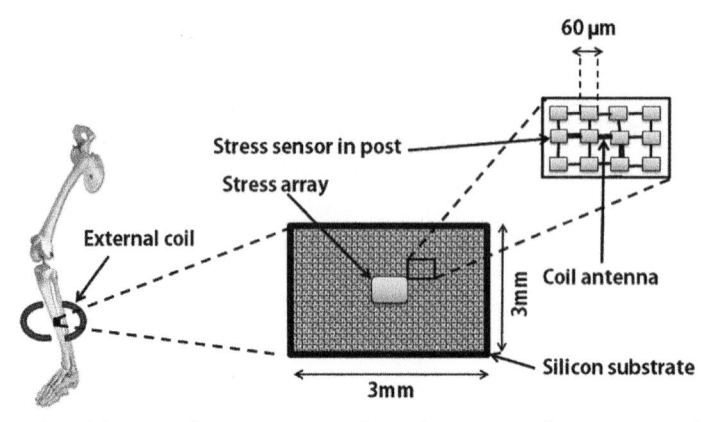

Figure 11.15 Implantable complementary metal oxide semiconductor—microelectromechanical systems—based multiaxis bone stress sensor.

may elicit toxic effects. The MEMS technology emerged as a potential tool for the fabrication of various systems that are capable of delivering precise quantities at the right time (on-demand drug delivery). These advanced systems are able to maintain the required therapeutic concentration of the drug at the site of administration as they are implanted as close to the treatment site as possible. Development and application of microfabricated implants for drug delivery have been reviewed in various articles [1,101,104,157—160]. Microsystems such as implantable pumps, smart pills, microporous materials, and microneedles have been extensively applied in drug delivery systems (Fig. 11.16).

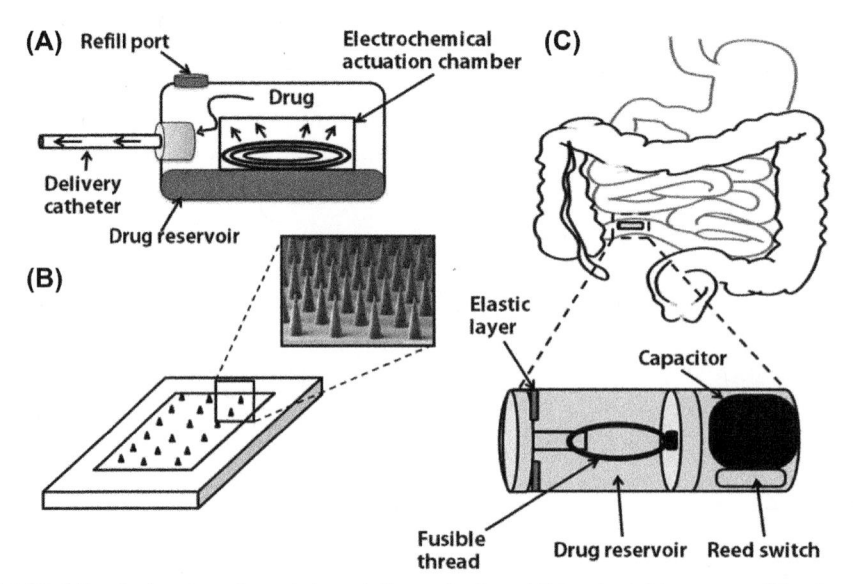

Figure 11.16 Microtechnology-based drug delivery devices. (A) implantable pumps, (B) microneedles, and (C) smart pills.

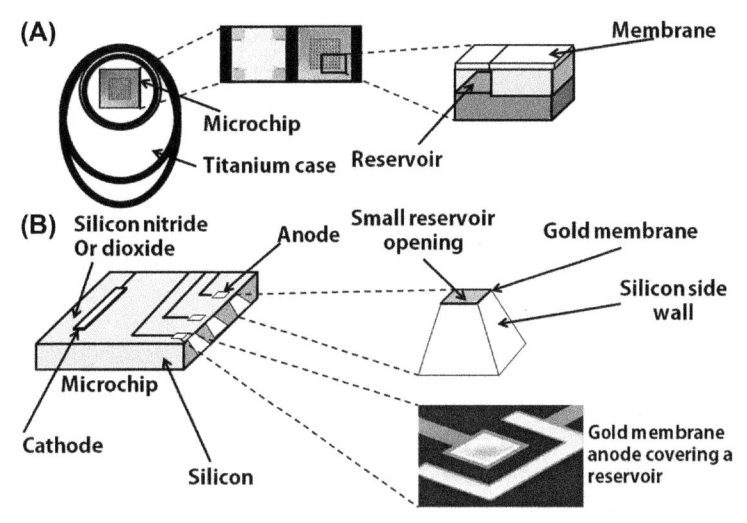

Figure 11.17 Microchip reservoir-based implantable drug delivery systems.

Prescott et al. [161] developed implantable microchips (4.5 × 5.5 × 1 cm^3) that contained 100 individually addressable reservoirs (300 nL) for controlled delivery of the peptide leuprolide acetate (Fig. 11.17A). Each reservoir present on a matrix of solid polyethylene glycol was filled with about 25 mg of lyophilized leuprolide. For in vivo investigation, these microdevices were implanted into the subcutaneous tissue of six male beagle dogs. The devices were programmed in such a way that selected reservoir will opened remotely for drug release. After device activation, blood was drawn at intervals starting 1 h before and continuing for 24 h. The averaged area under the curve and Cmax values ranged from 37 to 50 (ng h)/mL and 5 to 11 ng/mL, respectively. Results indicate that drug delivery from a microdevice is not restricted to solution-phase drug formulations. Formulation including stability-optimized and solid-phase drug can also be fabricated with these devices and released in vivo in a precise manner.

Santini et al. [162] developed a solid-state silicon microchip incorporated with micrometer-scale pumps, valves, and flow channels. This device (17 mm × 17 mm × 310 mm) contains 34 reservoirs and is able to provide controlled release of single or multiple drugs on demand (Fig. 11.17B). The device size may be reduced to 2 mm depending upon the specific application and site of implantation. An independent pulsatile release of two different molecules, such as Ca^{2+} ions and sodium fluorescein, was achieved from the device for several hours. Guan et al. [163] reported soft-lithographic processes employed for the fabrication of different types of microdevices. These devices include single and multiple reservoirs. The capsule-like microdevices are injectable drug-release depot systems and self-foldable microstructures for transmucosal drug delivery. Different microwell and micropillar structures (stamps) were used for the fabrication of the multiple-reservoir microstructures. The square

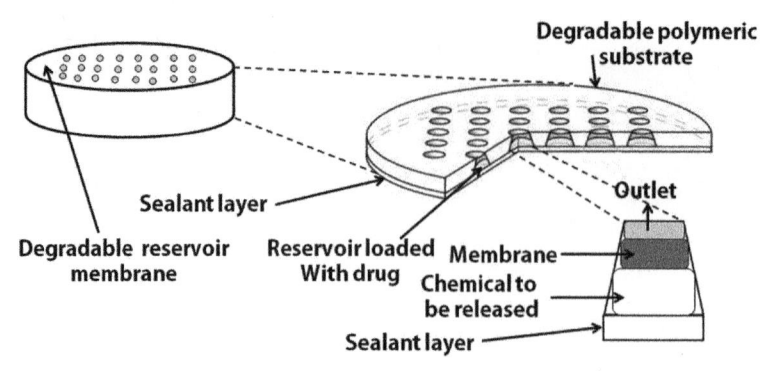

Figure 11.18 Diagram of polymeric microchip device.

microwells are 30 mm wide, 10.7 mm deep, with a 50-mm center-to-center distance. The cylinder-shaped micropillars are 7.0 mm in diameter, 3.4 mm high, with an 8.3-mm center-to-center distance.

Grayson et al. [8] developed microdevices based on PLGA polymer with size of about 11.9 mm in diameter and a 480–560 μm in thickness. The microreservoirs integrated on the device have volumes ranging from 116.4 to 195.7 nL, loaded with ^{14}C-dextran, ^{3}H-heparin, and ^{125}I-hGH (human growth hormone) (Fig. 11.18). Initially, the polymer degrades in a slow manner, which enables complete release of the drug in the controlled manner from the device. After complete polymer degradation, the main body of the microchip degrades, which minimizes the possibility of dose dumping. The prototype of the device contains 36 reservoirs of conical shape with a volume of 120–130 nL each. The molecular mass of the membrane decides the release rate of the drug from the device.

In another study, an electronic capsule-shaped MEMS-based drug delivery system was developed with a length of 30.0 mm, external diameter of 10.6 mm, and a net weight of 3.1 g (before the drug is loaded) [164]. The drug reservoir capacity of the capsule is up to 0.5 mL fluid drug. The main components of the system are a timer module for controlling drug release, a driving unit for releasing drug to the alimentary canal, a microfluidic chamber for the drug reservoir, and a power supply. The capsule was loaded with Mildronate (MET-88) and fed to beagle dogs with a 1-h timing schedule. The plasma concentration of MET-88 gradually increased due to continuous drug release with the concentration reaching a peak about 4 h after administration. Application of microtechnology-based devices for drug delivery has been reviewed in detail in various articles [101,159,165–174]. Table 11.3 summarizes microdevices for drug delivery applications.

4. NANOTECHNOLOGY-BASED IMPLANTABLE DEVICES AND BIONICS

NEMS are currently emerging as the next generation of miniature devices integrated with electrical and mechanical functionalities. The benefits associated with NEMS,

Table 11.3 Microdevices for drug delivery applications

Device	Mechanism	Structure	Size	References
Micropump	Electrostatic	Polysilicon	Not reported	[175]
	Piezoelectric	Si–Si	Not reported	[176]
	Piezoelectric	poly(methyl methacrylate) (PMMA)	Not reported	[177]
	Piezoelectric	Si–Si	160 mm	[178]
	Piezoelectric	Si–Si	Not reported	[179]
	Piezoelectric	Si–glass	24 mm × 75 mm	[56]
	Thermopneumatic	Glass–Si–Si	3000 mm^3	[180]
	Thermopneumatic	Glass–SU8–Si	105.3 mm^3	[181]
	Electrochemical	Glass–Si	Not reported	[182]
Microreservoir system	Electrochemical	Silicon nitride–coated silicon wafers	3.7 mm × 3.2 mm × 2.2 mm	[101]
Micropump	Osmosis	Polydimethylsiloxane (PDMS)	30 × 100 μm^2	[12]
Microreservoir system	Electromechanical	Pyrex plate with aluminum oxide reservoirs	Not reported	[183]
Microneedle	Electromechanical	Si–Si	50–100 μm	[184]
Micropump	Piezoelectric and mechanical	Ti-6Al-4V	6 mm × 5 mm	[185]
	Electromechanical	Polydimethylsiloxane and polyethylene glycol	6 mm × 9.5 mm	[186]
Microneedle	Electromechanical	PDMS, poly(lactic acid), and poly(lactic-ω-glycolic acid)	350–750 μm	[187]
Micropump	Electromechanical	Si–Si	0.36 mm diameter	[188]
	Electrostatic	Si–gold	7 mm × 4 mm × 1 mm	[20]
Microreservoir	Mechanical	PMMA	150 μm × 150 μm × 33 μm	[189]

such as low mass, potentially large quantum mechanical effects, high mechanical resonance frequencies, low power consumption, low fabrication costs, low force constants, and a high surface-to-volume ratio, make these devices highly suitable for sensing and drug delivery applications [190]. Two different general fabrication techniques such as (1) traditional electron beam lithography and (2) chemical properties of individual molecules for building such devices from the "bottom up" method are generally used to fabricate NEMS systems [191]. To improve physicochemical properties of the devices, nano and micro technologies were used in combination. In the following sections we describe the characteristics of different types of nanodevices and their applications. Table 11.4 lists different nanotechnology-based implantable devices available on the market or in clinical trials.

4.1 Sensing Systems

Lu et al. [199] reported on a tunable gold nanogap device as an electrochemical impedance biosensor. The device is fabricated with simple monolayer film deposition and in situ growth of gold nanoparticles on a traditional interdigitated array (IDA) microelectrode. Gold patterns on silicon wafer (doped with boron, resistivity $\sim 1-30\ \Omega\text{cm}$) with a 100-nm-thick oxide layer was used to fabricate the IDA microelectrode. Biotin-modified gold nanoparticles will be serving as the biosensing particles and are assembled

Table 11.4 Nanoscale biomedical implants available on the market or in clinical trials

Nanoimplant	Company	Indication	Current status	References
BrainGate 2	Cyberkinetics Neurotechnology Systems Inc.	Motor function impaired patients	Phase-II	[192]
Argus II (bionic eye)	Second Sight Medical Products Inc.	Retinitis pigmentosa	US FDA approved	[193]
Bio retina	Nano Retina Inc.	Age-related macular degeneration	Phase-III	[194]
NanoTite	Biomet 3i Inc.	Dental implant	US FDA approved	[195]
Comprehensive nano	Biomet Inc.	Bone conserving implant	Phase-II	[196]
FOCUS np	Envision Scientific Pvt. Ltd.	Blocked vascular vessels	Phase-III	[197]
Nano+	LepuMedical Technology Co. Ltd	Blocked vascular vessels	Phase-II/III	[198]

FDA, Food and Drug Administration.

between two interdigitated electrodes. The lowest detection limit of the biosensor actually measured is 1 pM, which is five times higher than several previously reported nanogap biosensors. In another study, a silky mesh tiny electronic device was developed that stimulates individual neurons. This injectable nanoimplant is only a few centimeters and can be injected directly into a target region through a hole in the top of the skull [200]. The implant is connected with nanowires (NWs) that poke out and can be connected to a computer to take recordings and stimulate cells. Lee et al. [201] reported on two types of circular diaphragms as pressure sensors, fabricated from Si and Si/SiO_2. These circular diaphragms are integrated with a hexagonal photonic crystal lattice with a triple-nanoring resonator as a nanoscale force. The diaphragm with the Si/SiO_2 can detect a pressure of 4.17 MPa. The results showed that the Si diaphragm—based sensor has higher sensitivity than the Si/SiO_2 diaphragm sensor. A carbon nanofiber based nanoimplant was developed for monitoring, diagnosis, and treatment of neural tissues [202]. The suitability of the proposed device for neural and orthopedic applications was determined via electrical and mechanical characterization. Experiments regarding cell adhesion indicated the suitability of these materials for neural (nerve cell) and osteoblast (bone-forming cell) functions. Du et al. [203] investigated nanohydroxyapatite/collagen composite implants as bone substitutes. The ultrastructural features of the implant, such as low crystallinity, biodegradability, and nanometer size, make it to more closely resemble bone marrow. Mozafari et al. [204] reported lead sulfite (PbS) hollow sphere quantum dots (QDs) for early cancer diagnosis, which are synthesized by a template-free green method. Results showed excellent photoluminescence quality with strong luminescence properties. Nanotechnology has also been introduced in the treatment of ophthalmic diseases. Ghaffari et al. [205] reviewed in detail the importance of nanomaterials in visual prosthesis, such as nanoparticles, NWs, multi- and single-walled carbon nanotubes (CNTs), polymer coatings, silicon lithographic elements, and nanodevices for ocular use.

Xiao et al. [206] investigated ultrananocrystalline diamond (UNCD) thin films as bioinert coatings for an implantable retinal microchip. These UNCD films are deposited on highly conductive Si substrates at different temperatures (from 400°C to 800°C). In vivo studies involving implantation of the UNCD-coated Si retinal microchips in the eye of pigmented rabbits for 6 months indicated the bioinert and biostable nature of the microchip. In another study, titanium dioxide (TiO_2) nanotubes (100 nm) were fabricated by electrochemical anodization [207]. The soft-tissue responses of TiO_2 nanotubes and TiO_2 control implants were evaluated by implanting them in the rat abdominal wall for 1 and 6 weeks. In vivo results indicate that the TiO_2 nanotubes elicit a favorable response in soft tissues. Cheng et al. [208] developed a new type of wireless nanogenerator (WLNG) based on biocompatible BZT-BCT [(Zr) TiO_3-(Ca) TiO_3] NWs. The developed WLNG works through compressing and releasing BZT-BCT NWs/PDMs nanocomposite by a changing magnetic field in wireless the noncontact mode. The proposed system opens a new avenue for a wireless and power-free biosensor. The developed system will be helpful in in vivo monitoring of physiological information, disease diagnosis, and health monitoring.

Piezoresistive nanomechanical membrane-type surface stress sensor (MSS) chips having a two-dimensional array of MSS on a single chip was developed for wide applications in the field of medicine, biology, security, and the environment [209]. Schwalb et al. [210] reported fabrication of strain-sensor elements by maskless lithography technique for NEMS applications based on the tunneling effect in nanogranular metals. Fabrication involved electron-beam-induced deposition employing the precursor trimethylmethyl cyclopentadienyl platinum [MeCpPt(Me)$_3$]. The technique makes 3-D application feasible due to a process that enables the deposition of the sensor material on nearly every smooth surface even on complex geometries. Titanium-based alloys are a common material in orthopedic implants because of their excellent mechanical properties and biocompatibility. However, the complex physiological environment may render such implants lose their natural properties and become incompatible or cytotoxic to cells and tissues. The nano-architectures on the surface of these alloys may improve both in vivo and in vitro biocompatibility of these alloys [211]. This can be achieved by various approaches, such as surface coating with nanofilms/layers by plasma immersion ion implantation and deposition, oxidation, hydrothermal, plasma spraying, electropolishing, magnetron sputtering, sol–gel process, surface nanocrystallization, and one-dimensional nanostructures, i.e., nanotubes and NWs or nanofibers.

In another study, materials, device architectures, and integration strategies including implantable silicon sensors have been reported for continuous monitoring of intracranial pressure and temperature in rats [212] (Fig. 11.19). These biosensors have the ability to completely dissolve into biocompatible end products immersed in biofluids such as CSF. The silicon nanomembrane and the magnesium foils are hydrolyzed at a rate of

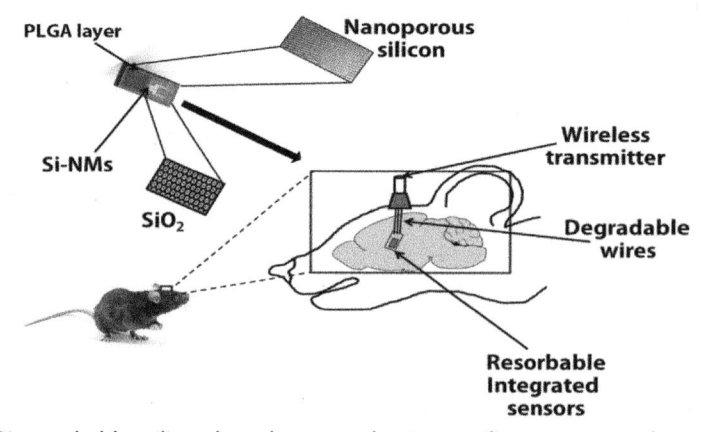

Figure 11.19 Bioresorbable, silicon-based sensors having a silicon nanomembrane (Si-NM) strain gage for continuous monitoring of intracranial pressure and temperature. *PLGA*, poly(lactic-*co*-glycolic acid).

23 nm/day, 8 nm/day, 9 µm/day, and 4 µm/day, in artificial CSF at physiological temperature (37°C). A separate study showed complete dissolution of PLGA membrane [75:25 (lactide:glycolide) composition] in biofluids within 4—5 weeks. These sensors were integrated with biodegradable molybdenum wires (10 µm thick) serving as interface to wireless communication systems before implantation into the rat brain. For data transmission through percutaneous wiring, these insulated wires were then connected to an externally mounted, miniaturized wireless transmitter potentiostat. Robinson et al. [213] reported on vertical NW electrode arrays as a scalable platform for intracellular interfacing to neuronal circuits. Such NW electrode arrays can intracellularly record and stimulate neuronal activity in dissociated cultures of rat cortical neurons. They can also be used to map multiple individual synaptic connections. Applications of nanotechnology in the fabrication of implantable biosensors have been previously reviewed in the literature [214—217].

4.2 Drug Delivery Devices

Nanotechnology-based drug delivery implants have been reviewed in various articles [216,218—220]. Table 11.5 lists various nanotechnology-based implantable systems for drug delivery applications.

Novel electrospun nanofibrous poly(D,L-lactide-co-ε-caprolactone) balloons were developed with electrospinning nanotechnique for the treatment of vertebral compression fractures [230]. Scanning electron microscopy (SEM) showed that the scaffolds consisted of smooth and randomly distributed nanofibers. The implant releases calcium in a sustained manner for 34 days, which can be beneficial for bone resorption, replacement with new bone, and restoration of vertebral body mass. Park et al. [48] reported on patterned carbon nanosyringe arrays (CNSAs), which consist of vertically orientated nanodimensional syringes of controllable height for intracellular delivery. These arrays facilitate successful intracellular delivery of plasmids and QDs into cancer and mesenchymal stem cells. For intracellular delivery, CNSAs were filled with a drop of water (100 µL) containing either plasmid (400 µg/mL) or quantum dots (1 nM) for 12 h. A 24-well cell culture plate (1×10^5 cells/well) was used to seed cells onto the CNSA for 12 h at 37°C in an atmosphere of 5% CO_2. SEM revealed that individual nanosyringes appear to pierce or deform the cell membrane of NIH3T3 cells. A novel polymer-free-composite drug-eluting coating was developed for stents composed of magnetic mesoporous silica nanoparticles (MMSNs) as well as CNTs with electrophoretic deposition [218]. A thin layer of CNT film acted as an inner buffer layer, and a second MMSNs/CNTs composite coating acted as a functional layer. The coating showed excellent mechanical flexibility and blood compatibility. In vitro studies showed drug release for about 2 weeks. The in vivo study revealed the obvious advantage of rapid reendotheliazation in the early stage by this system, which can reduce the risk of inflammatory reactions and late stent thrombosis.

Table 11.5 Nanotechnology-based implantable systems for drug delivery applications

Implant	Drug	Outcome	References
Titania nanotubes anodized from titanium	Gentamicin	Gentamicin-loaded nanotubes are effective in minimizing initial bacterial adhesion	[221]
PLGA/TiO$_2$ nanotubes on Ti implant surface	Ibuprofen	Increased drug release rate is observed with a combination of PLGA and TiO$_2$ nanotubes with a 100% release in 30 min to 5 days (low-molecular-weight PLGA) and 9 days (high-molecular-weight PLGA)	[222]
TiO$_2$ nanotube arrays on titanium surfaces	Vancomycin, silver	Drug loading is accelerated due to the larger surface area of the nanotubes. By adjusting the anodizing parameters and electrolyte composition, release kinetics can be modified	[223]
TiO$_2$ nanotube arrays loaded with antimicrobial peptides (AMPs) on titanium implants	HHC-36, broad-spectrum AMP	Nanotubes showed better AMP loading than the amorphous phase. The AMP/TiO$_2$ surface significantly inhibited *Staphylococcus aureus* growth and reduced bacterial adhesion	[224]
Silver (Ag)-implanted titanium with nanostructured surface	Silver	Generated a strong antimicrobial effect and promoted ontogenesis with increased cell attachment, viability, and osteogenic gene expression	[225]
Silver nanoparticles embedded in titanium implant	Silver	Found effective in inhibiting *S. aureus* and *Escherichia coli* while maintaining high activity on promoting proliferation of	[226]

Table 11.5 Nanotechnology-based implantable systems for drug delivery applications—cont'd

Implant	Drug	Outcome	References
Orthopedic carbon nanotube biosensor	Penicillin/ streptomycin	osteoblast-like cells line MG63 Reduced inflammation, promoted bone growth, and reduced fibroblast functions	[227]
Hyaluronic acid (HA)/ chitosan multilayer-coated neuronal implants	siRNA molecules	HA and chitosan sustained biodegradation and bioactivity of the siRNA NPs	[228]
Nanodecorated ocular implants	Cyclosporin A	Release from the formulation continues over 30–60 days. Cell viability was 77.4–99.0%. In vivo studies showed that healing is significantly faster in the presence of the implant formulation	[229]

NP, nanoparticle; *PLGA*, poly(lactic-*co*-glycolic acid); *siRNA*, small interfering RNA.

Hoare et al. [231] reported on nanocomposite membranes consisting of thermosensitive, poly(*N*-isopropylacrylamide)-based nanogels and magnetite nanoparticles. This construct provided "on-demand" drug delivery with the application of an oscillating magnetic field (Fig. 11.20). During multiple magnetic triggering cycles, the membrane retains its rigidity and this property can be extended to in vivo implantation, making reproducible drug delivery possible. These membranes are noncytotoxic, biocompatible, and can retain switchable flux properties after 45 days of subcutaneous implantation.

Titanium nanotube (TNT) arrays-based noninvasive and ultrasound-driven drug-releasing implants have been developed with drug-encapsulated polymeric micelles as drug carriers (Fig. 11.21) [232]. An implantable device consisting of TNT array as drug-releasing surface and polymeric micelles as drug carriers may have potential applications in bone therapies with local delivery of proteins, anticancer drugs, and bone growth factors. Indomethacin as a model drug was encapsulated in polymeric micelles, i.e., D-α-tocopheryl polyethylene glycol succinate 1000 as a drug carriers, and the drug release was evaluated in the presence of pulse length (1, 5, 10, and 15 pulses per min), amplitude (45, 90, 135, and 180 kPa), and probe-sample distance (2.0, 1.5, 1.0, and 0.5 cm). Results showed immediate and rapid drug-micelle pulsatile release, which was completed within 5 min to 2 h. SEM showed the structural stability of TNT with no signs of physical damage. Ultrasound-mediated drug-loaded micelle release from the

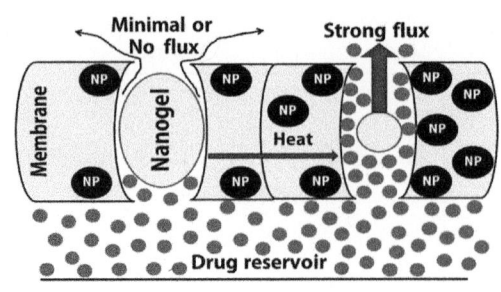

Figure 11.20 Schematic illustration of mechanism involved in stimulus-responsive membrane triggering. *NP*, nanoparticle.

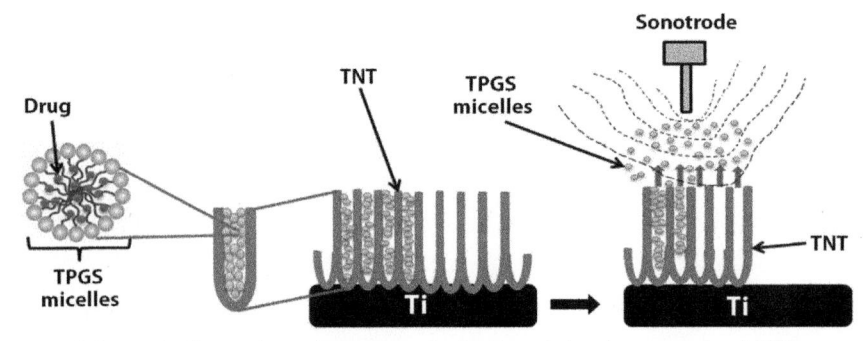

Figure 11.21 Schematic illustration of ultrasound-stimulated titania nanotube (TNT) arrays as drug delivery platform. *TPGS*, D-α-tocopheryl polyethylene glycol succinate 1000.

TNT surface involved a combination of cavitation and thermal processes. Mechanical vibration resulting from the forces may be produced by the ultrasound waves.

Zielinski et al. [233] developed silica nanoparticle (SiNP)-loaded biodegradable implants for laser tissue soldering of blood vessels in the brain. Nanoparticles were released into the surrounding brain tissue on degradation of the implant. Cell uptake of SiNPs in microglial cells and the effect on autophagy and inflammatory cytokines were investigated. SiNPs did not modulate cytokine secretion and autophagy, and the maximal uptake was reached after 4 h of incubation. Cell uptake is mainly through macropinocytosis and phagocytosis; however, there was a minor contribution of clathrin- and caveolin-independent endocytosis.

5. CONCLUSIONS AND FUTURE PERSPECTIVES

Over the past two decades, the medical device industries have been growing at a very fast rate. Many innovative strategies have been used for the development of various fascinating systems that are currently in clinical use. Researchers from various backgrounds, such as pharmaceutics, biotechnology, bioengineering, electronics, polymer chemistry, biophysics, and others, combined their expertise to develop systems that provide solutions to various medical complications. Improvements in micro- and nanofabrication technologies such as nanoimprint lithography have emerged as a powerful tool for the development of nanoscale devices for wide biological applications in a minimally invasive manner. These nanofabrication technologies have resulted in high-throughput, low-cost production, which leads to successful clinical applications. Micro- and nanotechnology-based implantable devices and bionics have exerted a significant impact on improving current therapeutic methods as biosensors, tissue engineering, as well as drug and gene delivery systems. Conventional therapeutic techniques are not able to treat effectively a wide range of diseased conditions, which require more advanced medical systems. These advanced systems provide precise early diagnosis and effective therapeutic management. Implantable devices have been extensively studied for cardiovascular, neural and retinal, bone, and dental applications as biosensors and drug delivery systems. Nanotechnology renders the development of small size devices implanted in a minimally invasive manner with lower chances of systemic toxicity. Recent advancements in micro- and nanotechnology have shown successful transformation of these devices from laboratory to market. Some of these already have FDA approval, whereas others are in clinical trials. A combination of micro- and nanofabrication techniques has resulted in implantable devices with better biocompatibility, longer stability, low toxicity, and low body rejection providing better case management.

REFERENCES

[1] Arsiwala A, Desai P, Patravale V. Recent advances in micro/nanoscale biomedical implants. J Control Release 2014;189:25−45.
[2] Elman NM, Ho Duc HL, Cima MJ. An implantable MEMS drug delivery device for rapid delivery in ambulatory emergency care. Biomed Microdevices 2009;11:625−31.
[3] Desai TA, Hansford D, Ferrari M. Characterization of micromachined silicon membranes for immunoisolation and bioseparation applications. J Membr Sci 1999;159:221−31.
[4] Desai TA, Hansford DJ, Kulinsky L, Nashat AH, et al. Nanopore technology for biomedical applications. Biomed Microdevices 1999;2:11−40.
[5] Maloney JM, Uhland SA, Polito BF, Sheppard Jr NF, Pelta CM, Santini Jr JT. Electrothermally activated microchips for implantable drug delivery and biosensing. J Control Release 2005;109:244−55.
[6] Rahimi S, Sarraf EH, Wong GK, Takahata K. Implantable drug delivery device using frequency-controlled wireless hydrogel microvalves. Biomed Microdevices 2011;13:267−77.
[7] Ahmed A, Bonner C, Desai TA. Bioadhesive microdevices with multiple reservoirs: a new platform for oral drug delivery. J Control Release 2002;81:291−306.
[8] Grayson ACR, Choi IS, Tyler BM, Wang PP, Brem H, Cima MJ, Langer R. Multi-pulse drug delivery from a resorbable polymeric microchip device. Nat Mater 2003;2:767−72.
[9] Chung AJ, Huh YS, Erickson D. A robust, electrochemically driven microwell drug delivery system for controlled vasopressin release. Biomed Microdevices 2009;11:861−7.
[10] Li PY, Givrad TK, Holschneider DP, Maarek JMI, Meng E. A parylene MEMS electrothermal valve. J Microelectromechanical Syst 2009;18:1184−97.
[11] Li PY, Givrad TK, Sheybani R, Holschneider DP, Maarek JM, Meng E. A low power, on demand electrothermal valve for wireless drug delivery applications. Lab Chip 2010;10:101−10.
[12] Yu-Chuan S, Lin L. A water-powered micro drug delivery system. J Microelectromechanical Syst 2004;13:75−82.
[13] Yu-Chuan S, Liwei L, Pisano AP. A water-powered osmotic microactuator. J Microelectromechanical Syst 2002;11:736−42.

[14] Yu-Hsien L, Yu-Chuan S. Miniature osmotic actuators for controlled maxillofacial distraction osteogenesis. J Micromechanics Microengineering 2010;20:065013.
[15] Evans AT, Chiravuri S, Gianchandani YB. A multidrug delivery system using a piezoelectrically actuated silicon valve manifold with embedded sensors. J Microelectromechanical Syst 2011;20:231—8.
[16] Evans AT, Park JM, Chiravuri S, Gianchandani YB. A low power, microvalve regulated architecture for drug delivery systems. Biomed Microdevices 2009;12:159—68.
[17] Rainov NG, Heidecke V, Burkert W. Long-term intrathecal infusion of drug combinations for chronic back and leg pain. J Pain Symptom Manage 2001;22:862—71.
[18] Tarik B, Alain Bosseb IMG, Jean-Paul G. Design and simulation of an electrostatic micropump for drug-delivery applications. J Micromechanics Microengineering 1997;7:186.
[19] Yih TC, Wei C, Hammad B. Modeling and characterization of a nanoliter drug-delivery MEMS micropump with circular bossed membrane. Nanomedicine 2005;1:164—75.
[20] Teymoori MM, Abbaspour-Sani E. Design and simulation of a novel electrostatic peristaltic micromachined pump for drug delivery applications. Sensors Actuators A Phys 2005;117:222—9.
[21] Geipel A, Goldschmidtboeing F, Jantscheff P, Esser N, Massing U, Woias P. Design of an implantable active microport system for patient specific drug release. Biomed Microdevices 2008;10:469—78.
[22] Geipel A, Goldschmidtböing F, Doll A, Jantscheff P, Esser N, Massing U, Woias P. An implantable active microport based on a self-priming high-performance two-stage micropump. Sensors Actuators A Phys 2008;145—146:414—22.
[23] Available from: http://www.debiotech.com; 2016.
[24] Gensler H, Sheybani R, Li PY, Mann RL, Meng E. An implantable MEMS micropump system for drug delivery in small animals. Biomed Microdevices 2012;14:483—96.
[25] Sheybani R, Gensler H, Meng E. Rapid and repeated bolus drug delivery enabled by high efficiency electrochemical bellows actuators. In: 16th International solid-state sensors, actuators and microsystems conference; 2011.
[26] Sheybani R, Meng E. High efficiency wireless electrochemical actuators: design, fabrication and characterization by electrochemical impedance spectroscopy. In: 2011 IEEE 24th international conference on micro electro mechanical systems (MEMS); 2011.
[27] Ha S-M, Cho W, Ahn Y. Disposable thermo-pneumatic micropump for bio lab-on-a-chip application. Microelectron Eng 2009;86:1337—9.
[28] Cooney CG, Towe BC. A thermopneumatic dispensing micropump. Sensors Actuators A Phys 2004;116:519—24.
[29] Spieth S, Schumacher A, Holtzman T, Rich PD, et al. An intra-cerebral drug delivery system for freely moving animals. Biomed Microdevices 2012;14:799—809.
[30] Samel B, Griss P, Stemme G. A thermally responsive PDMS composite and its microfluidic applications. J Microelectromechanical Syst 2007;16:50—7.
[31] Available from: http://www.alzet.com/; 2016.
[32] Available from: http://www.iprecio.com/; 2016.
[33] Rohloff CM, Alessi TR, Yang B, Dahms J, Carr JP, Lautenbach SD. DUROS technology delivers peptides and proteins at consistent rate continuously for 3 to 12 months. J Diabetes Sci Technol 2008;2:461—7.
[34] Available from: http://www.intarcia.com; 2016.
[35] Available from: https://professional.medtronic.com/; 2016.
[36] Available from: http://www.codmanpumps.com; 2016.
[37] Available from: http://www.flowonix.com; 2016.
[38] Available from: http://www.qmed.com; 2016.
[39] Ali SMU, Asif MH, Fulati A, Nur O, et al. Intracellular K(+) determination with a potentiometric microelectrode based on ZnO nanowires. IEEE Trans Nanotechnol 2011;10:913—9.
[40] Chu MX, Miyajima K, Takahashi D, Arakawa T, et al. Soft contact lens biosensor for in situ monitoring of tear glucose as non-invasive blood sugar assessment. Talanta 2011;83:960—5.
[41] Yu B, Long N, Moussy Y, Moussy F. A long-term flexible minimally-invasive implantable glucose biosensor based on an epoxy-enhanced polyurethane membrane. Biosens Bioelectron 2006;21:2275—82.

[42] Sun C, Chen X, Han Q, Zhou M, Mao C, Zhu Q, Shen J. Fabrication of glucose biosensor for whole blood based on Au/hyperbranched polyester nanoparticles multilayers by antibiofouling and self-assembly technique. Anal Chim Acta 2013;776:17—23.

[43] Shikida M, Yokota T, Naito J, Sato K. Fabrication of a stent-type thermal flow sensor for measuring nasal respiration. J Micromechanics Microengineering 2010;20:055029.

[44] Huang Y, Venkatraman SS, Boey FYC, Lahti EM, et al. In vitro and in vivo performance of a dual drug-eluting stent (DDES). Biomaterials 2010;31:4382—91.

[45] Chow EY, Chlebowski AL, Chakraborty S, Chappell WJ, Irazoqui PP. Fully wireless implantable cardiovascular pressure monitor integrated with a medical stent. IEEE Trans Biomed Eng 2010;57: 1487—96.

[46] Chow EY, Beier BL, Francino A, Chappell WJ, Irazoqui PP. Toward an implantable wireless cardiac monitoring platform integrated with an FDA-approved cardiovascular stent. J Interventional Cardiol 2009;22:479—87.

[47] Green SR, Kwon RS, Elta GH, Gianchandani YB. In vivo and in situ evaluation of a wireless magnetoelastic sensor array for plastic biliary stent monitoring. Biomed Microdevices 2013;15:509—17.

[48] Park S, Kim Y-S, Kim WB, Jon S. Carbon nanosyringe array as a platform for intracellular delivery. Nano Lett 2009;9:1325—9.

[49] Obataya I, Nakamura C, Han S, Nakamura N, Miyake J. Direct insertion of proteins into a living cell using an atomic force microscope with a nanoneedle. NanoBiotechnology 2005;1:347—52.

[50] Boo H, Jeong R-A, Park S, Kim KS, et al. Electrochemical nanoneedle biosensor based on multiwall carbon nanotube. Anal Chem 2006;78:617—20.

[51] Häfeli UO, Mokhtari A, Liepmann D, Stoeber B. In vivo evaluation of a microneedle-based miniature syringe for intradermal drug delivery. Biomed Microdevices 2009;11:943—50.

[52] Roxhed N, Gasser TC, Griss P, Holzapfel GA, Stemme G. Penetration-enhanced ultrasharp microneedles and prediction on skin interaction for efficient transdermal drug delivery. J Microelectromechanical Syst 2007;16:1429—40.

[53] Voskerician G, Shawgo RS, Hiltner PA, Anderson JM, Cima MJ, Langer R. In vivo inflammatory and wound healing effects of gold electrode voltammetry for MEMS micro-reservoir drug delivery device. IEEE Trans Biomed Eng 2004;51:627—35.

[54] Moore TL, Pitzer JE, Podila R, Wang X, et al. Multifunctional polymer-coated carbon nanotubes for safe drug delivery. Part Part Syst Charact 2013;30:365—73.

[55] Anis Y, Houkal J, Holl M, Johnson R, Meldrum D. Diaphragm pico-liter pump for single-cell manipulation. Biomed Microdevices 2011;13:651—9.

[56] Hsu Y-C, Lin S-J, Hou C-C. Development of peristaltic antithrombogenic micropumps for in vitro and ex vivo blood transportation tests. Microsyst Technol 2007;14:31—41.

[57] Reis J, Frias C, Canto e Castro C, Botelho ML, Marques AT, Simões JAO, Capela e Silva F, Potes J. A new piezoelectric actuator induces bone formation in vivo: a preliminary study. J Biomed Biotechnol 2012;2012:7.

[58] Fujita H, Van Dau T, Shimizu K, Hatsuda R, Sugiyama S, Nagamori E. Designing of a Si-MEMS device with an integrated skeletal muscle cell-based bio-actuator. Biomed Microdevices 2011;13:123—9.

[59] Lee KKC, Munce NR, Shoa T, Charron LG, Wright GA, Madden JD, Yang VXD. Fabrication and characterization of laser-micromachined polypyrrole-based artificial muscle actuated catheters. Sensors Actuators A Phys 2009;153:230—6.

[60] Proulx S, d'Arc Uwamaliya J, Carrier P, Deschambeault A, et al. Reconstruction of a human cornea by the self-assembly approach of tissue engineering using the three native cell types. Mol Vis 2010;16: 2192—201.

[61] Ceyssens F, van Kuyck K, Vande Velde G, Welkenhuysen M, Stappers L, Nuttin B, Puers R. Resorbable scaffold based chronic neural electrode arrays. Biomed Microdevices 2013;15:481—93.

[62] Vozzi G, Rechichi A, Dini F, Salvadori C, et al. PAM-microfabricated polyurethane scaffolds: in vivo and in vitro preliminary studies. Macromol Biosci 2008;8:60—8.

[63] Zhong Y, McConnell GC, Ross JD, DeWeerth SP, Bellamkonda RV. A novel Dexamethasone-releasing, anti-inflammatory coating for neural implants. In: Conference proceedings. 2nd international IEEE EMBS conference on neural engineering, 2005; 2005.

[64] Sahlin H, Contreras R, Gaskill DF, Bjursten LM, Frangos JA. Anti-inflammatory properties of micro-patterned titanium coatings. J Biomed Mater Res A 2006;77:43–9.

[65] Boucher W, Stern JM, Kotsinyan V, Kempuraj D, Papaliodis D, Cohen MS, Theoharides TC. Intravesical nanocrystalline silver decreases experimental bladder inflammation. J Urol 2008;179:1598–602.

[66] Ai F, Wang Q, Yuan WZ, Li H, Chen X, Yang L, Zhang Y, Pei S. Biocompatibility and anti-cracking performance of perfluorocarboxylic acid ionomer membranes for implantable biosensors. J Mater Sci 2012;47:5181–9.

[67] Sun C, Miao J, Yan J, Yang K, Mao C, Ju J, Shen J. Applications of antibiofouling PEG-coating in electrochemical biosensors for determination of glucose in whole blood. Electrochimica Acta 2013; 89:549–54.

[68] Kozai TD, Kipke DR. Insertion shuttle with carboxyl terminated self-assembled monolayer coatings for implanting flexible polymer neural probes in the brain. J Neurosci Methods 2009;184:199–205.

[69] Onuki Y, Bhardwaj U, Papadimitrakopoulos F, Burgess DJ. A review of the biocompatibility of implantable devices: current challenges to overcome foreign body response. J Diabetes Sci Technol 2008;2:1003–15.

[70] Anderson JM, Rodriguez A, Chang DT. Foreign body reaction to biomaterials. Seminars Immunol 2008;20:86–100.

[71] Ratner BD, Bryant SJ. Biomaterials: where we have been and where we are going. Annu Rev Biomed Eng 2004;6:41–75.

[72] Fournier E, Passirani C, Montero-Menei CN, Benoit JP. Biocompatibility of implantable synthetic polymeric drug carriers: focus on brain biocompatibility. Biomaterials 2003;24:3311–31.

[73] Sieminski AL, Gooch KJ. Biomaterial–microvasculature interactions. Biomaterials 2000;21:2233–41.

[74] Říhová B. Immunocompatibility and biocompatibility of cell delivery systems. Adv Drug Deliv Rev 2000;42:65–80.

[75] Babensee JE, Anderson JM, McIntire LV, Mikos AG. Host response to tissue engineered devices. Adv Drug Deliv Rev 1998;33:111–39.

[76] Williams DF. Tissue-biomaterial interactions. J Mater Sci 1987;22:3421–45.

[77] Fujioka K, Maeda M, Hojo T, Sano A. Protein release from collagen matrices. Adv Drug Deliv Rev 1998;31:247–66.

[78] Khor E, Lim LY. Implantable applications of chitin and chitosan. Biomaterials 2003;24:2339–49.

[79] de Vos P, Hoogmoed CG, Busscher HJ. Chemistry and biocompatibility of alginate-PLL capsules for immunoprotection of mammalian cells. J Biomed Mater Res 2002;60:252–9.

[80] Vercruysse KP, Prestwich GD. Hyaluronate derivatives in drug delivery 1998;15:43.

[81] Draye J-P, Delaey B, Van de Voorde A, Van Den Bulcke A, De Reu B, Schacht E. In vitro and in vivo biocompatibility of dextran dialdehyde cross-linked gelatin hydrogel films. Biomaterials 1998;19:1677–87.

[82] Anderson JM, Shive MS. Biodegradation and biocompatibility of PLA and PLGA microspheres. Adv Drug Deliv Rev 2012;64(Suppl.):72–82.

[83] Athanasiou KA, Niederauer GG, Agrawal CM. Sterilization, toxicity, biocompatibility and clinical applications of polylactic acid/polyglycolic acid copolymers. Biomaterials 1996;17:93–102.

[84] Shen M, Horbett TA. The effects of surface chemistry and adsorbed proteins on monocyte/macrophage adhesion to chemically modified polystyrene surfaces. J Biomed Mater Res 2001;57:336–45.

[85] Royals MA, Fujita SM, Yewey GL, Rodriguez J, Schultheiss PC, Dunn RL. Biocompatibility of a biodegradable in situ forming implant system in rhesus monkeys. J Biomed Mater Res 1999;45:231–9.

[86] Maruoka S, Matsuura T, Kawasaki K, Okamoto M, Yoshiaki H, Kodama M, Sugiyama M, Annaka M. Biocompatibility of polyvinylalcohol gel as a vitreous substitute. Curr Eye Res 2006;31:599–606.

[87] Mendes SC, Reis RL, Bovell YP, Cunha AM, van Blitterswijk CA, de Bruijn JD. Biocompatibility testing of novel starch-based materials with potential application in orthopaedic surgery: a preliminary study. Biomaterials 2001;22:2057–64.

[88] Kirkpatrick CJ, Bittinger F, Wagner M, Köhler H, van Kooten TG, Klein CL, Otto M. Current trends in biocompatibility testing. Proc Inst Mech Eng H 1998;212:75–84.

[89] Kotzar G, Freas M, Abel P, Fleischman A, Roy S, Zorman C, Moran JM, Melzak J. Evaluation of MEMS materials of construction for implantable medical devices. Biomaterials 2002;23:2737—50.
[90] Morrison C, Macnair R, MacDonald C, Wykman A, Goldie I, Grant MH. In vitro biocompatibility testing of polymers for orthopaedic implants using cultured fibroblasts and osteoblasts. Biomaterials 1995;16:987—92.
[91] Ciapetti G, Granchi D, Verri E, Savarino L, Cavedagna D, Pizzoferrato A. Application of a combination of neutral red and amido black staining for rapid, reliable cytotoxicity testing of biomaterials. Biomaterials 1996;17:1259—64.
[92] Ciapetti G, Cenni E, Pratelli L, Pizzoferrato A. In vitro evaluation of cell/biomaterial interaction by MTT assay. Biomaterials 1993;14:359—64.
[93] Pizzoferrato A, Ciapetti G, Stea S, Cenni E, Arciola CR, Granchi,Lucia D. Cell culture methods for testing biocompatibility. Clin Mater 1994;15:173—90.
[94] Johnston TP, Schoen FJ, Levy RJ. Prevention of calcification of bioprosthetic heart valve leaflets by Ca^{2+} diphosphonate pretreatment. J Pharm Sci 1988;77:740—4.
[95] Levy RJ, Wolfrum J, Schoen FJ, Hawley MA, Lund SA, Langer R. Inhibition of calcification of bioprosthetic heart valves by local controlled-release diphosphonate. Science 1985;228:190—2.
[96] Paolo D, Maria Chiara C, Antonella B, Arianna M. Micro-systems in biomedical applications. J Micromechanics Microengineering 2000;10:235.
[97] LaVan DA, McGuire T, Langer R. Small-scale systems for in vivo drug delivery. Nat Biotech 2003;21:1184—91.
[98] Williams DF. Corrosion of implant materials. Annu Rev Mater Sci 1976;6:237—66.
[99] Cima MJ. Microsystem technologies for medical applications. Annu Rev Chem Biomol Eng 2011;2:355—78.
[100] Ashraf MW, Tayyaba S, Afzulpurkar N. Micro electromechanical systems (MEMS) based microfluidic devices for biomedical applications. Int J Mol Sci 2011;12:3648—704.
[101] Nisar A, Afzulpurkar N, Mahaisavariya B, Tuantranont A. MEMS-based micropumps in drug delivery and biomedical applications. Sensors Actuators B Chem 2008;130:917—42.
[102] Nguyen N-T, Huang X, Chuan TK. MEMS-micropumps: a review. J Fluids Eng 2002;124:384—92.
[103] R KJ. Applications of MEMS in surgery. Proc IEEE 2004;92:43—55.
[104] Tsai N-C, Sue C-Y. Review of MEMS-based drug delivery and dosing systems. Sensors Actuators A Phys 2007;134:555—64.
[105] Bustillo JM, Howe RT, Muller RS. Surface micromachining for microelectromechanical systems. Proc IEEE 1998;86:1552—74.
[106] Schmidt MA. Wafer-to-wafer bonding for microstructure formation. Proc IEEE 1998;86:1575—85.
[107] Collins CC. Miniature passive pressure transensor for implanting in the eye. IEEE Trans Biomed Eng 1967;14:74—83.
[108] Luis JA, Roa Romero LM, Gómez-Galán JA, Hernández DN, Estudillo-Valderrama MÁ, Barbarov-Rostán G, Rubia-Marcos C. Design and implementation of a smart sensor for respiratory rate monitoring. Sensors 2014;14:3019—32.
[109] Mokwa W, Schnakenberg U. Micro-transponder systems for medical applications. IEEE Trans Instrum Meas 2001;50:1551—5.
[110] Puers R, Vandevoorde G, Bruyker DD, Puers R, Vandevoorde G. Electrodeposited copper inductors for intraocular pressure telemetry. J Micromechanics Microengineering 2000;10:124.
[111] Chen PJ, Rodger DC, Saati S, Humayun MS, Tai YC. Microfabricated implantable parylene-based wireless passive intraocular pressure sensors. J Microelectromechanical Syst 2008;17:1342—51.
[112] James T, Mannoor MS, Ivanov DV. BioMEMS — advancing the Frontiers of medicine. Sensors 2008;8:6077—107.
[113] Yu L, Kim BJ, Meng E. Chronically implanted pressure sensors: challenges and state of the field. Sensors 2014;14:20620—44.
[114] Chen LY, Tee BCK, Chortos AL, Schwartz G, et al. Continuous wireless pressure monitoring and mapping with ultra-small passive sensors for health monitoring and critical care. Nat Commun 2014;5.

[115] Cosman ER, Zervas NT, Chapman PH, Cosman BJ, Arnold MA. A telemetric pressure sensor for ventricular shunt systems. Surg Neurol 1979;11:287—94.
[116] Chapman PH, Cosman ER, Arnold MA. The relationship between ventricular fluid pressure and body position in normal subjects and subjects with shunts: a telemetric study. Neurosurgery 1990;26:181—9.
[117] Rogier AMR, Fred WL, Nicolaas FdR. Microsystem technologies for implantable applications. J Micromechanics Microengineering 2007;17:R50.
[118] Hierold C, Clasbrumme B, Behrend D, Scheiter T, et al. Implantable low power integrated pressure sensor system for minimal invasive telemetric patient monitoring. In: MEMS 98. Proceedings. The eleventh annual international workshop on micro electro mechanical systems, 1998; 1998.
[119] Eggers T, Marschner C, Marschner U, Clasbrummel B, Laur R, Binder J. Advanced hybrid integrated low-power telemetric pressure monitoring system for biomedical applications. In: MEMS 2000. The thirteenth annual international conference on micro electro mechanical systems; 2000.
[120] Flick BB, Orglmeister R. A portable microsystem-based telemetric pressure and temperature measurement unit. IEEE Trans Biomed Eng 2000;47:12—6.
[121] Aubert AE, Vrolix M, De Geest H, Van de Werf F. In vivo comparison between two tip pressure transducer systems. Int J Clin Monit Comput 1995;12:77—83.
[122] Miller HD. Pressure transducers. Patent 3, 623, 274, 874: Millar Instruments Inc. 1973.
[123] Smith RA, Millar HD. Reduced catheter tip measurement device. US Patent 5, 248 08/744,478: Millar Instruments Inc. 1999.
[124] Ji J, Cho ST, Zhang Y, Najafi K, Wise KD. An ultraminiature CMOS pressure sensor for a multiplexed cardiovascular catheter. IEEE Trans Electron Devices 1992;39:2260—7.
[125] Samaun, Wise KD, Angell JB. An IC piezoresistive pressure sensor for biomedical instrumentation. IEEE Trans Biomed Eng 1973;20:101—9.
[126] Tanerz L, Hök B. Miniaturized pressure sensor. US Patent 5, 375 721,508: Radi Medical Systems AB. 1993.
[127] Holland CE, Hesketh PJ. Miniature pressure sensor and pressure sensor arrays. 1992 [Google Patents].
[128] Esashi M, Shoji S, Matsumoto Y, Furuta K. Catheter-tip capacitive pressure sensor. Electron Commun Jpn 1990;73:79—87.
[129] Ritzema-Carter JLT, Smyth D, Troughton RW, Crozier IG, et al. Dynamic myocardial ischemia caused by circumflex artery stenosis detected by a new implantable left atrial pressure monitoring device. Circulation 2006;113:e705—6.
[130] Walton AS, Krum H. The heartpod implantable heart failure therapy system. Heart, Lung Circ 2005;14:S31—3.
[131] Magalski A, Adamson P, Gadler F, Böehm M, et al. Continuous ambulatory right heart pressure measurements with an implantable hemodynamic monitor: a multicenter, 12-month follow-up study of patients with chronic heart failure. J Cardiac Fail 2002;8:63—70.
[132] Parikh KH. Effect of Metroprolol CR/XL on pulmonary artery pressure in patients with heart failure measured using first in human implantable device responding to ultrasonic signal. J Am Coll Cardiol 2006;47:1871—81.
[133] Schnakenberg U, Krüger C, Pfeffer J-G, Mokwa W, vom Bögel G, Günther R, Schmitz-Rode T. Intravascular pressure monitoring system. Sensors Actuators A Phys 2004;110:61—7.
[134] Puers B, Van Den Bossche A, Peeters E, Sansen W. Proceedings of the 5th international conference on solid-state sensors and actuators and Eurosensors IIIAn implantable pressure sensor for use in cardiology. Sensors Actuators A Phys 1990;23:944—7.
[135] Ransbury T, Holbrook K. Intravascular implantable device having superior anchoring arrangement. 2012 [Google Patents].
[136] Meador JT, Miesel KA, Halperin LE, Robert II TT, Stylos L. Implantable medical device for sensing absolute blood pressure and barometric pressure. 2000 [Google Patents].
[137] Fonseca M, Allen M, Stern D, White J, Kroh J. Implantable wireless sensor for pressure measurement within the heart. 2005 [Google Patents].
[138] Cates AW, Goode PV, Mazar ST. Chronically-implanted device for sensing and therapy. 2007 [Google Patents].

[139] Heilman MS, Brandt AJ, Bowling LD, Russial JF. Portable device for sensing cardiac function and automatically delivering electrical therapy. 1990 [Google Patents].
[140] Siwapornsathain E, Lal A, Binard J. A telemetry and sensor platform for ambulatory urodynamics. In: 2nd Annual international IEEE-EMB special topic conference on microtechnologies in medicine & biology; 2002.
[141] Dakurah MN, Koo C, Choi W, Joung YH. Implantable bladder sensors: a methodological review. Int Neurourol J 2015;19:133−41.
[142] Jourand P, Puers R. The bladderPill: an in-body system logging bladder pressure. Sensors Actuators A Phys 2010;162:160−6.
[143] Kim A, Powell CR, Ziaie B. An implantable pressure sensing system with electromechanical interrogation scheme. IEEE Trans Biomed Eng 2014;61:2209−17.
[144] Lip, Le, Ijlra, Inra, et al. ENDOCOM: implantable wireless pressure sensor for the follow-up of abdominal aortic aneurysm stented. IRBM 2011;32:163−8.
[145] Mundt RB, Somps CJ, Hines JW. Advanced sensor systems for improved labor and fetal monitoring ISA EXPO 98. In: International conference and exposition for advancing measurement and control technologies, products, and Services, vol. 2. Houston (TX, USA): Automation and control issues and solutions; 1998. p. 79−89.
[146] Langenfeld H, Krein A, Kirstein M, Binner L. European pea clinical investigation, peak endocardial acceleration-based clinical testing of the "BEST" DDDR pacemaker. Pacing Clin Electrophysiol 1998;21:2187−91.
[147] Kudo H, Sawada T, Kazawa E, Yoshida H, Iwasaki Y, Mitsubayashi K. A flexible and wearable glucose sensor based on functional polymers with Soft-MEMS techniques. Biosens Bioelectron 2006;22:558−62.
[148] Hornig R, Eckmiller R. Optimizing stimulus parameters by modeling multi-electrode electrical stimulation for retina implants. In: Proceedings. Ijcnn '01. International joint conference on neural networks, 2001; 2001.
[149] Humayun MS, de Juan Jr E, Weiland JD, Dagnelie G, Katona S, Greenberg R, Suzuki S. Pattern electrical stimulation of the human retina. Vis Res 1999;39:2569−76.
[150] Zrenner E, Stett A, Weiss S, Aramant RB, et al. Can subretinal microphotodiodes successfully replace degenerated photoreceptors? Vis Res 1999;39:2555−67.
[151] Chow AY, Chow VY, Packo KH, Pollack JS, Peyman GA, Schuchard R. The artificial silicon retina microchip for the treatment of vision loss from retinitis pigmentosa. Archives Ophthalmol 2004;122:460−9.
[152] Wang J, Wise KD. A hybrid electrode array with built-in position sensors for an implantable MEMS-based cochlear prosthesis. J Microelectromechanical Syst 2008;17:1187−94.
[153] Young DJ, Zurcher MA, Semaan M, Megerian CA, Ko WH. MEMS capacitive accelerometer-based middle ear microphone. IEEE Trans Biomed Eng 2012;59:3283−92.
[154] Jackson N, Muthuswamy J. Flexible chip scale package and interconnect for implantable MEMS movable microelectrodes for the brain. J Microelectromechanical Syst 2009;18:396−404.
[155] Kim S, Tathireddy P, Normann RA, Solzbacher F. Thermal impact of an active 3-D microelectrode array implanted in the brain. IEEE Trans Neural Syst Rehabilitation Eng 2007;15:493−501.
[156] Fernando A, Lee W, Phil C, Mark M, Gary KF. Design of a multi-axis implantable MEMS sensor for intraosseous bone stress monitoring. J Micromechanics Microengineering 2009;19:085016.
[157] Nguyen N-T, Shaegh SAM, Kashaninejad N, Phan D-T. Design, fabrication and characterization of drug delivery systems based on lab-on-a-chip technology. Adv Drug Deliv Rev 2013;65:1403−19.
[158] Sheybani R, Schober SM, Meng E. 15-Drug delivery using wireless MEMS A2. In: Uttamchandani D, editor. Handbook of MEMS for wireless and mobile applications. Woodhead Publishing; 2013. p. 489−517.
[159] Gale BK, Eddings MA, Sundberg SO, Hatch A, Kim J, Ho T, Karazi SM. Low-cost MEMS technologies, in reference module in materials science and materials engineering. Elsevier; 2016.
[160] Meng E, Hoang T. MEMS-enabled implantable drug infusion pumps for laboratory animal research, preclinical, and clinical applications. Adv Drug Deliv Rev 2012;64:1628−38.

[161] Prescott JH, Lipka S, Baldwin S, Sheppard NF, et al. Chronic, programmed polypeptide delivery from an implanted, multireservoir microchip device. Nat Biotech 2006;24:437–8.
[162] Santini Jr JT, Cima MJ, Langer R. A controlled-release microchip. Nature 1999;397:335–8.
[163] Guan J, He H, Lee LJ, Hansford DJ. Fabrication of particulate reservoir-containing, capsulelike, and self-folding polymer microstructures for drug delivery. Small 2007;3:412–8.
[164] Zhuang Y, Hou W, Zheng X, Wang Z, et al. A MEMS-based electronic capsule for time controlled drug delivery in the alimentary canal. Sensors Actuators A Phys 2011;169:211–6.
[165] Vladisavljević GT, Khalid N, Neves MA, Kuroiwa T, Nakajima M, Uemura K, Ichikawa S, Kobayashi I. Industrial lab-on-a-chip: design, applications and scale-up for drug discovery and delivery. Adv Drug Deliv Rev 2013;65:1626–63.
[166] Gurman P, Miranda OR, Clayton K, Rosen Y, Elman NM. Clinical applications of biomedical microdevices for controlled drug delivery. Mayo Clin Proc 2015;90:93–108.
[167] Stevenson CL, Santini Jr JT, Langer R. Reservoir-based drug delivery systems utilizing microtechnology. Adv Drug Deliv Rev 2012;64:1590–602.
[168] Ziaie B, Baldi A, Lei M, Gu Y, Siegel RA. Hard and soft micromachining for BioMEMS: review of techniques and examples of applications in microfluidics and drug delivery. Adv Drug Deliv Rev 2004;56:145–72.
[169] Luttge R. Chapter 8-microfabrication for novel products in drug delivery: an example. In: Microfabrication for industrial applications. Boston: William Andrew Publishing; 2011. p. 235–72.
[170] Shawgo RS, Richards Grayson AC, Li Y, Cima MJ. BioMEMS for drug delivery. Curr Opin Solid State Mater Sci 2002;6:329–34.
[171] Lewis JR, Ferrari M. BioMEMS for drug delivery applications A2. In: Oosterbroek RE, Berg AVD, editors. Lab-on-a-Chip. Amsterdam: Elsevier; 2003. p. 373–89.
[172] Vasudev A, Bhansali S. 11-Microelectromechanical systems (MEMS) for in vivo applications. In: Implantable sensor systems for medical applications. Woodhead Publishing; 2013. p. 331–58.
[173] Li W. 14-MEMS as ocular implants. In: MEMS for biomedical applications. Woodhead Publishing; 2012. p. 396–431.
[174] Salazar RL, Camacho-Leon S, Olivares-Quiroz L, Hernandez J. Design and simulation of a high precision drug delivery system. Procedia Technol 2012;3:334–41.
[175] Judy JW, Tamagawa T, Polla DL. Surface-machined micromechanical membrane pump. In: Micro electro mechanical systems, 1991, MEMS '91, Proceedings. An investigation of micro structures, sensors, actuators, machines and robots. IEEE; 1991.
[176] Koch M, Harris N, Evans AGR, White NM, Brunnschweiler A. A novel micromachined pump based on thick-film piezoelectric actuation. In: International conference on solid state sensors and actuators, 1997. Transducers '97 Chicago., 1997; 1997.
[177] Junwu K, Zhigang Y, Taijiang P, Guangming C, Boda W. Design and test of a high-performance piezoelectric micropump for drug delivery. Sensors Actuators A Phys 2005;121:156–61.
[178] Guo-Hua F, Eun Sok K. Piezoelectrically actuated dome-shaped diaphragm micropump. J Microelectromechanical Syst 2005;14:192–9.
[179] Geipel A, Doll A, Goldschmidtboing F, Jantscheff P, Esser N, Massing U, Woias P. Pressure-independent micropump with piezoelectric valves for low flow drug delivery systems. In: 19th IEEE international conference on micro electro mechanical systems, 2006. MEMS 2006 Istanbul; 2006.
[180] Van de Pol FCM, Van Lintel HTG, Elwenspoek M, Fluitman JHJ. Proceedings of the 5th International Conference on solid-state sensors and actuators and Eurosensors IIIA thermopneumatic micropump based on micro-engineering techniques. Sensors Actuators A Phys 1990;21:198–202.
[181] Sung Rae H, Woo Young S, Do Han J, Geun Young K, Sang Sik Y, James Jungho P. Fabrication and test of a submicroliter-level thermopneumatic micropump for transdermal drug delivery. In: 3rd IEEE/EMBS special topic conference on microtechnology in medicine and biology, 2005; 2005.
[182] Suzuki H, Yoneyama R. A reversible electrochemical nanosyringe pump and some considerations to realize low-power consumption. Sensors Actuators B Chem 2002;86:242–50.
[183] Li Y, Hong Linh Ho D, Tyler B, Williams T, Tupper M, Langer R, Brem H, Cima MJ. In vivo delivery of BCNU from a MEMS device to a tumor model. J Control Release 2005;106:138–45.
[184] Xie Y, Xu B, Gao Y. Controlled transdermal delivery of model drug compounds by MEMS microneedle array. Nanomedicine 2005;1:184–90.

[185] Li Y-J, Lu C-C, Tsai W-L, Tai M-H. An intra-oral drug delivery system design for painless, long-term and continuous drug release. Sensors Actuators B Chem 2016;227:573—82.

[186] Cobo A, Sheybani R, Tu H, Meng E. A wireless implantable micropump for chronic drug infusion against cancer. Sensors Actuators A Phys 2016;239:18—25.

[187] Park JH, Yoon YK, Choi SO, Prausnitz MR, Allen MG. Tapered conical polymer microneedles fabricated using an integrated lens technique for transdermal drug delivery. IEEE Trans Biomed Eng 2007;54:903—13.

[188] Sewell WF, Borenstein JT, Chen Z, Fiering J, et al. Development of a microfluidics-based intracochlear drug delivery device. Audiology Neurotol 2009;14:411—22.

[189] Tao SL, Lubeley MW, Desai TA. Bioadhesive poly(methyl methacrylate) microdevices for controlled drug delivery. J Control Release 2003;88:215—28.

[190] Auciello O. Chapter 12-Science and technology of ultrananocrystalline diamond (UNCD™) film-based MEMS and NEMS devices and systems A2. In: Shenderova OA, Gruen DM, editors. Ultrananocrystalline diamond. 2nd ed. Oxford: William Andrew Publishing; 2012. p. 383—420.

[191] Berman D, Krim J. Surface science, MEMS and NEMS: progress and opportunities for surface science research performed on, or by, microdevices. Prog Surf Sci 2013;88:171—211.

[192] Available from: http://www.cyberkinetics.com/; 2016.

[193] Available from: http://www.2-sight.eu/en/patients-families-en; 2016.

[194] Available from: http://www.nano-retina.com/; 2016.

[195] Available from: http://www.biomet3i.com/; 2016.

[196] Available from: http://www.biomet.com.tr/tr-medical/extremities/Comprehensive-Nano; 2016.

[197] Available from: http://www.envisionscientific.com/; 2016.

[198] Available from: http://www.en.lepumedical.com/; 2016.

[199] Lu Y, Guo Z, Song J-J, Huang Q-A, Zhu S-W, Huang X-J, Wei Y. Tunable nanogap devices for ultra-sensitive electrochemical impedance biosensing. Anal Chim Acta 2016;905:58—65.

[200] Gibney E. Injectable brain implant spies on individual neurons. Nature 2015;522:137—8.

[201] Li B, Lee C. NEMS diaphragm sensors integrated with triple-nano-ring resonator. Sensors Actuators A Phys 2011;172:61—8.

[202] Thomas JW, Michael CW, Janice LM, Rachel LP, Jeremiah UE. Nano-biotechnology: carbon nanofibres as improved neural and orthopaedic implants. Nanotechnology 2004;15:48.

[203] Du C, Cui FZ, Feng QL, Zhu XD, de Groot K. Tissue response to nano-hydroxyapatite/collagen composite implants in marrow cavity. J Biomed Mater Res 1998;42:540—8.

[204] Mozafari M, Moztarzadeh F, Seifalian AM, Tayebi L. Self-assembly of PbS hollow sphere quantum dots via gas—bubble technique for early cancer diagnosis. J Luminescence 2013;133:188—93.

[205] Ghaffari M, Moztarzadeh S, Rahmanian F, Yazdanpanah A, Ramedani A, Mills DK, Mozafari M. Chapter 8-Nanobiomaterials for bionic eye: vision of the future A2. In: Grumezescu AM, editor. Engineering of nanobiomaterials. William Andrew Publishing; 2016. p. 257—85.

[206] Xiao X, Wang J, Liu C, Carlisle JA, et al. In vitro and in vivo evaluation of ultrananocrystalline diamond for coating of implantable retinal microchips. J Biomed Mater Res B Appl Biomater 2006;77B:273—81.

[207] Smith GC, Chamberlain L, Faxius L, Johnston GW, Jin S, Bjursten LM. Soft tissue response to titanium dioxide nanotube modified implants. Acta Biomater 2011;7:3209—15.

[208] Cheng L, Yuan M, Gu L, Wang Z, Qin Y, Jing T, Wang ZL. Wireless, power-free and implantable nanosystem for resistance-based biodetection. Nano Energy 2015;15:598—606.

[209] Yoshikawa G, Akiyama T, Loizeau F, Shiba K, et al. Two dimensional array of piezoresistive nanomechanical membrane-type surface stress sensor (MSS) with improved sensitivity. Sensors 2012;12:15873—87.

[210] Schwalb CH, Grimm C, Baranowski M, Sachser R, et al. A tunable strain sensor using nanogranular metals. Sensors 2010;10:9847—56.

[211] Wu S, Liu X, Yeung KWK, Guo H, Li P, Hu T, Chung CY, Chu PK. Surface nano-architectures and their effects on the mechanical properties and corrosion behavior of Ti-based orthopedic implants. Surf Coatings Technol 2013;233:13—26.

[212] Kang S-K, Murphy RKJ, Hwang S-W, Lee SM, et al. Bioresorbable silicon electronic sensors for the brain. Nature 2016;530:71—6.

[213] Robinson JT, Jorgolli M, Shalek AK, Yoon M-H, Gertner RS, Park H. Vertical nanowire electrode arrays as a scalable platform for intracellular interfacing to neuronal circuits. Nat Nano 2012;7:180—4.

[214] Young DJ, Zorman CA, Mehregany M. MEMS/NEMS devices and applications. In: Bhushan B, editor. Springer handbook of nanotechnology. Berlin, Heidelberg: Springer Berlin Heidelberg; 2004. p. 225–52.
[215] Cimalla V, Niebelschütz F, Tonisch K, Foerster C, et al. Nanoelectromechanical devices for sensing applications. Sensors Actuators B Chem 2007;126:24–34.
[216] Juanola-Feliu E, Colomer-Farrarons J, Miribel-Català P, Samitier J, Valls-Pasola J. Market challenges facing academic research in commercializing nano-enabled implantable devices for in-vivo biomedical analysis. Technovation 2012;32:193–204.
[217] Barkam S, Saraf S, Seal S. Fabricated micro-nano devices for in vivo and in vitro biomedical applications. Wiley Interdiscip Rev Nanomed Nanobiotechnol 2013;5:544–68.
[218] Wang Y, Zhang W, Zhang J, Sun W, Zhang R, Gu H. Fabrication of a novel polymer-free nanostructured drug-eluting coating for cardiovascular stents. ACS Appl Mater Interfaces 2013;5:10337–45.
[219] Lyndon JA, Boyd BJ, Birbilis N. Metallic implant drug/device combinations for controlled drug release in orthopaedic applications. J Control Release 2014;179:63–75.
[220] Streicher RM, Schmidt M, Fiorito S. Nanosurfaces and nanostructures for artificial orthopedic implants. Nanomedicine 2007;2:861–74.
[221] Popat KC, Eltgroth M, LaTempa TJ, Grimes CA, Desai TA. Decreased *Staphylococcus* epidermis adhesion and increased osteoblast functionality on antibiotic-loaded titania nanotubes. Biomaterials 2007;28:4880–8.
[222] Jia H, Kerr LL. Sustained Ibuprofen release using composite poly(lactic-*co*-glycolic acid)/titanium dioxide nanotubes from Ti implant surface. J Pharm Sci 2013;102:2341–8.
[223] Moseke C, Hage F, Vorndran E, Gbureck U. TiO_2 nanotube arrays deposited on Ti substrate by anodic oxidation and their potential as a long-term drug delivery system for antimicrobial agents. Appl Surf Sci 2012;258:5399–404.
[224] Ma M, Kazemzadeh-Narbat M, Hui Y, Lu S, Ding C, Chen DDY, Hancock REW, Wang R. Local delivery of antimicrobial peptides using self-organized TiO_2 nanotube arrays for peri-implant infections. J Biomed Mater Res A 2012;100A:278–85.
[225] Zheng Y, Li J, Liu X, Sun J. Antimicrobial and osteogenic effect of Ag-implanted titanium with a nanostructured surface. Int J Nanomedicine 2012;7:875–84.
[226] Cao H, Liu X, Meng F, Chu PK. Biological actions of silver nanoparticles embedded in titanium controlled by micro-galvanic effects. Biomaterials 2011;32:693–705.
[227] Sirivisoot S, Pareta RA. 7-Orthopedic carbon nanotube biosensors for controlled drug delivery A2. In: Webster T, editor. Nanomedicine. Woodhead Publishing; 2012. p. 149–79.
[228] Hartmann H, Hossfeld S, Schlossbauer B, Mittnacht U, et al. Hyaluronic acid/chitosan multilayer coatings on neuronal implants for localized delivery of siRNA nanoplexes. J Control Release 2013;168:289–97.
[229] Pehlivan SB, Yavuz B, Calamak S, Ulubayram K, et al. Preparation and in vitro/in vivo evaluation of cyclosporin A-loaded nanodecorated ocular implants for subconjunctival application. J Pharm Sci 2015;104:1709–20.
[230] Sun G, Wei D, Liu X, Chen Y, Li M, He D, Zhong J. Novel biodegradable electrospun nanofibrous P(DLLA-CL) balloons for the treatment of vertebral compression fractures. Nanomedicine 2013;9:829–38.
[231] Hoare T, Santamaria J, Goya GF, Irusta S, et al. A magnetically triggered composite membrane for on-demand drug delivery. Nano Lett 2009;9:3651–7.
[232] Aw MS, Losic D. Ultrasound enhanced release of therapeutics from drug-releasing implants based on titania nanotube arrays. Int J Pharm 2013;443:154–62.
[233] Zielinski J, Moller AM, Frenz M, Mevissen M. Evaluation of endocytosis of silica particles used in biodegradable implants in the brain. Nanomedicine 2016;12:1603–13.

CHAPTER 12

Solid Lipid Nanoparticles in Drug Delivery: Opportunities and Challenges

Ameya Deshpande, Majrad Mohamed, Saloni B. Daftardar, Meghavi Patel, Sai H.S. Boddu, Jerry Nesamony
The University of Toledo Health Science Campus, Toledo, OH, United States

Contents

1. Introduction	292
2. Components of Solid Lipid Nanoparticles	293
2.1 Lipid	293
2.2 Surfactant	295
3. Solid Lipid Nanoparticle Production Techniques	295
3.1 High-Pressure Homogenization	295
3.1.1 Hot Homogenization Technique	*296*
3.1.2 Cold Homogenization Technique	*296*
3.2 Microemulsion-Based Technique	297
3.3 Solvent Emulsification—Evaporation Technique	297
3.4 Solvent Displacement Technique	298
3.5 Emulsification—Diffusion Technique	298
4. Drug-Loading Capacity of Solid Lipid Nanoparticles	298
5. Drug Incorporation Models of Solid Lipid Nanoparticles	299
6. Drug Release From Solid Lipid Nanoparticles	300
6.1 Influence of Temperature	301
6.2 Influence of Surfactants	302
7. Applications of Solid Lipid Nanoparticles for Drug Delivery	302
7.1 Routes of Administration of SLNs	302
7.1.1 Oral Administration	*302*
7.1.2 Parenteral Route	*303*
7.1.3 Topical Administration	*304*
7.1.4 Pulmonary Administration	*305*
7.1.5 Rectal Administration	*305*
7.1.6 Ocular Administration	*306*
7.2 Application of Solid Lipid Nanoparticles for Delivery of Hydrophilic Drugs: PEG Coating	307
7.3 SLNs as Potential Carriers of Anticancer Agents	308
7.3.1 Significance of Solid Lipid Nanoparticles as Anticancer Carriers	*308*
7.3.2 Incorporation of Hydrophilic Anticancer Actives in Solid Lipid Nanoparticles	*310*
8. Stability Concerns of Solid Lipid Nanoparticles	310
8.1 Influence of Shear Forces and Lipid Concentration	311

    8.2 Influence of the Surface of the Packing Material   311
    8.3 Properties of the Lipids: SLNs Versus Bulk Material   312
    8.4 Stability and Storage Conditions   312
    8.5 Gelling Tendency: Temperature Versus Shear Forces   314
    8.6 Physical Stability   315
        8.6.1 Physical Stability due to Changes in Lipids   *315*
        8.6.2 Physical Stability due to Changes in Colloidal Lipid Dispersion   *318*
        8.6.3 Coalescence   *318*
    8.7 Chemical Stability   318
        8.7.1 Phospholipid Stability   *318*
        8.7.2 Triglycerides Stability   *319*
9. Toxicity Aspects of Solid Lipid Nanoparticles   319
10. Diagnostic Applications of Solid Lipid Nanoparticles   320
11. In Vivo Fate of Solid Lipid Nanoparticles   321
12. Conclusions   322
References   323

1. INTRODUCTION

In current drug discovery, more than 75% of potential drug candidates have low water solubility and belong to classes II and IV of the Biopharmaceutical Classification System [1]. The development of these new chemical entities into commercial drug products is often hampered by the hydrophobic nature of the compounds, resulting in drug precipitation and low drug bioavailability [2]. Potential strategies to overcome such problems are structure modification of the drug or incorporation of the drug into a carrier system. The in vivo fate of a drug depends on the drug delivery system in which it is incorporated [3]. Lipid-based formulations were first commercialized in the 1950s. Intralipid was introduced as a safe fat emulsion for parenteral nutrition, followed by Diazemuls, an injectable emulsion of diazepam. One possible reason for the popularity of lipid delivery systems is the reduced pain and inflammation at the site of injection [4]. A particular advantage offered by lipid colloidal carriers is the increase in bioavailability of poorly water-soluble drugs.

In recent years, lipid-based systems such as solid lipid nanoparticles (SLNs) have received increasing interest in drug formulation due to their ability to carry and solubilize lipophilic drugs. SLNs offer several advantages over other polymeric colloidal carrier systems. Table 12.1 summarizes the advantages and disadvantages of SLNs. SLNs have a mean diameter, as measured by photon correlation spectroscopy, ranging from 50 to 1000 nm. SLNs are formulated from emulsions that are used for parenteral administration by replacing the lipids in the liquid state with lipids in the solid state. SLNs are normally stabilized physically using surfactants. The major advantage that makes SLNs unique compared with polymeric nanoparticles is that they can be produced/manufactured using high-pressure homogenization (HPH) techniques used industrially for preparing emulsions. The emulsion production is generally equipped with temperature control units,

Table 12.1 Few advantages and disadvantages of solid lipid nanoparticles [88,152,153]

Advantages
Broad spectrum of route of administration
Good physical stability
Protection from degradation of incorporated labile drugs
Modulated (fast or sustained) release of the drug is possible
Targeted drug delivery
No use of organic solvents during preparation
Ease of scale-up
Excellent biocompatibility
No need of special solvents
Conventional emulsion production techniques could be employed
Raw materials used in the production of emulsions could be used
Can be sterilized by commercial sterilization methods

Disadvantages
Particle growth
Gelation tendency
Unexpected polymorphic transitions
Thermal degradation of heat-labile drugs
Sophisticated equipment

as elevated temperature sometimes favors emulsion production, which is equally applicable for producing SLNs by the hot homogenization technique [5]. This chapter provides an overview of various aspects of SLNs, stability problems associated with SLNs, and diagnostic applications of SLNs.

2. COMPONENTS OF SOLID LIPID NANOPARTICLES

2.1 Lipid

Because lipids are the main building material of SLNs, the selection of an appropriate lipid or mixture of lipids is an important element to consider when fabricating SLNs. Generally, lipids are a large and diverse group of organic substances; however, the lipid components used in the formation of SLNs have the common property of being solid both at room temperature and at body temperature. Different types of solid lipids behave differently, which consequently affects the properties and the intended use of nanocarriers themselves. The selection of a pertinent solid lipid or lipid blend for SLNs depends on several factors: (1) ability to produce particles in the submicron range, (2) biodegradability, (3) biocompatibility, (4) adequate drug-loading capacity, and (5) stability upon storage. Moreover, lipids can be classified on the basis of the lipid matrix formed, i.e., ordered, less ordered, and disordered matrices [6]. Thus the selection of lipids plays a crucial role in the formulation of stable SLNs. The purity and composition of lipids should be examined using several analytical techniques such as gas chromatography—mass spectrometry, Fourier transform infrared spectroscopy, and Raman spectroscopy. The apparent degradation of lipids can be quantified with the help of the spectra. Lipids tend to be metabolized easily. For example, a study pertaining to the lipolysis half-life of lipids revealed that Gelucire, which is a polyethylene glycol (PEG) ester, metabolizes easily, thereby exhibiting a low half-life of lipolysis. This could lead to problems such as precipitation and crystallization of drugs. Drug lipophilicity with respect to the selected lipid is an important aspect to be considered for a stable formulation. An ideal lipid phase should be sufficiently lipophilic to solubilize lipophilic drugs easily. The lipids most commonly used in the preparation of SLNs are listed in Table 12.2. For detailed information on the types of lipids used in SLNs, readers can refer to our earlier publication [7] and other references [8,9].

Table 12.2 Lipids commonly used in the preparation of solid lipid nanoparticles

Lipids	Matrix arrangement	Examples	Literature
Triglycerides	Highly ordered	Tricaprin	[154]
		Trilaurin	[49,114,155]
		Trimyristin	[49,114,156]
		Tripalmitin	[109,114]
		Tristearin	[15,154]
		Hydrogenated coco-glycerides	[157]
Hard fat types	–	Witepsol W 35	[15,48,158]
		Witepsol H 35	[15,32,44]
		Witepsol H 42	[32]
		Witepsol E 85	[44,157]
Acylglycerol mixtures	Less ordered	Glyceryl monostearate (Imwitor 900)	[87,97,156,159]
		Glyceryl behenate (Compritol 888 ATO)	[87]
		Glyceryl palmitostearate (Precirol ATO 5)	[160]

Table 12.3 Surfactants used in preparation of solid lipid nanoparticles

Emulsifiers	Literature
Poloxamer 188	[19,48,161]
Poloxamer 182	[157]
Polysorbate 20	[162,163]
Polysorbate 60	[164]
Polysorbate 80	[157]
Sodium cholate	[156,157,165,166]
Sodium glycocholate	[109,167]
Soybean lecithin	[44,49,167]
Soybean phosphatidylcholine	[165,166]
Sorbitan trioleate	[168]

2.2 Surfactant

Surfactants stabilize SLNs by decreasing the surface tension between water and lipids. The selection and concentration of surfactant used depends on the lipid and the route of administration. Surfactants are divided into three categories, depending on their charge as ionic, nonionic, and amphoteric surfactants. Table 12.3 lists a few examples of surfactants commonly used in SLNs. The toxicity of a surfactant is an important consideration, and not all surfactants can be used for preparation of all types of SLNs. For example, nonionic surfactants such as poloxamer 188 and lecithin are preferred for parenteral and ocular routes of administration.

3. SOLID LIPID NANOPARTICLE PRODUCTION TECHNIQUES

For several years, solid lipids have been used in the form of pellets to achieve delayed drug release [3]. In the early 1980s, Speiser and coworkers developed spray-dried and congealed micropellets [10] and nanopellets of lipids for oral administration [11]. Nanopellets developed by Speiser [11] often contained high amounts of microparticles. Domb produced liposphere by high shear mixing or ultrasonication [12]. But both the nanopellets and liposphere, produced by Speiser and Domb, respectively, were contaminated by microparticles. Since the last decade, several scientists have realized the potential of SLN technology, and their research efforts have brought about improvement in SLN synthesis.

3.1 High-Pressure Homogenization

Muller and Lucks were the first to prepare SLNs by applying HPH technique [13]. Homogenizers have been used commercially for several years now for the production of nanoemulsions for parenteral nutrition fluids such as Intralipid and Lipofundin [14]. Thus scaling up presents fewer problems when compared with other techniques, and it is highly cost-effective. Naturally, a lot of research has been done by several research groups utilizing this method to produce better SLNs. A homogeneous dispersion with narrow size distribution is desirable to increase the physical stability of the aqueous dispersion. In this technique, the liquid is forced at a high pressure (100–2000 bar) through a narrow gap of few microns. The resulting high shear stress and cavitation forces decrease the particle size. If the particles localized at different positions in the dispersion volume experience different forces then the degree of particle disruption will vary. The two basic production methods to HPH are the hot and the cold homogenization techniques.

3.1.1 Hot Homogenization Technique

In this method, the active ingredient is first dissolved in the lipid melt. A coarse preemulsion is made by dispersing the lipid melt into hot surfactant solution that is heated to a temperature above the melting point of the lipid, while applying stirring [15]. The preemulsion is then passed through a high-pressure homogenizer for 3–5 cycles and applying a pressure of about 500–1500 bar [16]. The obtained nanoemulsion is then allowed to cool to room temperature or lower. The lipid nanodroplets solidify while cooling and form an aqueous dispersion of SLNs. Homogenization pressure and the number of cycles should not be higher than that required to achieve the desired effects because this increases the cost of production and the chances of metal contamination, and in some cases, it would result in increase in particle size due to aggregation as a result of the high surface free energy of the particles [3]. This technique is performed at a high temperature and thus cannot be used for temperature-sensitive drugs. Moreover, it has been reported that the lipids remain as a supercooled melt for several months owing to their small particle size and the presence of an emulsifier. This method is also not suitable for hydrophilic drugs [5].

3.1.2 Cold Homogenization Technique

In this process, the active ingredient is first dissolved in the lipid at a temperature above the melting point of the lipid. The mixture is cooled rapidly with the help of liquid nitrogen or dry ice. The rapid cooling procedure helps in the homogeneous distribution of the active ingredient. This solidified mixture is milled to about 50–100 μm particles using a ball or mortar mill [14]. The lipid microparticles obtained by milling are suspended in a surfactant solution to obtain a suspension. This suspension is then passed through HPH at or below room temperature to obtain SLNs. The cold homogenization technique reduces the chances for temperature-induced drug degradation, and thus thermosensitive drugs can be used. Since the solid lipid is milled, the complexity arising due to lipid modification can be avoided [3]. Chances of drug distribution into the aqueous phase are limited, and hence this method can be used for hydrophilic drugs as well as lipophilic drugs. Lipid nanoparticles prepared via this technique possess a slightly larger particle size and polydispersity than particles obtained by the hot homogenization technique, using the same lipid at similar homogenization parameters (pressure, temperature, and the number of cycles). A higher number of homogenization cycles can be applied to reduce the particle size [17].

3.2 Microemulsion-Based Technique

Gasco and coworkers were the first to develop SLNs based on the dilution of microemulsions. Microemulsions are thermodynamically stable, clear, and isotropic mixtures, usually composed of an oil or lipid, emulsifier and/or coemulsifier, and water. Lipids used to prepare SLNs are solids at room temperature, and hence the microemulsion is prepared at a temperature above the melting point of the lipid. Both the lipid and the aqueous phase containing the emulsifier are mixed in appropriate ratios and stirred so that it will produce a microemulsion. The hot microemulsion is then diluted with cold water (2–8°C) while stirring. The ratio of the hot microemulsion to cold water is usually in the range of 1:25 to 1:50. It has been noted in the literature that a droplet structure is already present in the microemulsion, and therefore no external energy is required to achieve the small particle size. When the microemulsion is diluted by cold water, the lipid droplets solidify as the temperature decreases. The temperature gradient and pH value determine the quality of the product, in addition to the composition of the microemulsion. The major limitation of this technique is its sensitivity to minor changes in composition or thermodynamic variables, which can lead to phase transitions. The lack of robustness of the microemulsion technique can lead to high production costs. Moreover, solidification of lipids shifts the system to a thermodynamically unstable state. Due to the dilution of the microemulsion, the concentrations of particle content are below 1%; therefore a large amount of water has to be removed to process the SLNs to a final dosage form. The high concentration of surfactants used may produce toxicity. This necessitates removal of excess surfactants using ultracentrifugation, ultrafiltration, or dialysis.

3.3 Solvent Emulsification–Evaporation Technique

Sjöström and Bergenståhl were the first to describe the production of SLNs by solvent emulsification–evaporation technique [18]. The solid lipid is dissolved in a water-immiscible organic solvent such as cyclohexane, chloroform, ethyl acetate, or methylene chloride, and the drug is dissolved or dispersed in the solution [19]. This organic phase containing the drug is emulsified in an aqueous solution of a surfactant by mechanical stirring. The organic solvent is then removed from the emulsion under mechanical stirring or reduced pressure (40–60 mbar) [3,19]. Lipid nanoparticle dispersion is formed by the precipitation of the lipid phase in the aqueous surfactant medium. Particle aggregation can be avoided in this technique by removing the solvent at a faster rate [5]. This technique can be used to incorporate hydrophilic drugs by preparing a water/oil/water emulsion and dissolving the drug in the internal water phase [20,21]. Thermosensitive drugs can be incorporated via this technique, as it avoids thermal stress. Trace amounts of organic solvent remaining in the final product can potentially create toxicity problems. Moreover, increasing the lipid content decreases the efficiency of homogenization due to the high viscosity of the dispersed phase, and hence the dispersions are very dilute and have very low lipid particle content (0.1 g/L) [3]. A large quantity of water has to be removed during the final processing of the formulation [22,23].

3.4 Solvent Displacement Technique

Fessi et al. were the first to describe this technique for the preparation of polymeric nanoparticles by polymerization in solution [24]. This technique has been modified and used for the preparation of SLNs [25,26]. In this technique, the lipid and the active ingredient are dissolved in a water-miscible solvent such as ethanol, isopropanol, acetone, or methanol [27]. The mixture is then dispersed into an aqueous solution of a surfactant with mild mechanical stirring, producing a suspension of lipid nanoparticles [25]. The solvent is subsequently removed by distillation. Ultracentrifugation, ultrafiltration, or lyophilization can be used for isolating the lipid nanoparticles.

3.5 Emulsification—Diffusion Technique

Quintanar-Guerrero et al. were the first to describe this technique for the preparation of polymeric nanoparticles [28]. This technique has been modified by various research groups for the preparation of SLNs [29–31]. In this technique, the lipid is dissolved in a partially water-miscible solvent such as benzyl alcohol, isobutyric acid, or tetrahydrofuran, which is previously saturated with water at room temperature or at a controlled temperature. The mixture is then emulsified in an aqueous solution of a surfactant by mechanical stirring at the temperature used to dissolve the lipid producing an oil/water (o/w) emulsion. This o/w emulsion is then diluted with excess water at a controlled temperature, which causes the diffusion of solvent into the external phase and subsequent precipitation of lipid nanoparticles. The solvent can be removed either by distillation or by ultrafiltration. The concentration and the nature of the lipid and surfactant, stirring rate, and the processing temperature are critical variables in this technique [29].

4. DRUG-LOADING CAPACITY OF SOLID LIPID NANOPARTICLES

Various drugs have been investigated as potential agents for incorporation into SLNs. Some examples include timolol [32], deoxycorticosterone [33], doxorubicin [34], idarubicin [34], pilocarpine [35], thymopentin [36], diazepam [37], paclitaxel [38], retinol [39], acyclovir [14,40], tetracaine [14], etomidate [41], cyclosporin [42], azido thymidine palmitate [43], oxazepam [44], diazepam [44], cortisone betamethasone valerate [44], camptothecin [45], and piribedil [46]. Drug-loading capacity is an important parameter to investigate the suitability of a drug carrier system. The drug-loading capacity is related to the nature of the lipid and is generally expressed in terms of percentage. The drug-loading capacity varies depending on the drug incorporated in the SLNs. Drug-loading capacities ranging from 1% to 50% have been reported. Some of the factors that affect the drug-loading capacity of SLNs are drug solubility in lipid melt, miscibility of drug and lipid melt, structure of the lipid matrix, and polymeric state of the lipid [5]. However, it has been observed that the drug-loading capacities of lipid nanocarriers are comparatively lower due to low solubilization capacities of the molten lipids for the hydrophobic drug entities. Supercooled melts have been found to have higher drug-loading capacities when compared with crystallized nanoparticles. Hard fats have higher drug-loading capacities due to their crystalline nature when compared with pure monoacid triglycerides [44]. The drug solubility reduces when the lipid melt is cooled down. Hence, the solubility of drugs in the lipid should be higher than required. The drug solubility is enhanced in the presence of mono- or diglycerides and also by addition of solubilizers. A good drug-loading capacity is obtained when polydisperse lipids that are generally used in cosmetics are used in SLNs.

The chemical nature of the lipid is a key determining factor of drug-loading capacity in SLNs. Determination of crystallinity of the lipids and other excipients may prove to be beneficial for predicting the drug entrapment. Optimized drug incorporation and physical characterization of lipids and other excipients using analytical techniques such as nuclear magnetic resonance, powder X-ray diffraction, differential scanning calorimetry (DSC), and Fourier transform infrared spectroscopy are required [5]. The polymorphic form of a lipid also affects the drug-loading capacity. The polymorphic form, in which a lipid is present, differs depending on whether it is in the bulk form or if it is in the form of nanoparticles. It has been found that the lipid, when present as nanoparticles, recrystallizes at least partially if not fully into α form. In contrast, the bulk lipid is found to recrystallize into β form. The formation of the β form results in expulsion of the drug from the lipid matrix. This transformation is slower for long-chain triglycerides than for short-chain triglycerides. Dispersed lipids are found to recrystallize in the α form, whereas the bulk lipids are found to recrystallize in β'-modification, followed by transformation into the β form, if heated above the bulk melting temperature and then cooled under controlled conditions. SLNs may be optimized in a way to produce and maintain some fraction of the α form to achieve better entrapment and controlled release of the drug [5,47–50].

5. DRUG INCORPORATION MODELS OF SOLID LIPID NANOPARTICLES

The drug release pattern is defined by the drug incorporation models of SLNs, which have been categorized as follows (Fig. 12.1) [51]:

Solid solution model: When the cold homogenization technique is used to generate nanoparticles, the drug is molecularly dispersed in the lipid matrix and has strong interactions with the lipid matrix. No surfactant is required in this model.

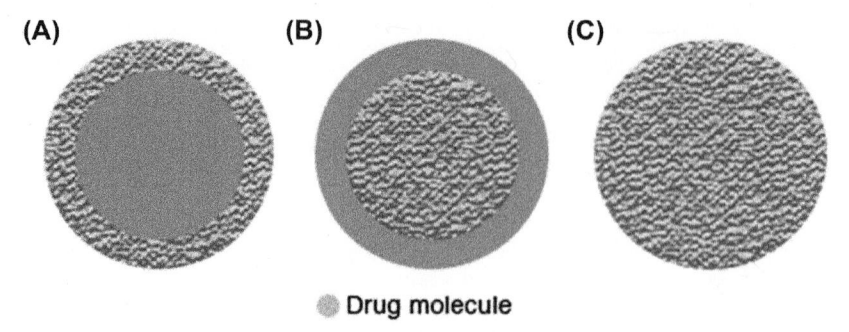

Figure 12.1 Drug incorporation models of solid lipid nanoparticles: (A) drug-enriched shell model, (B) drug-enriched core model, (C) solid solution model. *(Modified from Shah R, Eldridge D, Palombo E, Harding I. Lipid nanoparticles: production, characterization and stability. Springer; 2015.)*

Drug-enriched shell model: When the recrystallization temperature of lipid is attained, a solid lipid core is formed with drug molecules concentrating on the surface of SLNs.

Drug-enriched core model: Upon cooling, drug that is dissolved in a lipid melt at or near its saturation solubility precipitates before lipid recrystallization due to supersaturation. A membrane of recrystallized lipid is formed as the nanoemulsion is further cooled.

These models give an insight of modulating drug release by controlling the SLN structure during formulation. This in turn requires the necessary technical know-how for SLN production and fine tuning to achieve the desired drug release profile.

6. DRUG RELEASE FROM SOLID LIPID NANOPARTICLES

The release of the entrapped drug from the SLNs is governed by the following principles:
- An inverse relationship exists between the release of the drug and the partition coefficient of the drug.
- Smaller particle size promotes higher surface area, thereby leading to higher drug release.
- Homogeneous dispersion of the drug in the lipid matrix causes slow release of the drug.
- Lipid crystallinity and high drug mobility lead to rapid release of the drug from the SLNs [52].

Numerous studies have been carried out on the effect of formulation parameters and process conditions on the release of drug from SLNs. A crucial problem with SLNs is the initial burst release of drug. The burst release of drug from SLNs depends on the particle size and/or surface area. SLNs incorporated with tetracaine and etomidate demonstrated burst release with 100% release of the drug in less than 1 min (Fig. 12.2). This release pattern was attributed to the large surface area of nanoparticles and higher percentage

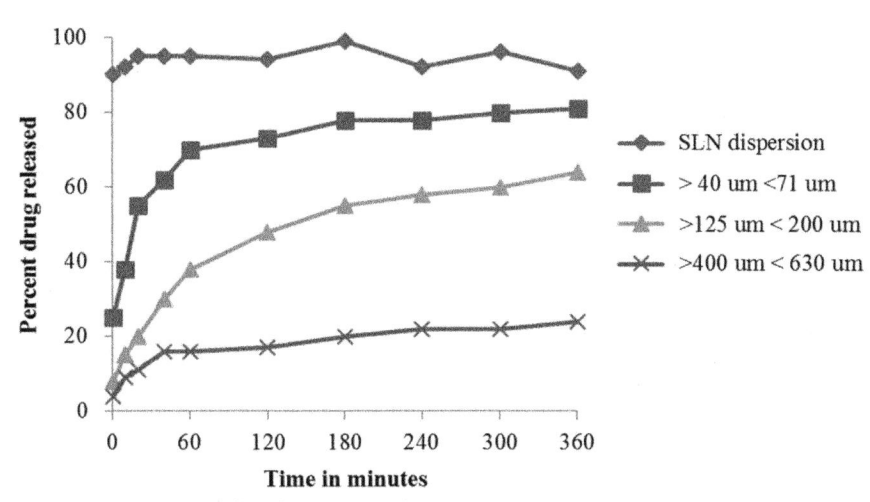

Figure 12.2 Drug release profile of etomidate from solid lipid nanoparticles (SLNs) and lipid microparticles of increasing particle size. *(Reproduced with permission from zur Mühlen A, Schwarz C, Mehnert W. Solid lipid nanoparticles (SLN) for controlled drug delivery—drug release and release mechanism. Eur J Pharm Biopharm 1998;45:149–155.)*

of drug in the outer layer of nanoparticles. The drug was found to be accumulated in the outer shell of nanoparticles with a relatively short distance of diffusion, which in turn resulted in a burst release. However, a prolonged drug release pattern was observed for lipid-soluble prednisolone-loaded SLNs. This could be explained with a "solid dispersion model" in which the drug is molecularly distributed into a lipid matrix. This study concluded that SLNs incorporated with lipophilic drugs follows prolonged release patterns [53]. Thus the desired drug release can be fabricated by modulating the process parameters. The parameters that affect the release of drug from SLNs are temperature, amount of drug incorporated, lipid structure, and drug structure, duration of production, processing equipment, lyophilization process, and sterilization process [52]. Among these, the two major parameters that influence the release of drug from the SLNs are temperature and presence of a surfactant.

6.1 Influence of Temperature

The release profile of SLNs generally follows a biphasic pattern. A burst release is observed initially followed by a prolonged release. Drug release investigations have proved that the highest burst release is observed at the highest temperatures of production and also if hot homogenization is used as the method of production. The burst release is found to decrease with decreasing production temperature and is negligible with the cold homogenization technique. The use of high temperature facilitates solubility of drug in the aqueous phase. Hence, use of lower production temperatures may eliminate burst release of the drug [52,53].

6.2 Influence of Surfactants

The amount of surfactant or surfactant mixture in the formulation also influences the burst release of the drug from SLNs. It has been found that at high surfactant concentrations the burst release of the drug is higher, whereas at lower concentrations of surfactants, the burst release is lower. This phenomenon is supported by the hot homogenization process in which redistribution of the drug occurs between the lipid and the aqueous phase during the heating process followed by a subsequent cooling process. As the dispersion of lipid and water is heated, the drug travels from melted lipid droplet to the aqueous phase. Then as the oil/water emulsion is being cooled, the solubility of the drug in the water continuously decreases with a decrease in the temperature leading to repartitioning of the drug into the lipid phase. Formation of the solid lipid core including the drug starts at the recrystallization temperature of the lipid. As the temperature further decreases, the pressure on the drug increases to repartition into the lipid phase because of the decrease in the solubility of the drug in water. But, as the lipid core is crystallized, the drug cannot incorporate into the lipid core [5]. This leads to supersaturation of the aqueous phase with the drug and results in formation of outer liquid layer of SLN enriched with the drug. Therefore hydrophilic drugs are observed to have higher burst release [53]. The use of surfactants facilitates the dissolution of drug in the aqueous phase. Hence, SLNs having low surfactant concentration or no surfactant may reduce burst release [52,53].

7. APPLICATIONS OF SOLID LIPID NANOPARTICLES FOR DRUG DELIVERY

The encapsulation of hydrophilic and lipophilic drugs by formulating them in SLNs results in their protection from degradation in the body and facilitates their prolonged release. Application of SLNs as a carrier system could be attributed to their unique features such as surface modification, enhanced permeation through biological membranes, increased resistance to chemical degradation, and ability to deliver two or more therapeutic agents.

7.1 Routes of Administration of SLNs
7.1.1 Oral Administration
SLNs may be administered orally after transformation into a traditional oral dosage form such as tablets, pellets, capsules, or powders. SLN dispersion can be used in place of a granulation fluid during wet granulation processes. SLNs can be directly tableted if the dispersion is transformed to powder form by spray drying or lyophilization. Dry SLN powder may be filled into hard gelatin capsules, or SLNs may be directly produced in liquid polyethylene glycol 600 and filled into soft gelatin capsule. Also, SLNs may be directly

commercialized as dry powders in sachet after spray drying or lyophilization since spray drying was found to be a more cost-effective method [5]. Various researchers have investigated SLNs for oral delivery of a variety of active compounds [54–58]. Cho et al. formulated SLNs incorporated with docetaxel, which has poor oral bioavailability [54]. SLNs were surface modified with tween 80 or D-alpha-tocopheryl poly(ethylene glycol 1000) succinate. The results indicated an increase in the oral bioavailability of docetaxel and thus SLNs may serve as an efficient oral drug delivery system for docetaxel [54]. SLNs of insulin were prepared using cetyl palmitate by Sarmento et al. and evaluated for oral delivery [55]. The SLNs were produced by a modified solvent emulsification–evaporation technique based on water/oil/water double emulsion. Oral administration of the formulated insulin-loaded SLNs to diabetic rats provided a considerable hypoglycemic effect during 24 h indicating SLNs to be a potential oral delivery system for insulin [55].

7.1.2 Parenteral Route

Drugs in the form of proteins and peptides are prone to enzymatic degradation and hence are not administered orally. To avoid frequent administration and to increase patient adherence, development of a controlled release parenteral formulation based on SLNs can provide an effective therapy [52]. The application of SLNs in parenteral delivery ranges from intraarticular delivery route to intravenous administration [5]. Various researchers have performed investigations on intravenous performance of SLNs [14,41]. Zara et al. investigated the effects of stealth and nonstealth SLNs incorporated with doxorubicin following intravenous administration [59]. The pharmacokinetics and tissue distribution of doxorubicin incorporated in SLNs were compared with commercial doxorubicin solution. The formulations were administered intravenously to conscious rabbits. Brain distribution of doxorubicin was obtained only with SLNs. The use of a stealth agent facilitated the distribution of doxorubicin to the brain. SLNs were found to significantly reduce the heart and liver distributions of doxorubicin. In one study, Manjunath et al. assessed the bioavailability of nitrendipine-loaded SLNs following intravenous and intraduodenal administration to rats [60]. Pharmacokinetic studies were performed following intravenous and intraduodenal administration of nitrendipine-loaded SLNs to conscious male Wistar rats, whereas the tissue distribution studies were carried out in Swiss albino mice after intravenous administration of nitrendipine-loaded SLNs and was compared with nitrendipine suspension. An increase in area under the curve and decrease in clearance was observed with nitrendipine-loaded SLNs when compared with the nitrendipine suspension. The effective bioavailability of the nitrendipine SLN was found to be higher after intraduodenal administration when compared with nitrendipine suspension, thus proving the suitability of SLNs as carrier system for improvement of bioavailability of nitrendipine. Generally corticosteroids are given to relieve arthritic inflammation; however, corticosteroids are poorly water soluble. They can be incorporated into a matrix of SLNs delivered via the intraarticular route. Upon administration,

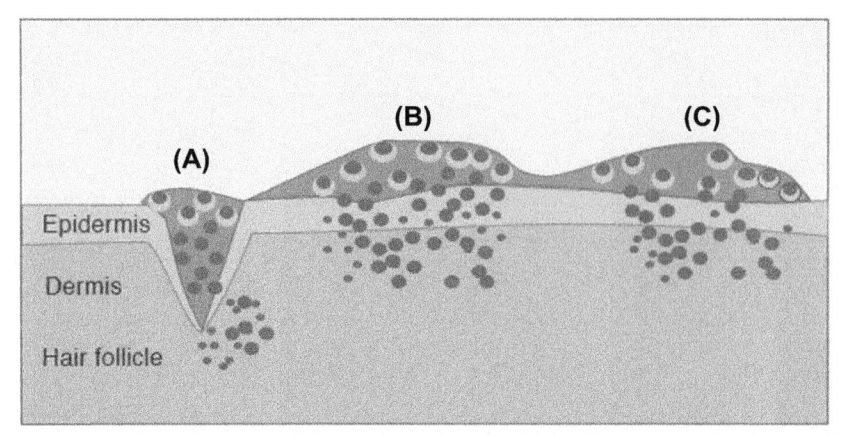

Figure 12.3 Proposed mechanism of drug release from solid lipid nanoparticles (SLNs) after transdermal administration. (A) Accumulation of SLNs in hair follicle; (B) penetration of drug and lipid into the skin; (C) drug release from SLNs and penetration into the skin. *(Modified from Zhang J, Purdon CH, Smith EW. Solid lipid nanoparticles for topical drug delivery. Am J Drug Deliv 2006;4:215–220.)*

macrophages can internalize the SLNs subsequently, causing the release of drug thereby reducing the inflammation of joints. Incorporation of drug into SLNs has been found to decrease its irritancy than injecting drug solution [61].

7.1.3 Topical Administration

Several investigations have attempted to show SLNs as enhanced transdermal delivery vehicles. SLNs easily adhere to the stratum corneum, forming a film with occlusive properties. The exact mechanism of transdermal delivery is not known; however, several mechanisms are possible as illustrated in Fig. 12.3. SLNs can penetrate through hair follicles, glands, and appendageal openings. Such accumulation provides continuous release of drug, thus reducing the frequency of drug administration. Another proposed mechanism may be attributed to drug partitioning from lipid particles and subsequent permeation into the skin. SLNs do not interact with stratum corneum. Upon disintegration of the lipid particles, both lipid as well as drug might independently permeate across stratum corneum [62]. SLN dispersions with low lipid content (<5%) are found to have small particle sizes. Higher viscosity and lipid concentrations are beneficial for dermal application. Hence, in most cases, it is necessary to incorporate the SLNs into an ointment or gel to obtain a formulation that could be applied to the skin. High lipid concentrations in SLNs may result in a semisolid form during SLN preparation that may be further utilized as a topical formulation. However, this approach can lead to an increase in particle size. Numerous studies have been performed on topical application of SLNs [2,45]. Lippacher et al. produced semisolid SLN dispersion by the HPH technique in a one-step process [63]. They were successful in obtaining SLNs in colloidal size range even with high volume concentration of dispersed lipids. The formulation obtained had viscoelastic properties similar to standard dermal formulations, which was proved by elastic responses obtained from oscillatory rheology experiments. The formulation demonstrated good particle size stability and gel structure stability.

7.1.4 Pulmonary Administration

Various researchers have investigated the utility of SLNs in pulmonary delivery [70–72]. Varshosaz et al. studied the biodistribution of amikacin-loaded SLNs following pulmonary delivery. This investigation was attempted to increase the concentration of amikacin for the treatment of cystic fibrosis lung infections. Drug-loaded cholesterol SLNs and free drug were administered to male rats through pulmonary and intravenous delivery routes, respectively. Pulmonary delivery reduced the drug side effects in kidneys and also prolonged the drug dosing interval since the drug was released in a sustained manner, thereby improving patient adherence [64] (Fig. 12.4). Sildenafil-loaded SLNs were developed for the treatment of pulmonary arterial hypertension by Paranjpe et al. [65]. They used phospholipids and triglycerides as the lipids and microchannel homogenization technique for production of SLNs. From wide-angle X-ray diffraction and differential scanning calorimetric studies it was found that polymorphic transitions occurred during SLN preparation thereby converting intermediate β' form to stable β form. The particle size analyses revealed that the blank SLNs maintained consistent particle sizes over a period of 6 months when compared with sildenafil-loaded SLNs. The drug-loaded SLNs showed increase in particle size after manufacturing and further increase within weeks of storage. Particle size was found to change as a function of emulsifier concentration after nebulization and redispersion of the SLNs. Particle sizes were smaller than 1 μm throughout.

7.1.5 Rectal Administration

Rectal administration is frequently used for pediatric patients. Parenteral and rectal routes of administration are preferred when quick therapeutic response is required. Rectally administered drugs are found to achieve better plasma levels and therapeutic effectiveness when compared with orally or intramuscularly administered drugs of similar dose [66]. Sznitowska et al. investigated the rectal administration of three different formulations of diazepam, which includes organic-aqueous diazepam rectal solution (containing ethanol, benzyl alcohol, and propylene glycol), submicron emulsion, and SLNs [67]. The submicron emulsion was prepared with 20% w/w medium-chain triglycerides oil, egg lecithin, and poloxamer, whereas the SLNs were prepared with 10% w/v cetyl palmitate and Plantacare 2000 (alkyl glucoside) was used as a nonionic surfactant. About 4 mg/mL of diazepam was incorporated in all the formulations and 2 mg/kg dose was administered to rabbits. The submicron emulsion was found to have similar pharmacokinetics as the solution. However, the relative bioavailability of SLNs was found to be as low as 47%, and hence they concluded that SLNs are not a potential carrier system for the rectal administration of diazepam [67]. This problem could be resolved by using lipids that melt at body temperature.

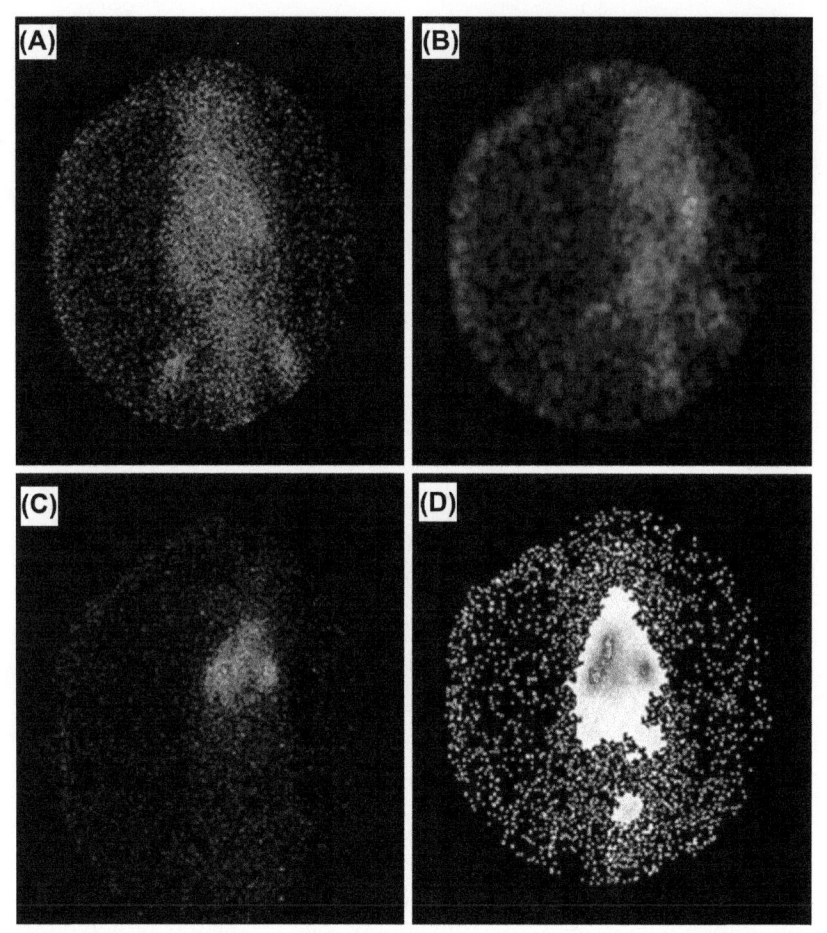

Figure 12.4 Gamma scintigraphy photographs of rats receiving amikacin-loaded SLNs: (A) intravenous (i.v.) after 0.5 h, (B) i.v. after 6 h, (C) pulmonary after 0.5 h, and (D) pulmonary after 6 h. *(Reproduced with permission from Varshosaz J, Ghaffari S, Mirshojaei S, Jafarian A, Atyabi F, Kobarfard F, Azarmi S. Biodistribution of amikacin solid lipid nanoparticles after pulmonary delivery. BioMed Res Int 2013;2013.)*

7.1.6 Ocular Administration

SLNs have been shown to improve interaction with ocular mucosa due to their biocompatible and mucoadhesive properties. Hence, SLNs prolong the drug duration in the cornea [18,42]. Cavalli et al. evaluated SLNs as drug delivery system for topical ocular administration of the drug tobramycin [68]. The formulated SLNs had an average diameter of less than 100 nm and a polydispersity index below 0.2. Longer retention times on the corneal surface and in the conjunctival sac were obtained with drug-free, fluorescent SLNs compared with an aqueous fluorescent solution. Tobramycin SLNs were found to produce significantly higher tobramycin bioavailability in the aqueous humor of rabbits that were topically administered with tobramycin SLNs containing 0.3% tobramycin when compared with an equal dose of tobramycin administered by standard commercial eye drops. Hence, it was concluded that SLNs are a promising drug delivery system for the ocular administration of tobramycin [68].

7.2 Application of Solid Lipid Nanoparticles for Delivery of Hydrophilic Drugs: PEG Coating

To avoid the uptake by phagocytic cells and to improve the biodistribution of drugs for a prolonged time, surface modification of SLNs using PEG polymers has been reported [69,70]. PEG polymers consist of hydrophilic and hydrophobic residues that help to incorporate the lipophilic SLN by shell formation surrounding it (Fig. 12.5) [52]. Thus PEG attaches covalently to SLNs and sterically stabilizes them with formation of a hydrophilic protective layer. This prevents aggregation of nanoparticles and improves the overall formulation stability. In a study, levothyroxine, a poorly soluble drug, was formulated into SLN by microemulsion technique. It was then coated using PEG-100-S. It was found that there was an increase in stability of SLN in varied pH of the gastrointestinal tract. There was a reduction in the zeta potential values from −40.0 to −23.0 mV for uncoated and PEG 100-S-coated SLN. This could be attributed to partial surface charge neutralization by PEG coating [71].

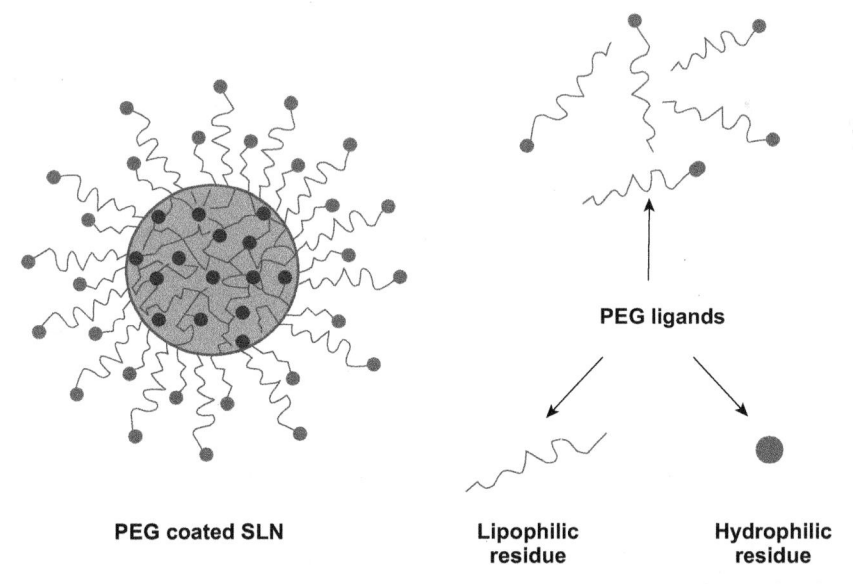

Figure 12.5 Polyethylene glycol (PEG)-coated solid lipid nanoparticle (SLN) and its molecular residues. *(Modified from Üner M, Yener G. Importance of solid lipid nanoparticles (SLN) in various administration routes and future perspectives. Int J Nanomedicine 2007;2:289.)*

7.3 SLNs as Potential Carriers of Anticancer Agents

Lipid nanoparticles have been used to incorporate various anticancer agents. These have been evaluated adequately for their in vitro and in vivo efficacies. SLNs have been demonstrated to have lesser side effects with an increase in the efficacy and residence time of cytotoxic drugs [72]. Use of chemotherapy for the treatment of solid tumors has faced challenges and the outcomes mostly remain unsatisfactory. The response rates of chemotherapy for pancreatic cancer, esophageal cancer, and ovarian cancer have been found to be as low as 20% [73]. At present, more than 85% of human cancers are solid tumors [74]. Cytotoxic drugs that are administered conventionally are highly unpredictable, as they are found to bind extensively to body tissues and serum proteins [73]. Delivery of the active ingredient specifically to tumor cells is very important for appropriate therapeutic activity, as if it is inadequate, regrowth of the tumor cells and/or development of resistant cells may occur. Cytotoxic drugs pose toxicity even to the nontarget cells, especially, rapidly dividing cells of bone marrow and gastrointestinal tract [73]. Use of chemotherapeutic agents results in many side effects (acute or chronic) such as alopecia, vomiting, depression, anemia, mouth sores, nausea, thrombocytopenia, and neutropenia due their poor specificity. They often lead to inconvenience and discomfort and in some cases may even cause death [75].

A significant portion of the new cancer cases found every year is drug resistant. Drug resistance occurs because the cancers either are inherently untreatable or are resistant to the broad spectrum of anticancer agents and their combinations. If particular tumor cells exhibit simultaneous resistance to a number of chemically and functionally different chemotherapeutic agents, they are said to be multidrug resistant [76]. Solid tumor cells are found to have more drug permeation barriers, which prevent the drug to attain adequate concentration inside the tumor cells and hence cancer cells prove to be more resistant to chemotherapy than normal cells [73]. Newer agents such as monoclonal antibodies, cytokines, viral/nonviral gene vectors, and genetically engineered cells have been developed for the delivery of anticancer drugs to the tumors. These agents, being large in size, pose a challenge to deliver to the tumor cells [74].

7.3.1 Significance of Solid Lipid Nanoparticles as Anticancer Carriers

SLNs are found to have "enhanced permeation and retention" (EPR) effect. Tumor tissues have pathophysiological and anatomical imperfections that are absent in the normal cells. Nanoparticles, proteins, polymer drug conjugates, and other macromolecules accumulate selectively in these solid tumor cells. This phenomenon is used to target the tumor cells and is called the EPR effect [77]. The vasculature of the tumor cells varies from that of the normal tissue cells. The tumor cells have irregular-shaped, dilated, leaky, and defective blood vessels. Also, they feature disorganized endothelial cells with large fenestrations with the absence of or abnormality in the perivascular cells and the basement membrane or smooth-muscle layer. A wide lumen and poor lymphatic drainage are the representative features of tumor tissues. These characteristics enable extensive passage of blood plasma components like macromolecules, nanoparticles, and lipid particles into the tumor tissue. These macromolecules are retained in the tumor because of the slow venous return in the tumor tissue and its poor lymphatic clearance leading to EPR [78].

Cytotoxic anticancer agents are found to be heterogeneous. As there are different classes of compounds that act as anticancer agents, there is diversity in their molecular structure and physicochemical properties. Polymeric material may not bind to this diverse group of anticancer actives. However, SLNs are versatile and have the ability to incorporate these cytotoxic agents. The newer variations of SLNs such as polymer–lipid hybrid nanoparticles and lipid–drug conjugate nanoparticles are capable of incorporating even hydrophilic drugs. A wide variety of lipids and hard fats can be utilized to prepare SLNs. Also, most of the emulsifiers approved by the drug regulatory agencies can be used to formulate SLNs [73]. Yang et al. performed a study to investigate the specific targeting of an anticancer drug camptothecin after incorporation into SLNs administered via intravenous administration and compared it with camptothecin solution [45]. They used the HPH technique to formulate the SLNs. They were successful in producing SLNs with a mean diameter of 196.8 nm and a zeta potential of -69.3 mV with prolonged in vitro drug release of up to 1 week. The area under the curve and mean residence time of the camptothecin SLNs in the tested organs such as the brain, heart, and reticuloendothelial cells containing organs were found to be much higher than the camptothecin solution. These data demonstrate SLN's potential as a sustained drug release and targeting drug delivery system [45].

Chen et al. investigated two types of long-circulating SLNs as colloidal carriers of paclitaxel formulated with Brij78 and Poloxamer F68, respectively [79]. Pharmacokinetics of these was compared with the injection of paclitaxel formulated in Cremophor EL in Kun Ming mice. It was found that the paclitaxel-loaded SLNs had longer half-lives compared with paclitaxel injection [79]. Paclitaxel was used against gliomas and other brain metastases [79]. Paclitaxel, being poorly permeable through the blood–brain barrier, and due to serious side effects of the paclitaxel solvent Cremophor ELR, was incorporated into cetyl alcohol/polysorbate nanoparticles. They used in situ rat brain perfusion model to evaluate the brain uptake of the nanoparticles. The drug brain uptake was found to increase significantly following entrapment of paclitaxel in nanoparticles [79]. Lee et al. developed a formulation of paclitaxel-loaded SLNs intended for parenteral administration [87]. Hot homogenization technique was used with trimyristin as a solid lipid core and egg phosphatidylcholine and PEGylated phospholipid as stabilizers. The particles were around 200 nm in size and had a zeta potential of 38 mV suggesting its applicability for parenteral use. Cytotoxicity was tested on the MCF-7 breast cancer cell line and the OVCAR-3 human ovarian cancer cell line and were found to be comparable with those of a commercially available Cremophor EL-based paclitaxel formulation [80].

Tamoxifen-loaded SLNs were investigated by Fontana et al. against breast cancer [81]. The SLNs were prepared by microemulsion and precipitation techniques. The formulated SLNs were found to have dimensions suitable for parenteral administration. The SLNs in the intact form demonstrated a prolonged release of drug following in vitro plasmatic drug release studies. Also, the in vitro antiproliferative studies carried out on MCF-7, human breast cancer cell line, indicated an antitumoral activity comparable with the free drug. The results indicated SLNs to be a potential carrier system for the prolonged delivery of drug via intravenous administration [81]. SLNs can be used to actively target tumors at a specific site such as brain tumors by modifying the physicochemical properties of the surface thereby modifying the biodistribution of the lipid nanoparticles [82,83].

7.3.2 Incorporation of Hydrophilic Anticancer Actives in Solid Lipid Nanoparticles

It is obvious that since lipids are the main constituent of SLNs, lipophilic drugs are more efficiently incorporated into SLNs. There are quite a few anticancer drugs that are hydrophilic and ionic in nature. The examples of water-soluble anticancer drugs include 5-fluorouracil and mitomycin C. Also, there are a few lipophilic anticancer agents that are better utilized in their salt form as they allow diluting and administering with the aqueous vehicles [73]. Bhandari et al. investigated the effect of use of different lipids and lipid combinations to enhance the entrapment efficiency of a hydrophilic drug isoniazid [84]. They were successful in proving that after the use of appropriate lipid combination in an appropriate ratio, the entrapment efficiency of a hydrophilic drug such as isoniazid could be significantly increased. They achieved an entrapment efficiency of approximately 84%, which is considerably higher than other reported data [84]. In a similar study, Shah et al. investigated the entrapment efficiency of a water-soluble drug, ciprofloxacin hydrochloride [85]. It was found that SLNs could be potentially utilized as hydrophilic drug carriers with improved entrapment efficiency and controlled release of the drug. Liu et al. used phospholipid complexes technology to incorporate hydrophilic drug diclofenac sodium in SLNs [86]. This technology was used to improve the solubility of diclofenac sodium in the lipid. They prepared SLNs by modified emulsion/solvent evaporation method. They were successful in formulating SLNs with small particle size of approximately 200 nm and a high entrapment efficiency of around 75%, incorporating the given hydrophilic drug diclofenac sodium [86].

8. STABILITY CONCERNS OF SOLID LIPID NANOPARTICLES

For a drug delivery system to be ideal, the system must have the following properties: sufficient drug loading, stable in environment conditions, controlled and targeted release, easy and inexpensive scale-up procedure, selective for the site, biodegradable, nontoxic, and nonimmunogenic. Thus merely achieving the knowledge of newer products does not necessarily confirm their successful commercialization. In this regard, SLNs happen to face many pharmaceutical and nonpharmaceutical challenges. SLNs are more stable formulations than liposomes and they confer prolonged drug release with no sterilization problems. Some SLN formulations are prone to gelation after certain period of storage time; usually this is avoided by changing the lipid composition and with the use of stabilizing surfactant mixtures [87]. Various factors affecting the stability of SLNs are briefly discussed in this section.

8.1 Influence of Shear Forces and Lipid Concentration

Shear forces, such as pushing through the needle of a syringe, promote gelation in some suboptimally stabilized formulations of SLN. In some studies, Compritol SLN was stored in a shaking bath at 20°C at a frequency of 70 cycles per minute to induce and observe the process in a controlled manner. The degree of crystallinity and particle size were determined every day over a period of 2 weeks. In dispersions with a lipid concentration of 10% particle aggregation could be detected after 3 days. The particle diameter increased from 0.77 ± 0.01 μm up to 23.34 ± 0.19 μm. The crystallinity increased with increasing time in the aqueous SLN dispersion and after solidification in the gel. The samples showed gelling within 5 days, and the resulting gel became increasingly solid with storage time. The lipid concentration was reduced from 10% to 5% and 2% to improve the stability of the SLN dispersion. The 10% stock SLN was diluted with deionized water and the ratio of lipid versus surfactant was the same. A reduction in aggregation was observed due to a lower probability of particle collision during the shaking process from a lower particle concentration [87]. The 5% SLN dispersion did not form a gel up to 2 weeks. The particle size increased after day 5, and solid particles were detected visually. The enthalpy increase was lower when compared with the 10% lipid concentration. The particle size of the 2% dispersion remained the same (280.1 ± 5.0 nm) at day 0 and 282.1 ± 3.9 nm after 14 days.

8.2 Influence of the Surface of the Packing Material

To study the effect of contact between the particles and the surface of the packing material, studies were done by varying the ratio of volume to contact surface in vials. Some glass vials were filled up to the top, and some were filled to only one-third capacity with a 10% Compritol SLN dispersion and stored in a shaking bath at 20°C and 70 cycles per minute. Gelation was accelerated and occurred 2 days quicker in the vials with a low volume to surface ratio. Aggregation and gelation of particles is not usually promoted by a particle—particle contact, but rather by a particle to vial surface contact. Droplets in emulsions coalesce through adherence to the wall of the container, and similarities exist in SLNs and oil-in-water emulsions since the inner lipid phase is stabilized by surfactants.

8.3 Properties of the Lipids: SLNs Versus Bulk Material

Energy input causes destabilization in Compritol SLNs at higher kinetic energy, leading to oscillation of lipid molecules promoting frequent collisions [87]. The number of particle contacts is further increased by shear forces that cause a partial ripping off and damage to the surfactant film on the surface of the particle, promoting aggregation. Freitas et al. showed that the fat fraction of Compritol SLNs is not completely solidified, as indicated from the recrystallization index. The enthalpy of the physical mixture of the excipients were compared with the recrystallization indices calculated from the enthalpy of SLNs by DSC. During storage conditions, the Compritol dispersion is stable at 8°C in the dark, recrystallization index increased slightly to about 87%. The gelling system showed higher crystallinity of 130%; this indicates that the whole fat fraction was solid. These changes are possibly because of the energetic changes occurring due to partial destruction of the surfactant film, and with particle collision, the lipid solidifies by bridging the particles.

8.4 Stability and Storage Conditions

SLNs and nanostructured lipid carriers (NLC) may contain additional colloidal structures, including mixed micelles, micelles, liposomes, and nanoemulsions [88]. SLNs/NLCs contain additional features such as various polymorphic modifications, supercooled melts, and nonspherical shapes and all these eventually affect the stability of the drug delivery system. During storage, there are several stability problems such as increase in particle size, gelation of the dispersion, and drug expulsion from the lipid matrix. Gelation occurs when networks and lipid bridges exist between the lipid particles [89]. In hot homogenization, the first product formed is supercooled melt, which usually has high drug-loading capacity, but because the lipid transforms to lipid crystals, there is a decrease in the lipid drug-loading capacity and eventually drug is expelled from the lipid matrix.

SLNs/NLCs physical stability is generally studied by evaluating measurements of particle size (photon correlation spectroscopy, laser diffraction), zeta potential (electrophoretic light scattering), and thermal analysis (DSC). Many studies have indicated that the physical stability of SLN dispersion is more than a year [44,90−92]. The study reported by Frietas et al. assessed the effect of light and temperature on the physical stability of SLN dispersions. The study shows that light and temperature enhanced particle growth and that gelation of the particles occurred within 7 days and 3 months storage in artificial light and day light, respectively. However, in the dark condition, the particle growth started after 4 months storage, zeta potentials decreased from −24.7 to below −18 mV when stored in light. They also found that the particle size was increased at elevated temperature that resulted in melting the lipids and modifying the lipid matrix. On the contrary, there was no significant change in particle size when stored in the refrigerator for more than 3 months. Also, upon particle growth the zeta potential decreased from −24.7

to −15 mV. Developing and optimizing storage conditions can improve and enhance the physical stability of SLN formulations [87]. Storage temperature has been found to have a profound effect on the quality of SLNs and it was found that SLNs stored at 5°C ± 3°C were stable beyond 1 year [90]. The particle size did not increase significantly after 1 year of storage, and the entrapment efficiency decreased by 9%. Total drug content was reduced by 3%, suggesting that the SLNs retained their potency beyond the 1-year study period. Long-term stability for SLNs can be performed by storing the formulation in three different environments, at 4°C, room temperature, and at 40°C. Approximately 10 mg SLNs was placed in a glass vial and diluted with 10 mL water and after vortexing and sonication the samples were subjected to particle size analysis [93].

The stability of an SLN formulation is dependent on components added to formulate the product, including the type of lipid used and the emulsifying agent [94]. Studies have shown that SLNs stored at refrigerated temperature 4°C ± 1°C were more stable as this storage did not significantly change the particle size and entrapment efficiency when compared with particles stored in room temperature [95]. The lipid transformations in SLNs can be produced by input of kinetic energy such as temperature and light. This leads to changes of the melting point of the lipid and causes transformation of β′ and α to β polymorph and this is usually accompanied by gel formation. However, formulations stored in the refrigerator in dark conditions were found to withstand transformations [89].

Chemical investigation of the stability of the lipids used in SLNs was performed by gas chromatography along with transmethylation of the lipids at the methyl esters of the fatty acids. The idea here was to extract the lipid from the aqueous SLN dispersions [96]. In the study performed by Radomska-Soukharev, the formulation incubated at 25°C, in which the lipid was made of triglycerides and Dynasan 118, showed the highest chemical stability [96]. Spray drying is used in SLNs to increase or prolong stability especially for preparations intended for intravenous administration. Spray drying was investigated for SLNs as an alternative method to lyophilization to convert liquid dispersions into a dry powder. For spray drying to be effective, the melting point of the lipid matrix should be greater than 70°C. Aqueous dispersions of SLNs can be converted by spray drying into a dry powder that can be stored for extended periods of time [97]. The spraying parameters and the chemical nature of the lipid phase, as well as the redispersion medium, influenced the particle size of the final dried SLN powder [97].

Lyophilization also has been found to enhance the stability of SLNs. Cryoprotectants such as sucrose, dextrose, trehalose, and mannitol were found to be beneficial to retain the integrity of SLNs during and after lyophilization. SLNs that are lyophilized in the absence of cryoprotectants produced severe particle aggregation [98]. Trehalose is considered to be the most effective cryoprotectant in terms of inhibiting SLN particle growth [99]. A study done by Ghaffari et al. showed that SLNs of 150 nm size increased to 190 nm after lyophilization. However, at a higher temperature, the stored, freeze-dried particles did not have any significant particle size enlargement. Amikacin-loaded SLNs were designed to target the *Pseudomonas aeruginosa* in order to reduce its dose or decrease the frequency of administration with the goal of reducing its side effects during long-term treatment. Amikacin-loaded SLNs stored in aqueous dispersion form without freeze-drying showed rapid particle growth at increasing temperatures. Zeta potential of SLNs lyophilized was higher than those before lyophilization and the polydispersity index after freeze-drying was less than 0.5. Activity of amikacin expressed no change after lyophilization, and the release profile of the drug did not change even when particles were stored at various temperatures. There was a burst release in all the conditions stored [98]. Based on various stability results, lyophilization is accepted as a suitable method to increase particle stability for long-term storage. Zeta potential of particles increased after freeze-drying, which may suggest that the risk of aggregation and enlargement of particles after redispersion is decreased. Release profile of amikacin SLNs increased with increasing temperature partly because the lipid melts at higher temperature and causes changes in the crystalline structure of the lipid. The lipid content of the SLN dispersion should not exceed 5% to prevent an increase in particle size. Lyophilization can compromise the protective effect of the surfactant [100]. SLN aggregation can be decreased by the addition of cryoprotectors and to obtain a better redispersion of the dry product. In the field of liposomes, the influences of the cryoprotectants have been widely investigated on the quality of the lyophilizates. Cryoprotectants favor the glassy state of the frozen sample and they decrease the osmotic activity of water and crystallization by preventing contact between discrete lipid nanoparticles [101–107]. They serve as a pseudohydration shell by interacting with the polar head groups of the surfactants. Morphology studies performed by Ghaffari et al. showed that particles lyophilized and redispersed did not change their particle size significantly and verified that the shape and size of the SLNs are not influenced by the freeze-drying method [108].

8.5 Gelling Tendency: Temperature Versus Shear Forces

In Compritol SLNs, the destabilization process and recrystallization behavior induced by temperature resulted in firm solid gels that are highly viscous by the effect of shear forces. DSC measurements over a period of 14 days on a 10% dispersion that was stored at 50°C demonstrated an increase in melting point and crystal fraction. At the higher temperature, the shoulder caused by incorporated water was detected after 1 week. The melting point of 72.3°C and the shape of the DSC curve were similar to that of the bulk lipid material after 2 weeks storage. However, Compritol samples containing 10% stored at room temperature in a shaker demonstrated a different crystallization behavior [87]. After 5 days, the water shoulder disappeared, and the enthalpy peaks at 50°C storage did not narrow much. The melting point increased from 68.9°C at day 0 to 70.0°C at day 14. The 5% lipid dispersions behaved similar to the freshly prepared SLNs from day 0 until day 7, except for the missing water shoulder on the DSC curve. The curve is more round and blunt, and the melting point increased to a higher temperature after 14 days.

8.6 Physical Stability

SLNs contain features such as various polymorphic modifications, supercooled melts, and nonspherical shapes, and all these eventually affect the stability of the drug delivery system. During storage, there are several stability problems such as an increase in particle size, gelation of the dispersion, and drug expulsion from the lipid matrix. The physical stability of SLNs is generally studied by evaluating measurements of particle size (photon correlation spectroscopy, laser diffraction), zeta potential (electrophoretic light scattering), and thermal analysis (DSC). Many studies have indicated that the physical stability of SLN dispersions is more than a year [87–89]. SLNs are prone to instabilities because of the complex crystallization behavior due to occurrence of polymorphic transitions. Such transitions can decide the location of drug entrapment with the drug either being integrated into the matrix or attached to the surface of the submicron particle. The following changes in lipids and colloidal lipid dispersion mostly affect the physical stability of SLNs.

8.6.1 Physical Stability due to Changes in Lipids
8.6.1.1 Gelation

Some SLN formulations are prone to gelation after a certain period of storage time. Gelation occurs when networks and lipid bridges exist between the lipid particles [19]. Usually, this is avoided by changing the lipid composition and with the use of stabilizing surfactant mixtures. It is desirable to use a specific formulation in some cases because of toxicological considerations and stabilization of incorporated drugs against chemical degradation. Certain surfactant mixtures produced drug accumulation in the outer shell of SLNs [87]. The lipid gelation process is accelerated with increasing storage temperature and with increasing light exposure. The addition of a coemulsifying surfactant with high mobility such as glycocholate can retard or prevent gelation [109].

The aqueous SLN dispersions are generally stable for up to 3 years, but some systems have shown an increase in particle size, subsequently leading to gelation. Freitas and Müller conducted a study to investigate the factors responsible for the destabilization of SLNs [89]. For this purpose, they formulated a poloxamer 188-stabilized Compritol SLN formulation. Its stability was tested as a function of three parameters viz. storage temperature, light exposure, and packing material (untreated and siliconized vials of glass quality I). They found that the energy introduction led to an increase in the particle size and gelation. Also, there was a reduction in the zeta potential from approximately −25 to −15 mV. The packing material did not impose any significant effects. They came to a conclusion that by optimizing the storage conditions, a stability of 3 years could be achieved for the less stable aqueous Compritol SLNs [89]. In another study, Freitas

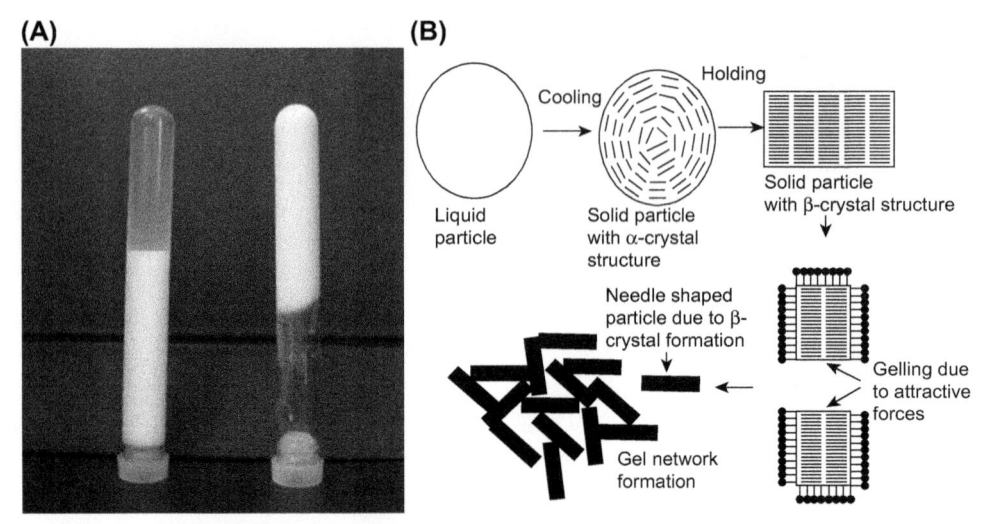

Figure 12.6 (A) Gel formation of solid lipid nanoparticles after cooling at 5°C, after holding for 5 min (left) and after holding for 60 min (right). (B) Schematic representation of gelation mechanism. *(Reproduced with permission from Helgason T, Awad T, Kristbergsson K, McClements DJ, Weiss J. Influence of polymorphic transformations on gelation of tripalmitin solid lipid nanoparticle suspensions. J Am Oil Chemists Soc 2008;85:501−511.)*

and Müller investigated the mechanism of gelation of aqueous dispersions of the SLNs [87]. They exposed Compritol SLNs to different temperatures, packing materials, and varying light exposure. Also, SLNs were subjected to stress by shear forces for short-term tests and a long-term study of 3 years. Thermal analysis and particle size analysis were used as the tools of analyses. They found that after SLN production by hot homogenization of the melted lipid, the Compritol SLNs crystallize in a mixture of stable β' with unstable polymorphs (α, sub α). There was a significant increase in the recrystallization index due to light, temperature, and shear forces because of transformation of the lipid to β' modification leading to formation of a gel. SLNs that have a mixture of polymorphic modifications are physically stable and an increase in their crystallinity index is slow when compared with SLNs containing single polymorph during storage. A similar study was conducted, examining the aggregation and gelation of tripalmitin SLNs. The rapid α to β polymorphic transitions attributed to the observed gelation of SLNs [110] (Fig. 12.6A and B).

8.6.1.2 Lipid Modification
SLN suspensions have complex additional stability aspects compared with other lipid systems because of their crystallization kinetics and the polymorphism of the dispersed lipid [3]. Solid lipids show crystallinity and have a definite melting point as they move from solid to liquid state [111], an important aspect that should be considered when formulating SLNs.

The matrix of SLNs is frequently composed of glycerides and the lipids that make SLNs solid at room temperature [112]. Fusion of the β form occurred at high temperature in long-chain triglycerides (tristearin, tripalmitin; 68°C and 60°C, respectively) and at lower temperature in short-chain triglycerides (trimyristin, trilaurin; 53°C and 43°C, respectively). The size characteristics of the structure can alter the solidification phenomenon [113,114]. Lipid nanocrystals melt at about 3–5°C lower than the bulk material as a result of their small particle size [115]. Triglycerides that are used in the preparation of nanoparticles are solid at room temperature and did not crystallize upon cooling to common storage temperatures. Particles remained without crystallization in the liquid form for a number of months. Westesen and Bunjes found that particles colloidally dispersed in trimyristin and trilaurin remained in the liquid state at room temperature for several months. When the dispersion was cooled below the critical crystallization temperature, no change occurred in particle crystallization. The particles can remain in a supercooled liquid state for a long period, and if this occurs, the emulsions of supercooled melts were formulated instead of SLNs [114]. The supercooled state of the droplets was not thermodynamically stable and upon long-term storage gradual crystallization cannot be excluded due to the fact that the properties of the product will change. Such gelling or the expulsion of the incorporated drug results because of the crystallization process that leads to instabilities in SLNs. When crystalline reorientation occurs, this can result in changes of the charge on the particle surface and eventually on the measured zeta potential, and the crystals can possess different charge densities. For glyceryl tribehenate SLNs, it resulted in an increase in zeta potential from -25 to -15 mV [89].

Polymorphism in SLNs is the ability to reveal different unit cell structure in crystals, originating from molecular conformations and molecular packing. Polymorphism is an important physical stability process that affects stability in solid dosage forms because various polymorphs have different thermodynamic properties such as melting points, X-ray diffraction, and solubility [111]. The main polymorphs in glycerides are the α, β′, and β forms; the α form can quickly transform to a form with better chain packing such as the β′ form. The transition of triglycerides of liquid melt from α to β via the β′ was the pathway to the optimum packing form of the molecules. During storage at elevated temperatures, this unstable form gradually transforms toward the most stable form while losing the initial spherical surface structure [116]. Polymorphism influenced the nanoparticle content, and the presence of oil allowed for higher drug loads [49,50]. Jenning showed that the in vitro results on skin showed that when water evaporates, it leads to solid modification changes of SLN dispersion causing drugs to be expelled from the lipids resulting in an increase in penetration of drug into the skin [117]. The problem of lipid modification is not always solved with assignments to α, β, or β′ form. The complexity increases as a result of many subspecies and the interactions of the lipid with the emulsifiers. Westesen's group demonstrated that the decisive factor for the physical properties of SLNs is the particle size [118].

8.6.2 Physical Stability due to Changes in Colloidal Lipid Dispersion
8.6.2.1 Ostwald Ripening
In an SLN suspension, the smaller particles can dissolve preferentially when compared with large particles in the suspension medium. The dissolved lipid then deposits on the larger particulate surfaces, thereby resulting in a growth in the particle size of the larger particles at the expense of the smaller particles. This phenomenon is called Ostwald ripening and is also seen in emulsions, causing an increase in the droplet size of the dispersed phase. SLNs are in general resistant to coalescence but are prone to creaming or gelling due to particle collision [115]. Ostwald ripening can be partially inhibited by narrowing particle size distribution, which minimizes the saturation solubility difference and drug concentration gradients within the medium. Stabilizers can reduce the interfacial tension between the solid particles and liquid medium, thereby preventing Ostwald ripening. Ostwald ripening can be mitigated by stabilizers as long as they do not enhance the drug solubility [119,120]. It depends on the granulometry of particles, in which species flux occurs from small to large droplets via the continuous phase.

8.6.3 Coalescence
Coalescence is an irreversible rupture of the emulsion resulting in phase separation. SLN dispersions tend to cream or gel after particle contact. By contrast, rigid solid particles are expected to be stable against coalescence. Coalescence occurs when two or more droplets merge to form a single larger droplet. This process leads to an irreversible breakdown, referred to as cracking of an emulsion [121]. In the absence of a primary maximum, rapid aggregation can take place, leading to the formation of a strong, irreversible aggregated structure. A network of three-dimensional aggregates with interconnections eventually fuses into a compact pack of particles, causing an irreversible caking of the dispersion [121].

8.7 Chemical Stability
8.7.1 Phospholipid Stability
Membranes in liposomes are primarily constituted of phospholipids, and these phospholipids consist of ester bonds, which are sensitive to hydrolysis [122]. The organization of the lipid assembly can change from lamellar to a micellar system because of the chemical hydrolysis of the liposomal phospholipids [123]. Lysophosphatidylcholine and fatty acids are formed [124] and membrane permeability is increased [125] when these transformations occur. The peroxidation of unsaturated acyl chains is generally accompanied by phospholipid degradation [125]. The permeability of the bilayer was increased by the lipid peroxidation. The degradation process resulted in a number of products with highly different chemical natures [122,125]. As a result of these degradation processes, phospholipid use in such formulations is very limited and is currently substituted with nonionic surfactants to circumvent degradation problems [125].

8.7.2 Triglycerides Stability

When triglyceride hydrolysis occurs, it degrades to mono- or diglycerides with free fatty acids. They are less susceptible to hydrolysis than the external phospholipids because of their internal location in SLNs.

9. TOXICITY ASPECTS OF SOLID LIPID NANOPARTICLES

SLNs are made from physiological compounds, and one can predict that they are well tolerated in living systems because the metabolic pathway to degrade the lipids exists in the body. However, the toxicity of the emulsifiers has to be evaluated. For peroral or transdermal administration and intramuscular or subcutaneous injection, appropriate surfactants have to be used. Particle size is not a critical issue for these administration routes because the performance of the SLN system might decrease because of low contents of microparticles, but will not cause toxic events. For parenteral administration, the absence of pyrogens must be assessed because SLNs may interfere with the pyrogen tests (limulus test) and cause gelation.

Originally, SLNs were designed for controlled release of drugs after intravenous injection. But because of the change in the lipid droplet (nanoemulsions) to a solid core (SLN), this should decrease drug delivery due to decreased drug diffusion coefficients. For intravenous injection, particle size distribution is a key issue due to the danger of capillary blockage; this could result in death due to fat embolism. The diameter of the capillaries is between 5 and 10 μm. For safety reasons, the particle size should be completely in the submicron range. On the other hand, nanoemulsions for parenteral nutrition in microparticles exceeding the size of the capillaries have been found in commercials [126,127]. Larger amounts of microdroplets are tolerated by human body, but this should not be the case with SLNs because a solid lipid is not deformable as oil in contrast to nanoemulsions. Blockage of capillary will occur if the particle size exceeds the size of the diameter of blood vessels. In the syringe needle, gelation of the low-viscosity SLN dispersion might occur, and this forms a viscous suspension with unacceptable particle size. Serious hurdles for the development of SLN dispersion suitable for intravenous injection in clinical practice are the solid state of the lipid and the danger of injection-induced gelation. Studies on the interaction of SLN with phagocytizing cells in vitro on human granulocytes have been performed [128,129]. To compare SLNs with polymer particles and to assess the influence of the SLN composition on the phagocytosis rate, a luminol-based chemiluminescence was used. The phagocytosis rate of the poloxamer-stabilized Compritol and cetyl palmitate SLN was lower in comparison with polystyrene nanoparticles [129–131]. To distinguish the small differences in SLN phagocytosis, an indirect chemiluminescence assay was developed [132]. Poloxamine 908 prevented the uptake of Compritol SLN more efficiently than poloxamer 407 [133].

10. DIAGNOSTIC APPLICATIONS OF SOLID LIPID NANOPARTICLES

With the advances in molecular imaging and nanotechnology, strategies in advancing cancer diagnostics, imaging, and drug delivery have been extended to SLNs [134,135]. Many studies have been done to combine therapeutic and diagnostic properties in a single particle [136−138]. The term coined for such integration is "theranostics." Such a combination might help in diagnosis of the disease at an early stage and enable prompt treatment. In addition to increasing in the efficacy and bioavailability of therapeutic or imaging agents, theranostic nanoparticles exhibit selective delivery to tumor cells resulting in enhanced image resolution and decrease in nontarget cell damage associated with chemotherapy [139]. Particulate systems allow sustained and targeted release of drugs with greater transport efficiency by endocytosis [140], synergistic performance, i.e., siRNA codelivery [141], and multimodality diagnosis [142−144], all-in-one single platform. SLNs have been identified as potential platforms for codelivery of diagnostic and therapeutic agent due to their small size and lipophilic nature. Magnetic resonance imaging (MRI) is the commonly used diagnostic technique [145]. The particles of iron oxide, gold, silver, and gadolinium are being explored in MRI to distinguish the damaged cells from the healthy ones.

A study demonstrated the use of SLN-loaded near-infrared quantum dots conjugated to $\alpha v \beta 3$ integrin-specific ligand, i.e., cyclic Arg-Gly-Asp (cRGD), for live animal imaging [146]. These SLNs were injected intravenously to nude mice with breast tumors. Optical imaging was used to study the whole animal biodistribution of SLNs. The results showed that active tumor targeting with cRGD significantly enhanced the distribution in the liver, spleen, and kidneys than the nontargeted SLNs. The authors also concluded that the spectral properties of quantum dots were enhanced by loading them in SLNs by improving the depth of light penetration through the tissue [146]. Another study attempted to develop a novel intravenous delivery system for simultaneous imaging and targeted therapy. Such a theranostic system comprised SLNs of methotrexate, a drug used in the treatment of rheumatoid arthritis, and superparamagnetic iron oxide nanoparticles as the contrast agent for MRI. The monoclonal antibody against the macrophage-specific cell surface receptor, CD64, which is overexpressed in rheumatoid arthritis, was functionalized with SLNs. The SLNs demonstrated low cytotoxicity at concentrations lesser than 500 μg/mL and showed consistent particle size (<250 nm) and zeta potential values (<16 mV), thereby suggesting their role as promising candidates for intravenous theranostic applications [147]. Bae et al. developed an "optically traceable" low-density lipoprotein (LDL)-mimetic SLN incorporated with anticancer combination therapy, paclitaxel and Bcl-2 siRNA [148]. To achieve in situ fluorescence imaging of SLNs delivered to cancer cells, highly fluorescent quantum dots were incorporated into the SLNs as a contrast agent. This codelivery of paclitaxel and Bcl-2 siRNA synergistically enhanced the anticancer activity of paclitaxel through siRNA-induced sensitization of cancer cells to apoptosis. Confocal laser scanning microscopy was used to investigate the cellular uptake of paclitaxel/siRNA complexes. As shown in Fig. 12.7, siRNA was internalized by the cancer cells 2 h after incubation. These results confirmed that paclitaxel/siRNA complexes dissociate inside the cells in just about 2 h after treatment suggesting the potential of LDL-mimetic SLNs as promising carriers for cancer therapy [148].

11. IN VIVO FATE OF SOLID LIPID NANOPARTICLES

The in vivo fate of SLNs will depend mainly on the following factors: the administration route and the SLN interaction with the biological surroundings, which is adsorption of biological material on the particle surface and desorption of SLN components into the

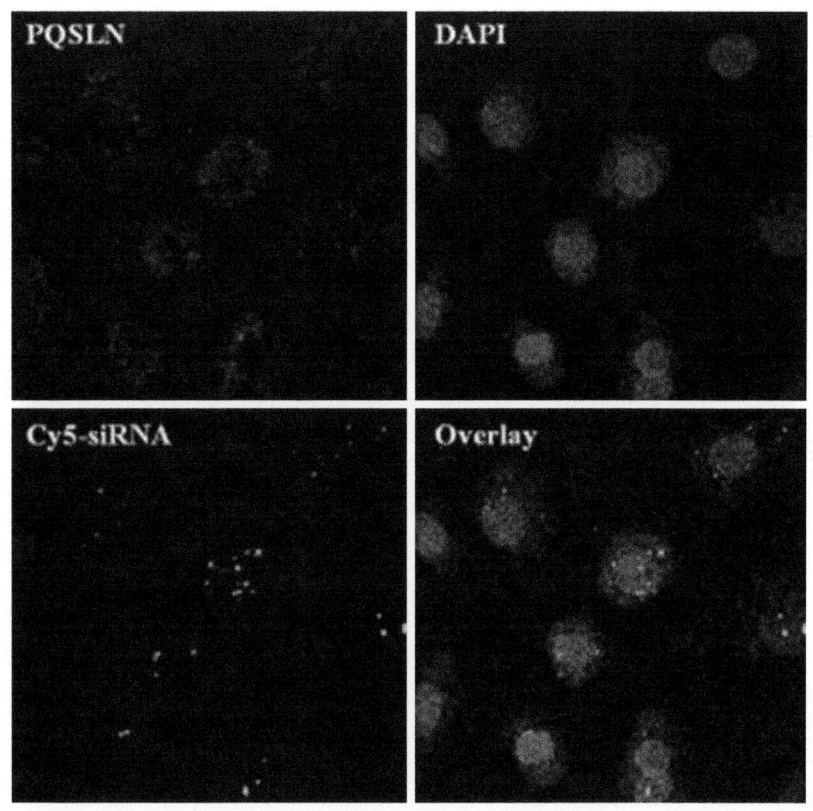

Figure 12.7 Intracellular distribution of paclitaxel/small interfering RNA (siRNA) complexes by confocal scanning microscopy. Green fluorescence (gray in print versions) resembles paclitaxel solid lipid nanoparticle and red region (white in print versions) resembles Cy5-labeled siRNA. *(Reproduced with permission from Bae KH, Lee JY, Lee SH, Park TG, Nam YS. Optically traceable solid lipid nanoparticles loaded with siRNA and paclitaxel for synergistic chemotherapy with in situ imaging. Adv Healthc Mater 2013;2:576−584.)*

biological surrounding. Also, lipid degradation by lipases and esterases via the enzymatic processes is very critical. Lipases are present in various organs and tissues and are the most important enzymes of SLN degradation. They split the ester linkage and form partial glycerides or glycerol and free fatty acids. The oil/water interface activates most lipases and the catalytic center is open [149,150]. Experiments done in vitro indicate that SLNs show different degradation velocities by the lipolytic enzyme pancreatic lipase, which serves as a function of their composition, the lipid matrix, and the stabilizing surfactant [151]. The length of the fatty acid chains in the triglycerides and the surfactants showed SLN degradation dependence. Longer fatty acid chains in the glycerides showed slow degradation. The surfactant effect on the degradation is to accelerate it such as cholic acid sodium salt and to hinder it because of steric stabilization such as poloxamer 407 and poloxamer 188. Tween 80 serves as a steric stabilizer, and results show that the hindering effect on the degradation process was less noticeable than that of poloxamer 407. This correlated with the number of ethylene glycol chains in the molecule that result in the degradation of the SLN through suppressing the lipase/colipase complex.

12. CONCLUSIONS

SLNs have emerged as a promising drug delivery system in recent years. Many drugs having therapeutic activity are highly lipophilic in nature. Incorporation and delivery of such lipophilic active ingredients at the target site have always been a concern. SLNs have been found to have several desirable characteristics required for the delivery of such lipophilic agents to the target site of action. SLNs also efficiently deliver hydrophilic drugs. When compared with other colloidal carrier systems, SLNs are found to be highly stable, being present in the solid form. SLNs share the advantages of both polymeric nanoparticles and nanoemulsions. SLNs, being composed of biocompatible lipids, have shown negligible toxicity after administration or application. Production scale-up of SLNs is easy and economical when compared with that of other colloidal systems. Site-specific delivery and sustained drug delivery are two typical advantages of SLNs. SLNs have been proved to be a potential carrier system for tumor targeting. Cytotoxic drugs are particularly more reactive, unstable, toxic, and structurally and physicochemically diverse when compared with other drug classes. SLNs can accommodate all these different classes of compounds into its solid core.

Stability of drug nanoparticles remains a very challenging issue during pharmaceutical product development. Stability is affected by various factors such as the dosage form, dispersion medium, delivery route, production technique, and the nature of drug molecule: whether it has small or large biomolecules. For SLNs to occupy a considerable place in the pharmaceutical market, it is essential that the pharmaceutical industries along with the academic research groups specialized in the development of new drug delivery systems engage in novel formulation technology and enhance their scale-up production and establish these formulations in the market. Further work has to be undertaken to understand the interaction of SLNs with their biological surroundings such as adsorption/desorption processes, enzymatic degradation, agglomeration, and interaction with endogenous lipid carrier systems. SLN administration through intravenous injection is the most challenging route because it requires absolute control of the particle size. The primary application of SLNs appears to be the dermal route of administration since results from such studies so far are encouraging and promising. To conclude, SLNs are complex systems with obvious advantages when compared with other colloidal carriers. More studies have to be done in terms of understanding the structure and dynamics of SLNs on a molecular level in ex vivo and in vivo conditions. It is expected that in the near future, the modified forms of SLNs such as nanoparticulate lipid carriers (NLC), stealth SLNs, and targeted SLNs with combination drugs will be optimized, thereby reducing side effects and increasing the efficacy to serve as potential carriers of antitumor drugs.

REFERENCES

[1] Di L, Fish PV, Mano T. Bridging solubility between drug discovery and development. Drug Discov Today 2012;17:486—95.
[2] Amidon GL, Lennernäs H, Shah VP, Crison JR. A theoretical basis for a biopharmaceutic drug classification: the correlation of in vitro drug product dissolution and in vivo bioavailability. Pharm Res 1995;12:413—20.
[3] Mehnert W, Mäder K. Solid lipid nanoparticles: production, characterization and applications. Adv Drug Deliv Rev 2001;47:165—96.
[4] Parhi R, Suresh P. Preparation and characterization of solid lipid nanoparticles—a review. Curr Drug Discov Technol 2012;9:2—16.
[5] MuÈller RH, MaÈder K, Gohla S. Solid lipid nanoparticles (SLN) for controlled drug delivery— a review of the state of the art. Eur J Pharm Biopharm 2000;50:161—77.
[6] Pathak K, Keshri L, Shah M. Lipid nanocarriers: influence of lipids on product development and pharmacokinetics. Crit Rev Ther Drug Carr Syst 2011;28.
[7] Lakkadwala S, Nguyen S, Lawrence J, Nauli SM, Nesamony J. Physico-chemical characterisation, cytotoxic activity, and biocompatibility studies of tamoxifen-loaded solid lipid nanoparticles prepared via a temperature-modulated solidification method. J Microencapsul September 1, 2014;31(6): 590—9.
[8] Shah R, Eldridge D, Palombo E, Harding I. Composition and structure. In: Lipid nanoparticles: production, characterization and stability. Springer; 2015. p. 11—22.
[9] Svilenov H, Tzachev C. Solid lipid nanoparticles—a promising drug delivery system. In: Nanomedicine. Manchester: One Central Press; 2014. p. 187—237.
[10] Eldem T, Speiser P, Hincal A. Optimization of spray-dried and-congealed lipid micropellets and characterization of their surface morphology by scanning electron microscopy. Pharm Res 1991;8: 47—54.
[11] Speiser P. Lipidnanopellets als Trägersystem für Arzneimittel zur peroralen Anwendung, European Patent EP, 167825; 1990.
[12] Domb AJ, Maniar M. Liposheres for controlled delivery of substances, in, EP Patent 0,502,119; 1996.
[13] Lucks S, Müller R. Medication vehicles made of solid lipid particles (solid lipid nanospheres-SLN), in, EP Patent 0,605,497; 1999.
[14] zur Mühlen A, Schwarz C, Mehnert W. Solid lipid nanoparticles (SLN) for controlled drug delivery—drug release and release mechanism. Eur J Pharm Biopharm 1998;45:149—55.

[15] Ahlin P, Kristl J, Smid-Korbar J. Optimization of procedure parameters and physical stability of solid lipid nanoparticles in dispersions. Acta Pharm 1998;48:259—67.
[16] Schwarz C, Mehnert W, Müller R. Influence of production parameters of solid lipid nanoparticles (SLN) on the suitability for intravenous injection. Eur J Pharm Biopharm 1994;40:24S.
[17] Friedrich I, Müller-Goymann C. Characterization of solidified reverse micellar solutions (SRMS) and production development of SRMS-based nanosuspensions. Eur J Pharm Biopharm 2003;56:111—9.
[18] Sjöström B, Bergenståhl B. Preparation of submicron drug particles in lecithin-stabilized o/w emulsions I. Model studies of the precipitation of cholesteryl acetate. Int J Pharm 1992;88:53—62.
[19] Siekmann B, Westesen K. Investigations on solid lipid nanoparticles prepared by precipitation in o/w emulsions. Eur J Pharm Biopharm 1996;42:104—9.
[20] Garcia-Fuentes M, Torres D, Alonso M. Design of lipid nanoparticles for the oral delivery of hydrophilic macromolecules. Colloids Surf B Biointerfaces 2003;27:159—68.
[21] Yassin AEB, Anwer MK, Mowafy HA, El-Bagory IM, Bayomi MA, Alsarra IA. Optimization of 5-flurouracil solid-lipid nanoparticles: a preliminary study to treat colon cancer. Int J Med Sci 2010;7:398.
[22] Sjöström B, Bergenståhl B, Kronberg B. A method for the preparation of submicron particles of sparingly water-soluble drugs by precipitation in oil-in-water emulsions. II: influence of the emulsifier, the solvent, and the drug substance. J Pharm Sci 1993;82:584—9.
[23] Sjöstrom B, Kronberg B, Carlfors J. A method for the preparation of submicron particles of sparingly water-soluble drugs by precipitation in oil-in-water emulsions. I: influence of emulsification and surfactant concentration. J Pharm Sci 1993;82:579—83.
[24] Fessi C, Devissaguet JP, Puisieux F, Thies C. Process for the preparation of dispersible colloidal systems of a substance in the form of nanoparticles. 1992 [Google Patents].
[25] Hu F, Yuan H, Zhang H, Fang M. Preparation of solid lipid nanoparticles with clobetasol propionate by a novel solvent diffusion method in aqueous system and physicochemical characterization. Int J Pharm 2002;239:121—8.
[26] Dubes A, Parrot-Lopez H, Abdelwahed W, Degobert G, Fessi H, Shahgaldian P, Coleman AW. Scanning electron microscopy and atomic force microscopy imaging of solid lipid nanoparticles derived from amphiphilic cyclodextrins. Eur J Pharm Biopharm 2003;55:279—82.
[27] Schubert M, Müller-Goymann C. Solvent injection as a new approach for manufacturing lipid nanoparticles—evaluation of the method and process parameters. Eur J Pharm Biopharm 2003;55: 125—31.
[28] Quintanar-Guerrero D, Allemann E, Fessi H, Doelker E. Pseudolatex preparation using a novel emulsion-diffusion process involving direct displacement of partially water-miscible solvents by distillation. Int J Pharm 1999;188:155—64.
[29] Trotta M, Debernardi F, Caputo O. Preparation of solid lipid nanoparticles by a solvent emulsification-diffusion technique. Int J Pharm 2003;257:153—60.
[30] Shahgaldian P, Gualbert J, Aïssa K, Coleman AW. A study of the freeze-drying conditions of calixarene based solid lipid nanoparticles. Eur J Pharm Biopharm 2003;55:181—4.
[31] Shahgaldian P, Quattrocchi L, Gualbert J, Coleman AW, Goreloff P. AFM imaging of calixarene based solid lipid nanoparticles in gel matrices. Eur J Pharm Biopharm 2003;55:107—13.
[32] Cavalli R, Gasco M, Morel S. Behaviour of timolol incorporated in liospheres in the presence of a series of phosphate esters. STP Pharma Sci 1992;2:514—8.
[33] Gasco M, Morel S, Carpignano R. Optimization of the incorporation of deoxycorticosterone acetate in liospheres. Eur J Pharm Biopharm 1992;38:7—10.
[34] Cavalli R, Caputo O, Gasco MR. Solid liospheres of doxorubicin and idarubicin. Int J Pharm 1993; 89:R9—12.
[35] Cavalli R, Morel S, Gasco M, Chetoni P. Preparation and evaluation in vitro of colloidal liospheres containing pilocarpine as ion pair. Int J Pharm 1995;117:243—6.
[36] Morel S, Ugazio E, Cavalli R, Gasco MR. Thymopentin in solid lipid nanoparticles. Int J Pharm 1996;132:259—61.
[37] Cavalli R, Caputo O, Carlotti ME, Trotta M, Scarnecchia C, Gasco MR. Sterilization and freeze-drying of drug-free and drug-loaded solid lipid nanoparticles. Int J Pharm 1997;148:47—54.

[38] Cavalli R, Caputo O, Gasco MR. Preparation and characterization of solid lipid nanospheres containing paclitaxel. Eur J Pharm Sci 2000;10:305—9.
[39] Jenning V, Schäfer-Korting M, Gohla S. Vitamin A-loaded solid lipid nanoparticles for topical use: drug release properties. J Control Release 2000;66:115—26.
[40] Lukowski G, Pflegel P. Electron diffraction of solid lipid nanoparticles loaded with aciclovir. Pharmazie 1997;52:642—3.
[41] Schwarz C, Freitas C, Mehnert W, Muller R. Sterilization and physical stability of drug-free and etomidate-loaded solid lipid nanoparticles. Proc Int Symp Control Release Bioact Mater 1995: 766—7.
[42] Penkler LJ, Müller RH, Runge SA, Ravelli V. Pharmaceutical cyclosporin formulation with improved biopharmaceutical properties, improved physical quality and greater stability, and method for producing said formulation. 2003 [Google Patents].
[43] Heiati H, Tawashi R, Phillips N. Drug retention and stability of solid lipid nanoparticles containing azidothymidine palmitate after autoclaving, storage and lyophilization. J Microencapsul 1998;15: 173—84.
[44] Westesen K, Bunjes H, Koch M. Physicochemical characterization of lipid nanoparticles and evaluation of their drug loading capacity and sustained release potential. J Control Release 1997;48: 223—36.
[45] Yang SC, Lu LF, Cai Y, Zhu JB, Liang BW, Yang CZ. Body distribution in mice of intravenously injected camptothecin solid lipid nanoparticles and targeting effect on brain. J Control Release 1999; 59:299—307.
[46] Demirel M, Yazan Y, Müller R, Kilic F, Bozan B. Formulation and in vitro-in vivo evaluation of piribedil solid lipid micro-and nanoparticles. J Microencapsul 2001;18:359—71.
[47] Jenning V, Mäder K, Gohla SH. Solid lipid nanoparticles (SLN) based on binary mixtures of liquid and solid lipids: a 1 H-NMR study. Int J Pharm 2000;205:15—21.
[48] Westesen K, Siekmann B, Koch MH. Investigations on the physical state of lipid nanoparticles by synchrotron radiation X-ray diffraction. Int J Pharm 1993;93:189—99.
[49] Bunjes H, Westesen K, Koch MH. Crystallization tendency and polymorphic transitions in triglyceride nanoparticles. Int J Pharm 1996;129:159—73.
[50] Jenning V, Thünemann AF, Gohla SH. Characterisation of a novel solid lipid nanoparticle carrier system based on binary mixtures of liquid and solid lipids. Int J Pharm 2000;199:167—77.
[51] Shah R, Eldridge D, Palombo E, Harding I. Lipid nanoparticles: production, characterization and stability. Springer; 2015.
[52] Üner M, Yener G. Importance of solid lipid nanoparticles (SLN) in various administration routes and future perspectives. Int J Nanomedicine 2007;2:289.
[53] Müller RH, Radtke M, Wissing SA. Solid lipid nanoparticles (SLN) and nanostructured lipid carriers (NLC) in cosmetic and dermatological preparations. Adv Drug Deliv Rev 2002;54: S131—55.
[54] Cho H-J, Park JW, Yoon I-S, Kim D-D. Surface-modified solid lipid nanoparticles for oral delivery of docetaxel: enhanced intestinal absorption and lymphatic uptake. Int J Nanomedicine 2014;9:495.
[55] Sarmento B, Martins S, Ferreira D, Souto EB. Oral insulin delivery by means of solid lipid nanoparticles. Int J Nanomedicine 2007;2:743.
[56] Padhye S, Nagarsenker MS. Simvastatin solid lipid nanoparticles for oral delivery: formulation development and in vivo evaluation. Indian J Pharm Sci 2013;75:591.
[57] Sangsen Y, Likhitwitayawuid K, Sritularak B, Wiwattanawongsa K, Wiwattanapatapee R. Novel solid lipid nanoparticles for oral delivery of oxyresveratrol: effect of the formulation parameters on the physicochemical properties and in vitro release. Int J Med Pharm Sci Eng 2013;7:506—13.
[58] Yang S, Zhu J, Lu Y, Liang B, Yang C. Body distribution of camptothecin solid lipid nanoparticles after oral administration. Pharm Res 1999;16:751—7.
[59] Zara GP, Cavalli R, Bargoni A, Fundarò A, Vighetto D, Gasco MR. Intravenous administration to rabbits of non-stealth and stealth doxorubicin-loaded solid lipid nanoparticles at increasing concentrations of stealth agent: pharmacokinetics and distribution of doxorubicin in brain and other tissues. J Drug Target 2002;10:327—35.

[60] Manjunath K, Venkateswarlu V. Pharmacokinetics, tissue distribution and bioavailability of clozapine solid lipid nanoparticles after intravenous and intraduodenal administration. J Control Release 2005; 107:215−28.
[61] Wise DL. Handbook of pharmaceutical controlled release technology. CRC Press; 2000.
[62] Zhang J, Purdon CH, Smith EW. Solid lipid nanoparticles for topical drug delivery. Am J Drug Deliv 2006;4:215−20.
[63] Lippacher A, Müller R, Mäder K. Liquid and semisolid SLN dispersions for topical application: rheological characterization. Eur J Pharm Biopharm 2004;58:561−7.
[64] Varshosaz J, Ghaffari S, Mirshojaei S, Jafarian A, Atyabi F, Kobarfard F, Azarmi S. Biodistribution of amikacin solid lipid nanoparticles after pulmonary delivery. BioMed Res Int 2013;2013.
[65] Paranjpe M, Finke J, Richter C, Gothsch T, Kwade A, Büttgenbach S, Müller-Goymann C. Physicochemical characterization of sildenafil-loaded solid lipid nanoparticle dispersions (SLN) for pulmonary application. Int J Pharm 2014;476:41−9.
[66] Nair R, Arunkumar K, Vishnu Priya K, Sevukarajan M. Recent advances in solid lipid nanoparticle based drug delivery systems. J Biomed Sci Res 2011;3:368−84.
[67] Sznitowska M, Gajewska M, Janicki S, Radwanska A, Lukowski G. Bioavailability of diazepam from aqueous-organic solution, submicron emulsion and solid lipid nanoparticles after rectal administration in rabbits. Eur J Pharm Biopharm 2001;52:159−63.
[68] Cavalli R, Gasco MR, Chetoni P, Burgalassi S, Saettone MF. Solid lipid nanoparticles (SLN) as ocular delivery system for tobramycin. Int J Pharm 2002;238:241−5.
[69] YuDA T, Maruyama K, Iwatsuru M. Prolongation of liposome circulation time by various derivatives of polyethyleneglycols. Biol Pharm Bull 1996;19:1347−51.
[70] Zhang Y, Zhang J. Surface modification of monodisperse magnetite nanoparticles for improved intracellular uptake to breast cancer cells. J Colloid Interface Sci 2005;283:352−7.
[71] Kashanian S, Rostami E. PEG-stearate coated solid lipid nanoparticles as levothyroxine carriers for oral administration. J Nanoparticle Res 2014;16:1−10.
[72] Joshi MD, Müller RH. Lipid nanoparticles for parenteral delivery of actives. Eur J Pharm Biopharm 2009;71:161−72.
[73] Wong HL, Bendayan R, Rauth AM, Li Y, Wu XY. Chemotherapy with anticancer drugs encapsulated in solid lipid nanoparticles. Adv Drug Deliv Rev 2007;59:491−504.
[74] Shenoy V, Vijay I, Murthy R. Tumour targeting: biological factors and formulation advances in injectable lipid nanoparticles. J Pharm Pharmacol 2005;57:411−21.
[75] Lowenthal RM, Eaton K. Toxicity of chemotherapy. Hematol/Oncol Clin N Am 1996;10:967−90.
[76] Krishna R, Mayer LD. Multidrug resistance (MDR) in cancer: mechanisms, reversal using modulators of MDR and the role of MDR modulators in influencing the pharmacokinetics of anticancer drugs. Eur J Pharm Sci 2000;11:265−83.
[77] Matsumura Y, Maeda H. A new concept for macromolecular therapeutics in cancer chemotherapy: mechanism of tumoritropic accumulation of proteins and the antitumor agent SMANCS. Cancer Res 1986;46:6387−92.
[78] Iyer AK, Khaled G, Fang J, Maeda H. Exploiting the enhanced permeability and retention effect for tumor targeting. Drug Discov Today 2006;11:812−8.
[79] Chen D-B, Yang T-Z, Lu W-L, Zhang Q. In vitro and in vivo study of two types of long-circulating solid lipid nanoparticles containing paclitaxel. Chem Pharm Bull 2001;49:1444−7.
[80] Lee M-K, Lim S-J, Kim C-K. Preparation, characterization and in vitro cytotoxicity of paclitaxel-loaded sterically stabilized solid lipid nanoparticles. Biomaterials 2007;28:2137−46.
[81] Fontana G, Maniscalco L, Schillaci D, Cavallaro G, Giammona G. Solid lipid nanoparticles containing tamoxifen characterization and in vitro antitumoral activity. Drug Deliv 2005;12:385−92.
[82] Shaji J, Jain V. Int J Pharm Pharm Sci 2010;2:8−17.
[83] Béduneau A, Saulnier P, Benoit J-P. Active targeting of brain tumors using nanocarriers. Biomaterials 2007;28:4947−67.
[84] Rohit B, Pal KI. A method to prepare solid lipid nanoparticles with improved entrapment efficiency of hydrophilic drugs,. Curr Nanosci 2013;9:211−20.
[85] Shah M, Agrawal Y, Garala K, Ramkishan A. Solid lipid nanoparticles of a water soluble drug, ciprofloxacin hydrochloride. Indian J Pharm Sci 2012;74:434.

[86] Liu D, Chen L, Jiang S, Zhu S, Qian Y, Wang F, Li R, Xu Q. Formulation and characterization of hydrophilic drug diclofenac sodium-loaded solid lipid nanoparticles based on phospholipid complexes technology. J Liposome Res 2014;24:17–26.
[87] Freitas C, Müller RH. Correlation between long-term stability of solid lipid nanoparticles (SLN) and crystallinity of the lipid phase. Eur J Pharm Biopharm 1999;47:125–32.
[88] Wissing SA, Kayser O, Müller RH. Solid lipid nanoparticles for parenteral drug delivery. Adv Drug Deliv Rev 2004;56:1257–72.
[89] Freitas C, Müller RH. Effect of light and temperature on zeta potential and physical stability in solid lipid nanoparticle (SLN) dispersions. Int J Pharm 1998;168:221–9.
[90] Kakkar V, Singh S, Singla D, Kaur IP. Exploring solid lipid nanoparticles to enhance the oral bioavailability of curcumin. Mol Nutr Food Res 2011;55:495–503.
[91] Shahgaldian P, Da Silva E, Coleman AW, Rather B, Zaworotko MJ. Para-acyl-calix-arene based solid lipid nanoparticles (SLNs): a detailed study of preparation and stability parameters. Int J Pharm 2003;253:23–38.
[92] Westesen K. Novel lipid-based colloidal dispersions as potential drug administration systems – expectations and reality. Colloid Polym Sci 2000;278:608–18.
[93] Shegokar R, Singh KK, Müller RH. Production & stability of stavudine solid lipid nanoparticles—from lab to industrial scale. Int J Pharm 2011;416:461–70.
[94] Tsai M-J, Huang Y-B, Wu P-C, Fu Y-S, Kao Y-R, Fang J-Y, Tsai Y-H. Oral apomorphine delivery from solid lipid nanoparticles with different monostearate emulsifiers: pharmacokinetic and behavioral evaluations. J Pharm Sci 2011;100:547–57.
[95] Paliwal R, Rai S, Vaidya B, Khatri K, Goyal AK, Mishra N, Mehta A, Vyas SP. Effect of lipid core material on characteristics of solid lipid nanoparticles designed for oral lymphatic delivery. Nanomedicine Nanotechnol Biol Med 2009;5:184–91.
[96] Radomska-Soukharev A. Stability of lipid excipients in solid lipid nanoparticles. Adv Drug Deliv Rev 2007;59:411–8.
[97] Freitas C, Müller RH. Spray-drying of solid lipid nanoparticles (SLN). Eur J Pharm Biopharm 1998;46:145–51.
[98] Solmaz G, Jaleh V, Afrooz S, Fatemeh A. Stability and antimicrobial effect of amikacin-loaded solid lipid nanoparticles. Int J Nanomedicine 2010;6.
[99] Kramer T, Kremer DM, Pikal MJ, Petre WJ, Shalaev EY, Gatlin LA. A procedure to optimize scale-up for the primary drying phase of lyophilization,. J Pharm Sci 2009;98:307–18.
[100] Torchilin VP. Nanoparticulates as drug carriers. Imperial College Press; 2006.
[101] Crowe LM, Womersley C, Crowe JH, Reid D, Appel L, Rudolph A. Prevention of fusion and leakage in freeze-dried liposomes by carbohydrates. Biochim Biophys Acta Biomembr 1986;861:131–40.
[102] Bensouda Y, Cavé G, Seiller M, Puisieux F. Freeze-drying of emulsions—influence of congealing on granulometry research of a cryoprotective agent. Pharm Acta Helvetiae 1989;64:40–4.
[103] Madden TD, Bally MB, Hope MJ, Cullis PR, Schieren HP, Janoff AS. Protection of large unilamellar vesicles by trehalose during dehydration: retention of vesicle contents. Biochim Biophys Acta 1985;817:67–74.
[104] Strauss G, Schurtenberger P, Hauser H. The interaction of saccharides with lipid bilayer vesicles: stabilization during freeze-thawing and freeze-drying,. Biochim Biophys Acta 1986;858:169–80.
[105] Hauser H, Strauss G. Stabilization of small, unilamellar phospholipid vesicles by sucrose during freezing and dehydration. Adv Exp Med Biol 1988;238:71–80.
[106] Vemuri S, Yu C-D, Degroot JS, Wangsatornthnakun V, Venkataram S. Effect of sugars on freeze-thaw and lyophilization of liposomes. Drug Dev Ind Pharm 1991;17:327–48.
[107] Shulkin PM, Seltzer SE, Davis MA, Adams DF. Lyophilized liposomes: a new method for long-term vesicular storage. J Microencapsul 1984;1:73–80.
[108] Ghaffari S, Varshosaz J, Saadat A, Atyabi F, Ghaffari S, Varshosaz J, Saadat A, Atyabi F. Stability and antimicrobial effect of amikacin-loaded solid lipid nanoparticles. Int J Nanomedicine 2011;6:35.
[109] Westesen K, Siekmann B. Investigation of the gel formation of phospholipid-stabilized solid lipid nanoparticles. Int J Pharm 1997;151:35–45.
[110] Helgason T, Awad T, Kristbergsson K, McClements DJ, Weiss J. Influence of polymorphic transformations on gelation of tripalmitin solid lipid nanoparticle suspensions. J Am Oil Chemists Soc 2008;85:501–11.

[111] Martin AN, Swarbrick J, Cammarata A. Physical pharmacy: physical chemical principles in the pharmaceutical sciences. Lea & Febiger; 1983.
[112] Lippacher A, Müller RH, Mäder K. Investigation on the viscoelastic properties of lipid based colloidal drug carriers. Int J Pharm 2000;196:227–30.
[113] Bunjes H, Koch MHJ, Westesen K. Effect of particle size on colloidal solid triglycerides. Langmuir 2000;16:5234–41.
[114] Westesen K, Bunjes H. Do nanoparticles prepared from lipids solid at room temperature always possess a solid lipid matrix? Int J Pharm 1995;115:129–31.
[115] Heurtault B, Saulnier P, Pech B, Proust J-E, Benoit J-P. Physico-chemical stability of colloidal lipid particles. Biomaterials 2003;24:4283–300.
[116] Eldem T, Speiser P, Altorfer H. Polymorphic behavior of sprayed lipid micropellets and its evaluation by differential scanning calorimetry and scanning electron microscopy. Pharm Res 1991; 8:178–84.
[117] Jenning V, Gysler A, Schäfer-Korting M, Gohla SH. Vitamin A loaded solid lipid nanoparticles for topical use: occlusive properties and drug targeting to the upper skin. Eur J Pharm Biopharm 2000; 49:211–8.
[118] Unruh T, Bunjes H, Westesen K, Koch MH. Observation of size-dependent melting in lipid nanoparticles. J Phys Chem B 1999;103:10373–7.
[119] Tadros TF. Applied surfactants: principles and applications. John Wiley & Sons; 2006.
[120] McClements DJ. Food emulsions: principles, practices, and techniques. CRC Press; 2015.
[121] Kulshreshtha AK, Singh ON, Wall GM. Pharmaceutical suspensions, from formulation development to manufacturing. New York: Springer; 2010.
[122] Grit M, Crommelin DJA. Chemical stability of liposomes: implications for their physical stability. Chem Phys Lipids 1993;64:3–18.
[123] Zuidam NJ, Gouw HK, Barenholz Y, Crommelin DJ. Physical (in) stability of liposomes upon chemical hydrolysis: the role of lysophospholipids and fatty acids. Biochim Biophys Acta 1995; 1240:101–10.
[124] Zuidam NJ, Crommelin DJA. Differential scanning calorimetric analysis of dipalmitoylphosphatidylcholine-liposomes upon hydrolysis. Int J Pharm 1995;126:209–17.
[125] Kreuter J. Colloidal drug delivery systems. CRC Press; 1994.
[126] Mehta RC, Head LF, Hazrati AM, Parr M, Rapp R, DeLuca P. Fat emulsion particle-size distribution in total nutrient admixtures. Am J Health-Syst Pharm 1992;49:2749–55.
[127] Puntis J, Wilkins K, Ball P, Rushton D, Booth I. Hazards of parenteral treatment: do particles count? Arch Dis Child 1992;67:1475–7.
[128] Müller R, Maassen S, Schwarz C. Solid lipid nanoparticles (SLN) as potential carrier for human use: interaction with human granulocytes. J Control Release 1997;47:261–9.
[129] Blunk T, Hochstrasser DF, Sanchez JC, Müller BW, Müller RH. Colloidal carriers for intravenous drug targeting: plasma protein adsorption patterns on surface-modified latex particles evaluated by two-dimensional polyacrylamide gel electrophoresis. Electrophoresis 1993;14:1382–7.
[130] Müller R, Maaben S, Weyhers H, Mehnert W. Phagocytic uptake and cytotoxicity of solid lipid nanoparticles (SLN) sterically stabilized with poloxamine 908 and poloxamer 407. J Drug Target 1996;4:161–70.
[131] Illum L, Davis S, Müller R, Mak E, West P. The organ distribution and circulation time of intravenously injected colloidal carriers sterically stabilized with a blockcopolymer—poloxamine 908. Life Sci 1987;40:367–74.
[132] Rudt S, Müller R. In vitro uptake of polystyrene latex particles and parenteral fat emulsions by human granulocytes. Int J Pharm 1993;99:1–6.
[133] Muller R, Olbrich C. Solid lipid nanoparticles: phagocytic uptake, in vitro cytotoxicity and in vitro biodegradation. Drugs Made Ger 1999;42:49–53.
[134] Prabhu P, Patravale V. The upcoming field of theranostic nanomedicine: an overview,. J Biomed Nanotechnol 2012;8:859–82.
[135] Schroeder A, Heller DA, Winslow MM, Dahlman JE, Pratt GW, Langer R, Jacks T, Anderson DG. Treating metastatic cancer with nanotechnology. Nat Rev Cancer 2012;12:39–50.

[136] McCarroll J, Teo J, Boyer C, Goldstein D, Kavallaris M, Phillips P. Potential applications of nanotechnology for the diagnosis and treatment of pancreatic cancer. Front Physiol 2014;5:2.

[137] de Barros ALB, Soares DCF. Theranostic nanoparticles: imaging and therapy combined. J Mol Pharm Org Process Res 2014. http://dx.doi.org/10.4172/2329-9053.1000e113.

[138] Muthu MS, Leong DT, Mei L, Feng S-S. Nanotheranostics — application and further development of nanomedicine strategies for advanced theranostics. Theranostics 2014;4:660—77.

[139] Ferrari M. Cancer nanotechnology: opportunities and challenges. Nat Rev Cancer 2005;5:161—71.

[140] Muthu MS, Singh S. Targeted nanomedicines: effective treatment modalities for cancer, AIDS and brain disorders. Nanomedicine 2009;4:105—18.

[141] Zhao J, Mi Y, Feng S-S. siRNA-based nanomedicine. Nanomedicine 2013;8:859—62.

[142] Mei L, Zhang Z, Zhao L, Huang L, Yang X-L, Tang J, Feng S-S. Pharmaceutical nanotechnology for oral delivery of anticancer drugs. Adv Drug Deliv Rev 2013;65:880—90.

[143] Lammers T, Aime S, Hennink WE, Storm G, Kiessling F. Theranostic nanomedicine. Acc Chem Res 2011;44:1029—38.

[144] Ma X, Zhao Y, Liang X-J. Theranostic nanoparticles engineered for clinic and pharmaceutics. Acc Chem Res 2011;44:1114—22.

[145] Ahmed N, Fessi H, Elaissari A. Theranostic applications of nanoparticles in cancer. Drug Discov Today 2012;17:928—34.

[146] Shuhendler AJ, Prasad P, Leung M, Rauth AM, DaCosta RS, Wu XY. A novel solid lipid nanoparticle formulation for active targeting to tumor $\alpha v \beta 3$ integrin receptors reveals cyclic RGD as a double-edged sword,. Adv Healthc Mater 2012;1:600—8.

[147] Albuquerque J, Moura CC, Sarmento B, Reis S. Solid lipid nanoparticles: a potential multifunctional approach towards rheumatoid arthritis theranostics. Molecules 2015;20:11103—18.

[148] Bae KH, Lee JY, Lee SH, Park TG, Nam YS. Optically traceable solid lipid nanoparticles loaded with siRNA and paclitaxel for synergistic chemotherapy with in situ imaging. Adv Healthc Mater 2013;2: 576—84.

[149] Borgstrom B. Importance of phospholipids, pancreatic phospholipase A2, and fatty acid for the digestion of dietary fat. Gastroenterology 1980;78:954—62.

[150] Borgström B, Donnér J. The polar interactions between pancreatic lipase, colipase and the triglyceride substrate. FEBS Lett 1977;83:23—6.

[151] Olbrich C, Müller R. Enzymatic degradation of SLN—effect of surfactant and surfactant mixtures. Int J Pharm 1999;180:31—9.

[152] Saupe A, Rades T. Solid lipid nanoparticles. In: Nanocarrier technologies. Springer; 2006. p. 41—50.

[153] Ekambaram P, Sathali AAH, Priyanka K. Solid lipid nanoparticles: a review. Sci Rev Chem Commun 2012;2:80—102.

[154] Domb AJ. Long acting injectable oxytetracycline—liposphere formulations. Int J Pharm 1995;124: 271—8.

[155] Heiati H, Tawashi R, Shivers RR, Phillips NC. Solid lipid nanoparticles as drug carriers. I. Incorporation and retention of the lipophilic prodrug 3′-azido-3′-deoxythymidine palmitate. Int J Pharm 1997;146:123—31.

[156] Müller RH, Rühl D, Runge SA. Biodegradation of solid lipid nanoparticles as a function of lipase incubation time. Int J Pharm 1996;144:115—21.

[157] Almeida AJ, Runge S, Müller RH. Peptide-loaded solid lipid nanoparticles (SLN): influence of production parameters. Int J Pharm 1997;149:255—65.

[158] Siekmann B, Westesen K. Submicron-sized parenteral carrier systems based on solid lipids. Pharm Pharmacol Lett 1992;1:123—6.

[159] Cavalli R, Peira E, Caputo O, Gasco MR. Solid lipid nanoparticles as carriers of hydrocortisone and progesterone complexes with β-cyclodextrins. Int J Pharm 1999;182:59—69.

[160] Müller RH, Rühl D, Runge S, Schulze-Forster K, Mehnert W. Cytotoxicity of solid lipid nanoparticles as a function of the lipid matrix and the surfactant. Pharm Res 1997;14:458—62.

[161] Zur Mühlen A, Zur Mühlen E, Niehus H, Mehnert W. Atomic force microscopy studies of solid lipid nanoparticles. Pharm Res 1996;13:1411—6.

[162] Pardeike J, Weber S, Haber T, Wagner J, Zarfl H, Plank H, Zimmer A. Development of an itraconazole-loaded nanostructured lipid carrier (NLC) formulation for pulmonary application. Int J Pharm 2011;419:329—38.

[163] Cavalli R, Caputo O, Marengo E, Pattarino F, Gasco M. The effect of the components of microemulsions on both size and crystalline structure of solid lipid nanoparticles (SLN) containing a series of model molecules. Pharmazie 1998;53:392–6.

[164] Cavalli R, Marengo E, Rodriguez L, Gasco MR. Effects of some experimental factors on the production process of solid lipid nanoparticles. Eur J Pharm Biopharm 1996;42:110–5.

[165] Li Y-Z, Sun X, Gong T, Liu J, Zuo J, Zhang Z-R. Inhalable microparticles as carriers for pulmonary delivery of thymopentin-loaded solid lipid nanoparticles. Pharm Res 2010;27:1977–86.

[166] Liu J, Gong T, Fu H, Wang C, Wang X, Chen Q, Zhang Q, He Q, Zhang Z. Solid lipid nanoparticles for pulmonary delivery of insulin. Int J Pharm 2008;356:333–44.

[167] Chattopadhyay P, Shekunov BY, Yim D, Cipolla D, Boyd B, Farr S. Production of solid lipid nanoparticle suspensions using supercritical fluid extraction of emulsions (SFEE) for pulmonary delivery using the AERx system. Adv Drug Deliv Rev 2007;59:444–53.

[168] Rudolph C, Schillinger U, Ortiz A, Tabatt K, Plank C, Müller RH, Rosenecker J. Application of novel solid lipid nanoparticle (SLN)-gene vector formulations based on a dimeric HIV-1 TAT-peptide in vitro and in vivo. Pharm Res 2004;21:1662–9.

CHAPTER 13

Microneedles in Drug Delivery

Rubi Mahato
Fairleigh Dickinson University, Florham Park, NJ, United States

Contents

1. Introduction	331
2. Skin Structure and Barrier to Transdermal Delivery	331
3. Microneedles	333
3.1 Solid Microneedles	334
3.2 Hollow Microneedles	337
3.3 Coated Microneedles	339
3.4 Dissolving Microneedles	341
3.5 Hydrogel-Forming Microneedles	343
4. Selection of Microneedle Designs for Applications	346
5. Commercial Microneedle Devices	346
References	349

1. INTRODUCTION

There is a need for a drug delivery system that can efficiently deliver the drug to the target site with minimum invasion and pain. Transdermal delivery can solve this problem to some extent since it has the advantage of avoidance of first-pass metabolism associated with oral route, and less or no painful delivery compared with injections. However, transdermal route has its own limitation due to the outer layer of skin, the stratum corneum (SC) that acts as a barrier and limits the permeation only to small lipophilic molecules.

Delivery of macromolecules across the skin is primarily mediated by hypodermic injection or intramuscular injection. These two routes possess several disadvantages, such as patient incompliance, needle phobia, pain, and accidental needle-stick injury. A novel strategy to overcome these limitations and problems is to use microneedles (MNs).

2. SKIN STRUCTURE AND BARRIER TO TRANSDERMAL DELIVERY

Skin is the largest organ of the human body and performs a wide variety of functions. It protects us from microbes and infections, as well as protects organs and fluids. This structure helps regulate body temperature, and permits the sensation of touch, heat, cold, and pressure. Skin has three distinctive layers; the outer most layer is called epidermis, which

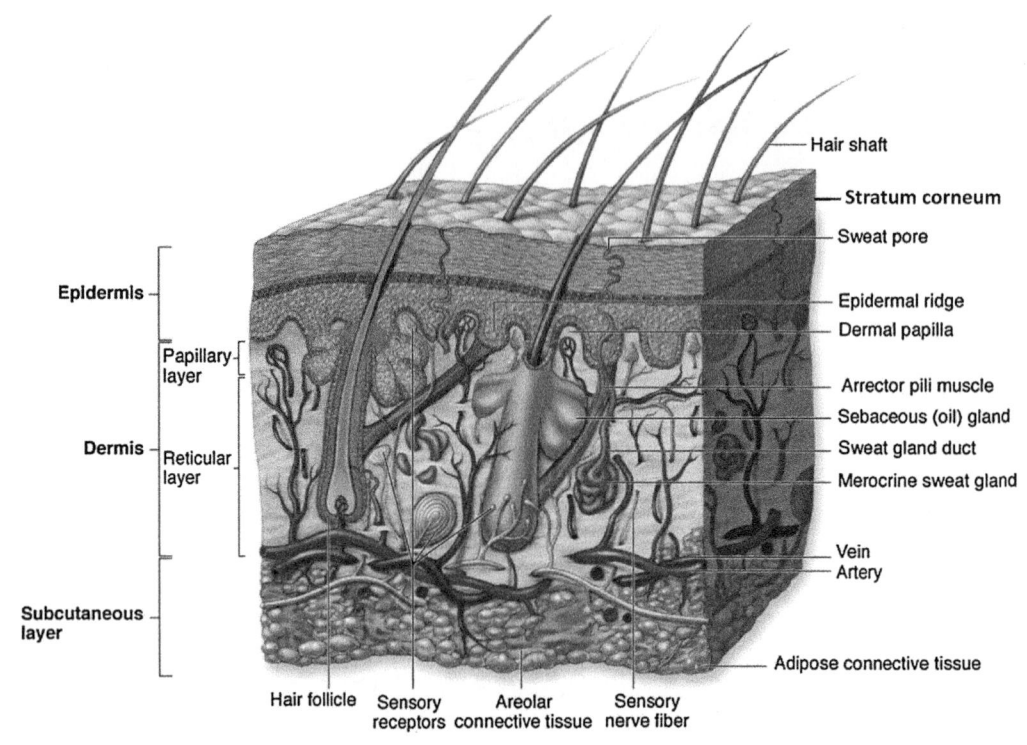

Figure 13.1 Structure of the skin showing different layers of skin (stratum corneum, epidermis, dermis, and hypodermis) and skin appendages (hair follicles, arrector pili muscle, sweat gland, sebaceous gland, and blood capillaries). *(Mescher AL, Junqueira's basic histology: Text and Atlas. 12th ed. Reprinted with permission (Copyright The McGraw-Hill Companies, Inc.).)*

is composed of the SC, beneath lies the middle dermis, and the deepest layer is the hypodermis (also known as subcutis) (Fig. 13.1) [1].

The outermost layer of the epidermis is the SC. It is composed of 15–20 layers of densely packed dead, flattened corneocytes (keratinocytes) (Fig. 13.2) embedded in three lipid components: ceramides, cholesterol, and fatty acids [2]. Due to the brick and mortar structural arrangement of SC it acts as a barrier to almost all macromolecules and hydrophilic drugs [3,4]. The major mechanism of drug transport across this layer is passive diffusion, which limits drug delivery to the highly lipophilic molecules under 500 Da. In addition, the rate of diffusion depends on the molecular weight and concentration gradient [5–7]. According to one study reported by Andrew et al., the transdermal delivery of molecules is limited by the full epidermis, not just SC, in that these researchers found that the removal of full epidermis increases the skin permeability by one- to twofold greater than that achieved by removal of SC alone [8].

The dermis is made up of 1- to 2-mm-thick connective tissue, including collagen and elastic fibers. It also contains macrophages and adipocytes throughout the layer [9]. This

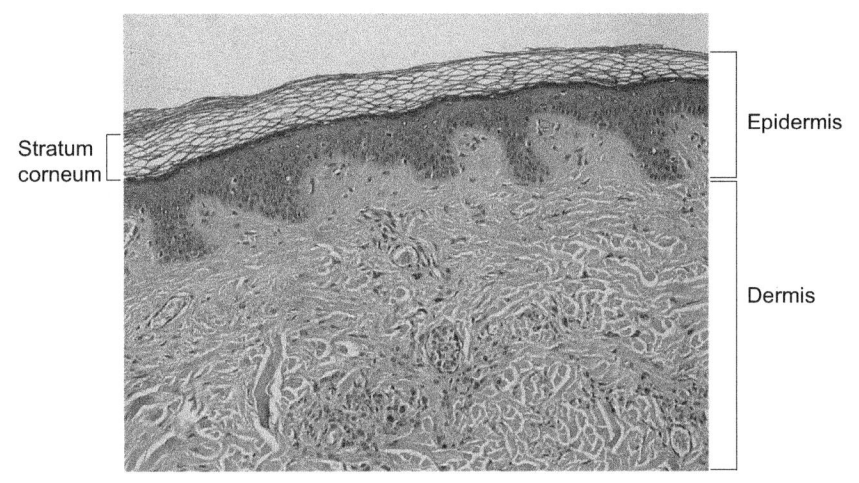

Figure 13.2 Histological cross-section of skin, stained with hematoxylin and eosin, showing stratum corneum, epidermis, and dermis.

layer expresses blood vessels, lymphatics, nerves, and various skin appendages such as hair follicles, sebaceous glands, and sweat glands [10].

The deepest layer of skin is hypodermis (subcutaneous). It has a thickness of up to several millimeters. This layer is made up of connective tissue and fibrous collagen, and it is the major site for fat storage [11].

3. MICRONEEDLES

MNs, as the name suggest, are micron-sized needles that are used for transdermal drug delivery and vaccinations. Since MN can enhance the permeation of small molecules, macromolecules, and vaccines across the skin, these needles have been widely researched to replace the traditional needle injections [12]. MNs are ideal delivery systems due to their painlessness and minimally invasive nature. Due to the small and thin projectile of needles MNs do not penetrate deep enough to stimulate the nerve endings and blood capillaries, making them painless [13]. MNs are preassembled for self-administration for patients, and are generally disposable in nature. This process avoids the need of skilled personnel and the chances of cross-contamination. In addition, MNs that are formulated to contain therapeutic agents such as proteins, small molecules, and vaccines are stable at room temperature, avoiding the problem of storage. MNs are being explored for ocular drug delivery, where the drug is delivered to the cornea, sclera, and suprachoroidal space. MNs are generally made from metal, ceramic, silicon, or polymeric materials. Based on design MNs can be classified into five different categories: solid, hollow, coated, dissolving, and hydrogel-forming (Fig. 13.4) [14,15]. MNs can be designed in various forms,

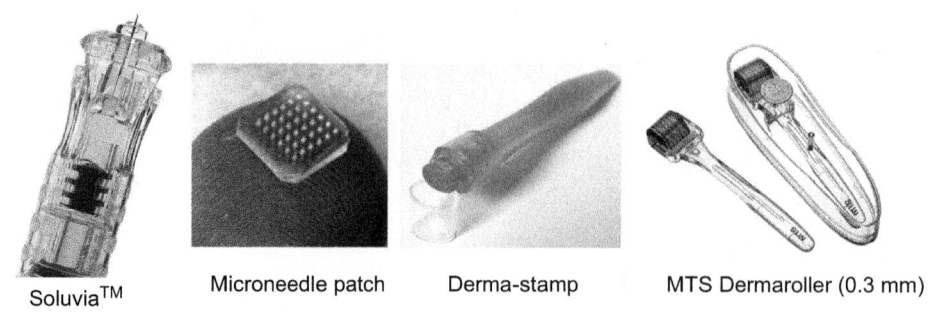

Figure 13.3 Various forms of microneedles (single, patch, stamp, and roller).

such as a single needle with an applicator, a patch where an array of MNs is assembled on a patch, a stamp with few MNs, or a roller where many MNs are mounted on a cylindrical surface that rolls over the skin (Fig. 13.3).

3.1 Solid Microneedles

Transdermal delivery using solid microneedles (SMNs) is a two-step process; in the first step MN arrays are applied to the skin and then removed, this process creates microchannels; in the second step a conventional drug formulation or a transdermal drug patch is applied (Fig. 13.4A). This approach is called *poke and patch* [17]. SMN is technically simple to deliver and it does not require drug coating or encapsulation as with coated microneedles (CMNs) or dissolving microneedles (DMNs). Drug permeation from the formulation occurs by passive diffusion through the created microchannels. Topical semisolid dosage forms such as ointment, gel, cream, and lotions can be efficiently delivered through SMNs. This device is generally fabricated using biocompatible metals such as stainless steel and titanium, silicon, polymers, or ceramics (Fig. 13.5). SMN produces high drug permeability across the skin, with negligible tissue damage compared with conventional injections. Besides pharmaceutical or medical application, SMN is also applied for the delivery of cosmetic agents. For cosmetic application, SMN is made into stamp, pen, or roller instead of a conventional patch, for example, Derma-stamp, Dermapen, Dermaroller, and similar devices to pretreat the skin before applying collagen, serum, acne medication, or other cosmetic products [18,19]. These devices have been designed to induce skin's natural ability to produce collagen, reduce wrinkle, treat burn scar and scars caused by sunburn, acne, and stretch mark, as well as for skin tightening [20].

For pharmaceutical applications, SMN can be used for the delivery of vaccines, small molecules, biotherapeutic agents such as insulin, growth hormones, proteins, and peptides, as well as anticancer drugs. A study by Nalluri et al. showed that permeability of drug molecules across the skin increased with increase in the size of MN, in that they

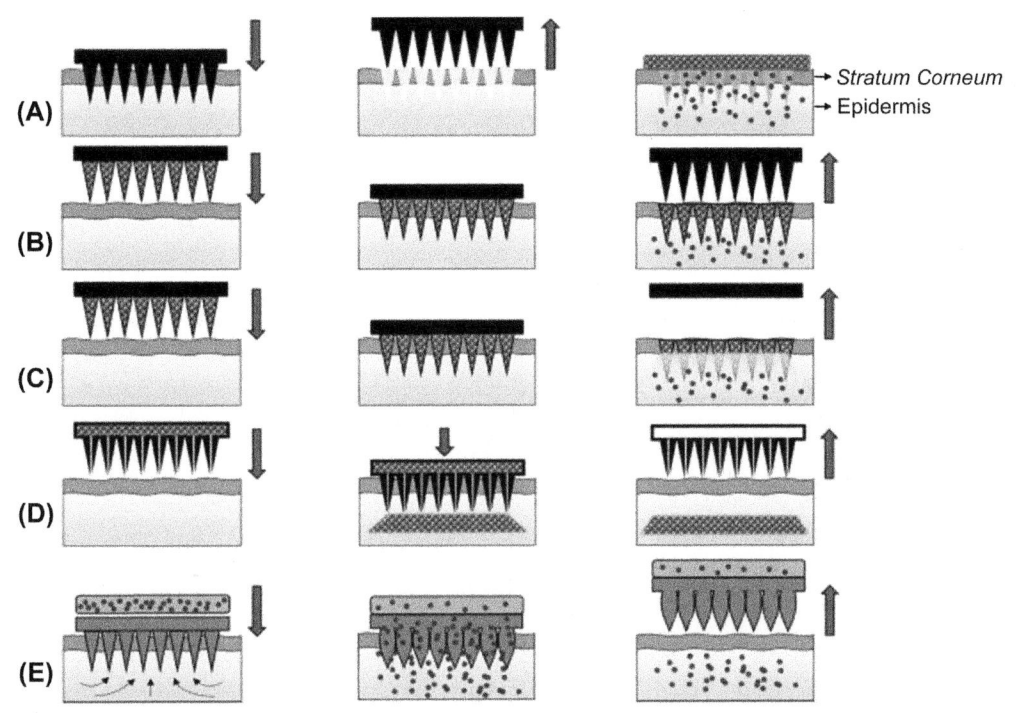

Figure 13.4 A schematic representation of five different microneedle (MN) types applied to facilitate drug delivery transdermally. (A) Solid MNs for enhancing the permeability of a drug formulation by creating microholes across the skin. (B) Coated MNs for rapid dissolution of the coated drug into the skin. (C) Dissolvable MNs for rapid or controlled release of the drug incorporated within the microneedles. (D) Hollow MNs used to puncture the skin and enable release of a liquid drug through active infusion or diffusion of the formulation through the needle bores. (E) Hydrogel-forming MNs take up interstitial fluids from the tissue, thereby inducing diffusion of the drug located in a patch through the swollen microprojections [16]. *(Adapted with permission from Larrañeta E, et al. Microneedle arrays as transdermal and intradermal drug delivery systems: materials science, manufacture and commercial development, Mater Sci Eng R Rep 2016;104:1–32, Available from: http://dx.doi.org/10.1016/j.mser.2016.03.001.)*

used MN patch with the needle length of 0.6, 0.9, 1.2, and 1.5 mm. The permeability or diffusion coefficient values observed with these MNs were in the order of 1.5 > 1.2 > 0.9 > 0.6 mm MN > passive permeation [21]. In addition, a comparison of the effectiveness of MN array patch with that of Dermaroller MN roller suggested that array patch was superior to the rollers with similar length MN in enhancing drug permeation. The researchers attributed this effect to the higher density of MN and force of application onto the skin. SMN's ability to enhance vaccine delivery across the skin was proved by immune response induced against diphtheria toxoid vaccine and influenza vaccine in combination with cholera toxin as an adjuvant. The result obtained was comparable with that achieved by subcutaneous injection of either vaccine [22].

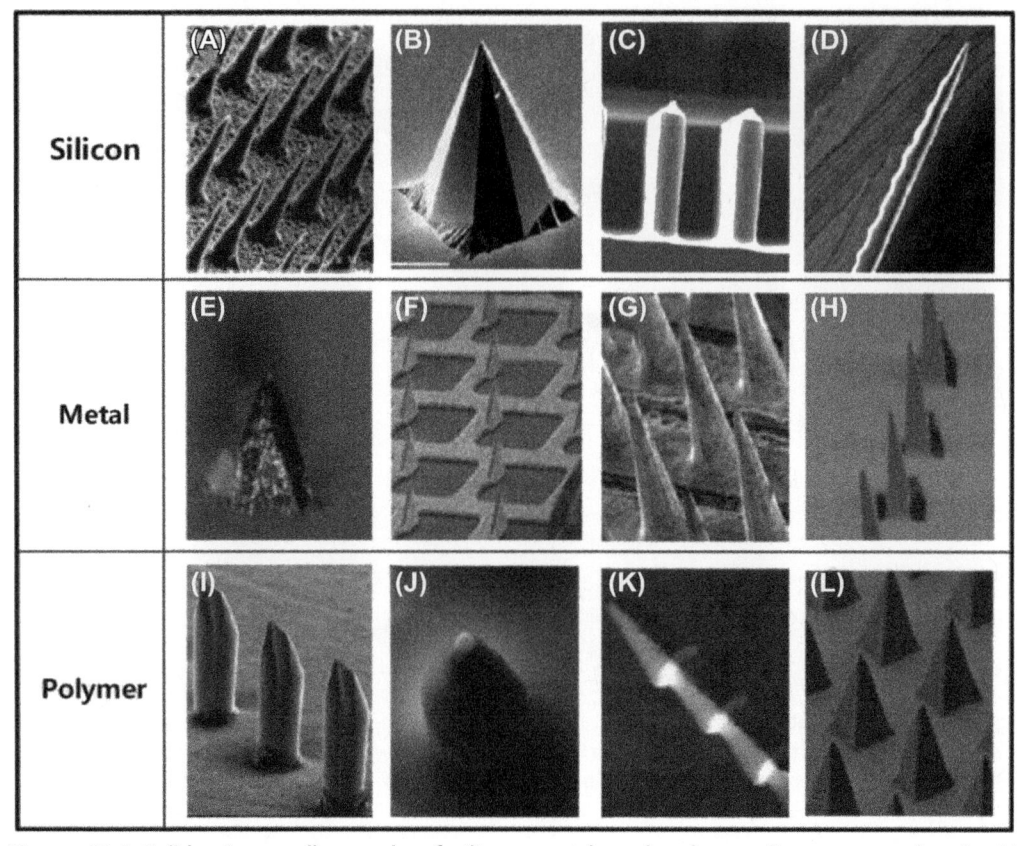

Figure 13.5 Solid microneedles made of silicon, metal, and polymer. *(Images reproduced with permission from Kim YC, Park JH, Prausnitz MR. Microneedles for drug and vaccine delivery. Adv Drug Deliv Rev 2012;64(14):1547–68 (Copyright 2012 Elsevier).)*

Formation of microchannels in the skin layer by SMN is useful for delivery of small- as well as large-molecular-weight drugs, but is especially beneficial for the particles. A high-molecular-weight drug with poor water solubility, such as docetaxel, loaded in elastic liposomes was applied to the skin pretreated with SMNs. This strategy significantly enhanced the transdermal delivery of the drug. The lag time obtained following the application of elastic liposomes through MN-treated skin was shortened by nearly 70% relative to conventional liposomes [23]. Insulin delivery efficiency was significantly enhanced with SMN before the topical application of an insulin solution in diabetic rat, this treatment resulted in reduced blood glucose level [24].

SMNs have also been applied in combination with other permeation enhancement techniques. One such study by Chen et al. reported the use of iontophoresis to enhance the transdermal delivery of insulin encapsulated in nanovesicles through the holes created in skin by SMN arrays. This approach resulted in reduction of blood glucose level and the effect was comparable with that obtained after subcutaneous injection of insulin [25]. In other studies SMN was utilized in combination with iontophoresis to administer human growth hormone [26] and oligonucleotide [27], and also used in combination with sonophoresis to deliver bovine serum albumin into the skin [28].

The main limitation of SMN is its two-step application process, which may not be very convenient for the patients. Because of this, precise dosing cannot be assured. Moreover, there is limited drug permeation enhancement through SMNs, especially for high-molecular-weight viscous liquid drug formulations. For example, when PEGylated naltrexone (polyethylene glycol-naltrexone) and propylene glycol water mixture were prepared to deliver naltrexone across the MN-treated skin, the enhanced permeation was not achieved because of the increased viscosity of the formulation [29,30]. Besides, there are other disadvantages associated with SMN. SMNs in cosmetology, such as Dermaroller and Derma-stamp, are used for multiple times and may also be shared among different individuals. This strategy may lead to skin contamination and infection. These side effects can be prevented by thoroughly cleaning the MNs after each treatment.

3.2 Hollow Microneedles

Hollow microneedles (HMNs), as the name suggests, consists of hollow needles that act as conduit structure that are specifically used to inject fluid and liquid formulations (Fig. 13.4D). Therefore the mechanism of drug delivery through HMN is termed as *poke and flow*. HMN allows the delivery of molecules in a continuous fashion, where drug solution can flow through the MN bore by different methods such as diffusion, pressure, or electrically driven flow. Because of these features HMN allows the modulation of flow rate for a rapid bolus injection, i.e., a slow infusion or a time-varying delivery rate [32]. In addition, delivering larger amounts of drug substances are possible in comparison with solid, coated, and dissolving MNs [33]. However, there are disadvantages associated with the drug formulation delivered by HMN, such as low stability, reduced shelf life, and low patient compliance compared with other types of MNs. The main limitation of HMN is the potential for needle clogging during skin insertion [34]. Moreover, the clogging arises from the flow resistance due the compression of dense dermal tissue around the MN tips during insertion [35]. The clogging of MN can be prevented by a very sharp MN with bore-opening on the side of MN instead of the tip [36], whereas partial retraction of MNs may relieve skin compaction and improve the flow conductivity, while the MN tip remains embedded in the skin [35]. Another disadvantage of HMN is the potential for leakage in the surrounding area. Generally there are two types of HMNs, one that utilizes a single MN, which mimics the conventional hypodermic needle, and the other an array of multiple hollow MNs. The array-type HMNs can deliver the formulation to a wide surface area all at once, but if one of the MNs has a leak, then pressure cannot be applied equally to all of the needles, leading to uneven flow through the MNs [31].

HMNs are made from a range of materials such as silicon, metal, glass, polymer, and ceramic (Fig. 13.6) [14]. HMNs are suitable for delivering any drug substances as long as these compounds are stable in liquid formulations. The deliverable drugs include small molecules such as lidocaine and nicotine, macromolecules, and biotherapeutic drugs such as peptides, proteins, DNA, and RNA. In one study, lidocaine was injected into the human skin with a single HMN, and the anesthetic effect produced was compared with that produced by conventional intradermal injection. Although both methods developed similar effect, HMN elicited significantly less pain; therefore patients expressed strong preference for MNs [37]. Hollow MNs have been applied for insulin delivery to adolescents and children with type 1 diabetes. That study reported that intradermal insulin delivery with a single HMN device was able to reduce the glucose level with less insertion pain compared with conventional subcutaneous injection [38]. HMNs have also been used for vaccine delivery, where the MNs were first examined for influenza vaccination in rats. The intradermal injection via HMN enabled 100-fold dose sparing effect by using inactivated virus vaccine, and up to fivefold dose sparing effect with DNA vaccine relative to intramuscular delivery [39].

Advancement in MNs has developed the new designs of MNs for ocular drug delivery. As reported in one study, HMN was successfully applied to inject soluble molecules, as well as nano- and microparticles, into the sclera of the eye. The intrascleral injection was influenced by scleral thickness, infusion pressure, MN retraction depth, and

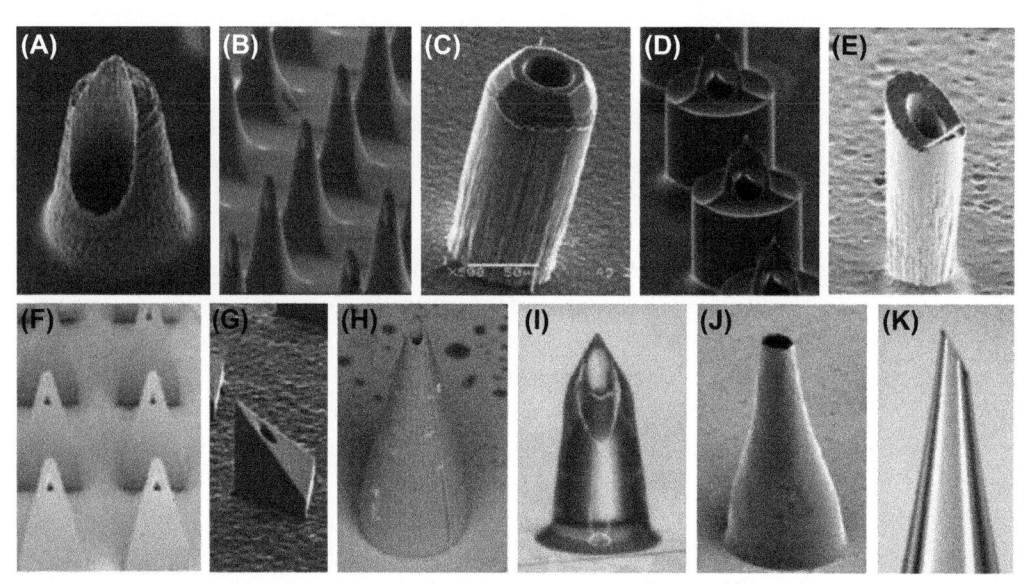

Figure 13.6 Hollow microneedles made of silicon, metal, polymer, and glass. *(Images reproduced with permission from Kim YC, Park JH, Prausnitz MR. Microneedles for drug and vaccine delivery. Adv Drug Deliv Rev 2012;64(14):1547–68 (Copyright 2012 Elsevier).)*

concomitant use of enzymes [40]. A microinjector has been developed by a company called Clearside Biomedical. This microinjector can be used to inject the fluid into the suprachoroidal space, the space between sclera and choroid of eye, so that the medication can flow circumferentially around the eye. The microinjector is a 30-gage HMN with the length of <1.2 mm, and is designed to focus on diseases affecting the choroid and retina, especially diseases associated with macular edema.

In contrast to drug delivery applications, HMNs have also been developed to extract body fluids. The glass and silicon HMNs were used to collect interstitial fluid, whereas stainless steel HMNs were used for blood sampling [31].

3.3 Coated Microneedles

SMN, in addition to being a piercing structure, can also be considered as carrier to carry and deposit the drug molecules onto the skin and other tissues. This can be achieved by coating the SMN with a drug formulation suitable for coating, and subsequent dissolution into the skin after insertion (Fig. 13.4B). This approach can be termed as *coat and poke*. With this design and mechanism this type of MN allows a simple one-step application process, where the dose can be quickly delivered into the tissue upon insertion of the MN. However, the amount of drug that can be administered by this approach is limited to the amount that can be coated onto the finite surface area of the MN structure, and generally the quantity is less than 1 mg for small MN arrays [41]. Therefore coated MNs are mostly recommended for potent drug substances. In addition, several factors need to be taken into consideration for a CMN delivery system to be effective, which include uniform, efficient, and stable MN coating formulations and procedures, effective skin penetration performance, and targeted and efficient drug deposition [42]. CMN is prepared by coating the drugs on solid MN generally made of silicon, metal, ceramic, and polymer (Fig. 13.7) [16]. MNs can be coated by various techniques, such as dipping or spraying the MNs with aqueous drug formulation, inkjet printing, and layer-by-layer coating with drug formulation. For an effective skin insertion, the mechanical strength and adhesive properties of a dried coating should be strong enough to maintain the coating adherent to the MN during insertion into the skin.

CMNs have been employed for quicker delivery of small molecule drugs such as vitamin B [24], lidocaine [43], and pilocarpine [44]; macromolecules such as protein and peptide (insulin, ovalbumin, bovine serum albumin) [41,45,46] and DNA (plasmid DNA, antisense oligonucleotides) [27,47,48]; and vaccines [48–51]. Although CMNs have been applied to different types and sizes of drug molecules, these structures have been the most studied technique for vaccination with MNs. Among them influenza vaccination with CMN takes the first place. Studies have shown improved immune responses after transdermal delivery of inactivated influenza virus with MN patches [50,52,53]. Vaccine in CMN may be stabilized by adding the viscosity enhancer trehalose. Partial or total vaccine activity was retained by adding trehalose and carboxymethyl cellulose (CMC), respectively [54]. MNs coated with stabilized vaccine or virus-like part vaccine

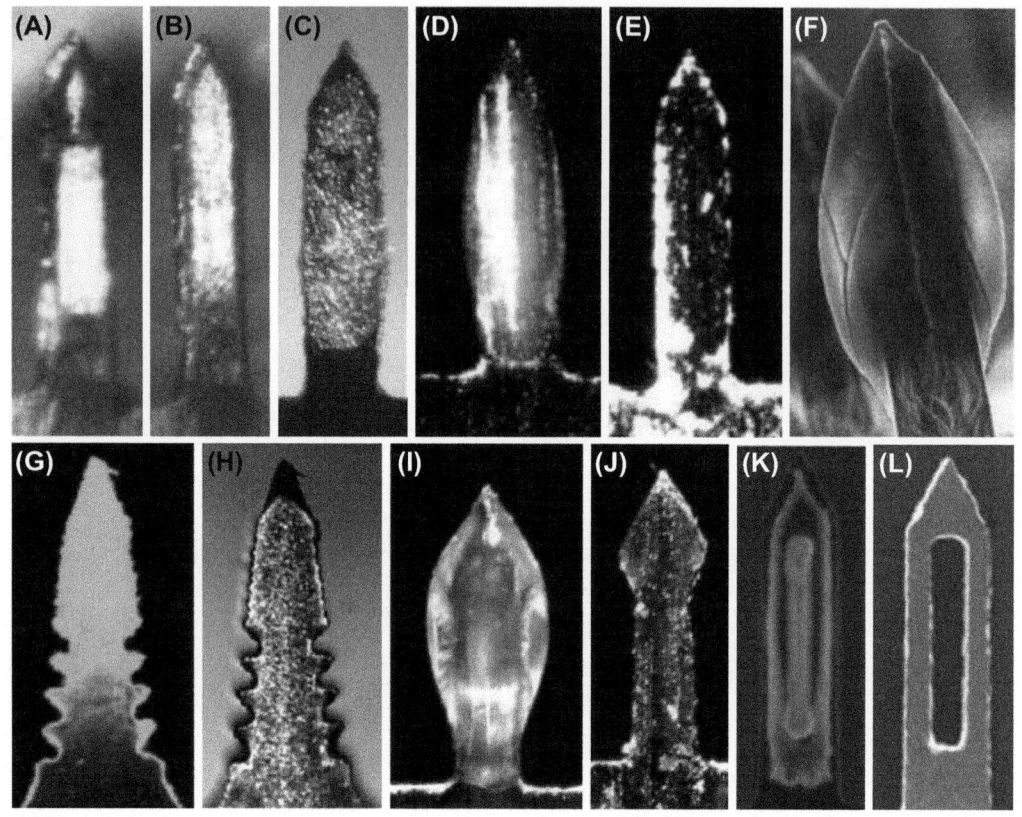

Figure 13.7 Coated microneedles made of metal and polymer after (A,C,D,F,G,I,K) and before (B,E,H,J,L) coating. *(Images reproduced with permission from Kim YC, Park JH, Prausnitz MR. Microneedles for drug and vaccine delivery. Adv Drug Deliv Rev 2012;64(14):1547–68 (Copyright 2012 Elsevier).)*

against seasonal influenza (H1 strain) or avian influenza (H5 strain) produced stronger immunogenicity and enabled dose sparing compared with intramuscular route [55–57]. In addition, CMN can also be indicated for measles vaccine [58], bacillus Calmette-Guérin vaccine [59], and hepatitis B [49] and hepatitis C vaccines [48].

As a proof-of-concept study, Chong et al. evaluated the gene-silencing efficiency of small interfering RNA (siRNA) delivered to skin via coated steel MN. This article reported that Lamin A/C siRNA retained its full activity after being released from MN and deposited into the skin. Furthermore, these researchers evaluated the in vivo gene-silencing efficiency of anti-CBL/hMGFP[1] siRNA delivered by CMN in a

---

[1] siRNA targeting CBL and hMGFP [transgenic click beetle luciferase/humanized monster green fluorescent protein (Tg CBL/hMGFP)] expressed by transgenic reporter mouse.

transgenic reporter (luciferase/GFP) mouse skin model. The results showed a decrease in fluorescence intensity at the site treated with MN, where hMGFP mRNA was reduced to 38—49% [42]. Another study by a group of researchers used Nanopatch microprojection arrays with ultrahigh density of much finer projections to deliver the siRNA to the skin. These microprojection arrays were coated with liposome-encapsulated chemokine (C-X-C motif) ligand 1 (CXCL1)-specific siRNA. Upon insertion the microprojections coated with siRNA penetrated 74 μm into mouse ear skin, the distance from SC to the dermis, and a strong response was elicited where CXCL1 was reduced by 75% up to 20 h after treatment [60].

CMNs have also been delivered with anticancer drugs intratumorally. In one such study by Ma et al., anticancer drug doxorubicin (DOX) was encapsulated in poly (lactide-*co*-glycolide) (PLGA) nanoparticles (NPs) and these NPs were coated on in-plane MNs. Upon insertion of MNs DOX diffused into the tissue and produced cytotoxicity, whereas hypodermic injection of different volumes into a porcine buccal tissue showed significant leakage of the injected volume (about 25%). In summary, this study showed that drug-coated microneedles can uniformly and effectively deliver the therapeutic agents to localized oral cancers [61]. In another study, CMNs were utilized to deliver three anticancer drugs, 5-fluorouracil, curcumin, and cisplatin, simultaneously by transdermal delivery. These drugs were encapsulated within the hydrophilic graft copolymer Soluplus [62]. The drug release rates depended on the drug—polymer ratio, lipophilicity of drug, and skin thickness. Soluplus assisted the drug release especially for the water-insoluble curcumin and cisplatin due to its solubilizing capacity. However, an additional antitumor efficacy analysis is needed for this CMN.

3.4 Dissolving Microneedles

DMNs have been developed with an idea that MNs completely dissolve in the skin after insertion, thereby leaving behind no biohazardous sharps waste after use (Fig. 13.4C). This mechanism of drug delivery is termed as *poke and dissolve*. The major advantages of DMN drug delivery system include limited drug loss during the encapsulation and absorption process, precise dosing possible as MN dissolves in skin, and patch- or pump-free technique. DMNs are made of safe, inert, water-soluble materials, which include (1) polymers such as hyaluronic acid (HA), CMC, poly(vinyl) alcohol, poly(vinyl pyrrolidone), PLGA, and chondroitin sulfate and (2) carbohydrates such as dextran, dextrin, sucrose, and maltose to name a few (Fig. 13.8) [31]. The advantages of using polymers are that these materials possess good biocompatibility and hydrophilicity and are amenable to fast degradation at physiological pH. Carbohydrates also possess high biocompatibility, and impart stability to biomolecules, rendering them ideal delivery carriers for biotherapeutics such as protein, peptides, and nucleic acids. One study by

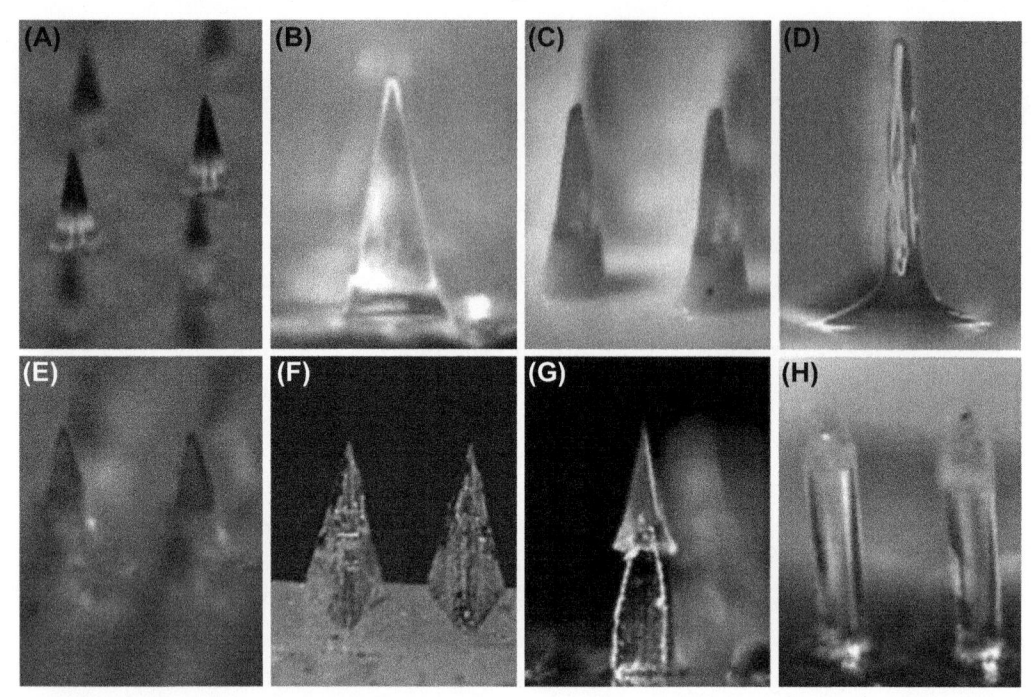

Figure 13.8 Dissolving microneedles made of water-soluble polymers and biodegradable polymers. *(Images reproduced with permission from Kim YC, Park JH, Prausnitz MR. Microneedles for drug and vaccine delivery. Adv Drug Deliv Rev 2012;64(14):1547–68 (Copyright 2012 Elsevier).)*

Loizidou et al. reported that CMC/maltose-based DMN possesses higher mechanical strength and drug permeation ability than CMC/trehalose-based DMN [63].

After insertion the MNs dissolve in skin interstitial fluid thereby releasing the cargo over time. The drug release kinetics depends on the dissolution rate of the constituent polymers. Therefore the rate of delivery can be controlled by adjusting the polymeric constituent. DMNs have been selected for delivering human growth hormone, erythropoietin, insulin, low-molecular-weight heparin, leuprolide acetate, desmopressin, lidocaine, ovalbumin, and vaccines [14,31,64]. Most DMNs reported in the literature need to be inserted into the skin for at least for 5 min to fully dissolve. To shorten this time, arrowhead MNs encapsulating drug are designed to separate from the shaft within seconds and remain embedded in the skin for subsequent dissolution and drug release (Fig. 13.8G) [65]. In contrast, drug-encapsulated biodegradable polymer MNs must be inserted and remain embedded in the skin for at least several days to fully release the drug due to polymeric degradation. This system can provide controlled drug delivery in skin for up to months [66]. However, disadvantages of this biodegradable MN are (1) significantly low mechanical strength at high drug load, which limits the loading to less than 10%, and (2) exposure of the encapsulated drugs to elevated temperature during MN fabrication (that involves melted polymer), which may degrade heat-sensitive drugs.

Sometimes MNs may not fully insert into the skin. In those cases it is desirable to encapsulate the drug only in the tip of the MN. One such study was performed by Fukushima et al., where the researchers developed two-layered DMNs with sequential applications of different compositions of polymer solutions, and the drug was loaded in the tip (around 60% of the length from top) of the MN (Fig. 13.8A) [67]. Drug substances may also be loaded into the MN tip either with a highly concentrated polymer solution to increase viscosity or by introducing an air bubble at the base of the needle that prevented back diffusion [68]. The same research group also added a pedestal at the base of the MN to provide higher aspect ratio MNs capable of inserting more fully into the skin and with sufficient mechanical strength to avoid failure during insertion. MicroHyala, a DMN patch made of HA containing trivalent influenza hemagglutinins, was developed against three strains of influenza: A/H1N1, A/H3N2, and B. The device produced equal or stronger effect than vaccine given by subcutaneous injection [69]. Similarly, Matsuo et al. reported that the vaccination efficacy of tetanus and diphtheria, malaria, and influenza-loaded DMN made of MicroHyala is comparable with or stronger than subcutaneous and intramuscular injections. The researchers also observed that tetanus and diphtheria toxoids and malaria vaccine administered by transcutaneous immunization achieved comparable immunogenicity and protection as subcutaneous injection in mouse and rat models. However, influenza hemagglutinin induced similar immune response to intramuscular and intradermal injections with an adjuvant (alum) and a stronger response than intranasal injection with another adjuvant (cholera toxin) [70]. In separate studies, insulin and human growth hormone embedded in DMNs retained their activities for at least 1 month, at temperatures ranging from $-80°C$ to $+40°C$ [67,71,72].

The major limitation with DMNs is the deposition of polymer in skin, possibly making these systems undesirable since they are likely to be used as multiple dosing or used repeatedly for a long period [73]. The limited drug loading capacity, thereby lower delivered dose is problematic. Additionally, there is a high risk for MN fracture or deformation of the geometry during application [12].

3.5 Hydrogel-Forming Microneedles

Hydrogel-forming microneedles (HGMNs) are generally composed of a swelling material or aqueous polymer gels. In HGMN, drugs/biotherapeutics can either be integrated with the MN matrix or stored in the reservoir backing. In either case as MNs are inserted into the skin layer they absorb the interstitial fluid and swell. As a result the MN cross-linked structure becomes porous through which drug is easily released (Fig. 13.4E). For simplicity this mechanism can be called as *poke and gel*. Yu et al.

developed a novel glucose-responsive insulin delivery patch where glucose-responsive vesicles were loaded with insulin and glucose oxidase enzyme. These vesicles were loaded at the tip of hypoxia-sensitive hyaluronic acid (HS-HA) MN. The principle behind this system is that a local hypoxic microenvironment is caused by the enzymatic oxidation of glucose in the hyperglycemic state. It promotes the reduction of HS-HA, which rapidly triggers the dissociation of vesicles and subsequently releases the insulin. This smart insulin patch effectively regulates the blood glucose in a mouse model of chemically induced type 1 diabetes (Fig. 13.9A and B) [74].

HGMN made with a drug reservoir attached to the baseplate of the array provides the advantage of higher drug-loading capacity compared with DMN and CMN. In case of reservoir-backing HGMN, after insertion the MN array swells, producing continuous, unblockable, hydrogel conduits from patch-type drug reservoirs to the dermal microcirculation through which the drug from the reservoir diffuses into the skin (Fig. 13.5E) [75,76]. Because of this mechanism, the MNs initially act as a tool to penetrate the SC barrier; however, upon swelling MNs become a rate-controlling membrane. In one

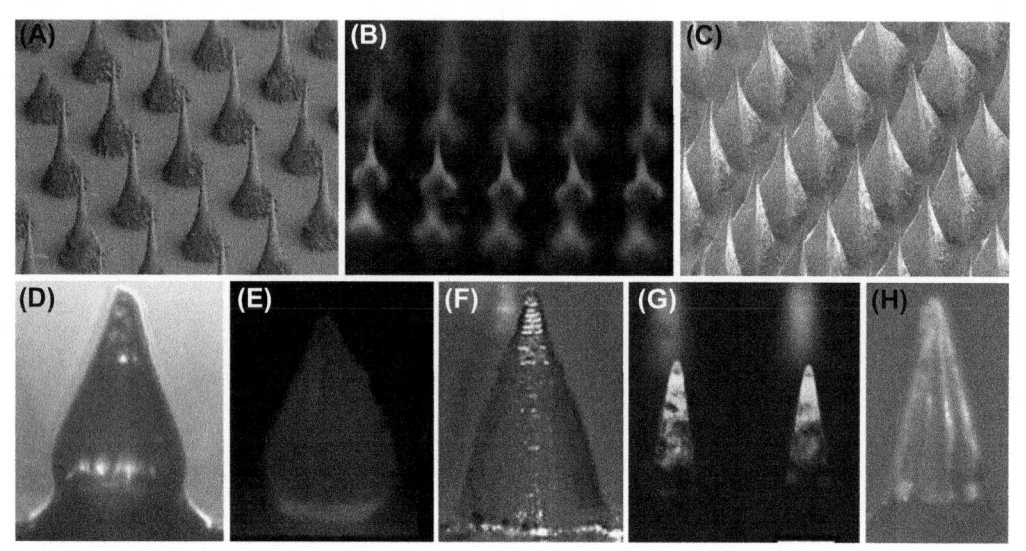

Figure 13.9 Hydrogel-forming microneedles made of biopolymers, synthetic polymers, and swelling materials. *(Reproduced with permission from (A and B) Yu J, et al. Microneedle-array patches loaded with hypoxia-sensitive vesicles provide fast glucose-responsive insulin delivery. Proc Natl Acad Sci USA 2015; 112(27):8260–65; (C) Ye Y, et al. Microneedles integrated with pancreatic cells and synthetic glucose-signal amplifiers for smart insulin delivery. Adv Mater 2016;28(16):3115–21; (D–F) Lutton RE, et al. A novel scalable manufacturing process for the production of hydrogel-forming microneedle arrays. Int J Pharm 2015;494(1):417–29; (G) Kim M, Jung B, and Park J-H. Hydrogel swelling as a trigger to release biodegradable polymer microneedles in skin. Biomaterials 2012;33(2):668–78; (H) Donnelly RF, et al. Hydrogel-forming microneedle arrays exhibit antimicrobial properties: potential for enhanced patient safety. Int J Pharm 2013;451(1–2):76–91.)*

study, Gu's research group developed a smart insulin-delivering MN patch to modulate insulin secretion from pancreatic β-cell in response to elevated blood glucose levels. In that, "glucose-signal amplifier" vesicles were integrated in the tip of the MN and the pancreatic β-cell-embedded capsules were positioned on the back of the MN patch. It was called live (cell based) and synthetic glucose responsive system (L-S GRS). This L-S GRS system rapidly lowers the elevated blood glucose level and maintains it at that level for 6 h without causing hyperglycemic or hypoglycemic state [77].

HGMNs may overcome the disadvantages of all other types of previously developed MNs. Solid, noncoated MN that requires a two-step application process may not be suitable for patient use [78,79] (Fig. 13.5A). In that MN-induced holes normally close very quickly (<1 h). Although the rate of hole closure can be slowed by heavy occlusion, it cannot be prevented [80]. Moreover, silicon or metal MN can cause skin problems [78]. In case of CMN precise coating of MN is difficult. Moreover, coated MNs deliver only a very small quantity of drug as a bolus [79,81–83] (Fig. 13.4B). Biomolecules can be significantly degraded by the heating used to produce polymeric DMN from molten polymers or carbohydrates [81–84] (Fig. 13.4C). Hollow MNs have only one outlet and can become blocked by compressed dermal tissue [81–83] (Fig. 13.4D).

In a study done by Donelly et al., an aqueous blend containing 15% w/w poly(methylvinylether/maleic acid) (PMVE/MA) and 7.5% w/w poly(ethyleneglycol) 10,000 (PEG) was utilized to fabricate HGMN with laser-engineered silicone micromold templates. A study of five mechanical tests was performed on MN, which includes axial and transverse deformation, skin penetration, MN base plate deformation, and break. This study reported that axial forces could reduce the MN height, but did not completely fail the MN indicating residual viscoelasticity. At a greater force the MN baseplate bent, indicating that the baseplate had considerable strength and conformability, which is important on a micron scale since the skin is not perfectly flat. Therefore some degree of flexibility in baseplate can ensure all MN to penetrate the skin when applied. Moreover, this study observed that even at a very low insertion force the MNs may completely penetrate the SC of porcine skin (400 μm thick). In addition, hydrogel MN arrays remained fully intact after application in vitro and in vivo, indicating the retention of strong mechanical strength of the swollen hydrogel. It is required since there should not be any local or systemic reaction if the needle breaks and a portion is left within the skin [73,75]. The same research group also observed that HGMN can generate controlled drug delivery across the skin. The rates and extents of permeation were independent of molecular weight and log P values.

In another study by the same group, the researchers compared the efficiency of drug delivery by HGMN with that by DMN and observed that puncturing the skin with HGMN resulted in approximately a twofold increase in 5-aminolevulinic acid (ALA) and mesotetra (*N*-methyl-4- pyridyl) porphine tetra tosylate (TMP) delivery relative to DMN [73]. Various polymeric compositions were evaluated to investigate rapidly swelling materials so as to compose superswelling hydrogel MN, which would be sufficiently hard in its dry state and can easily penetrate the skin, but once swollen, should maintain the structural integrity and be reasonably robust during handling. A group of researchers developed copolymer (Gantrez AN-139) of methyl vinyl ether and maleic anhydride (PMVE/MAH), and copolymer (Gantrez S-97) of methyl vinyl ether and maleic acid (PMVE/MA). HGMNs were then prepared with varying concentrations of the copolymer, PEG 10,000, and the modifying agent, sodium carbonate (Na_2CO_3). The investigators observed that hydrogel MN casted from aqueous blends of 20% w/w Gantrez S-97, 7.5% w/w PEG 10,000, and 3% w/w Na_2CO_3 produced superswelling hydrogels. The researchers in this study employed lyophilized wafer for drug reservoir instead of flexible polymeric patch. A hygroscopic reservoir generated extensive swelling of the MNs due to absorption of water from skin interstitial fluid by osmosis through the HGMN. The moisture helped in the dissolution of lyophilized drugs in the reservoir, leading to drug diffusion. This system was robust, effectively penetrated the skin, and caused excessive swelling of MN, but could be removed intact after application [76].

Studies done on HGMN show that it can efficiently deliver small molecule drugs such as methylene blue, caffeine, theophylline, metronidazole, lidocaine hydrochloride, ibuprofen sodium, ALA, and TMP, as well as macromolecules such as peptides and protein like insulin and ovalbumin [73,75,76,85]. Therefore HGMN offers a promising approach for effective drug delivery.

4. SELECTION OF MICRONEEDLE DESIGNS FOR APPLICATIONS

Many MN designs and delivery strategies have been developed. For a given application, it is important to find the best MN design. In general, drug delivery strategies can be divided into four major categories, each with different strengths and weaknesses: (1) skin pretreatment with MNs followed by drug application as a topical formulation or patch for slow delivery over time, (2) drug coating on or encapsulation in MNs for bolus delivery into the skin, (3) bolus or extended release of large dose from reservoir patch through swollen (hydrogel forming) MN, and (4) injection of a liquid drug formulation through one or more HMNs for bolus injection or controlled infusion over time (Table 13.1). For detailed explanation, please refer to a review publication by Kim et al. [31,87].

5. COMMERCIAL MICRONEEDLE DEVICES

Many pharmaceutical industries and research laboratories are involved in the development of MN devices and delivery systems. The exploration in this field began through three isolated efforts operated in parallel at Becton Dickinson (BD), Alza Corporation, and

Table 13.1 Characteristics of different microneedle-based drug delivery system designs

Microneedle design	Simplicity of design and manufacturing	Simplicity of use by patient	Maximum possible drug dose	Control over drug delivery profile
Microneedle pretreatment	++++	+++	+++	++
Microneedle patch	++	++++	+	++
Microneedle with reservoir patch	+++	++++	++	+++
Hollow microneedle	+	+	++++	++++

Adapted and modified with permission from Kim YC, Park JH, Prausnitz MR. Microneedles for drug and vaccine delivery. Adv drug Deliv Rev 2012;64(14):1547—68.

Georgia Institute of Technology. Most of the MN devices discussed here are still in clinical trials, and only a few of them are currently available (Fig. 13.10). The first commercialized MN was developed by BD to administer the vaccine and the product was marketed as **Soluvia**. It is a prefillable microinjection system integrated with a very short hollow steel needle. It allows a drug or vaccine to be accurately delivered intradermally [89]. This product has been widely used for intradermal injection of influenza vaccine by Sanofi Pasteur, and is marketed with different names (IDflu, **Intanza**, Fluzone).

Nanopass Technologies, an Israel-based company, developed **MiconJet**, a HMN system for intradermal injection. It is a single-use MN device composed of four hollow silicon needles shorter than 500 μm in length attached to a plastic device that can be connected with any standard syringe to inject drugs, biologics, and vaccines approved for this route [90].

Clearside's **SCS microinjector** is a single-use 30-gage HMN that comes with varying needle lengths <1.2 mm. It is designed to inject the drug solution into the suprachoroidal space to spread the drug around to the back of the eye. This microinjector is designed for the delivery of drugs to the choroid and retina, especially for diseases associated with macular edema. This product is currently in phase III clinical trial (Clearside Biomedical) [91,92].

Micro-Trans represents MN arrays patch, which enables drug delivery into the dermis without limitations of drug size, structure, charge, or the patient's skin characteristics (Valeritas) [93].

Corium's **MicroCor** system delivers drugs and vaccines from an integrated transdermal system in a one-step, user-friendly format. The system integrates the active drug ingredients and vaccines directly into arrays of biodegradable MNs, which penetrate the outer layers of the skin to release the drug for local or systemic absorption. The MNs can be in lengths up to 200 μm (or longer), offering significant flexibility in the depth of drug delivery (SC to dermis) and duration of delivery (bolus to sustained administration).

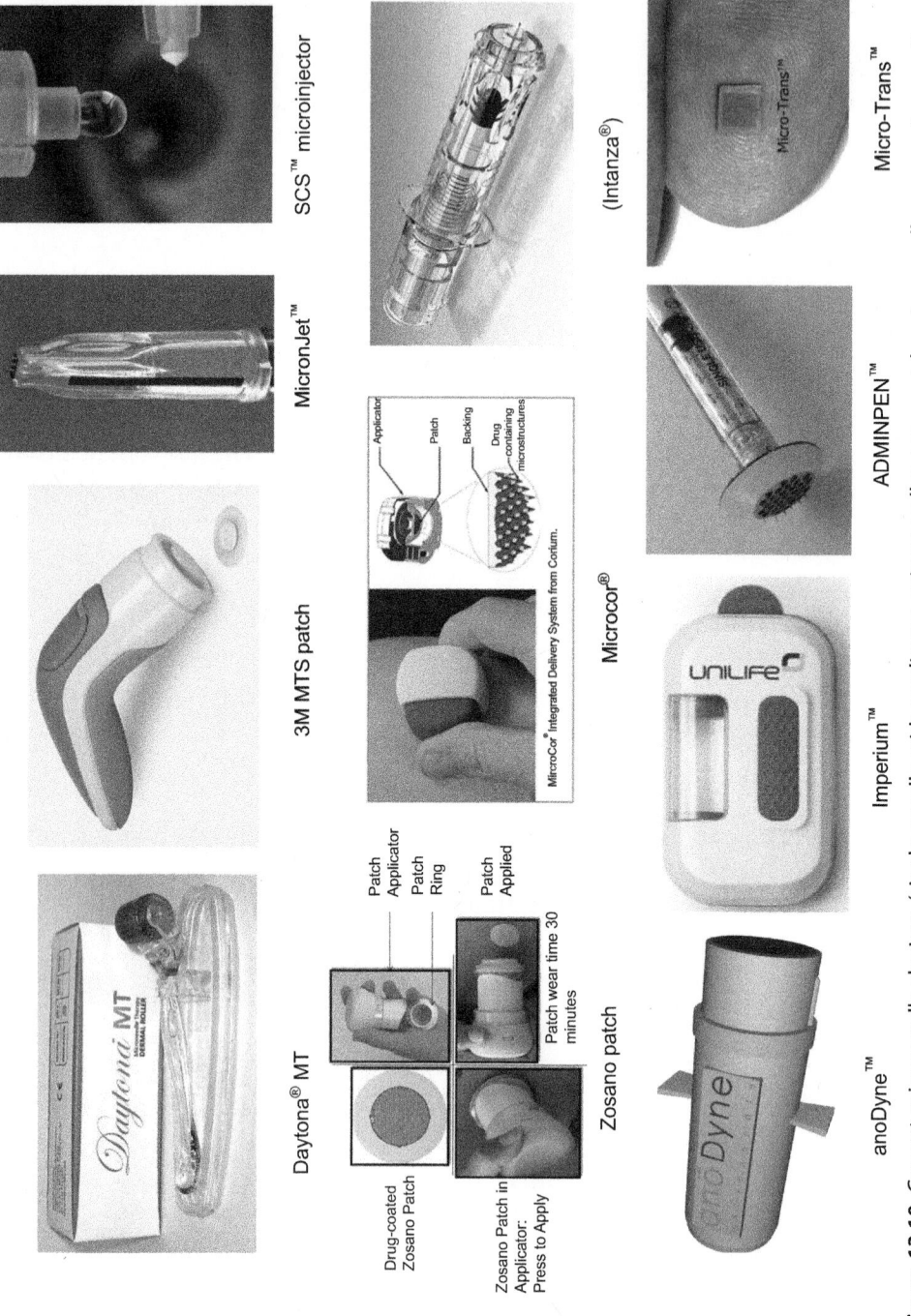

Figure 13.10 Current microneedle devices (single needle with applicator, microneedles array patch, microneedles pen, microneedle pump patch, and microneedle roller).

This active transdermal technology allows large molecules, such as peptides, proteins, and vaccines, to be delivered efficiently through the skin. It also provides faster skin permeation of small molecules (Corium) [94].

The **3M Microneedle transdermal system** consists of a coated MN to deliver water-soluble, polar, and ionic molecules, such as lidocaine, through the skin. This system has successfully delivered drugs to the skin within seconds with a rapid onset of local anesthesia [7].

Zosano patch (formerly known as Macroflux) was designed for the enhanced delivery of biopharmaceuticals such as protein, peptide, vaccines, and other biologics. Coated titanium microprojections array are designed for bolus delivery into the skin. The MN patch comes with a reusable applicator (Zosano Pharma) [95].

Unilife's **Imperium** is the world's first prefilled, disposable, multiday wearable insulin patch pump. Because it is prefilled and preassembled like an insulin pen, only three intuitive steps are required to commence continuous subcutaneous insulin infusion. On-demand bolus delivery is available to the user via the simple push of a button. Imperium can include wireless connectivity systems, such as Bluetooth LE, to integrate with smartphone apps for patient reminders and status updates (Unilife) [96].

anoDyne MN is a prefilled, single-use disposable device for insulin delivery that comes in the size of a thumb. It is easy to use, virtually painless, and can be self-administered almost anywhere on the body. Moreover, it comes with color-coded dose indicators. Since it is disposable the tiny needle retracts after it is pushed into the skin, then it pulls back and locks into place so it cannot be reused (anoDyne) [97].

Daytona MT Dermal Roller is a precision engineered handheld roller MN device that helps to combat the appearance of scars, wrinkles, stretch marks, cellulite, uneven skin tone, and even hair loss. The use of Daytona MT Dermal Roller encourages collagen production within the skin and helps to reduce the appearance of skin imperfections (Daytona Pharmaceutical Laboratory) [98].

ADMINPEN pen-injector device is based on MN array technology called AdminPatch. A simple low-cost molded plastic part is attached on the back surface of the AdminPatch to provide a fluidic connection of ADMINPEN device, which is externally connected to a liquid drug reservoir. This device can be attached to any standard commercially available syringe with a luer-lock connector. ADMINPEN allows more effective and painless delivery of many vaccines (such as Ebola, Flu, and cancer vaccines), particle-based vaccines, liquid medical drugs, cosmetics, and hair growth supplements (AdminMed) [99].

REFERENCES

[1] Krieg T, Bickers DR, Miyachi Y. Therapy of skin diseases: a worldwide perspective on therapeutic approaches and their molecular basis. Berlin Heidelberg: Springer; 2010.
[2] Bissett DL. Common cosmeceuticals. Clin Dermatol 2009;27(5):435—45.

[3] Polat BE, Blankschtein D, Langer R. Low-frequency sonophoresis: application to the transdermal delivery of macromolecules and hydrophilic drugs. Expert Opin Drug Deliv 2010;7(12):1415—32.
[4] Bouwstra JA, et al. Structural investigations of human stratum corneum by small-angle X-ray scattering. J Invest Dermatol 1991;97(6):1005—12.
[5] Prausnitz MR, Mitragotri S, Langer R. Current status and future potential of transdermal drug delivery. Nat Rev Drug Discov 2004;3(2):115—24.
[6] Arora A, Prausnitz MR, Mitragotri S. Micro-scale devices for transdermal drug delivery. Int J Pharm 2008;364(2):227—36.
[7] Alkilani AZ, McCrudden MT, Donnelly RF. Transdermal drug delivery: innovative pharmaceutical developments based on disruption of the barrier properties of the stratum corneum. Pharmaceutics 2015;7(4):438—70.
[8] Andrews SN, Jeong E, Prausnitz MR. Transdermal delivery of molecules is limited by full epidermis, not just stratum corneum. Pharm Res 2013;30(4):1099—109.
[9] Moore TL, et al. Seventeen-point dermal ultrasound scoring system—a reliable measure of skin thickness in patients with systemic sclerosis. Rheumatology 2003;42(12):1559—63.
[10] McGrath JA, Uitto J. The filaggrin story: novel insights into skin-barrier function and disease. Trends Mol Med 2008;14(1):20—7.
[11] Jepps OG, et al. Modeling the human skin barrier—towards a better understanding of dermal absorption. Adv Drug Deliv Rev 2013;65(2):152—68.
[12] Rejinold NS, et al. Biomedical applications of microneedles in therapeutics: recent advancements and implications in drug delivery. Expert Opin Drug Deliv 2016;13(1):109—31.
[13] Schoellhammer CM, Blankschtein D, Langer R. Skin permeabilization for transdermal drug delivery: recent advances and future prospects. Expert Opin Drug Deliv 2014;11(3):393—407.
[14] Larraneta E, et al. Microneedles: a new Frontier in nanomedicine delivery. Pharm Res 2016;33(5):1055—73.
[15] Ita K. Transdermal delivery of drugs with microneedles—potential and challenges. Pharmaceutics 2015;7(3):90—105.
[16] Larrañeta E, et al. Microneedle arrays as transdermal and intradermal drug delivery systems: materials science, manufacture and commercial development. Mater Sci Eng R Rep 2016;104:1—32.
[17] van der Maaden K, Jiskoot W, Bouwstra J. Microneedle technologies for (trans)dermal drug and vaccine delivery. J Control Release 2012;161(2):645—55.
[18] Badran MM, Kuntsche J, Fahr A. Skin penetration enhancement by a microneedle device (dermaroller) in vitro: dependency on needle size and applied formulation. Eur J Pharm Sci 2009;36(4—5):511—23.
[19] Lewis W. Is microneedling really the next big thing?. 2014.
[20] Aust MC, et al. Percutaneous collagen induction therapy: an alternative treatment for scars, wrinkles, and skin laxity. Plast Reconstr Surg 2008;121(4):1421—9.
[21] Nalluri BN, et al. In vitro skin permeation enhancement of sumatriptan by microneedle application. Curr Drug Deliv 2015;12(6):761—9.
[22] Ding Z, et al. Microneedle arrays for the transcutaneous immunization of diphtheria and influenza in BALB/c mice. J Control Release 2009;136(1):71—8.
[23] Qiu Y, et al. Enhancement of skin permeation of docetaxel: a novel approach combining microneedle and elastic liposomes. J Control Release 2008;129(2):144—50.
[24] Martanto W, et al. Transdermal delivery of insulin using microneedles in vivo. Pharm Res 2004;21(6):947—52.
[25] Chen H, et al. Iontophoresis-driven penetration of nanovesicles through microneedle-induced skin microchannels for enhancing transdermal delivery of insulin. J Control Release 2009;139(1):63—72.
[26] Cormier M, Daddona PE. Macroflux technology for transdermal delivery of therapeutic proteins and vaccines. Drugs Pharm Sci 2003;126:589—98.
[27] Lin W, et al. Transdermal delivery of antisense oligonucleotides with microprojection patch (macroflux) technology. Pharm Res 2001;18(12):1789—93.

[28] Han T, Das DB. Permeability enhancement for transdermal delivery of large molecule using low-frequency sonophoresis combined with microneedles. J Pharm Sci 2013;102(10):3614–22.
[29] Milewski M, et al. In vitro permeation of a pegylated naltrexone prodrug across microneedle-treated skin. J Control Release 2010;146(1):37–44.
[30] Milewski M, Stinchcomb AL. Vehicle composition influence on the microneedle-enhanced transdermal flux of naltrexone hydrochloride. Pharm Res 2011;28(1):124–34.
[31] Kim YC, Park JH, Prausnitz MR. Microneedles for drug and vaccine delivery. Adv Drug Deliv Rev 2012;64(14):1547–68.
[32] Yuen C, Liu Q. Hollow agarose microneedle with silver coating for intradermal surface-enhanced Raman measurements: a skin-mimicking phantom study. J Biomed Opt 2015;20(6):061102.
[33] Roxhed N, Griss P, Stemme G. Membrane-sealed hollow microneedles and related administration schemes for transdermal drug delivery. Biomed Microdevices 2008;10(2):271–9.
[34] Gardeniers HJ, et al. Silicon micromachined hollow microneedles for transdermal liquid transport. J Microelectromechanical Syst 2003;12(6):855–62.
[35] Martanto W, et al. Mechanism of fluid infusion during microneedle insertion and retraction. J Control Release 2006;112(3):357–61.
[36] Griss P, Stemme G. Side-opened out-of-plane microneedles for microfluidic transdermal liquid transfer. J Microelectromechanical Syst 2003;12(3):296–301.
[37] Gupta J, et al. Rapid local anesthesia in human subjects using minimally invasive microneedles. Clin J Pain 2012;28(2):129.
[38] Norman JJ, et al. Faster pharmacokinetics and increased patient acceptance of intradermal insulin delivery using a single hollow microneedle in children and adolescents with type 1 diabetes. Pediatr Diabetes 2013;14(6):459–65.
[39] Alarcon JB, et al. Preclinical evaluation of microneedle technology for intradermal delivery of influenza vaccines. Clin Vaccine Immunol 2007;14(4):375–81.
[40] Jiang J, et al. Intrascleral drug delivery to the eye using hollow microneedles. Pharm Res 2009;26(2):395–403.
[41] Gill HS, Prausnitz MR. Coating formulations for microneedles. Pharm Res 2007;24(7):1369–80.
[42] Chong RH, et al. Gene silencing following siRNA delivery to skin via coated steel microneedles: in vitro and in vivo proof-of-concept. J Control Release 2013;166(3):211–9.
[43] Zhang Y, et al. Development of lidocaine-coated microneedle product for rapid, safe, and prolonged local analgesic action. Pharm Res 2012;29(1):170–7.
[44] Jiang J, et al. Coated microneedles for drug delivery to the eye. Invest Ophthalmol Vis Sci 2007;48(9):4038–43.
[45] Chen X, et al. Dry-coated microprojection array patches for targeted delivery of immunotherapeutics to the skin. J Control Release 2009;139(3):212–20.
[46] Marin A, Andrianov AK. Carboxymethylcellulose–chitosan-coated microneedles with modulated hydration properties. J Appl Polym Sci 2011;121(1):395–401.
[47] Saurer EM, et al. Layer-by-layer assembly of DNA-and protein-containing films on microneedles for drug delivery to the skin. Biomacromolecules 2010;11(11):3136–43.
[48] Gill HS, et al. Cutaneous vaccination using microneedles coated with hepatitis C DNA vaccine. Gene Ther 2010;17(6):811–4.
[49] Andrianov AK, et al. Poly [di (carboxylatophenoxy) phosphazene] is a potent adjuvant for intradermal immunization. Proc Natl Acad Sci USA 2009;106(45):18936–41.
[50] Kim Y-C, et al. Formulation and coating of microneedles with inactivated influenza virus to improve vaccine stability and immunogenicity. J Control Release 2010;142(2):187–95.
[51] Corbett HJ, et al. Skin vaccination against cervical cancer associated human papillomavirus with a novel micro-projection array in a mouse model. PLoS One 2010;5(10):e13460.
[52] Kim Y-C, et al. Improved influenza vaccination in the skin using vaccine coated microneedles. Vaccine 2009;27(49):6932–8.
[53] Kim Y-C, et al. Enhanced memory responses to H1N1 influenza vaccination in the skin using vaccine coated-microneedles. J Infect Dis 2010;201(2):190–8.

[54] Choi H-J, et al. Effect of osmotic pressure on the stability of whole inactivated influenza vaccine for coating on microneedles. PLoS One 2015;10(7):e0134431.
[55] Kim Y-C, et al. Influenza immunization with trehalose-stabilized virus-like particle vaccine using microneedles. Procedia Vaccinol 2010;2(1):17—21.
[56] Quan F-S, et al. Dose sparing enabled by skin immunization with influenza virus-like particle vaccine using microneedles. J Control Release 2010;147(3):326—32.
[57] Song J-M, et al. Improved protection against avian influenza H5N1 virus by a single vaccination with virus-like particles in skin using microneedles. Antivir Res 2010;88(2):244—7.
[58] Edens C, et al. Measles vaccination using a microneedle patch. Vaccine 2013;31(34):3403—9.
[59] Hiraishi Y, et al. Bacillus Calmette-Guerin vaccination using a microneedle patch. Vaccine 2011;29(14):2626—36.
[60] Haigh O, et al. CXCL1 gene silencing in skin using liposome-encapsulated siRNA delivered by microprojection array. J Control Release 2014;194:148—56.
[61] Ma Y, et al. Drug coated microneedles for minimally-invasive treatment of oral carcinomas: development and in vitro evaluation. Biomed Microdevices 2015;17(2):44.
[62] Uddin MJ, et al. Inkjet printing of transdermal microneedles for the delivery of anticancer agents. Int J Pharm 2015;494(2):593—602.
[63] Loizidou EZ, et al. Structural characterisation and transdermal delivery studies on sugar microneedles: experimental and finite element modelling analyses. Eur J Pharm Biopharm 2015;89:224—31.
[64] Ito Y, et al. Dissolving microneedles to obtain rapid local anesthetic effect of lidocaine at skin tissue. J Drug Target 2013;21(8):770—5.
[65] Chu LY, Prausnitz MR. Separable arrowhead microneedles. J Control Release 2011;149(3):242—9.
[66] Park J-H, Allen MG, Prausnitz MR. Polymer microneedles for controlled-release drug delivery. Pharm Res 2006;23(5):1008—19.
[67] Fukushima K, et al. Two-layered dissolving microneedles for percutaneous delivery of peptide/protein drugs in rats. Pharm Res 2011;28(1):7—21.
[68] Chu LY, Choi SO, Prausnitz MR. Fabrication of dissolving polymer microneedles for controlled drug encapsulation and delivery: bubble and pedestal microneedle designs. J Pharm Sci 2010;99(10):4228—38.
[69] Hirobe S, et al. Clinical study and stability assessment of a novel transcutaneous influenza vaccination using a dissolving microneedle patch. Biomaterials 2015;57:50—8.
[70] Matsuo K, et al. Transcutaneous immunization using a dissolving microneedle array protects against tetanus, diphtheria, malaria, and influenza. J Control Release 2012;160(3):495—501.
[71] Ito Y, et al. Feasibility of microneedles for percutaneous absorption of insulin. Eur J Pharm Sci 2006;29(1):82—8.
[72] Liu S, et al. The development and characteristics of novel microneedle arrays fabricated from hyaluronic acid, and their application in the transdermal delivery of insulin. J Control Release 2012;161(3):933—41.
[73] Donnelly RF, et al. Hydrogel-forming and dissolving microneedles for enhanced delivery of photosensitizers and precursors. Photochem Photobiol 2014;90(3):641—7.
[74] Yu J, et al. Microneedle-array patches loaded with hypoxia-sensitive vesicles provide fast glucose-responsive insulin delivery. Proc Natl Acad Sci USA 2015;112(27):8260—5.
[75] Donnelly RF, et al. Hydrogel-forming microneedle arrays for enhanced transdermal drug delivery. Adv Funct Mater 2012;22(23):4879—90.
[76] Donnelly RF, et al. Hydrogel-forming microneedles prepared from "super swelling" polymers combined with lyophilised wafers for transdermal drug delivery. PLoS One 2014;9(10):e111547.
[77] Ye Y, et al. Microneedles integrated with pancreatic cells and synthetic glucose-signal amplifiers for smart insulin delivery. Adv Mater 2016;28(16):3115—21.
[78] Prausnitz MR. Microneedles for transdermal drug delivery. Adv Drug Deliv Rev 2004;56(5):581—7.
[79] Schuetz YB, et al. Emerging strategies for the transdermal delivery of peptide and protein drugs. Expert Opin Drug Deliv 2005;2(3):533—48.
[80] Kalluri H, Banga AK. Formation and closure of microchannels in skin following microporation. Pharm Res 2011;28(1):82—94.

[81] Donnelly RF, Raj Singh TR, Woolfson AD. Microneedle-based drug delivery systems: microfabrication, drug delivery, and safety. Drug Deliv 2010;17(4):187–207.
[82] Singh TR, et al. Microporation techniques for enhanced delivery of therapeutic agents. Recent Pat Drug Deliv Formul 2010;4(1):1–17.
[83] Garland MJ, et al. Microneedle arrays as medical devices for enhanced transdermal drug delivery. Expert Rev Med Devices 2011;8(4):459–82.
[84] Donnelly RF, et al. Processing difficulties and instability of carbohydrate microneedle arrays. Drug Dev Ind Pharm 2009;35(10):1242–54.
[85] Caffarel-Salvador E, et al. Potential of hydrogel-forming and dissolving microneedles for use in paediatric populations. Int J Pharm 2015;489(1–2):158–69.
[86] Lutton RE, et al. A novel scalable manufacturing process for the production of hydrogel-forming microneedle arrays. Int J Pharm 2015;494(1):417–29.
[87] Kim M, Jung B, Park J-H. Hydrogel swelling as a trigger to release biodegradable polymer microneedles in skin. Biomaterials 2012;33(2):668–78.
[88] Donnelly RF, et al. Hydrogel-forming microneedle arrays exhibit antimicrobial properties: potential for enhanced patient safety. Int J Pharm 2013;451(1–2):76–91.
[89] Laurent PE, et al. Evaluation of the clinical performance of a new intradermal vaccine administration technique and associated delivery system. Vaccine 2007;25(52):8833–42.
[90] Tuan-Mahmood TM, et al. Microneedles for intradermal and transdermal drug delivery. Eur J Pharm Sci 2013;50(5):623–37.
[91] Patel SR, et al. Suprachoroidal drug delivery to the back of the eye using hollow microneedles. Pharm Res 2011;28(1):166–76.
[92] SCS microinjector (internet), Available from: http://clearsidebio.com/news/product-fact-sheet/.
[93] Miro-tran (internet), Available from: https://www.valeritas.com/technologies/micro-trans.
[94] MicroCor (internet), Available from: http://www.stratagentlifesciences.com/Tech_MicroCor.html.
[95] Zosano patch (internet), Available from: http://www.zosanopharma.com/index.php/20091103117/Research/Research-General/Technology-Platform.html.
[96] Imperium (internet), Available from: http://www.unilife.com/product-platforms/insulin-delivery/imperium.
[97] anoDyne (internet), Available from: http://anodyne.life.
[98] Daytona MT dermal roller (internet), Available from: http://www.daytonalabs.com/daytona_mt.
[99] AdminPen (internet), Available from: http://www.adminmed.com/technology.

CHAPTER 14

Nanotechnology-Based Medical and Biomedical Imaging for Diagnostics

Kishore Cholkar[1], Nupoor D. Hirani[1], Chandramouli Natarajan[2]
[1]Ingenus Pharmaceuticals/RiconPharma LLC, Denville, NJ, United States; [2]University of Missouri—Kansas City, Kansas City, MO, United States

Contents

1. Introduction	355
2. Fluorescence-Based Imaging and Diagnostics	356
3. Nanocarriers in Biological Imaging	359
3.1 Inorganic Nanomaterials	359
3.1.1 Magnetic Nanoparticles	*359*
3.1.2 Gold Nanoparticles	*359*
3.1.3 Silica Nanoparticles	*361*
3.1.4 Quantum Dots	*361*
3.1.5 Surface-Enhanced Raman Scattering	*362*
3.2 Lipid Nanocarriers	363
3.2.1 Gadolinium Nanoparticles	*363*
3.2.2 Radiolabeled Nanoparticles	*363*
3.2.3 Radiolabeled Liposomes	*364*
3.2.4 Radiolabeled Iron Oxide Nanoparticles	*365*
3.2.5 Gold Nanoparticles	*366*
3.2.6 Gold Nanoshells	*366*
3.2.7 Radiolabeled Nanomicelles	*366*
4. Photoacoustic and Ultrasound Imaging	367
5. Conclusions	369
References	370

1. INTRODUCTION

High-resolution imaging techniques developed in the past decade enables visualization and quantification of molecules of interest. Moreover, these imaging techniques have gained momentum in transforming diagnosis and clinical medicine to new horizons. On the other hand, nanotechnology coupled with imaging techniques may offer solutions to a multitude of challenges in clinics for incomprehensible diseased-state biology. Nanotechnology involves strategies that consolidate materials in a nanometer scale either by sizing up from atoms or by refining or sizing down large materials into nanoparticles [1]. The advantage of nanometer size is it allows interactions with biomolecules on cell surface and organelles. Such interactions may provide a broad scope in disease diagnosis and treatment such as, but not limited to, cancer, inflammation, infectious diseases, and penetration of the blood—brain barrier. Biological (static and dynamic) and physiochemical barriers may limit nanotechnology approaches at preclinical and clinical stages. Nanomaterials such as gold, iron oxide, and lipid-based nanocarriers have been extensively studied for in vivo distribution, evasion of reticuloendothelial system, and pharmacokinetics. Imaging techniques such as confocal microscopy, fluorescence, X-ray, radionuclides, and positron emission techniques have been applied. In this chapter, discussion is focused on nanomaterials that utilize fluorescence, magnetic, electromagnetic, and radioactive properties. Applications of such nanomaterials to elicit a wide range of biomolecular interactions can overcome challenges in diagnostics and imaging.

2. FLUORESCENCE-BASED IMAGING AND DIAGNOSTICS

Fluorescence technique is widely applied in imaging and diagnosis. The applications include study of an enzyme activity, identification of tumor/cancer cell, and other disorders. Moreover, fluorescence technique may be applied to study the phenotypic changes in intracellular organelles like mitochondria and nucleus [2]. Recent work utilized fluorescent dyes for intracellular targeted drug delivery [3]. Structural organization of tissues is complex and nonhomogeneous. Selection of an appropriate fluorescent dye for specific target, imaging and diagnosis within the tissue is pivotal. For example, erythrocytes are commonly infected with *Plasmodium falciparum*, the parasite responsible for malaria [4]. Fluorescence confocal microscopy has been used to diagnose and differentiate infected erythrocytes from normal. Such differentiation of infected erythrocytes from noninfected ones was demonstrated with calcein fluorescent dye relative to changes in volume and area (Fig. 14.1).

Fluorescence-based in situ hybridization aka FISH is another technique that is most reliable, precise, and very sensitive. FISH technique is designed for understanding cytogenetic abnormalities, detecting aberrations, and monitoring diseases during treatment. It is regularly used for prenatal testing to examine the chances of trisomy 21, aka "Down syndrome" [5]. In this technique, FISH develops three bright colored spots on a cell, where each spot indicates chromosome 21 (Fig. 14.2). Cells from amniotic fluid are studied for any submicroscopic deletions that are beyond the resolution of an extended chromosome study. This technique is occasionally applied in amniocentesis during late pregnancy to assess the growth of the fetus. Another rapid FISH technique, FastFISH, has been developed to study the abnormalities related to chromosomes 13, 18, 21, X, Y and DiGeorge syndrome with centromere evaluation probe and locus specific identifier probe. FastFISH study may require less than 2 h to determine chromosomal abnormalities [6]. Fluorescent probes have been utilized to assess rare aberrations. Fig. 14.3 is an example of rare deletion of mixed lineage leukemia (MLL) located at gene 11q23 [7]. This type of mutation may be de novo or a therapy-related hematologic disorder. In normal cells, fluorescent probe normally colocalizes and produces two yellow fusion signals. However, MLL gene deletion displays a characteristic

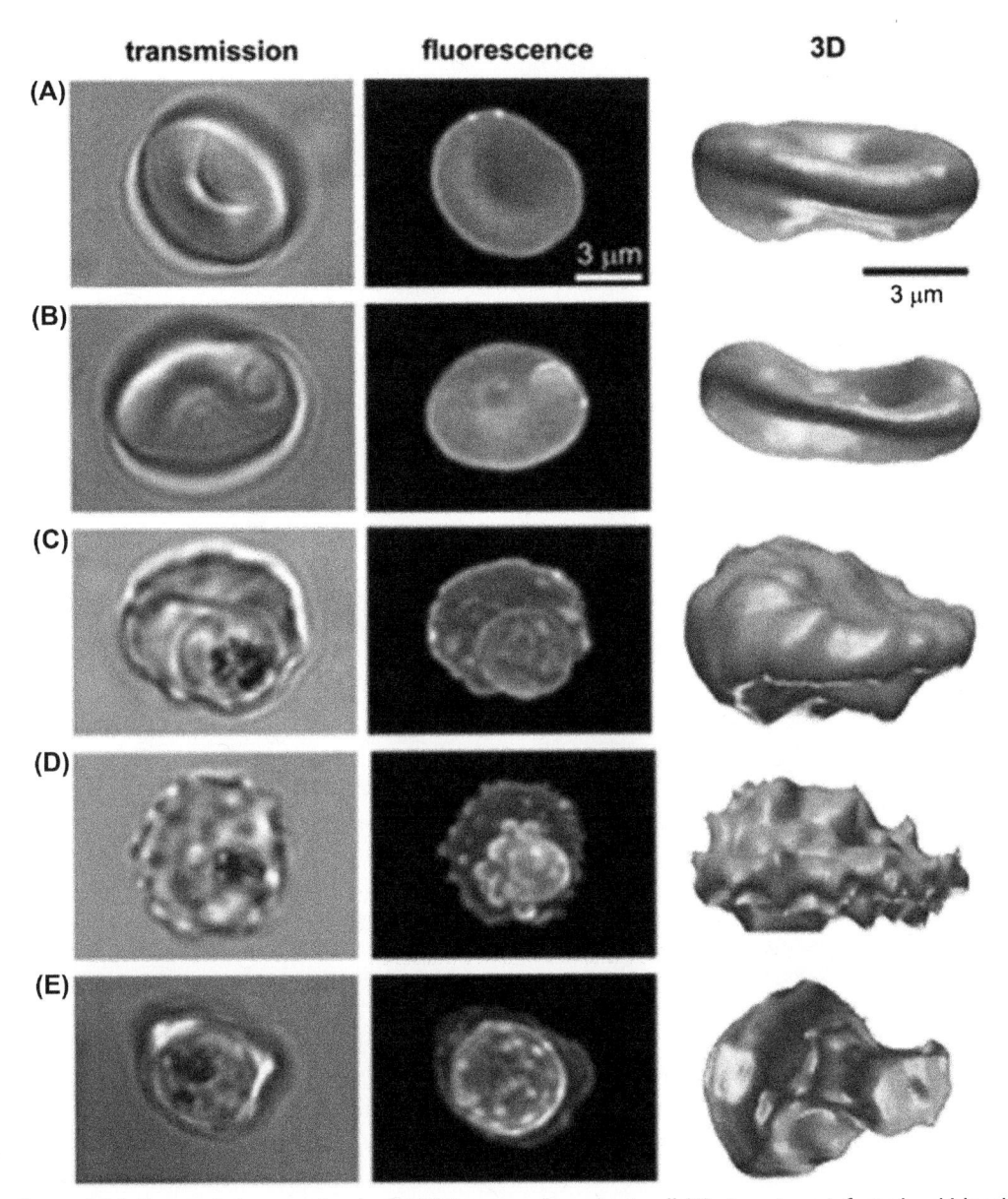

Figure 14.1 Transmission, confocal, and 3D images of a cohort cell (A), ring-stage infected red blood cell (IRBC) (B), trophozoite-stage IRBC (C), and schizont-stage IRBC (D and E). Fluorescence images are maximum intensity projections of the deconvolved confocal 3D image stacks. The selected images are representative of a total of 119 cells analyzed. Panels D and E show typical phenotypes exhibited by schizont-stage IRBCs.

Figure 14.2 Fluorescence in situ hybridization probes for chromosomes 21 (*red signal*, black in print versions), 18 (*yellow or fused red/green signal*, white in print versions), and 12 (*green signal*, light gray in print versions) were used to identify cells with trisomy 21 (left) and both trisomy 18 and trisomy 21 (right).

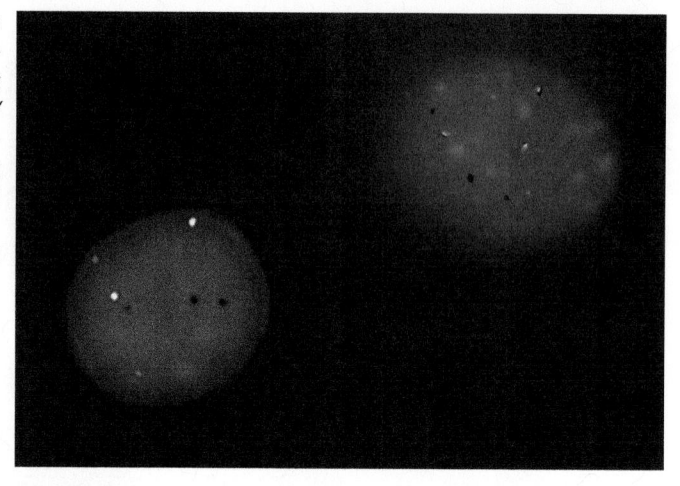

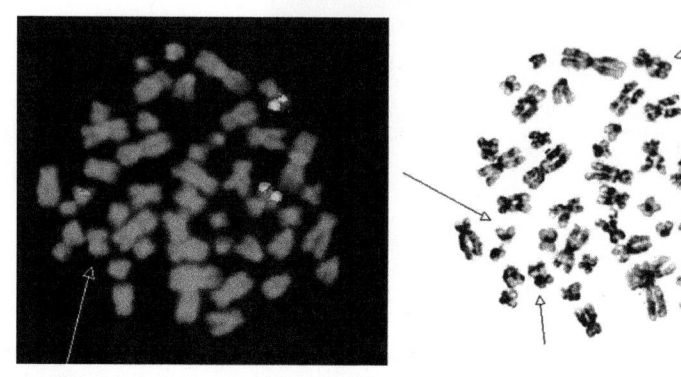

Figure 14.3 G-banded metaphase spread [47,XY,+11,t(11,21)(q23; q22)] on the *right with arrows* showing the two normal copies of chromosome 11 and derivative chromosomes 11 and 21. Mixed lineage leukemia break-apart probe fluorescence in situ hybridization analysis on the same metaphase cell (left) showing the two normal copies of chromosome 11 (*yellow*, white in print versions), the red derivative chromosome 21 [der(21)] signal, and the derivative chromosome 11 (*arrow*).

tricolor (red–green–yellow) fusion signal pattern (Fig. 14.3, left). In such a scenario, the FISH technique is advantageous where all recurrent and MLL deletions may be simultaneously detected. Fig. 14.3 demonstrates a G-band metaphase (right) MLL gene deletion. It is detected with karyotyping to identify the derivatives of chromosome 21 and 11 along with two normal copies of chromosome 11. On the other hand, FISH-treated cells demonstrate clear detection of the aforementioned condition (left) as a fluorescent colored spot indicating each chromosome of interest. These results indicate that the FISH technique can precisely ascertain the chromosomal aberration. Moreover, this technique provides an in-depth and better understanding of the underlying mechanism of the metaphase cells [7] (Fig. 14.3). Several dyes and fluorescent techniques have been developed to study chromosomal aberrations. For example, spectral karyotyping and multiplex FISH have been employed to uniquely color chromosomes. However, RX-FISH is another dye that requires a cross-species color banding [8].

A limitation of the fluorescence technique is photobleaching, which occurs due to photochemical destruction of fluorophores. Photobleaching faints the fluorescence signal leading to development of unclear images and improper quantitative analysis [9]. This may be avoided with proper selection of neutral-density filters and with a reduced amount of light. Super-resolution microscopy, aka nanoscopy, may help overcome such limitations [10]. Imaging in three dimension (3D) and live cell imaging can be prepared with fluorescence to investigate cellular processes. Optics, cameras, fluorescent probes and algorithms are helpful in improving the resolution.

3. NANOCARRIERS IN BIOLOGICAL IMAGING

Nanocarriers have been mostly explored for target-specific drug delivery as systems/ vehicles. Primarily, such vehicles have been exploited as transporters for anticancer drugs. Examples of nanocarriers include, but are not limited to, liposomes, nanomicelles, nanoparticles, iron oxide, and gold and carbon-based materials. Such delivery systems can be designed for controlled drug release [11]. In the following sections we focused our discussion on inorganic and lipid-based carrier systems in imaging and diagnosis.

3.1 Inorganic Nanomaterials
3.1.1 Magnetic Nanoparticles

Magnetic nanoparticles, paramagnetic contrast agents (CAs), and superparamagnetic iron oxide nanoparticles (SPIOs) have been employed for various soft-tissue imaging. SPIOs may be size tailored and functionalized for targeted imaging. Magnetic nanoparticles are considered as an excellent diagnostic tracers for magnetic resonance and disease management [12]. Magnetic resonance imaging (MRI) has been utilized for imaging soft tissues, especially brain tumors. For individualized therapy, MRI is preferred for guidance and monitoring delivery of therapeutic agents, including antibodies, peptides, aptamers, genes, or therapeutic agents to target tissues [13]. Studies demonstrate that iron oxide nanoparticles induce cytotoxicity and genotoxicity by elevating oxidative stress and DNA damage in human breast cancer cell [14].

3.1.2 Gold Nanoparticles

Gold nanoparticles are indicated in the treatment of rheumatoid arthritis as anti-inflammatory agents. On the other hand, radioactive gold microparticles are directed to cancer therapy as local radioisotope [14]. Silica-coated gold nanoparticles can deliver excess heat and active agent simultaneously to the tumor cells to achieve superior efficacy [15]. Similarly, gadolinium-loaded dendrimer-entrapped gold nanoparticles (Gd-Au DENPs) contain gold nanoparticles and gadolinium entrapped within the same nanoparticle carrier system. These dual-loaded inorganic nanoparticles may aid in simultaneous magnetic resonance (MR) and computed tomography (CT) imaging of kidney, heart, liver, and other biological systems [16]. A combination of gold nanoparticles with X-ray has been prepared to induce DNA damage and cytotoxicity of tumor cells. Fig. 14.4 demonstrates model tumor cells and illustrates the mean displacement of gold nanoparticles from the nuclear boundary. Moreover, the size of the cell nuclei can be mapped (Fig. 14.4) by calculating the intensity of gold, which is directly proportional to the ionization of gold particles causing DNA damage.

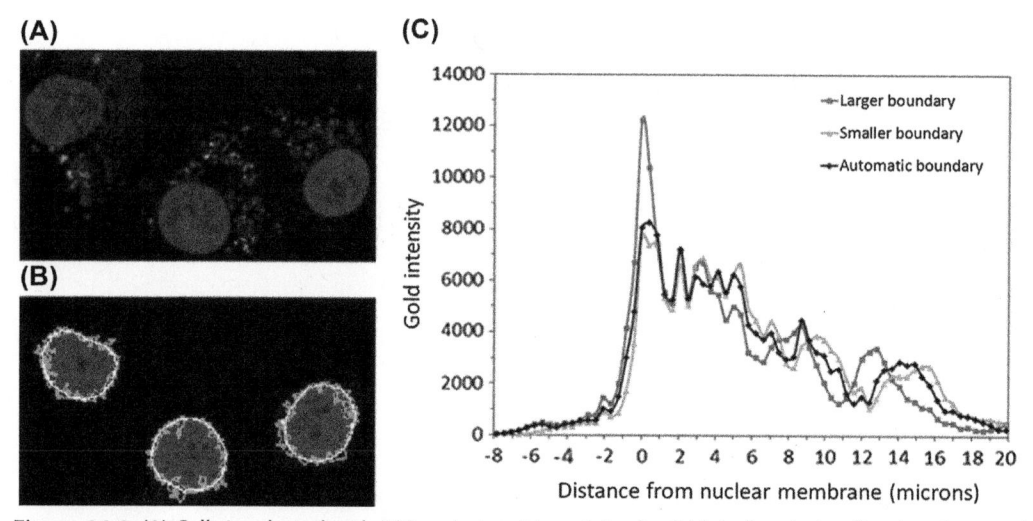

Figure 14.4 (A) Cells incubated with 500 μg/mL gold particles for 24 h before being fixed and stained with 4′,6-diamidino-2-phenylindole (DAPI). Image contains both the surface plasmon resonance signal from two-photon interaction with gold particles (*orange*, black in print versions) and nuclei regions (*blue*, dark gray in print versions). The gold nanoparticles are observed in the cytoplasmic regions with some of the gold particles accumulating close to the nuclear boundary regions. (B) Nuclei boundaries produced in image analysis by a varying binary threshold. The automatic threshold determined by ImageJ (*white*) in comparison with a lower threshold (*green*, white in print versions) and higher threshold (*red*, light gray in print versions). (C) Integrated gold signal of 20 cells for increasing distance from the nuclear membrane for the three thresholds chosen in (B). The automatic threshold outline (*black line*) produces a maximum gold intensity at 0.5 μm outside the nuclear membrane. The gold intensity reduces significantly across the membrane (distance = 0) and the gold signal within the nucleus (distances < 0) is consistent with the assumption that all of the gold is outside the nucleus, instead reflecting the measured point spread function for the gold image of 0.5 μm. The integration was done taking account of the number of pixels in the image at each distance from the nuclear membrane. Hence to a good approximation the intensity is equivalent to the relative density of gold nanoparticles.

3.1.3 Silica Nanoparticles

Silica (silicon dioxide) nanoparticles facilitate surface properties such as geometry and porosity to be utilized in therapeutics and diagnostic fields. Silica nanoparticles can deliver hydrophilic drugs to target tissues. However, extensive research is currently being conducted to utilize silica nanoparticles for diagnostic, therapeutic, and imaging purposes. Mesoporous silica nanoparticles have been evaluated as controlled drug delivery system and gene transfection carriers [17]. For in vitro targeting, therapy, and imaging, studies have been conducted with silica nanoparticles to deliver hydrophobic drugs [18–21]. Fig. 14.5 demonstrates silica nanoparticles encapsulated with combinations of organic doping dyes as barcoding tags. These nanoparticles have been utilized with multiple signaling as fluorescence resonance energy transfer (FRET). This technology can mediate emissions of multiple colors based on the ratios of the encapsulated organic dyes when excited with a single wavelength. FRET helps in understanding a complex biological signaling system [22]. The US Food and Drug Administration approved the first clinical trial with multimodal silica nanoparticles (7 nm diameter). Such particles have a unique combination of biological, structural, and optical properties for tumor (melanoma) targeting [23].

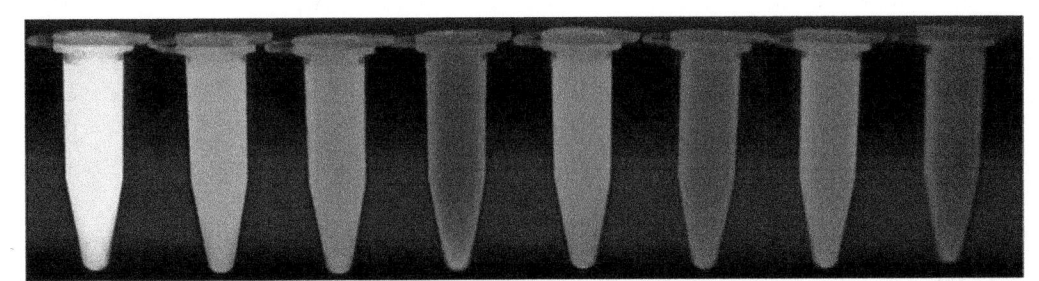

Figure 14.5 Nanoparticle samples with different doping dye combinations under 300 nm ultraviolet illumination. Dye doping ratio (in order): 1:0:0, 0:1:0, 1:0:1, 4:1.5:3, 0.5:0.5:0.5, 2:2:2, 0:1:1, 0.5:0.5:4.

3.1.4 Quantum Dots

Quantum dots (QDs) are composed of semiconducting material with high surface to volume ratios. QDs emit fluorescence based on the size of the valence band and conduction band of the material. Different types of QDs are available based on structure and composition. Core type QD is composed of a single material, whereas core–shell type is composed of two materials, a small region of one material embedded in another with a wider band gap. Alloy QDs allow tuning of multiple components. QDs are brighter, can emit the whole spectrum, and the degradation is very minimal compared with the traditional organic dyes used for biomedical analysis [24]. Studies have shown that successful gene delivery can be developed for the treatment of lung cancer with carbon QD as theranostic nanocarriers [25] (Fig. 14.6). QDs have been explored and

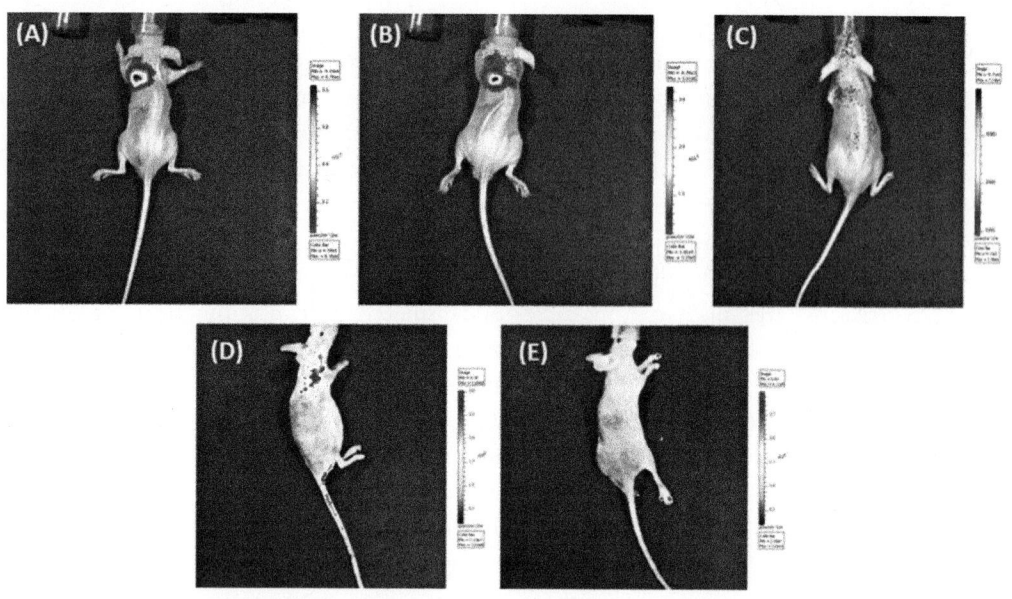

Figure 14.6 Monitoring luciferase inhibition in vivo with bioluminescent imaging. Representative images show the reduction in lung tumor size following intratracheal instillation of fc-rPEI-Cdots nanoagents in luciferase-expressing H460 lung carcinoma. Panels (A—C) depict bioluminescent images of the lungs before and after treatment. (B) 7 days, (C) 10 days after two times inhaled administration. After aerosol delivery, the fc-rPEI-Cdots/pooled siRNA nanoagents (D) can accumulated at lung region when compared to PBS (E).

demonstrated with multidisciplinary applications. For example, graphene quantum dot (GQD) contains one or more lateral dimensional sheets of carbon nanomaterials. GQD is suitable as drug carrier, biosensors, and for cell imaging because of their photostability, low toxicity, and biocompatibility [26—29]. Similarly, fluorescence has been utilized in sensing temperature of human-derived neuronal cell lines, SH-SY5Y, because of nonhomogenous heat production in neurites relative to normal cells [30].

3.1.5 Surface-Enhanced Raman Scattering

Surface-enhanced Raman scattering (SERS) is commonly applied in biological studies and microanalysis with a laser beam [31]. A small amount of circulating tumor cells, RNA, nucleic acid, lipids, and proteins present in blood samples may be detected with SERS. Cancer diagnosis and nanoscale hexagonal columns (NHCs) can also be diagnosed with SERS [32—36]. Studies demonstrated that negatively charged silver NHCs can be applied in SERS. This technology can sense positively charged histone tails of the methylated cell-free DNA from patients with cancer [37]. Apart from silver NHCs, silicone amorphous nanomaterials have been utilized for biosensing applications with SERS [38].

SERS also provides single molecule detection by amplifying Raman signal intensity, which renders it suitable for multicolor imaging in multiplex detection in complex molecular studies [39—46]. Because of high sensitivity, this technique can be applied for early detection and quantification of hemozoin, which is an indicator of parasitemia levels in malarial patients (*P. falciparum*) [47]. Surface-enhanced spatially offset Raman spectroscopy has been utilized with SERS active nanoparticles. In vivo imaging of the skull is performed with non-invasive, real-time spectroscopic measurements of neurochemicals [48].

3.2 Lipid Nanocarriers
3.2.1 Gadolinium Nanoparticles
Gadolinium-loaded nanoparticles (GdNPs) are the most promising theranostic agents. GdNPs can be very promising as diagnostics (molecular imaging), therapeutics (molecular therapy), and a combination on a single platform. Clinical MR scans utilize CAs such as gadolinium. In proton MR, gadolinium (Gd^{3+})-based T_1 CAs are applied to reduce the spin-lattice relaxation time of water. Moreover, these agents increase the signal from protons, which produce effected voxel to appear "brighter" in T_1-weighted image. Higher resolution and signal to noise ratio are provided by T_1-weighted sequences. Accelerating the longitudinal molar relaxivity (r1) of T_1 CA prolongs rotational correlation time (τ_r, i.e., the tumbling time of the CA in the bulk water). Higher molecular weight Gd-based agents like Gd functionalized polymer, peptide amphiphiles, or viral capsid, dendrimer, liposomes, nanoparticles, nanomicelles, zeolites, fullerenes, carbon nanotubes, clays, and QDs have been explored [49—53]. Such gadolinium complexes are impeded by cell membrane translocation and are not suitable for targeting. Moreover, Gd-based complexes are associated with difficulty and reproducibility of their fabrications [54]. Till now, only a few gadolinium-based smart MR probes have been developed as responsive to β-galactosidase or myeloperoxidase [55—59]. Kang et al., have developed gadolinium nanoparticles (50—60 nm) conjugated with bifunctional chelates. Two of these have been abbreviated as $Gd@SiO_2$-DO_3A and Gd_2SiO_2-DO_2A-BTA. In vivo studies demonstrated that the latter gadolinium nanoparticles exhibited stronger intracellular uptake and cytotoxicity in tumor cells such as SK-HEP1, MDA-MB-231, HeLa, and Hep-3B [60]. In another study, Chun et al. demonstrated intracellular controlled self-assembly of gadolinium nanoparticles [61]. These nanoparticles can act as smart molecular MR CAs. In another study, Li et al. prepared a construct integrating an active gemcitabine metabolite (gemcitabine 5-monophosphate) by coordinating with Gd(III). It self-assembles into nanoparticles and can be applied as theranostics [62]. Such combination demonstrated a stronger T_1 contrast signal and simultaneously enhanced retention in mice. Moreover, this combination significantly inhibited tumor growth in mice.

3.2.2 Radiolabeled Nanoparticles
Radiolabeled nanoparticles represent a class of agents that possess long circulation time, high plasma stability, and great potential for clinical applications in early diagnosis of cancer and cardiovascular diseases. Radiotracer-based imaging technology generates

either single-photon emission computed tomography (SPECT) or positron-emission tomography (PET) for targeted in vivo imaging. Both technologies are highly sensitive, specific, and useful in accurate quantification. In contrast, other in vivo imaging techniques may be of limited application because of tissue-specific penetration [63]. Table 14.1 summarizes available high-resolution imaging techniques and their sensitivity. On the other hand, Table 14.2 summarizes properties of radionuclides such as half-life and type of radiation emitted from the radionuclide.

Table 14.1 Some features of imaging technology used in acquiring anatomical and molecular probing [63]

Imaging techniques	Resolution	Detection range	Molecular sensitivity	Penetration
PET	1–2 mm	10^{-11} to 10^{-12}	ng	Unlimited depth
SPECT	0.3–1 mm	10^{-11} to 10^{-11}	ng	Unlimited depth
FMT	1–3 mm	10^{-6} to 10^{-12}	µg	<5 cm
MRI	50–250 µm	10^{-3} to 10^{-5}	µg to mg	Unlimited depth
X-ray, CT	25–150 µm		mg	Unlimited depth
Ultrasound	30–500 µm	10^{-6} to 10^{-9}	µg to mg	Limited (mm to cm)

CT, computed tomography; FMT, fluorescence molecular tomography; MRI, magnetic resonance imaging; PET, positron-emission tomography; SPECT, single-photon emission computed tomography.

Table 14.2 Characteristics of radionuclides used in various imaging modalities [63]

Radionuclide tracer	Radiation	Half-life	Imaging modality
F-18	Positron	1.83 h	PET
Cu	β	12.7 h	PET/CT
Re	β, γ	16.9 h	SPECT/CT
I-123	Auger, γ	13.2 h	PET/CT
In	Auger, γ	67.2 h	PET/CT
Ga	γ	78.3 h	SPECT
Tc	γ	6.0 h	SPECT
I-131	γ, β	8.0 days	PET/SPECT

CT, computed tomography; PET, positron-emission tomography; SPECT, single-photon emission computed tomography.

3.2.3 Radiolabeled Liposomes

Liposomes labeled with radioisotopes have the advantage of permeating through inflamed and infected sites. Dam et al. documented the application of ^{99m}Tc–polyethylene glycol (PEG) liposomes in scintigraphic detection of infection and inflammation. These liposomes exploit the inherent nature of the enhanced permeability at infection and inflammatory sites [64]. Li et al. prepared surface-targeted indium-loaded liposomes against LOX-1 (low density lipoprotein receptor) to acquire molecular images of atherosclerotic plaques in ApoE$^{-/-}$ mice. The specificity of these liposomes was confirmed by injecting mice with liposomes coated with nonspecific IgG. These control liposomes did not show any traceable signal in atherosclerotic plaques [65].

Harrington et al. demonstrated the application of ^{111}In-pentetic acid or diethylenetriaminepentaacetic acid (DTPA)-labeled PEGylated liposomes in cancer diagnosis. Patients with cancer were subjected to scintigraphic imaging studies by administering radiolabeled PEGylated liposomes. Interestingly, results demonstrated liposome uptake in tumor. Moreover, a correlation has been established between tumor images and tumor volume [66]. In another study, Chang et al., demonstrated bio-distribution of Re-N,N-bis (2-mercaptoethyl) N′ N′-diethylenediamine (BMEDA)—labeled PEGylated liposomes in mice colon tumor model [67]. However, this study has been associated with a limitation of short half-life of positron emitters. To overcome such limitations, Peterson and team demonstrated rapid encapsulation of ^{64}Cu-loaded PEGylated liposomes. The researchers demonstrated the application of ^{64}Cu-liposomes for quantitative in vivo imaging of healthy and tumor-bearing mice with PET. Such remote loading technique appears to be a powerful tool for characterizing in vivo performance of liposome-based nanomedicine. Moreover, such technique may significantly improve diagnosis and yield an effective treatment [68].

3.2.4 Radiolabeled Iron Oxide Nanoparticles

Magnetic properties of iron oxide nanoparticles render them as an ideal candidate for MRI, PET, and SPECT imaging technologies [69—71]. Lee et al. prepared radiolabeled iron oxide nanoparticle conjugated to a RGD peptide (arginine, glycine, aspartic acid) functionalized with (1,4,7,10-tetraazacyclododecane)-1,4,7,10-tetraacetate (DOTA) (chelator) for labeling with ^{64}Cu. Mice bearing human glioblastoma exhibited the highest uptake at the tumor site at 4 h after injection. The specificity of this construct was examined by blocking RGD receptors, αvβ3 integrin, with unconjugated nanoparticles [72].

A trifunctional modality comprising PET/near-infrared fluorescence (NIRF)/MRI functional iron oxide nanoparticles has been reported by Xie et al. This study documented that ^{64}Cu-DOTA and Cy 5.5 CLIO (cross-linked iron oxide nanoparticles) were injected into a sub-cutaneous xenograft U87MG tumor-bearing mice. Delineation of tumors was reported in all three modalities. However, PET imaging revealed high muscle to tumor ratio relative to NIRF results [73]. Nahrendorf et al. studied dextranated DTPA-modified magnetofluorescent 20-nm nanoparticles. These particles with ^{64}Cu radionuclide were injected into ApoE$^{-/-}$ atherosclerotic mice. Bio-distribution suggested 260% and 392% higher levels in aortas and carotid arteries, respectively, in comparison with wild-type mice [74]. In another study by Nahrendorf et al., fluorine-18 (F^{18})-labeled macrophage-targeted nanoparticles were utilized for PET-CT detection of inflammation in aortic aneurysm (AA)-induced ApoE$^{-/-}$ mice. Aneurismal aortic sections revealed significantly higher uptake relative to wild-type aorta. Atherosclerotic plaques with macrophage infiltration exhibited lower PET signal than AA. The investigators also performed ex vivo imaging to validate in vivo PET data. Moreover, the researchers reported higher uptake of F^{18}-labeled macrophage-targeted CLIO nanoparticles. For ex vivo imaging by autoradiography and fluorescence reflective microscopic studies, nanoparticles were labeled with near-infrared fluorochrome [75].

3.2.5 Gold Nanoparticles

Several studies have documented the applications of gold nanoparticles in PET/CT imaging [76–79]. These particles are labeled with radioactive agents such as positron or gamma emitters. This approach exploits the sensitive nature of PET combined with the accuracy of CT in localization. Morales-Avila et al. documented the efficacy of 99-m technetium gold nanoparticles conjugated to RGD peptides for imaging metastatic tumor. This non-invasive study conducted in C6 human glioma tumor-bearing athymic mice demonstrated high specificity in imaging tumor $\alpha v\beta 3$ expression [80]. The integrin's role in tumor metastasis and angiogenesis has been documented. This target-specific approach may be a potential tool for oncologists to design highly effective individualized therapeutic regimen for patients with cancer.

3.2.6 Gold Nanoshells

Gold nanoshells (NS) are spherical nanoparticles comprising a dielectric core and a metal shell. The plasmon resonance frequency is determined by the relative size of the core and the metal shell [81]. The unique size, shape, and optical properties of the gold NS render these shells ideal candidate for cancer detection and treatment. Xie et al. studied a radiolabeled gold nanoshell. This construct was injected into nude mice induced with head and neck squamous carcinoma xenograft. PET/CT imaging revealed accumulation of ^{64}Cu-labeled nanoparticles in the tumor site 20 and 40 h after injection. This construct was labeled with PEG2k-DOTA for chelation of Cu^{64} and surface modification, to a diameter of 174 nm and surface charge of -5 mV [82]. The authors obtained high radiolabeling efficiency (81.3%), stability (3 h), and high-resolution PET images [82].

Shao et al. reported the efficacy of I-125-labeled gold nanorods (NR) in arthritic-induced mice. These nanorods were conjugated with anti-intercellular adhesion molecule 1 antibody, which is overexpressed in arthritic disease. PEGylation of gold NR resulted in longer circulation time. It leads to higher accumulation at inflamed joints yielding better treatment [83].

3.2.7 Radiolabeled Nanomicelles

Nanomicelles are lipid-based or polymer-based amphiphilic molecules comprising a hydrophobic core and a hydrophilic shell. These constructs are formed spontaneously above a certain concentration termed as critical micellar concentration [84]. The physical and chemical properties of micelles can be found elsewhere [85]. Zhang et al. documented images obtained on SPECT scanning of peptide-conjugated polymeric nanomicelles. This construct is targeted against a prostate cancer molecule known as EPHB4 receptor [86]. In another study, the same group prepared annexinA5-conjugated nanomicelles labeled with I^{125} and indocyanine Cy7-like dye to detect apoptosis. Such Cy7-like dye expresses near-infrared fluorescent properties that can facilitate acquiring optical images. Annexin A5 is a strong binder of phosphatidyl serine residues that are expressed on the cell surface during the early stages of apoptosis. Mice bearing EL5 lymphomas treated with antilymphoma agents were injected with the annexin A5-conjugated construct and subjected to SPECT and optical imaging. The authors reported significant accumulation of the construct in drug-treated mice compared with untreated mice, indicating early apoptosis [87]. In another study conducted by Xiao et al. on U87MG tumor-bearing mice injected with $\alpha v \beta 3$ specific multifunctional polymeric micelles were reported. These particles are prepared with hyperbranched amphiphilic block copolymer. It is conjugated to cRGD peptide for targeting, a Cu-64 chelator [1,4,7-triazacyclononane-triacetic acid (NOTA)] for labeling, PET imaging, and an anticancer agent (doxorubicin). Mice injected with these multifunctional nanomicelles showed higher accumulation at the tumor site relative to the control mice (treated with a blocking dose of cRGD peptide) indicating $\alpha v \beta 3$ specificity [86].

4. PHOTOACOUSTIC AND ULTRASOUND IMAGING

Photoacoustic (PA) imaging can provide real-time changes with high spatial resolution. This technology combines the contrast and spectral sensitivities of optical imaging with the resolution and tissue penetration abilities of ultrasound. Materials absorb light energy and convert it into heat energy by a nonradiative relaxation mechanism. On exposure to heat the materials expand due to their thermoelastic properties generating a pressure wave. This pressure wave in turn helps detection, in the course of its dissemination process through the surrounding environment onto the surface. The conversion of light into heat energy results in generation of sound waves and thus the term, photoacoustic [88]. Bayer et al. tuned gold nanorods (GNR) by coating the construct with amorphous silica, which improves thermal stability and PA signal generation efficiency [89–91]. The optical absorption spectra of GNR can be tuned to exhibit different absorption wavelengths that help distinguish multiple CAs through multiwavelength PA imaging [91]. Similarly, Rich et al. demonstrate the potential clinical utility of PA imaging for visualization of cancer in salivary gland [92]. Silica-coated GNR (SIO_2-GNR) with peak absorption wavelengths at 780 and 830 nm were targeted to cells expressing two receptors, EGFR and HER2. Cells incubated with target-specific SIO_2-GNR were inserted into a phantom tissue and imaged with PA technology. The authors reported enhanced PA signal in cells targeted with SIO_2-GNR relative

Table 14.3 Different types of gold nanoparticles used for photoacoustic imaging

Type	Size, shape, and symmetry	Absorption spectrum	Characteristics	Reference
Gold nanoshells	Dielectric core coated by a metallic shell; Core 50 nm, shell 3.2 nm	600–900 nm [visible–near infrared (NIR) region]	1. Minimal absorption and maximal optical penetration 2. Resistance to thermal denaturation and bleaching	[63], [94], [95]
Gold nanorods	Cylindrical shape, width 20 nm, length 6.6 nm	600–900 nm (visible–NIR region)	Effective in targeting specific cellular receptors	[95]
Gold nanocages	Cuboidal; inner edges length of 50 nm, thickness of wall 6 nm	600–900 nm (visible–NIR region)	1. Gold nanocages can enhance images on integration with optical coherence tomography for resolving tissue microanatomy 2. Immunotargeting moieties capable of photothermal destruction of cancer cells in vitro	[95], [96], [97]
Indocyanine green doped	100 nm	700–2500 nm (NIR region)	1. Photosensitizer (PS) that can produce singlet oxygen via energy transfer from dye to oxygen molecule 2. PS effective in photodynamic therapy 3. Dye encapsulated in nanoparticles prolong circulation time	[95], [98]

to non-SIO$_2$-GNR-coated construct [91]. Description of PA signal detection with a custom-built system that acquires images by a combination of ultrasound and PA signals can be found elsewhere [91].

Bayer et al. demonstrated the efficacy of PA technology in vivo by injecting SIO$_2$-GNR particles into a breast cancer murine model overexpressing HER2 and $\alpha v \beta 3$ receptors. The researchers reported high-resolution 3D anatomical images of the tumor region with a combination of PA and ultrasound technology. Interestingly, this study determined tumor growth by functional PA imaging of blood oxygen saturation. By assessing the levels of oxygen saturation, hypoxic regions within tumor region can be mapped with this robust technology [88]. This imaging system has the potential to provide unique information on prognosis and individualized response to therapy.

Agarwal et al. prepared GNRs conjugated to tumor necrosis factor (TNF-α) antibody and radiolabeled with I^{125} to monitor anti-rheumatic drug delivery. A combination of dual modalities, PA and nuclear imaging through one CA comprising GNRs, is able to capture images of deep and mineralized tissue joints of rat tail in situ. This technology has the capability to track GNRs down to a concentration of 10 pm with a minimal radiolabeling of 5 µCi [77]. Chamberland et al., demonstrated PA tomography (PAT) of joints to monitor drug delivery non-invasively [93]. GNRs conjugated to molecules that inhibit TNF (etanercept) were injected intraarticularly in mice. PAT of tail joints ex vivo was performed to acquire images of GNR-conjugated etanercept molecules. The system was able to capture images down to concentrations of 1 pm in phantom tissues and 10 pM in biological samples with high spatial resolution and excellent signal-to-noise ratio [93]. An overview on different types of gold nanoparticles used in PA imaging and their properties are summarized Table 14.3.

5. CONCLUSIONS

Disease diagnostics and molecular imaging are challenging subjects to pharmacologists and drug delivery scientists. The advent of nanotechnology and imaging techniques has helped us to understand the disease prognosis and yielding an efficient treatment. Imaging techniques have been a significantly improving science. A combination of nanotechnology and imaging improved the specificity, accuracy, and sensitivity for molecular imaging. Moreover, such combination is being applied in diagnosis and treatment of cancer or heart and brain diseases. For example, iron oxide nanoparticles and MRI. To improve selectivity, targeted nanocarriers with imaging techniques have been investigated. These techniques may be used to load therapeutic agents that can improve diagnosis and treatment of ailments. In the near future, such combination of technologies may lead to better, selective, and sensitive treatment modalities.

REFERENCES

[1] Jabir NR, Tabrez S, Ashraf GM, Shakil S, Damanhouri GA, Kamal MA. Nanotechnology-based approaches in anticancer research. Int J Nanomedicine 2012;7:4391–408.
[2] Chowdhury SR, Djordjevic J, Albensi BC, Fernyhough P. Simultaneous evaluation of substrate-dependent oxygen consumption rates and mitochondrial membrane potential by TMRM and safranin in cortical mitochondria. Biosci Rep 2016;36(1):e00286.
[3] Graef F, Gordon S, Lehr CM. Anti-infectives in drug delivery—overcoming the gram-negative bacterial cell envelope. In: Current topics in microbiology and immunology; March 5, 2016. p. 1–22.
[4] Esposito A, Choimet JB, Skepper JN, Mauritz JM, Lew VL, Kaminski CF, et al. Quantitative imaging of human red blood cells infected with *Plasmodium falciparum*. Biophys J 2010;99(3):953–60.
[5] Olmos-Serrano JL, Kang HJ, Tyler WA, Silbereis JC, Cheng F, Zhu Y, et al. Down Syndrome developmental brain transcriptome reveals defective oligodendrocyte differentiation and myelination. Neuron 2016;89(6):1208–22.
[6] Choolani M, Ho SS, Razvi K, Ponnusamy S, Baig S, Fisk NM, et al. FastFISH: technique for ultra-rapid fluorescence in situ hybridization on uncultured amniocytes yielding results within 2 h of amniocentesis. Mol Hum Reprod 2007;13(6):355–9.
[7] Wolff DJ, Bagg A, Cooley LD, Dewald GW, Hirsch BA, Jacky PB, et al. Guidance for fluorescence in situ hybridization testing in hematologic disorders. J Mol Diag 2007;9(2):134–43.
[8] Azofeifa J, Fauth C, Kraus J, Maierhofer C, Langer S, Bolzer A, et al. An optimized probe set for the detection of small interchromosomal aberrations by use of 24-color FISH. Am J Hum Genet 2000;66(5):1684–8.
[9] Song L, Hennink EJ, Young IT, Tanke HJ. Photobleaching kinetics of fluorescein in quantitative fluorescence microscopy. Biophys J 1995;68(6):2588–600.
[10] Huang B, Bates M, Zhuang X. Super-resolution fluorescence microscopy. Annu Rev Biochem 2009;78:993–1016.
[11] Qian WY, Sun DM, Zhu RR, Du XL, Liu H, Wang SL. pH-sensitive strontium carbonate nanoparticles as new anticancer vehicles for controlled etoposide release. Int J Nanomedicine 2012;7:5781–92.
[12] Mahmoudi M, Sahraian MA, Shokrgozar MA, Laurent S. Superparamagnetic iron oxide nanoparticles: promises for diagnosis and treatment of multiple sclerosis. ACS Chem Neurosci 2011;2(3):118–40.
[13] Lee JH, Kim JW, Cheon J. Magnetic nanoparticles for multi-imaging and drug delivery. Mol Cells 2013;35(4):274–84.
[14] Bhattacharyya S, Kudgus RA, Bhattacharya R, Mukherjee P. Inorganic nanoparticles in cancer therapy. Pharm Res 2011;28(2):237–59.
[15] Lee J, Chatterjee DK, Lee MH, Krishnan S. Gold nanoparticles in breast cancer treatment: promise and potential pitfalls. Cancer Lett 2014;347(1):46–53.
[16] Li K, Wen S, Larson AC, Shen M, Zhang Z, Chen Q, et al. Multifunctional dendrimer-based nanoparticles for in vivo MR/CT dual-modal molecular imaging of breast cancer. Int J Nanomedicine 2013;8:2589–600.
[17] Slowing II, Vivero-Escoto JL, Wu CW, Lin VS. Mesoporous silica nanoparticles as controlled release drug delivery and gene transfection carriers. Adv Drug Deliv Rev 2008;60(11):1278–88.
[18] Zhao Y, Sun X, Zhang G, Trewyn BG, Slowing II, Lin VS. Interaction of mesoporous silica nanoparticles with human red blood cell membranes: size and surface effects. ACS Nano 2011;5(2):1366–75.
[19] Tang F, Li L, Chen D. Mesoporous silica nanoparticles: synthesis, biocompatibility and drug delivery. Adv Mater 2012;24(12):1504–34.
[20] Hudson SP, Padera RF, Langer R, Kohane DS. The biocompatibility of mesoporous silicates. Biomaterials 2008;29(30):4045–55.
[21] Liu Y, Mi Y, Zhao J, Feng SS. Multifunctional silica nanoparticles for targeted delivery of hydrophobic imaging and therapeutic agents. Int J Pharm 2011;421(2):370–8.

[22] Wang L, Tan W. Multicolor FRET silica nanoparticles by single wavelength excitation. Nano Lett 2006;6(1):84–8.
[23] Benezra M, Penate-Medina O, Zanzonico PB, Schaer D, Ow H, Burns A, et al. Multimodal silica nanoparticles are effective cancer-targeted probes in a model of human melanoma. J Clin Invest 2011;121(7):2768–80.
[24] Jin Y, Jia C, Huang SW, O'Donnell M, Gao X. Multifunctional nanoparticles as coupled contrast agents. Nat Commun 2010;1:41.
[25] Wu YF, Wu HC, Kuan CH, Lin CJ, Wang LW, Chang CW, et al. Multi-functionalized carbon dots as theranostic nanoagent for gene delivery in lung cancer therapy. Sci Rep 2016;6:21170.
[26] Abdullah Al N, Lee JE, In I, Lee H, Lee KD, Jeong JH, et al. Target delivery and cell imaging using hyaluronic acid-functionalized graphene quantum dots. Mol Pharm 2013;10(10):3736–44.
[27] Wang Z, Xia J, Zhou C, Via B, Xia Y, Zhang F, et al. Synthesis of strongly green-photoluminescent graphene quantum dots for drug carrier. Colloids Surf B Biointerfaces 2013;112:192–6.
[28] Wang X, Sun X, Lao J, He H, Cheng T, Wang M, et al. Multifunctional graphene quantum dots for simultaneous targeted cellular imaging and drug delivery. Colloids Surf B Biointerfaces 2014;122:638–44.
[29] Shen J, Zhu Y, Yang X, Li C. Graphene quantum dots: emergent nanolights for bioimaging, sensors, catalysis and photovoltaic devices. Chem Commun 2012;48(31):3686–99.
[30] Tanimoto R, Hiraiwa T, Nakai Y, Shindo Y, Oka K, Hiroi N, et al. Detection of temperature difference in neuronal cells. Sci Rep 2016;6:22071.
[31] Stosch R, Henrion A, Schiel D, Guttler B. Surface-enhanced Raman scattering based approach for quantitative determination of creatinine in human serum. Anal Chem 2005;77(22):7386–92.
[32] Lin D, Feng S, Pan J, Chen Y, Lin J, Chen G, et al. Colorectal cancer detection by gold nanoparticle based surface-enhanced Raman spectroscopy of blood serum and statistical analysis. Opt Express 2011;19(14):13565–77.
[33] Feng S, Chen R, Lin J, Pan J, Chen G, Li Y, et al. Nasopharyngeal cancer detection based on blood plasma surface-enhanced Raman spectroscopy and multivariate analysis. Biosens Bioelectron 2010;25(11):2414–9.
[34] Chen Y, Chen G, Feng S, Pan J, Zheng X, Su Y, et al. Label-free serum ribonucleic acid analysis for colorectal cancer detection by surface-enhanced Raman spectroscopy and multivariate analysis. J Biomed Opt 2012;17(6):067003.
[35] Lin J, Chen R, Feng S, Pan J, Li Y, Chen G, et al. A novel blood plasma analysis technique combining membrane electrophoresis with silver nanoparticle-based SERS spectroscopy for potential applications in noninvasive cancer detection. Nanomedicine 2011;7(5):655–63.
[36] Wang X, Qian X, Beitler JJ, Chen ZG, Khuri FR, Lewis MM, et al. Detection of circulating tumor cells in human peripheral blood using surface-enhanced Raman scattering nanoparticles. Cancer Res 2011;71(5):1526–32.
[37] Ito H, Hasegawa K, Hasegawa Y, Nishimaki T, Hosomichi K, Kimura S, et al. Silver nanoscale hexagonal column chips for detecting cell-free DNA and circulating nucleosomes in cancer patients. Sci Rep 2015;5:10455.
[38] Powell JA, Venkatakrishnan K, Tan B. Programmable SERS active substrates for chemical and biosensing applications using amorphous/crystalline hybrid silicon nanomaterial. Sci Rep 2016;6:19663.
[39] Zhang R, Zhang Y, Dong ZC, Jiang S, Zhang C, Chen LG, et al. Chemical mapping of a single molecule by plasmon-enhanced Raman scattering. Nature 2013;498(7452):82–6.
[40] Acuna GP, Moller FM, Holzmeister P, Beater S, Lalkens B, Tinnefeld P. Fluorescence enhancement at docking sites of DNA-directed self-assembled nanoantennas. Science 2012;338(6106):506–10.
[41] Matschulat A, Drescher D, Kneipp J. Surface-enhanced Raman scattering hybrid nanoprobe multiplexing and imaging in biological systems. ACS Nano 2010;4(6):3259–69.
[42] Gellner M, Kompe K, Schlucker S. Multiplexing with SERS labels using mixed SAMs of Raman reporter molecules. Anal Bioanal Chem 2009;394(7):1839–44.

[43] Lee S, Chon H, Yoon SY, Lee EK, Chang SI, Lim DW, et al. Fabrication of SERS-fluorescence dual modal nanoprobes and application to multiplex cancer cell imaging. Nanoscale 2012;4(1):124–9.

[44] Li Y, Qi X, Lei C, Yue Q, Zhang S. Simultaneous SERS detection and imaging of two biomarkers on the cancer cell surface by self-assembly of branched DNA-gold nanoaggregates. Chem Commun 2014;50(69):9907–9.

[45] Maitia KK, Samantab A, Vendrella M, Soha K-S, Parka S-J, Olivoa M, Changa Y-T. Multiplex targeted in vivo cancer detection using sensitive near-infrared SERS nanotags. Nanotoday April 2012;7(2):85–93.

[46] Kang H, Jeong S, Park Y, Yim J, Jun B-H, Kyeong S, et al. Near-infrared SERS nanoprobes with plasmonic Au/Ag hollow-shell assemblies for in vivo multiplex detection. Adv Funct Mater 2013;23:3719–27.

[47] Chen K, Yuen C, Aniweh Y, Preiser P, Liu Q. Towards ultrasensitive malaria diagnosis using surface enhanced Raman spectroscopy. Sci Rep 2016;6:20177.

[48] Sharma B, Ma K, Glucksberg MR, Van Duyne RP. Seeing through bone with surface-enhanced spatially offset Raman spectroscopy. J Am Chem Soc 2013;135(46):17290–3.

[49] Ananta JS, Godin B, Sethi R, Moriggi L, Liu X, Serda RE, et al. Geometrical confinement of gadolinium-based contrast agents in nanoporous particles enhances T_1 contrast. Nat Nanotechnol 2010;5(11):815–21.

[50] Karfeld-Sulzer LS, Waters EA, Kohlmeir EK, Kissler H, Zhang X, Kaufman DB, et al. Protein polymer MRI contrast agents: longitudinal analysis of biomaterials in vivo. Magn Reson Med 2011;65(1):220–8.

[51] Chen WT, Thirumalai D, Shih TT, Chen RC, Tu SY, Lin CI, et al. Dynamic contrast-enhanced folate-receptor-targeted MR imaging using a Gd-loaded PEG-dendrimer-folate conjugate in a mouse xenograft tumor model. Mol Imaging Biol 2010;12(2):145–54.

[52] Yang H, Lu C, Liu Z, Jin H, Che Y, Olmstead MM, et al. Detection of a family of gadolinium-containing endohedral fullerenes and the isolation and crystallographic characterization of one member as a metal-carbide encapsulated inside a large fullerene cage. J Am Chem Soc 2008;130(51):17296–300.

[53] Bridot JL, Faure AC, Laurent S, Riviere C, Billotey C, Hiba B, et al. Hybrid gadolinium oxide nanoparticles: multimodal contrast agents for in vivo imaging. J Am Chem Soc 2007;129(16):5076–84.

[54] Silva GA. Neuroscience nanotechnology: progress, opportunities and challenges. Nat Rev Neurosci 2006;7(1):65–74.

[55] Ronald JA, Chen JW, Chen Y, Hamilton AM, Rodriguez E, Reynolds F, et al. Enzyme-sensitive magnetic resonance imaging targeting myeloperoxidase identifies active inflammation in experimental rabbit atherosclerotic plaques. Circulation 2009;120(7):592–9.

[56] Querol M, Bogdanov Jr A. Amplification strategies in MR imaging: activation and accumulation of sensing contrast agents (SCAs). J Magn Reson Imaging 2006;24(5):971–82.

[57] Chen JW, Pham W, Weissleder R, Bogdanov Jr A. Human myeloperoxidase: a potential target for molecular MR imaging in atherosclerosis. Magn Reson Med 2004;52(5):1021–8.

[58] Bogdanov Jr A, Matuszewski L, Bremer C, Petrovsky A, Weissleder R. Oligomerization of paramagnetic substrates result in signal amplification and can be used for MR imaging of molecular targets. Mol Imaging 2002;1(1):16–23.

[59] Louie AY, Huber MM, Ahrens ET, Rothbacher U, Moats R, Jacobs RE, et al. In vivo visualization of gene expression using magnetic resonance imaging. Nat Biotechnol 2000;18(3):321–5.

[60] Kang MK, Lee GH, Jung KH, Jung JC, Kim HK, Kim YH, et al. Gadolinium nanoparticles conjugated with therapeutic bifunctional chelate as a potential T_1 theranostic magnetic resonance imaging agent. J Biomed Nanotechnol 2016;12(5):894–908.

[61] Cao CY, Shen YY, Wang JD, Li L, Liang GL. Controlled intracellular self-assembly of gadolinium nanoparticles as smart molecular MR contrast agents. Sci Rep 2013;3:1024.

[62] Li L, Tong R, Li M, Kohane DS. Self-assembled gemcitabine-gadolinium nanoparticles for magnetic resonance imaging and cancer therapy. Acta Biomater 2016;33:34—9.
[63] de Barros AB, Tsourkas A, Saboury B, Cardoso VN, Alavi A. Emerging role of radiolabeled nanoparticles as an effective diagnostic technique. EJNMMI Res 2012;2(1):39.
[64] Dams ET, Oyen WJ, Boerman OC, Storm G, Laverman P, Kok PJ, et al. ^{99m}Tc-PEG liposomes for the scintigraphic detection of infection and inflammation: clinical evaluation. J Nucl Med 2000;41(4): 622—30.
[65] Li D, Patel AR, Klibanov AL, Kramer CM, Ruiz M, Kang BY, et al. Molecular imaging of atherosclerotic plaques targeted to oxidized LDL receptor LOX-1 by SPECT/CT and magnetic resonance. Circ Cardiovasc Imaging 2010;3(4):464—72.
[66] Harrington KJ, Mohammadtaghi S, Uster PS, Glass D, Peters AM, Vile RG, et al. Effective targeting of solid tumors in patients with locally advanced cancers by radiolabeled pegylated liposomes. Clin Cancer Res 2001;7(2):243—54.
[67] Chang YJ, Chang CH, Chang TJ, Yu CY, Chen LC, Jan ML, et al. Biodistribution, pharmacokinetics and microSPECT/CT imaging of 188Re-bMEDA-liposome in a C26 murine colon carcinoma solid tumor animal model. Anticancer Res 2007;27(4B):2217—25.
[68] Petersen AL, Binderup T, Rasmussen P, Henriksen JR, Elema DR, Kjaer A, et al. ^{64}Cu loaded liposomes as positron emission tomography imaging agents. Biomaterials 2011;32(9):2334—41.
[69] Rossin R, Pan D, Qi K, Turner JL, Sun X, Wooley KL, et al. ^{64}Cu-labeled folate-conjugated shell cross-linked nanoparticles for tumor imaging and radiotherapy: synthesis, radiolabeling, and biologic evaluation. J Nucl Med 2005;46(7):1210—8.
[70] Shokeen M, Fettig NM, Rossin R. Synthesis, in vitro and in vivo evaluation of radiolabeled nanoparticles. Q J Nucl Med Mol Imaging 2008;52(3):267—77.
[71] Devaraj NK, Keliher EJ, Thurber GM, Nahrendorf M, Weissleder R. ^{18}F labeled nanoparticles for in vivo PET-CT imaging. Bioconjug Chem 2009;20(2):397—401.
[72] Lee HY, Li Z, Chen K, Hsu AR, Xu C, Xie J, et al. PET/MRI dual-modality tumor imaging using arginine-glycine-aspartic (RGD)-conjugated radiolabeled iron oxide nanoparticles. J Nucl Med 2008; 49(8):1371—9.
[73] Xie J, Chen K, Huang J, Lee S, Wang J, Gao J, et al. PET/NIRF/MRI triple functional iron oxide nanoparticles. Biomaterials 2010;31(11):3016—22.
[74] Nahrendorf M, Zhang H, Hembrador S, Panizzi P, Sosnovik DE, Aikawa E, et al. Nanoparticle PET-CT imaging of macrophages in inflammatory atherosclerosis. Circulation 2008;117(3):379—87.
[75] Nahrendorf M, Keliher E, Marinelli B, Leuschner F, Robbins CS, Gerszten RE, et al. Detection of macrophages in aortic aneurysms by nanoparticle positron emission tomography-computed tomography. Arterioscler Thromb Vasc Biol 2011;31(4):750—7.
[76] Xie H, Diagaradjane P, Deorukhkar AA, Goins B, Bao A, Phillips WT, et al. Integrin $\alpha_v\beta_3$-targeted gold nanoshells augment tumor vasculature-specific imaging and therapy. Int J Nanomedicine 2011;6: 259—69.
[77] Agarwal A, Shao X, Rajian JR, Zhang H, Chamberland DL, Kotov NA, et al. Dual-mode imaging with radiolabeled gold nanorods. J Biomed Opt 2011;16(5):051307.
[78] Guerrero S, Herance JR, Rojas S, Mena JF, Gispert JD, Acosta GA, et al. Synthesis and in vivo evaluation of the biodistribution of a ^{18}F-labeled conjugate gold-nanoparticle-peptide with potential biomedical application. Bioconjug Chem 2012;23(3):399—408.
[79] Shao X, Agarwal A, Rajian JR, Kotov NA, Wang X. Synthesis and bioevaluation of ^{125}I-labeled gold nanorods. Nanotechnology 2011;22(13):135102.
[80] Morales-Avila E, Ferro-Flores G, Ocampo-Garcia BE, De Leon-Rodriguez LM, Santos-Cuevas CL, Garcia-Becerra R, et al. Multimeric system of ^{99m}Tc-labeled gold nanoparticles conjugated to c [RGDfK(C)] for molecular imaging of tumor $\alpha_v\beta_3$ expression. Bioconjug Chem 2011;22(5): 913—22.
[81] Pyayt AL, Fattal DA, Li Z, Beausoleil RG. Nanoengineered optical resonance sensor for composite material refractive-index measurements. Appl Opt 2009;48(14):2613—8.
[82] Xie H, Wang ZJ, Bao A, Goins B, Phillips WT. In vivo PET imaging and biodistribution of radiolabeled gold nanoshells in rats with tumor xenografts. Int J Pharm 2010;395(1—2):324—30.

[83] Shao X, Zhang H, Rajian JR, Chamberland DL, Sherman PS, Quesada CA, et al. ^{125}I-labeled gold nanorods for targeted imaging of inflammation. ACS Nano 2011;5(11):8967–73.
[84] Gupta AS. Nanomedicine approaches in vascular disease: a review. Nanomedicine 2011;7(6):763–79.
[85] Talelli M, Rijcken CJ, van Nostrum CF, Storm G, Hennink WE. Micelles based on HPMA copolymers. Adv Drug Deliv Rev 2010;62(2):231–9.
[86] Zhang R, Xiong C, Huang M, Zhou M, Huang Q, Wen X, et al. Peptide-conjugated polymeric micellar nanoparticles for Dual SPECT and optical imaging of EphB4 receptors in prostate cancer xenografts. Biomaterials 2011;32(25):5872–9.
[87] Zhang R, Lu W, Wen X, Huang M, Zhou M, Liang D, et al. Annexin A5-conjugated polymeric micelles for dual SPECT and optical detection of apoptosis. J Nucl Med 2011;52(6):958–64.
[88] Bayer CL, Luke GP, Emelianov SY. Photoacoustic imaging for medical diagnostics. Acoust Today 2012;8(4):15–23.
[89] Jain PK, Lee KS, El-Sayed IH, El-Sayed MA. Calculated absorption and scattering properties of gold nanoparticles of different size, shape, and composition: applications in biological imaging and biomedicine. J Phys Chem B 2006;110(14):7238–48.
[90] Chen YS, Frey W, Kim S, Homan K, Kruizinga P, Sokolov K, et al. Enhanced thermal stability of silica-coated gold nanorods for photoacoustic imaging and image-guided therapy. Opt Express 2010;18(9):8867–78.
[91] Bayer CL, Chen YS, Kim S, Mallidi S, Sokolov K, Emelianov S. Multiplex photoacoustic molecular imaging using targeted silica-coated gold nanorods. Biomed Opt Express 2011;2(7):1828–35.
[92] Rich LJ, Seshadri M. Photoacoustic imaging of salivary glands. Biomed Opt Express 2015;6(9):3157–62.
[93] Chamberland DL, Agarwal A, Kotov N, Brian Fowlkes J, Carson PL, Wang X. Photoacoustic tomography of joints aided by an Etanercept-conjugated gold nanoparticle contrast agent-an ex vivo preliminary rat study. Nanotechnology 2008;19(9):095101.
[94] Hirsch LR, Stafford RJ, Bankson JA, Sershen SR, Rivera B, Price RE, et al. Nanoshell-mediated near-infrared thermal therapy of tumors under magnetic resonance guidance. Proc Natl Acad Sci USA 2003;100(23):13549–54.
[95] Yang X, Stein EW, Ashkenazi S, Wang LV. Nanoparticles for photoacoustic imaging. Wiley Interdiscip Rev Nanomed Nanobiotechnol 2009;1(4):360–8.
[96] Cang H, Sun T, Li ZY, Chen J, Wiley BJ, Xia Y, et al. Gold nanocages as contrast agents for spectroscopic optical coherence tomography. Opt Lett 2005;30(22):3048–50.
[97] Chen J, Saeki F, Wiley BJ, Cang H, Cobb MJ, Li ZY, et al. Gold nanocages: bioconjugation and their potential use as optical imaging contrast agents. Nano Lett 2005;5(3):473–7.
[98] Kim G, Huang SW, Day KC, O'Donnell M, Agayan RR, Day MA, et al. Indocyanine-green-embedded PEBBLEs as a contrast agent for photoacoustic imaging. J Biomed Opt 2007;12(4):044020.

CHAPTER 15

Drug and Gene Delivery Materials and Devices

Ann-Marie Ako-Adounvo, Beatriz Marabesi, Rayssa Costa Lemos, Ayuk Patricia, Pradeep K. Karla

Howard University, Washington, DC, United States

Contents

1. Introduction	375
2. Advances in Delivery Systems	376
2.1 Nanomaterials	379
2.1.1 Nano Drug Delivery Systems	*379*
3. Gene Delivery	383
3.1 Viral Vector Approach	383
3.2 Nonviral Vector Approach	384
3.3 Physical Approach	384
4. Gene Therapy Products	385
5. Conclusion and Future Direction	385
Acknowledgment	386
References	386

1. INTRODUCTION

Delivery mechanism has a significant impact on the therapeutic efficacy of drugs [1–3]. Drugs must be efficiently delivered to the target site to achieve the desired therapeutic concentrations and pharmacodynamic response. However, complex biological drug barriers can pose challenges for nano drug delivery systems. A prominent study by Xu et al. assessed the complexity of pharmacological and biochemical barriers preventing the effective delivery of small interfering RNA (siRNA)-loaded lipid nanoparticles [4]. Prominent physiologic and biochemical drug barriers include blood—brain barrier, intestinal epithelium, skin, blood—ocular barrier, metabolizing enzymes, and efflux transporters [5–13]. Another challenge encountered in the development of drug delivery vehicles for genes and complex drug molecules is the poor shelf life. The high cost associated with the development of new drugs has led to the increase in research that identifies novel strategies to deliver old drugs [14]. Circumventing the barriers for improved therapeutic efficacy and reduced side-effect profile is one of the primary aims driving drug delivery technology research. In addition, the research is focused on developing stable drug delivery vehicles with improved shelf life. Primary factors considered in the development of drug delivery technology include the type of drug polymer vehicle, intended drug target site, type of formulation, desired efficacy, drug release profile, and safety [15]. Current drug delivery research emphasizes on nanocarriers as an effective delivery technology for the delivery of drugs and small molecules.

Ideal polymeric delivery vehicles should be biocompatible and have affinity for the therapeutic agent for optimal drug-loading efficacy [16]. Furthermore, the materials should be stable, readily available, and support large-scale manufacture. The drug delivery system may be modified further to achieve site-specific targeting and controlled drug release [16—18]. In addition, a delivery system may be expected to protect the drug from enzyme metabolism and other intra/extracellular factors contributing to drug loss [19].

Remarkable advances in polymer technology led to the increase in the use of polymers for drug and gene delivery [18]. The research advances contributed to the development of nanomedicine as a specialty drug delivery technology. Formulations with structured polymeric materials of submicron sizes were successfully used to deliver small molecules and polynucleotides for the treatment of various types of cancers, human immunodeficiency virus infection, diabetes, among many other disease states. The success of nanotherapeutics is attributed to the submicron size. A drug molecule with poor aqueous solubility exhibits improved solubility when its particle size is reduced to submicrons. This reduction in particle size is shown to impart a high surface area to volume ratio. Nanocarriers in drug delivery systems are demonstrated to penetrate capillaries and overcome biological barriers enabling successful delivery and accumulation at target sites [20—21]. Additional demonstrated benefits include reduced systemic toxicity and clearance.

This chapter focuses on the use of nanomaterials for drug, gene delivery and provides information on novel materials investigated for the formulation development. A summary of prominent patent disclosures in the area of nanomedicine, with emphasis in drug/gene delivery, is presented in Table 15.1. Novel nanotherapeutics such as liposomes, nanoparticles, polymeric micelles, nanocapsules, and nanotubes will be discussed briefly in the chapter. The discussion focuses on prominence of nanomaterials in gene therapy and various drug delivery technologies designed for gene delivery. In addition, a summary of US Food and Drug Administration (FDA)-approved and marketed nanopharmaceuticals and gene therapy products is presented in Table 15.2.

2. ADVANCES IN DELIVERY SYSTEMS

Prominent challenges for delivering therapeutic agents via nonsystemic conventional methods include: (1) difficulty in crossing biological barriers, (2) susceptibility to degradation, and (3) rapid clearance. Rapid advancements in nanotechnology have led to its application in many fields including nanomedicine (diagnostics, therapeutics, imaging, etc.). Particle size is a key characteristic in nanotherapy and is demonstrated to significantly impact absorption, distribution, and efficacy. Furthermore, nanoparticles are demonstrated to overcome the above challenges [22—25].

Table 15.1 Prominent patented nanomaterials for drug and gene delivery

Nanocarrier	Indication	Patent number	Publication year	References
PLA-PEG copolymers	Cancer treatment and imaging	WO2013127949 A1	2013	[32]
Gelatin and PLGA	Cancer treatment	CN102697737 A	2014	[33]
mPEG-PLGA-PLL	Cancer treatment	CN102793671 A	2012	[34]
PLGA	Cancer treatment	CN102525936 A	2014	[35]
PLGA	Delivery of therapeutic agents	US8114883 B2	2012	[36]
PLGA	Cancer treatment	CN102697795 A	2014	[37]
PLA-PEG-DTPA-Gd	Magnetic resonance	CN101612407 B	2011	[38]
PEG-b-PLA	Steroids deficit treatment	WO2013063279 A1	2013	[39]
Polysaccharide gels	Body tissue treatment	US8110561 B2	2012	[40]
Cyclodextrin	Delivery of therapeutic agents	US8128954 B2	2012	[41]
PEGylated-terminated PAMAM	Liver-specific delivery of therapeutic agents	WO2011072290 A3	2011	[42]
Hydroxyl-terminated PAMAM	Cancer treatment and diagnosis	WO2011053618 A3	2011	[43]
PAMAM	Cancer treatment and diagnosis	EP2488172 A2	2012	[44]
Carbosilane	Antiviral, antibacterial, or antifungal treatment	EP2537880 A2	2012	[45]
PPI	Cancer treatment	WO2012024396 A3	2012	[46]
Cystamine core PAMAM	Cancer treatment	WO2012018383 A2	2012	[47]
Legumin-coated immunoliposome	Cancer treatment	WO2012031175 A2	2012	[48]
SLNs	Glaucoma treatment	CN102793672 A	2012	[49]
Immunoliposome	Cancer treatment	WO2010103118 A1	2010	[50]

Continued

Table 15.1 Prominent patented nanomaterials for drug and gene delivery—cont'd

Nanocarrier	Indication	Patent number	Publication year	References
Cationic liposome	Delivery of therapeutic agents	WO2011149733 A3	2012	[51]
Prostaglandin-coated liposome	Delivery of therapeutic agents, cancer treatment	WO2012021107 A2	2012	[52]
Carbon-coated iron nanoparticles	Liver cancer	CN101347455 A	2009	[53]
Metallic nanoparticles	Cancer	EP2559429 A2	2013	[54]
CNTs	Delivery of therapeutic agents, cancer	WO2012031164 A2	2012	[55]
MWCNTs	Immunotherapy, cancer	CN101537015 A	2013	[56]
MWCNTs	Cancer	WO2013110150 AI	2013	[57]
CMC- Ac-PEG	Cancer treatment	WO2012103634 AI	2012	[58]
POE	Eye-related diseases, cancer	US20130209566 AI	2013	[59]
Albumin	Photodynamic therapy	WO2011071968 A3	2011	[60]
HPMA-HMA and HPMA-TBA	Occluding normal or malformation of blood vessels	US20120195826 AI	2014	[61]
Albumin	Treating, preventing cancer	US20130280336 AI	2013	[62]
PLA, PLGA or PGA	Delivery of therapeutic agents	WO2012015481 AI	2012	[63]
PAMAM	Therapeutic treatment	EP2552458 AI	2013	[64]
Anti-TNF-α-coated immunolipose	Inflammatory diseases	US20130115269 AI	2013	[65]
Cationic liposome	Cancer treatment, inflammatory diseases	WO2013135800 AI	2013	[66]
Liposome	Magnetic resonance imaging	WO2011061541 AI	2011	[67]

Table 15.1 Prominent patented nanomaterials for drug and gene delivery—cont'd

Nanocarrier	Indication	Patent number	Publication year	References
SLNs	Delivery of therapeutic agents	WO2013105101 AI	2014	[68]
PEGylated liposome	Delivery of therapeutic agents, imaging	WO2013135892 AI	2013	[69]
Liposome	Delivery of therapeutic agents, cancer treatment	US20130136790 AI	2014	[70]
HA CNs	Cancer treatment	WO2010078941 AI	2010	[71]
AuNPs	Cancer	US20120027861 AI	2012	[72]
Iron oxide nanoparticles	Imaging and cancer	US20130189367 AI	2013	[73]
Iron oxide nanoparticles	Cancer	WO2010134087 AI	2010	[74]

AuNP, gold nanoparticle; *CMC*, carboxy methyl cellulose; *CN*, calcium nanoparticles; *CNT*, carbon nanotube; *DTPA*, diethylene triamine penta acetate; *HA*, hydroxyapatite; *HMA*, hexyl methacrylate; *HPMA*, hydroxy propyl methacrylate; *MWCNT*, multiwalled carbon nanotube; *PAMAM*, poly(amido amine); *PEG*, poly(ethylene glycol); *PGA*, poly(alycolic acid); *PLA*, poly lactic acid; *PLGA*, poly(lactic-co-glycolic acid); *PLL*, poly(L-lysine); *POE*, poly(ortho ester); *PPI*, poly(propylene imine); *SLN*, solid lipid nanoparticles; *TBA*, tert-butyl acrylate; *TNF*, tumor necrosis factor.

2.1 Nanomaterials

The properties and mechanism of a nanodevice/delivery system is significantly influenced by the material(s) used in their manufacture. These materials can be broadly classified as biodegradable, nonbiodegradable, natural, synthetic, or inorganic. Examples of such materials include phospholipids and polymers such as poly(lactic-co-glycolic acid), poly lactic acid (PLA), chitosan, poly(ethylene imine), polymethacrylates, dendrimers, poly(ethylene glycol) (PEG), poly(ethylene oxide), poly(ε-caprolatone), among several others. Also, inorganic materials such as gold, calcium phosphate, silica, iron oxides, graphene, and silicon have been explored. Nanomaterials designed from the abovementioned materials and their application in drug and gene delivery have been extensively reviewed in the literature [26–30].

The use of novel materials resulted in a few prominent patent disclosures. Martins et al. present a comprehensive review [31] of the patents; a summary of the prominent ones is presented in Table 15.1 [32–74].

2.1.1 Nano Drug Delivery Systems

Well-known nano drug delivery systems include nanoparticles, nanocapsules, micelles, liposomes, polymer–drug conjugates, colloidal dispersions, nanogels, and nanotubes

Table 15.2 Prominent FDA-approved nanopharmaceuticals

Brand name	Approval	Active ingredient	Indication	References
Liposome				
Abelcet	1995	Amphotericin B	Fungal infections	[77,87,88]
AmBisome	1997	Liposomal amphotericin B	Fungal infections, leishmaniasis	[77,87,88]
DaunoXome	1996	Liposomal daunorubicin citrate	HIV-associated Kaposi sarcoma	[77,87,88]
Depocyt(e)	1999	Liposomal cytosine arabinoside	Lymphomatous meningitis	[77,87,88]
DepoDur	2004	Morphine	Analgesia	[87,77]
Doxil	1995	PEGylated-stabilized liposomal doxorubicin	AIDS-related Kaposi sarcoma, refractory ovarian cancer, multiple myeloma	[77,87,88]
Eligard	2002	Leuprolide acetate and PLGH polymer formulation	Advanced prostate cancer	[87,88]
Estrasorb topical emulsion	2003	Estradiol	Moderate to severe symptoms of hot flashes and night sweats associated with menopause	[87,77]
Visudyne	2006	Verteporfin	Choroidal neovascularization due to age-related macular degeneration, pathologic myopia, or presumed ocular histoplasmosis	[77,87,88]
Survanta	1991	Beractant (bovine lung homogenate)	Respiratory distress syndrome (RDS)	[87,77]
Curosurf	1999	Poractant Alfa	RDS in premature infants	[87,77]
Polymeric nanoparticles				
Abraxane	2005	Paclitaxel albumin-stabilized	Metastatic breast cancer, non—small cell lung cancer (NSCLC) and pancreatic cancer	[77,87,88]
Adagen	1993	PEGylated adenosine deaminase enzyme	Severe combined immunodeficiency disease	[77,87,88]

Table 15.2 Prominent FDA-approved nanopharmaceuticals—cont'd

Brand name	Approval	Active ingredient	Indication	References
Alimta	2004	Pemetrexed	Nonsquamous NSCLC, malignant pleural mesothelioma	[87,88]
Amphotec	1996	Liposomal amphotericin B	Invasive aspergillosis	[77,87,88]
Cimzia	2008	PEGylated Fab' fragment of a humanized anti–TNF-alpha antibody	Crohn disease, rheumatoid arthritis	[87,88]
Copaxone	1996	Glatiramer acetate	Multiple sclerosis	[87]
Elestrin	2006	Estradiol	Treatment of moderate to severe vasomotor symptoms due to menopause	[87]
Estrasorb	2003	Estradiol	Treatment of moderate to severe vasomotor symptoms associated with menopause	[87,77]
Macugen	2004	Pegaptanib (PEGylated anti-VEGF aptamer)	Wet age-related macular degeneration	[77,87,88]
Mircera	2007	Methoxy PEG-epoetin beta	Symptomatic anemia associated with CKD	[87,88]
Neulasta	2002	PEGylated filgrastim	Chemotherapy-associated neutropenia	[77,87,88]
Oncaspar	1994	PEGylated L-asparaginase	Acute lymphocytic leukemia	[87,77]
Ontak	1999	Interleukin-2 diphtheria toxin fusion protein	Cutaneous T-cell lymphoma	[77,87,88]
Pegasys	2002	Peginterferon alpha-2a	Hepatitis B and C	[77,87,88]
PegIntron	2001	Peginterferon alfa-2b	Hepatitis C	[77,87,88]
Renagel	2000	Amine-loaded polymer	Serum phosphorus control in patients with CKD on dialysis	[87,88]
Somavert	2003	PEGylated human growth hormone receptor antagonist	Acromegaly	[77,87,88]

Continued

Table 15.2 Prominent FDA-approved nanopharmaceuticals—cont'd

Brand name	Approval	Active ingredient	Indication	References
Nanocrystal				
Emend	2003	Aprepitant nanocrystal particles	Chemotherapy-related nausea and vomiting	[77,87,88]
Rapamune	1999	Sirolimus	Prevention of rejection (antirejection medicine) in people who have received a kidney transplant	[87,77]
Tricor	2004	Fenofibrate	Hypercholesterolemia, mixed dyslipidemia, hypertriglyceridemia	[77,87,88]
TRIGLIDE	2005	Fenofibrate	Reduction of LDL-C, Total-C, triglycerides, and Apo B in adult patients with primary hypercholesterolemia or mixed dyslipidemia (Fredrickson types IIa and IIb)	[87]
Visudyne	2000	Liposomal verteporfin	Wet age-related macular degeneration, pathologic myopia, ocular histoplasmosis syndrome	[77,87,88]
Solid lipid nanoparticles				
Amphotec	2006	Colloidal suspension of lipid-based amphotericin B	Invasive aspergillosis in patients who are refractory to or intolerant of conventional amphotericin B	[77,87,88]

CKD, chronic kidney disease; *FDA*, US Food and Drug Administration; *HIV*, human immunodeficiency virus; *LDL-C*, low-density lipoprotein—cholesterol; *PLGH*, poly(DL-lactide-co-glycolide) with a carboxylic acid end group; *TNF*, tumor necrosis factor; *VEGF*, vascular endothelial growth factor.

[75–78]. Liposomes, micelles, and polymer—drug conjugates are the widely explored nano drug delivery systems. The development of polymeric liposomes as drug delivery systems dates back to the 1970s [79–81]. The first FDA-approved (1995) nanopharmaceutical, Doxil [82], is based on liposomal drug delivery technology. Doxil is a PEGylated liposomal encapsulation of the anticancer drug doxorubicin for the treatment of AIDS-related Kaposi sarcoma [83,84]. In addition, many of the nanopharmaceuticals currently available for clinical use are liposomal-based delivery systems [85]. Over the past few decades, there has been a gradual rise in the number of commercially available pharmaceutical products that have employed nanocarriers as delivery systems, with quite a number in the pipeline or clinical trials [18]. This increase in nanobased commercially available pharmaceutical products reflects the success of nanomedicine. As of 2014, there were ~43 nanopharmaceutical drug formulations approved by the FDA [79]. Several publications [17,77,79,86] have reviewed FDA-approved and marketed nanopharmaceutical products, prominent of which are summarized in Table 15.2.

3. GENE DELIVERY

The goal of gene therapy is to deliver genetic material to in vivo targets (cells) for treating genetic disorders or to program cells with new functions (i.e., expression of new proteins) [89]. Since the inception of the first human gene therapy trial in 1990 [90,91], there has been an expanding interest on drug delivery tools for improved delivery of genes. Delivery vehicles are shown to play a vital role in the effectiveness of gene therapy and transfection process [92]. Gene delivery materials can be categorized into viral, nonviral, or physical [91,93–95]. An RNA viral vector, retrovirus, was used in the first gene therapy clinical trial involving two unrelated pediatric subjects, both born with adenosine deaminase deficiency [90].

3.1 Viral Vector Approach

As of 2015, the utilization of viral vectors for gene delivery accounted for ~70% of gene therapy clinical trials conducted worldwide [96]. Virus replicates inside the living cells of a host organism and contains either RNA or DNA as genetic material. Although viruses do not have the ability to self-multiply, they are known to utilize the host cell's machinery postinfection to divide and produce more replicas [97]. Viral vectors utilized for gene delivery are genetically engineered by stripping their gene for replication and replacing it with the therapeutic gene (gene of interest) [98]. The process still preserved the virus's ability to transfect host cells [91].

Key properties for selecting a viral vector include: (1) safe to handle, (2) exhibit low toxicity in infected cells, (3) stable enough to ensure reproducibility of the work, (4) possess the ability to be modified for cell-type specificity, (5) ability to incorporate a marker gene to aid identification, (6) an appreciable foreign gene carrying capacity, (7) efficiency in transfection and transduction. Commonly used viral vectors include adenovirus, adenoassociated viruses, retroviruses, herpes simplex virus, poxvirus, lentivirus, and vaccinia virus. Base on clinical trial information regarding vector usage, adenovirus and retrovirus are the most prominent of the viral vectors, accounting for >40% of all vectors used in gene therapy clinical trials [96]. It is worth noting that each viral vector system possesses its own distinctive benefits and restrictions, and hence requires an additional assessment to determine the applications for which each is best suited [99,100]. Retroviruses are single-stranded RNA-based viruses with a genome capacity of 7–11 kb [95,101] available for the incorporation of transgene up to

10 kb [101,102]. Retroviral vectors are highly effective in dividing cells and can pass through the nuclear pores of the dividing cells [103,104]. Furthermore, retroviruses are best suited for therapies where permanent gene transfer is preferred [105,99]. Unfortunately, because retroviral vectors integrate quiet well into the genome of the host cell, there is a possibility of insertional mutagenesis in addition to pathogenicity and immunogenicity [105,91]. Furthermore, the use of retroviral vector systems can result in unspecific or random infection of target cells [106].

Adenoviruses are nonenveloped, linear double-stranded DNA viruses that were isolated from human adenoid tissue cultures in 1953 [107–109]. With a large viral genome (36–38 kilobases), adenoviruses can be genetically engineered to have a very high capacity transgene insertion. For example, the high-capacity "gutless" Helper-dependent adenovirus has a transgene capacity of ∼37 kb [95,110]. However, despite the high transgene capacity, host immune response and subsequent transient gene expression significantly limit the use of adenoviral vector systems as delivery vehicles [95]. Further limitations associated with viral vector use include their propensity to elicit immune response, transgene capacity limitations, and high cost of production [111]. Hence, nonviral approaches were explored in recent years.

3.2 Nonviral Vector Approach

Nonviral vector approach was developed as an alternative to conventional viral-based vectors. Nonviral vector systems investigated for gene delivery include cationic lipids and cationic polymers [112–114]. Such vectors form condensed complexes (lipoplexes, where cationic lipids are utilized; or polyplexes, where cationic polymers are utilized) via electrostatic interactions with the negatively charged gene [115]. A review by Al-Dosari and Gao lists lipids and polymers commonly used for gene transfer [93]. One of the limitations associated with cationic vectors aimed for systemic gene delivery is its short in vivo circulation time as they are targeted by host mononuclear phagocyte system (MPS). This was overcome by surface modification of nonviral vector systems with hydrophilic polymers such as PEG escaping the recognition by MPS. The flexibility for surface-modification was further utilized to achieve increased target specificity [116,117].

Despite the above-mentioned benefits, nonviral vector-based gene delivery has low transfection efficiency compared with viral vectors, and sometimes resulted in short-lived gene expression [93,118]. For increased efficiency in transfection and safety without the use of vectors, the delivery of genes by physical methods was investigated.

3.3 Physical Approach

The physical approach for gene transfer is non–vector mediated and does not involve the use of nanocarriers (expect in the case of "gene gun"). This includes techniques such as electroporation (in which an electrical field is used to perturb the cell membrane, making it transiently permeable to surrounding gene in solution) [119,120], and sonoporation (utilizes ultrasound waves to generate transient nanomeric pores in the cell membrane to facilitate the permeation of genetic material) [121–123]. Other physical methods or delivery devices include microinjection [124,125] and microprojectile gene transfer or "gene gun" (which propels naked DNA-coated nanoparticle into target cells) [126,127]. The principles, applications, advantages, and limitations of these and other physical methods and devices for gene transfer have been extensively reviewed in a number of articles [93,95,103,128].

4. GENE THERAPY PRODUCTS

After more than two decades of the first gene therapy trial in human [90,91], the first commercial gene therapy product, Gendicine, manufactured by SiBiono was approved in 2003 by China's State Food and Drug Administration for the treatment of head and neck squamous cell carcinoma [129–132]. The product utilizes recombinant adenovirus as vector to deliver wild-type p53 gene, the expression of which is known to transfer antitumor abilities into the nucleus of tumor cells [116,117]. A Biologics License Application (BLA) for a similar (to Gendicine) therapy, Advexin [133], an orphan-designated therapy by Introgen for the treatment of head and neck cancer as well as Li-Fraumeni syndrome, was turned down by the US FDA in September 2008.

In 2007 another gene therapy product, Rexin-G, which was the first targeted injectable gene therapy product, was approved by regulatory authorities in the Philippines for the treatment of all solid tumors [134]. Rexin-G employs a retroviral-based vector to deliver "a gene for a dominant-negative mutant form of human cyclin G1 which stops cell cycle by blocking endogenous cyclin-G1 protein" [79].

In November 2012, another gene therapy product by UniQure, Glybera (alipogene tiparvovec), was approved by the European Medicines Agency for the treatment of lipoprotein lipase (LPL) deficiency [135]. This marks the first gene therapy product to be granted a BLA in Europe. The product employs adenoassociated virus as a vector to convey a functional replica of the LPL gene to skeletal muscle [135]. UniQure's application for Glybera approval in the United States was turned down by the FDA as the regulatory body suggested further clinical trials [136,137]. UniQure plans to carry out additional clinical trials for Glybera in early 2016, to be incorporated in a BLA submission to the FDA.

5. CONCLUSION AND FUTURE DIRECTION

The chapter emphasizes the potential of nanosystems in the delivery of pharmaceutical, biological, and gene molecules. The chapter further provides a summary of FDA-approved and commercialized nanopharmaceuticals, potential gene therapy products, and important patent inventions in nanotherapeutics. With the advances in nanomaterial research, major strides were made in the area of drug and gene delivery research. These research advances and promising clinical outcomes solidified the area of "Nanomedicine" with several FDA-approved nanopharmaceuticals in the market and many in various stages of clinical development. Nano drug delivery systems have significantly improved the stability, toxicity profile, and therapeutic effectiveness of several drugs. Further drug molecules in nanoparticle size range were found to have improved solubility and ability to circumvent biological barriers. Furthermore, the surfaces of various nanocarriers have been engineered with ligands for site-specific targeting and improved pharmacokinetic parameters.

Nanocarriers for nonviral gene delivery were found to be safer (low immunogenic potential) and easy to modify than traditional viral vectors. In addition, nanocarriers enabled larger size of genetic material to be loaded. However, the low transfection efficiency of nonviral gene delivery has been a limiting factor. Gene therapy products have been approved for human use across the globe and all existing products are based on viral or virus-associated vectors.

It is worth noting that despite the success achieved in nanomedicine, many potential nanobased delivery systems failed to progress for commercialization. Few limitations include the insufficient understanding of the transport and the mechanisms that underline their uptake, biodistribution, and pharmacokinetics. Current research efforts in the nano drug delivery field emphasizes on the development of up-scalable, consistently reproducible, efficient, and highly specific nano drug delivery systems with low toxicity.

ACKNOWLEDGMENT

The research release time is funded by Howard University Research Innovations BRIDGE Grant (Pradeep Karla, PI) and Howard University RCMI grant (William Southerland, PI).

REFERENCES

[1] Sharma HS, Ali SF, Tian ZR, Patnaik R, Patnaik S, Sharma A, Boman A, et al. Nanowired-drug delivery enhances neuroprotective efficacy of compounds and reduces spinal cord edema formation and improves functional outcome following spinal cord injury in the rat. Acta Neurochir Suppl 2010; 106:343—50.
[2] Kim H, Kim Y, Lee J. Liposomal formulations for enhanced lymphatic drug delivery. Asian J Pharm Sci 2013;8:96—103.
[3] Yuan X, Marcano DC, Shin CS, Hua X, Isenhart LC, Pflugfelder SC, et al. Ocular drug delivery nanowafer with enhanced therapeutic efficacy. ACS Nano 2015;9(2):1749—58.
[4] Xu Y, Ou M, Keough E, Roberts J, Koeplinger K, Lyman M, et al. Quantitation of physiological and biochemical barriers to siRNA liver delivery via lipid nanoparticle platform. Mol Pharm 2014;11: 1424—34.
[5] Groothuis DR. The blood—brain and blood-tumor barriers: a review of strategies for increasing drug delivery. Neuro-Oncology 2000;2(1):45—59.
[6] Pardridge WM. Blood—brain barrier delivery. Drug Discov Today 2007;12(1—2):54—61.

[7] Abbott NJ, Romero IA. Transporting therapeutics across the blood–brain barrier. Mol Med Today 1996;2(3):106–13.

[8] Gan LSL, Thakker DR. Applications of the Caco-2 model in the design and development of orally active drugs: elucidation of biochemical and physical barriers posed by the intestinal epithelium. Adv Drug Deliv Rev 1997;23(1–3):77–98.

[9] Rojanasakul Y, Wang LY, Bhat M, Glover DD, Malanga CJ, Ma JKH. The transport barrier of epithelia: a comparative study on membrane permeability and charge selectivity in the rabbit. Pharm Res 1992;9(8):1029–34.

[10] Benet LZ, Izumi T, Zhang Y, Silverman JA, Wacher VJ. Intestinal MDR transporter proteins and P-450 enzymes as barrier to oral drug delivery. J Control Release 1999;62(1–2):25–31.

[11] Wacher VJ, Wu CY, Benet LZ. Overlapping substrate specificities and tissue distribution of cytochrome P450 3A and P-glycoprotein: implications for drug delivery and activity in cancer chemotherapy. Mol Carcinog 1995;13(3):129–34.

[12] Urtti A. Challenges and obstacles of ocular pharmacokinetics and drug delivery. Adv Drug Deliv Rev 2006;58(11):1131–5.

[13] Barar J, Javadzadeh AR, Omidi Y. Ocular novel drug delivery: impacts of membranes and barriers. Expert Opin Drug Deliv 2008;5(8):567–81.

[14] Tiwari G, Tiwari R, Sriwastawa B, Bhati L, Pandey S, Pandey P, et al. Drug delivery systems: an updated review. Int J Pharm Investig 2012;2(1):2–11.

[15] Agrawal PA. Perspective on drug discovery, development and delivery. J Drug Discov Dev Deliv 2014;1(1):2.

[16] Slowing II, Vivero-Escoto JL, Wu C-W, Lin VS-Y. Mesoporous silica nanoparticles as controlled release drug delivery and gene transfection carriers. Adv Drug Deliv Rev 2008;60:1278–88.

[17] Zhang Y, Chan HF, Leong KW. Advanced material and processing for drug delivery: the past and the future. Adv Drug Deliv Rev 2013;65:104–20.

[18] Zhang L, Gu FX, Chan JM, Wang AZ, Langer RS, Farokhzad OC. Nanoparticles in medicine: therapeutic applications and developments. Clin Pharmacol Ther 2008;83(5):761–9.

[19] Alonso MJ. Nanomedicines for overcoming biological barriers. Biomed Pharmacother 2004;58: 168–72.

[20] Blanco E, Shen H, Ferrari M. Principles of nanoparticle design for overcoming biological barriers to drug delivery. Nat Biotechnol 2015;33:941–51.

[21] Jordan C, Shuvaev VV, Bailey M, Muzykantov VR, Dziubla TD. The role of carrier geometry in overcoming biological barriers to drug delivery. Curr Pharm Des 2015.

[22] Shi XY, Fan XG. Advances in nanoparticle system for delivering drugs across the biological barriers. J China Pharm Univ 2002;33(3):169–72.

[23] Desai MP, Labhasetwar V, Walter E, Levy RJ, Amidon GL. The mechanism of uptake of biodegradable microparticles in Caco-2 cells is size dependent. Pharm Res 1997;14:1568–73.

[24] Desai MP, Labhasetwar V, Amidon GL, Levy RJ. Gastrointestinal uptake of biodegradable microparticles: effect of particle size. Pharm Res 1996;13:1838–45.

[25] Gao K, Jiang X. Influence of particle size on transport of methotrexate across blood–brain barrier by polysorbate 80-coated polybutylcyanoacrylate nanoparticles. Int J Pharm 2006;310:213–9.

[26] Nam K, Nam HY, Park JS. Dendrimer-based nanomaterials. In: Torchilin V, Amiji MM, editors. Handbook of materials for nanomedicine. Pan Stanford Publishing; 2010. p. 235–53.

[27] Loh XJ, Lee TC, Dou Q, Deen GR. Utilizing inorganic nanocarriers for gene delivery. Biomater Sci 2016;4:70–86.

[28] Gascón AR, del Pozo-Rodriguez A, Solinis MÁ. Non-viral delivery systems in gene therapy. In: Molina FM, editor. Gene therapy – tools and potential applications. InTech; 2013. p. 1–33.

[29] Martinho N, Damgé C, Reis CP. Recent advances in drug delivery systems. J Biomater Nanobiotechnol 2011;2:510–26.

[30] Kumari A, Yadav SK, Yadav SC. Biodegradable polymeric nanoparticles based drug delivery systems. Colloids Surf B Biointerfaces 2010;75(1):1–18.

[31] Martins D, Rosa D, Fernandes AR, Baptista PV. Nanoparticle drug delivery systems: recent patents and applications in nanomedicine. Recent Pat Nanomed 2013;3(2):105–18.

[32] Bazile D, Couvreur P, Lakkireddy HR, Mackiewicz N, Nicolas J. Functional PLA-PEG copolymers, the nanoparticles thereof, their preparation and use for targeted drug delivery and imaging. 2013. WO2013127949 A1.
[33] Jessie A, Guillaume WM. Tumor-targeting drug-loaded particles. 2012. CN102697737A.
[34] Wen D, Yourong D, Yunfei W, Peifeng L. Human recombinant epidermal growth factor (hrEGF)-modified cisplatin-loaded polymeric nanoparticles and preparation method and application thereof. 2012. CN102793671A.
[35] Jiansong J, Hongxing F, Jingjing S, Hui L, Chenying L. Compound epirubicin hydrochloride polylactic-co-glycolic acid (PLGA) nanoparticles and preparation method thereof. 2012. CN102525936A.
[36] Taft D, Tzannis S, Dai WG, Ottensmann S, Bitler S, Zheng Q, Bell A. Polymer formulations for delivery of bioactive materials. 2012. US8114883 B2.
[37] Yiyi S, Ling Z, Dong L, Jia Y. Anti-tumor combined medicament. 2014. CN102697795A.
[38] Na Z, Zhijin C, Zaijun L, Chunhong M, Dexin Y. Polymer nanoparticle magnetic resonance contrast agent and preparing method thereof. 2011. CN 101612407 B.
[39] Prud'homme RK, Figueroa CE. A high-loading nanoparticle-based formulation for water-insoluble steroids. 2013. WO2013063279 A1.
[40] Cohen S, Leor J. Injectable cross-linked polymeric preparations and uses thereof. 2012. US8110561 B2.
[41] Davis ME, Wright KW, Mack B. Biodegradable drug-polymer delivery system. 2012. US8128954 B2.
[42] El-Sayed MEH, Ensminger W, Shewach D. Targeted dendrimer-drug conjugates. 2011. WO2011072290 A3.
[43] Baker JR, Zhang Y. Hydroxyl-terminated dendrimers. 2011. WO 2011053618 A3.
[44] Baker JR, Huang B. Dendrimer compositions and methods of synthesis. 2012. EP 2488172 A2.
[45] De La Mata J, Ramirez RG, Fernandez MA, Fernandez JSN, Lopez PO, Jimenez LC, Moreno BR, Garrido EA, Lobera MJS. Carbosilane dendrimers and the use thereof as antiviral agents. 2012. EP 2537880 A2.
[46] Minko T, Rodriguez LR, Garbuzenko O, Taratula O, Shah V. Compositions and methods for delivering nucleic acid molecules and treating cancer. 2012. WO 2012024396 A3.
[47] Anderson ML, Gunaratne PH, Jayarathne LC. Interior functionalized hyperbranched dendron-conjugated nanoparticles and uses thereof. 2012. WO 2012018383 A2.
[48] Chen S, Chen T, Liao D, Liu Z, Lu D, Luo Y, Reisfeld RA, Xiang R. Nanoparticle-based tumor-targeted drug delivery. 2012. WO 2012031175 A2.
[49] Rui L, Qunwei X, Fengzhen W, Qing Z, Sunmin J, Hongliang X. Chitosan-modified methazolamide solid lipid nanoparticles and preparation method thereof. 2012. CN102793672A.
[50] Rochlitz C, Mamot C, Wicki A, Christofori G. Chemotherapeutic composition for the treatment of cancer. 2010. WO 2010103118 A1.
[51] Budzik BW, Colletti SL, Seifried DD, Stanton MG, Tian L. Novel amino alcohol cationic lipids for oligonucleotide delivery. 2012. WO 2011149733 A3.
[52] Chiang Y, Boey F, Chattopadhyay S, Natarajan JV, Venkatraman S, Wong T. A liposomal formulation for ocular drug delivery. 2012. WO 2012021107 A2.
[53] Haiyan Z, Yiming C, Jin C. Carbon-encapsulated iron nanoparticles and use thereof as vector of medicament for treating liver cancer. 2009. CN101347455A.
[54] Kim S, Nam J. Anticancer drug delivery system using pH-sensitive metal nanoparticles. 2013. EP 2559429 A2.
[55] Aria AI, Beizai M, Gharib M. Drug delivery by carbon nanotube arrays. 2012. WO 2012031164 A2.
[56] Haiyan X, Jie M, Hua K. Application of carbon nano-tubes in immunity accelerators for preparing anti-tumor immunotherapy medicaments. 2013. CN101537015A.
[57] Tostes GR, Ladeira LO, Furtado CA, Batista FGPC. Anti-tumour vaccine formulation based on carbon nanotubes and the use thereof. 2013. WO 2013110150 A1.
[58] Ernsting MJ, Li SD, Tang WL. Cellulose-based nanoparticles for drug delivery. 2012. WO 2012103634 A1.

[59] Jablonski M, Palamoor M. Nanoparticle composition and methods to make and use the same. 2013. US 20130209566 A1.
[60] Langer K, Wacker M, Röder B, Pruess A, Albrecht V, Gräfe S, Wiehe A, Von BH, Wagner S. Nanoparticle carrier systems based on human serum albumin for photodynamic therapy. 2011. WO 2011071968 A3.
[61] Baylatry MT, Bisdorf-Bresson A, Labarre D, Laurent A, Moine L, Saint-Maurice JP, Slimani K, Wassef M. Injectable biomaterial. 2014. US 8673264 B2.
[62] Desai NP, Soon-Shiong P, Trieu V. Nanoparticle comprising rapamycin and albumin as anticancer agent. 2013. US 20130280336 A1.
[63] Banerjee A, Pugh C, Storms W, Wright C. Functional biodegradable polymers. 2012. WO 2012015481 A1.
[64] Kannan RM, Kannan S, Romero R, Navath R, Menjoge A. Injectable dendrimer hydrogel nanoparticles. 2013. EP 2552458 A1.
[65] Smith HJ, Smith JR. Anti-tumor necrosis factor alpha (TNF-a) antibody used as a targeting agent to treat arthritis and other diseases. 2013. US 20130115269 A1.
[66] Jensen SS, Andresen TL, Henriksen JR, Johansen PT. Cationic liposomal drug delivery system for specific targeting of human cd14$^+$ monocytes in whole blood. 2013. WO 2013135800 A1.
[67] Kamaly N, Kalber TL, Kenny GD, Thanou M, Miller AD, Bell J. Liposome nanoparticles for tumor magnetic resonance imaging. 2011. WO 2011061541 A1.
[68] Kaur IP, Bhandari R. Solid lipid nanoparticles entrapping hydrophilic/amphiphilic drug and a process for preparing the same. 2014. WO 2013105101 A8.
[69] Kett V, Yusuf H, McCarthy H, Chen KH. Liposomal delivery system. 2013. WO 2013135892 A1.
[70] Bally M, Ramsay E. Liposomes with improved drug retention for treatment of cancer. 2014. US 8709474 B2.
[71] Schwiertz J, Ganesan K, Epple M, Wiehe A, Gräfe S, Gitter B, Albrecht V. Calcium phosphate-based nanoparticles as carrier-systems for photodynamic therapy. 2012. WO 2010078941 A1.
[72] Shieh DB, Yeh CS, Chen DH, Wu YN, Wu PC. Nano-carrier, complex of anticancer drug and nano-carrier, pharmaceutical composition thereof, method for manufacturing the complex, and method for treating cancer by using the pharmaceutical composition. 2012. US 20120027861 A1.
[73] Zhang M, Mok H. Nanovectors for targeted gene silencing and cytotoxic effect in cancer cells. 2013. US 20130189367 A1.
[74] Sahoo SK, Dilnawaz F, Singh AS. Water dispersible glyceryl monooleate magnetic nanoparticle formulation. 2010. WO 2010134087 A1.
[75] Rawat M, Singh D, Saraf S, Saraf S. Nanocarriers: promising vehicle for bioactive drugs. Biol Pharm Bull 2006;29(9):1790—8.
[76] Lacerda L, Bianco A, Prato M, Kostarelos K. Carbon nanotube as nanomedicines: from toxicity to pharmacology. Adv Drug Deliv Rev 2006;58(14):1460—70.
[77] Ochekpe NA, Olorunfemi PO, Ngwuluka NC. Nanotechnology and drug delivery. Part 2: nanostructures for drug delivery. Trop J Pharm Res 2009;8(3):275—87.
[78] Mudshinge SR, Deore AB, Patil S, Bhalgat CM. Nanoparticles: emerging carriers for drug delivery. Saudi Pharm J 2011;19:129—41.
[79] Weissig V, Pettinger TK, Murdock N. Nanopharmaceuticals (part 1): products on the market. Int J Nanomed 2014;9:4357—73.
[80] Forssen EA, Tökes ZA. Use of anionic liposomes for the reduction of chronic doxorubicin-induced cardiotoxicity. Proc Natl Acad Sci USA 1981;78(3):1873—7.
[81] Forssen EA, Tökes ZA. Improved therapeutic benefits of doxorubicin by entrapment in anionic liposomes. Cancer Res 1983;43(2):546—50.
[82] Barenholz Y. Doxil®—the first FDA-approved nano-drug: lessons learned. J Control Release 2012;160(2):117—34.
[83] Simpson JK, Miller RF, Spittle MF. Liposomal doxorubicin for treatment of AIDS-related Kaposi's sarcoma. Clin Oncol (R Coll Radiol) 1993;5(6):372—4.

[84] Northfelt DW, Dezube BJ, Thommes JA, Levine R, Von Roenn JH, Dosik GM, et al. Efficacy of pegylated-liposomal doxorubicin in the treatment of AIDS-related Kaposi's sarcoma after failure of standard chemotherapy. J Clin Oncol 1997;15(2):653—9.
[85] Ryan SM, Brayden DJ. Progress in the delivery of nanoparticle constructs: towards clinical translation. Curr Opin Pharmacol 2014;18:120—8.
[86] Bamrungsap S, Zhao Z, Chen T, Li C, Fu T, Tan W. Nanotechnology in therapeutics: a focus on nanoparticles as drug delivery systems. Nanomedicine (London) 2012;7(8):1253—71.
[87] Kailash CP, Sandip SC, Snezana A, Krutika KS. Nanostructured materials in drug and gene delivery: a review of the state of the art. Crit Rev Ther Drug Carr Syst 2011;28(2):101—70.
[88] Ventola CL. The nanomedicine revolution. Part 2: current and future clinical applications. Pharm Ther 2012;37(10):582—91.
[89] Stone D. Novel viral vector systems for gene therapy. Viruses 2010;2(4):1002—7.
[90] Blaese RM, Culver KW, Miller AD, Carter CS, Fleisher T, Clerici M, et al. T lymphocyte-directed gene therapy for ADA—SCID: initial trial results after 4 years. Science 1995; 270(5235):475—80.
[91] Basarkar A, Singh J. Nanoparticulate systems for polynucleotide delivery. Int J Nanomed 2007;2(3): 353—60.
[92] Hu WS, Pathak VK. Design of retroviral vectors and helper cells for gene therapy. Pharmacol Rev 2000;52(4):493—511.
[93] Al-Dosari MS, Gao X. Nonviral gene delivery: principle, limitations, and recent progress. AAPS J 2009;11(4):671—81.
[94] Walther W, Stein U. Viral vectors for gene transfer: a review of their use in the treatment of human diseases. Drugs 2000;60(2):249—71.
[95] Kamimura K, Suda T, Zhang G, Lui D. Advances in gene delivery systems. Pharm Med 2011;25(5): 293—306.
[96] http://www.wiley.com/legacy/wileychi/genmed/clinical/ (Gene therapy clinical trial Worldwide. J Gene Med. Website updated: July 2015).
[97] Lodish H, Berk A, Zipursky SL, et al. Molecular cell biology. 4th ed. New York: W.H. Freeman; 2000 Available from: http://www.ncbi.nlm.nih.gov/books/NBK21475/.
[98] Thomas CE, Ehrhardt A, Kay MA. Progress and problems with the use of viral vectors for gene therapy. Nat Rev Genet 2003;4(5):346—58.
[99] Mancheño-Corvo P, Martin-Duque P. Viral gene therapy. Clin Transl Oncol 2006;8(12):858—67.
[100] Siemens DR, Crist S, Austin CJ, Tataglia J, Ratliff T. Comparison of viral vectors: gene transfer efficiency and tissue specificity in bladder cancer model. J Urol 2003;170(3):979—84.
[101] Barquinero J, Eixarch H, Perez-Melgosa M. Retroviral vectors: new applications for an old tool. Gene Ther 2004;11(1):S3—9.
[102] Daniel R, Smith JA. Integration site selection by retroviral vectors: molecular mechanism and clinical consequences. Hum Gene Ther 2008;19:557—68.
[103] Nayerossadat N, Maedeh T, Ali PA. Viral and nonviral delivery systems for gene delivery. Adv Biomed Res 2012;1:27. http://dx.doi.org/10.4103/2277-9175.98152.
[104] Bushman FD. Retroviral integration and human gene therapy. J Clin Invest 2007;117(8):2083—6.
[105] Anson DS. The use of retroviral vectors for gene therapy — what are the risks? A review of retroviral pathogenesis and its relevance to retroviral vector-mediated gene delivery. Genet Vaccines Ther 2004;2:9. http://dx.doi.org/10.1186/1479-0556-2-9.
[106] Yi Y, Noh MJ, Lee KH. Current advances in retroviral gene therapy. Curr Gene Ther 2011;11(3): 218—28.
[107] Rowe WP, Huebner RJ, Gilmore LK, Parrott RH, Ward TG. Isolation of a cytopathogenic agent from human adenoids undergoing spontaneous degeneration in tissue culture. Proc Soc Exp Biol Med 1953;84(3):570—3.
[108] Campos SK, Barry MA. Current advances and future challenges in adenoviral vector biology and targeting. Curr Gene Ther 2007;7:189—204.
[109] Majhen D, Ambriovic-Ristov A. Adenoviral vectors — how to use them in cancer gene therapy? Virus Res 2006;119(2):121—33.

[110] Volper C, Kochanek S. Adenoviral vectors for gene transfer and therapy. J Gene Med 2004;6(S1): S164−71.
[111] Azzam T, Domb AJ. Current developments in gene transfection agents. Curr Drug Deliv 2004;1(2): 165−93.
[112] Godbey WT, Mikos AG. Recent progress in gene delivery using non-viral transfer complexes. J Control Release 2001;72(1−3):115−25.
[113] Zhi D, Zhang S, Cui S, Zhao Y, Wang Y, Zhao D. The headgroup evolution of cationic lipids for gene delivery. Bioconjug Chem 2013;24(4):487−519.
[114] Eliyahu H, Barenholz Y, Domb AJ. Polymers for DNA delivery. Molecules 2005;10:34−64.
[115] Tros de Ilarduya C, Sun Y, Düzgüneş N. Gene delivery by lipoplexes and polyplexes. Eur J Pharm Sci 2010;40(3):159−70.
[116] Nelson CE, Kintzing JR, Hanna A, Shannon JM, Gupta MK, Duvall CL. Balancing cationic and hydrophobic content of PEGylated siRNA polyplexes enhances endosome escape, stability, blood circulation time, and bioactivity in vivo. ACS Nano 2013;7(10):8870−80.
[117] Ogris M, Brunner S, Schüller S, Kircheis R, Wagner E. PEGylated DNA/transferrin−PEI complexes: reduced interaction with blood components, extended circulation in blood and potential for systemic gene delivery. Gene Ther 1999;6:595−605.
[118] Robbins PD, Ghivizzani SC. Viral vectors for gene therapy. Pharmacol Ther 1998;80(1):35−47.
[119] Neumann E, Schaefer-Ridder M, Wang Y, Hofschneider PH. Gene transfer into mouse lyoma cells by electroporation in high electric fields. EMBO J 1987;1(7):841−5.
[120] André F, Mir LM. DNA Electrotransfer: its principles and an updated review of its therapeutic applications. Gene Ther 2004;(Suppl. 1):S33−42.
[121] Kim HJ, Greenleaf JF, Kinnick RR, Bronk JT, Bolander ME. Ultrasound-mediated transfection of mammalian cells. Hum Gene Ther 1996;7(11):1339−46.
[122] Miao CH, Brayman AA, Loeb KR, Ye P, Zhou L, Mourad P, Crum LA. Ultrasound enhances gene delivery of human factor IX plasmid. Hum Gene Ther 2005;16(7):893−905.
[123] Taniyama Y, Tachibana K, Hiraoka K, Aoki M, Yamamoto S, Matsumoto K, Nakamura T, et al. Gene Ther 2002;9(6):372−80.
[124] Capecchi MR. High efficiency transformation by direct microinjection of DNA into cultured mammalian cells. Cell 1998;22(2 Pt. 2):479−88.
[125] Auerbach AB. Production of functional transgenic mice by DNA pronuclear microinjection. Acta Biochim Pol 2004;51(1):9−31.
[126] Williams RS, Johnston SA, Riedy M, DeVit MJ, McElligott SG, Sanford JC. Introduction of foreign genes into tissues of living mice by DNA-coated microprojectiles. Proc Natl Acad Sci USA 1991; 88(7):2726−30.
[127] Trimble C, Lin CT, Hung CF, Pai S, Juang J, He L, et al. Comparison of the CD8[+] T cell responses and antitumor effects generated by DNA vaccine administered through gene gun, biojector, and syringe. Vaccine 2003;21(25−26):4036−42.
[128] Mehier-Humbert S, Guy RH. Physical methods for gene transfer: improving the kinetics of gene delivery into cells. Adv Drug Deliv Rev 2005;57(5):733−53.
[129] Pearson S, Jia H, Kandachi K. China approves first gene therapy. Nat Biotechnol 2004;22:3−4. http://dx.doi.org/10.1038/nbt0104-3.
[130] Wilson JM. Gendicine: the first commercial gene therapy product. Hum Gene Ther 2005;16(9): 1014−5.
[131] Peng Z. Current status of gendicine in China: recombinant human Ad-p53 agent for treatment of cancers. Hum Gene Ther 2005;16(9):1016−27.
[132] Wang Z, Sun Y. Targeting p53 for novel anticancer therapy. Transl Oncol 2010;3(1):1−12.
[133] Gabrilovich DI. INGN 201 (Advexin): adenoviral p53 gene therapy for cancer. Expert Opin Biol Ther 2006;6(8):823−32.
[134] Gordon EM, Hall FL. Rexin-G, a targeted genetic medicine for cancer. Expert Opin Biol Ther 2010;10(5):819−32.
[135] Kastelein JJP, Ross CJD, Hayden MR. From mutation identification to therapy: discovery and origin of the first approved gene therapy in the Western World. Hum Gene Ther 2013;24:472−8.

[136] http://www.fiercebiotech.com/story/uniqure-mulls-options-1m-gene-therapy-after-fda-demands-extra-trial/2015-08-27 (UniQure mulls options for $1M gene therapy after FDA demands extra trial; by Nick Paul Taylor, August 27, 2015).

[137] http://labiotech.eu/fda-shelves-uniqures-glybera-will-the-gene-therapy-once-reach-the-us-market/ (FDA shelves UniQure's Glybera — will the gene therapy once reach the US market?; Article dated: August 28, 2015).

INDEX

'*Note*: Page numbers followed by "f" indicate figures and "t" indicate tables.'

A

Absorptive-mediated transcytosis (AMT), 70–71
N-Acetyl-glucosamine units, 7–8
Adenocarcinoma, 160–161
Adipose tissue–derived progenitor cells, 94–95
ADMINPEN pen-injector device, 348f, 349
Adult stem cells, 85
Alzet pump, 250–252, 257f
L-Amino acid transporter (LAT), 65
Amphiphilic block copolymers, 46
Amphiphilic monomers, 46
Amphiphilic polymers, 6–7
anoDyne, 349
Anticancer carriers, 308–310
Aquasomes, 154
Aqueous buffer solution, 170–171
Artificial silicon retina (ASR) microchip, 267–268, 268f

B

Bioactive factor molecules, 7–8, 8f
Biodegradable polymeric nanoparticles
  advantages, 120
  carbon nanotubes (CNTs), 126–127, 127f, 128t–131t
  emulsion polymerization method, 122–124, 123f
  in vivo cytotoxicity, 125–126, 125f
  iron nanoparticles. *See* Iron nanoparticles
  laboratory-scale nanoparticle preparation methods, 120–121
  macromolecules, 126
  nonaqueous phase separation method, 122
  paclitaxel delivery, 127, 132f
  particle size, 125–126, 125f
  preparation, 120
  salting out/emulsion diffusion method, 122, 122f
  solvent evaporation method, 121, 121f
  spontaneous emulsification/solvent diffusion method, 121
  spray drying, 124, 124f
  supercritical fluid technology, 124
  SWNTs, CXR4 expression levels, 127, 132f
  types, 120f

Biodegradable polymers, 1–2, 30
Biomechanical endocardial sorin transducer (BEST) sensor, 267
Biomedical implants (BMIs), 249–250
  Alzet pump, 250–252, 257f
  antiinflammatory agents, 257–258
  applications, 250–252, 259t–261t
  biocompatibility and biofunctionality, 257–258
  Duros pumps, 250–252, 258f
  immune system, 252, 261f
  immunological responses, 252
  International Organization for Standardization (ISO) 10993, 257–258
  iPrecio microinfusion pumps, 250–252, 257f
  osmotic pumps, 250, 256f
  passive and active reservoir, 250, 256f
  peristaltic pump, 250, 257f
  reciprocating pump, 250, 257f
  spring-powered pump, 250, 256f
  synchromed II micropumps, 250–252, 258f
  types, 250
Biopharmaceutics Classification System, 50–52
Biosensors, 209
Block copolymer (BCP), 2–3
Blood–brain barrier (BBB), 60
  absorptive-mediated transcytosis (AMT), 70–71
  active targeting strategies, 70
  blood–brain tumor barrier (BBTB) targeting strategies, 72–73
  blood–cerebrospinal fluid (BCSF) barrier, 61, 61f
  brain drug delivery, 62. *See also* Brain drug delivery
  brain endothelial capillary cells (BCECs), 60–61
  capillary endothelial cells, 69
  composition, 60–61
  exosomes, 74, 75f
  macrophages, 73–74
  mesenchymal stem cells, 73
  receptor-mediated transcytosis, 71–72
  structural components, 69, 70f
  tight junctions (TJs), 60–61
  transporter-mediated transcytosis, 71

393

Blood—brain tumor barrier (BBTB) targeting strategies, 72—73
Blood—cerebrospinal fluid (BCSF) barrier, 61, 61f
Bone tissue engineering, 203—204
Bovine serum albumin (BSA), 207—208
Brain drug delivery, 60
　classification, 62
　invasive methods
　　convection enhanced drug delivery (CED), 62
　　permeability modulation, 62—63
　　transcranial injections, 62
　　ultrasound-mediated drug delivery (USMD), 63
　　vascular permeability, optical modulation, 63—64
　noninvasive methods
　　chemical derivatization, 64—65
　　chronic disorders, 64
　　intranasal drug delivery, 66—67
　　nanocarriers, 64
　　prodrug lipidization, 65
　　transporter-targeted prodrugs, 65—66, 66t
Brain endothelial capillary cells (BCECs), 60—61

C
Carbidopa, 65—66
Carbohydrate-responsive systems, 200
Carbohydrates, 34
Carbon nanotubes (CNTs), 152—153, 222
　biodegradable polymeric nanoparticles, 126—127, 127f, 128t—131t
　peptide and protein therapeutics (PPTs), 152—153
Cardiac tissue engineering, 204—205
Carrier-mediated transport, 65
Casting technique, 249—250, 251f
Cationic proteins/cell-penetrating peptides (CPPs), 70—71
Caveolae-independent pathways, 172—173
Caveolae-mediated endocytosis, 172
CD44 membrane receptor, 99
Cell penetrating peptides (CPPs), 157
Chitin, 7—8
Chitosan-based micro/nanoparticles, 30
Clathrin-independent pathways, 172—173
Clathrin-mediated endocytosis (CME), 171
CLIC/GEEC pathway, 173

Coated microneedles (CMN)
　anticancer drugs, 341
　metal and polymer, 339, 340f
　preparation, 339
　proof-of-concept study, 340—341
　small molecule drugs, 339—340
Cold homogenization technique, 296—297
Complementary metal oxide semiconductor (CMOS), 264—265
Computed tomography (CT), 48—49
Confocal microscopy, 180—181, 181f
Convection enhanced drug delivery (CED), 62
Coprecipitation, 133
Critical micellar concentration (CMC), 45—46

D
Daytona MT Dermal Roller, 349
Dendrimers, 30—31
Detergent removal methods, 112
Direct dissolution method, 47
Dissolving microneedles (DMNs)
　disadvantages, 342—343
　drug release kinetics, 342—343
　limitation, 343
　mechanism, 341—342
　MicroHyala, 343
　water-soluble and biodegradable polymers, 341—342, 342f
L-DOPA, 65—66
Drug-enriched core model, 300, 300f
Drug-enriched shell model, 300, 300f
Drug-loaded nanomicelles, 47
Duros pumps, 250—252, 258f

E
Early endocytic vesicles, 174
Electrospun nanofibers
　applications, 190, 191f
　　biomedical application, 209
　　biosensors, 209
　　bovine serum albumin (BSA), 207—208
　　cancer therapy, 208—209
　　dentistry, 205—206
　　drug release rate, 207
　　enzyme-linked immunosorbent assay (ELISA), 210
　　glucose oxidase (GOD), 210
　　ocular injuries, 206—207

PLLA fiber/chitosan microsphere composites, 208
tissue engineering. *See* Tissue engineering
transdermal drug delivery system, 208
drug-loaded NFs, 190
electrospinning process, 191f
applied voltage, 194
collector types, 195
components, 190
concentration, 192
conductivity, 192—194
electrostatic repulsive force, 190—192
flow rate, 194
humidity and temperature, 194—195
morphology and properties, 192, 193t
needle tip and collector distance, 194
polymer molecular weight, 192
polymer solution parameters, 192
surface tension, 190—192
Taylor cone, 190—192
viscosity, 194
stimuli-responsive nanofibers
applications, 195, 196t—198t, 201
carbohydrate-responsive systems, 200
enzyme-responsive systems, 200
light-activated systems, 195—199
multiresponsive systems, 201
oxidative stress—responsive nano fiber systems, 200
pH-responsive systems, 195
thermoresponsive systems, 199—200
triggered drug release, 195, 199f
ultrasound-responsive systems, 200
Embryonic stem cells, 85
Emulsification—diffusion technique, 298
Emulsion polymerization method, 122—124, 123f
Encapsulation process, 47
ENDOCOM, 265—267, 266f
Enhanced permeability and retention (EPR) effect, 2, 308—309
Enzyme-linked immunosorbent assay (ELISA), 210
Enzyme-responsive systems, 200
Exosomes, 74, 75f

F

FDA-approved nanopharmaceuticals, 376, 380t—382t
Flotillin-mediated endocytosis, 173
Fluorescence-based in situ hybridization aka FISH, 356—359, 358f
Fluorescence confocal microscopy, 356, 357f
Fluorescence-mediated molecular tomography (FMT), 76
Fluorescent dyes, 34—35
Freeze-drying technique, 7—8
Functional moieties
antigen-binding sites, 33
carbohydrates, 34
epitope-binding sites, 33
fluorescent dyes, 34—35
nucleic acids, 33—34
peptides, 32—33
proteins, 33

G

Gadolinium-diethylene triamine pentaacetic acid (Gd-DTPA), 90
Gadolinium-loaded nanoparticles (GdNPs), 363
Gamma scintigraphy, 230
Gel forming pentablock copolymer, 6, 9f
Gene delivery
genetic disorders, 383
nanomaterials, 376, 377t—379t
nonviral vector approach, 384
physical approach, 384—385
viral vector approach, 383—384
Gene therapy products, 385
Glucose sensors
glucose oxidase (GOD), 234
immobilized enzyme film glucose biosensors, 234, 235f
insulin, 233
nanoparticle/carbon nanotube, 236f
advantage, 235—236
gold nanoparticles, 235
implantable biosensor, 237—238
multiwall carbon nanotubes (MWCNTs), 236
nafion (NF), 235—236
nanobiocomposite, 237
nanofibrous composite electrode, 236—237
nonenzymatic glucose biosensors, 238—239
response time, 237
nonenzymatic glucose biosensors, 233—234
Glucose transporters (GLUT), 71
Glycosylation, 148—149

Gold nanoparticles (AuNPs), 32, 159–160, 221–222
    inorganic nanomaterials, 359–360, 360f
    lipid nanocarriers, 366
    macropinocytosis, 183–185, 183f, 184t
    peptide and protein therapeutics (PPTs), 159–160
Gold nanoshells, 366

H

HeartPOD, 265–267, 266f
High-pressure homogenization (HPH) technique
    cold homogenization technique, 296–297
    hot homogenization technique, 296
    nanoemulsions, 295–296
    shear stress and cavitation forces, 295–296
Hollow microneedles (HMNs)
    array-type HMNs, 337–338
    disadvantages, 337–338
    fluid and liquid formulations, 337–338
    materials, 338, 338f
    microinjector, 338–339
    ocular drug delivery, 338–339
Hot embossing technique, 249–250, 251f
Hot homogenization technique, 115–116, 296, 309
Hydrogel-forming microneedles (HGMNs)
    advantages, 344–345
    cross-linked structure, 343–344
    disadvantages, 345
    hypoxia-sensitive hyaluronic acid (HS-HA) MN, 343–344
    materials, 343–344, 344f
    mechanical tests, 345
    pancreatic β-cell-embedded capsules, 344–345
    polymeric compositions, 345–346
    small molecule drugs, 346
Hydrophilic anticancer actives, 310
Hyperbranched polymers (HBPs), 3

I

Immobilized enzyme film glucose biosensors, 234, 235f
Imperium, 349
Implantable biosensor, 237–238
Implantable bladder pressure sensor, 265–267, 266f
Implantable hemodynamic monitoring (IHM) device, 265
Implantable telemetric endosystem (ITES), 263–264
Inorganic micro/nanocarriers
    gold nanoparticles (AuNPs), 32
    magnetic nanoparticles, 32
    quantum dots (QDs), 31–32
Inorganic nanomaterials
    gold nanoparticles, 359–360, 360f
    magnetic nanoparticles, 359
    quantum dots (QDs), 361–362, 362f
    silica nanoparticles, 361, 361f
    surface-enhanced Raman scattering (SERS), 362–363
International Organization for Standardization (ISO) 10993, 257–258
Intracellular trafficking, 171, 172f, 178–179, 179f
    phases, 174, 176f
Intracranial pressure (ICP), 263–264, 264f
Intranasal drug delivery, 66–67
Intraocular pressure (IOP) sensors, 262–263, 263f
Intravascular pressure monitoring system, 265–267, 266f
iPrecio microinfusion pumps, 250–252, 257f
Iron nanoparticles, 133f
    applications
        antiproliferative activity, 134, 138f
        blood–brain barrier, 137
        methotrexate (MTX)-magnetic nanoparticles, 134, 137f
        therapeutic agents, 134, 137t
        vascular endothelium, 137
    coprecipitation, 133
    hydrothermal synthesis, 134
    microemulsion, 134
    passive targeting technique, 127–133
    preparation methods, 133–134
    sonochemical synthesis, 134, 135t, 136f, 136t
    thermal decomposition, 133
Iron oxide nanoparticles, 365–366

L

Late endosomes, 174–175, 176f
Light-activated systems, 195–199
Lipid-based micro/nanocarriers
    liposome, 28–29
    microemulsion, 29
    solid-lipid nanoparticles (SLNs), 29–30
Lipid film hydration method, 109–110, 110f

Lipid nanocarriers
    gadolinium-loaded nanoparticles (GdNPs), 363
    gold nanoparticles, 366
    gold nanoshells, 366
    iron oxide nanoparticles, 365–366
    nanomicelles, 366–367
    radiolabeled liposomes, 364–365
    radiolabeled nanoparticles, 363–364, 364t
Liposomes, 28–29, 153–154, 223, 224f
    bilamellar liposome structure, 108–109, 109f
    cryoprotectants, 114
    detergent removal methods, 112
    gadolinium-DTPA, 113–114, 113f
    large unilamellar vesicles (LUVs), 109
    lipid film hydration method, 109–110, 110f
    mononuclear phagocyte system (MPS), 109
    passive loading method
        hydrophobic/hydrophilic drugs, 110–111
        mechanical dispersion–extrusion method, 111
        mechanical dispersion–freeze-thaw technique, 111
        mechanical dispersion–sonication method, 111
        solvent dispersion–ethanol injection method, 112
        solvent dispersion–ether injection method, 111
        solvent dispersion–reverse phase evaporation method, 112
        trapping efficiency, 110–111
    phospholipid molecules, 108–109
    small unilamellar vesicles (SUVs), 109
    solid lipid nanoparticles (SLNs), 118t. See also Solid lipid nanoparticles (SLNs)
    stability, 114
    topotecan (TPT) distribution, 112–113, 113f
    types, 109, 109f
Lysosomes, 177, 177f

M

Macromolecular delivery systems
    CD44 membrane receptor, 99
    chemical transfection agents, 96–97
    drug resistance proteins, 98
    FITC-conjugated mesoporous silica nanoparticles, 97–98
    methyltransferase expression, 99
    nonviral gene delivery system, 97–98
    residual posttreatment tumors, 98
    viral vectors, 96–97
    wild-type p53 gene, 99
Macropinocytosis
    cell nucleus, 179–180
    confocal microscopy, 180–181, 181f
    early endocytic vesicles, 174
    gold nanoparticles, 183–185, 183f, 184t
    GTPases and kinases, 173–174
    intracellular trafficking, 178–179, 179f
        phases, 174, 176f
    late endosomes, 174–175, 176f
    lysosomes, 177, 177f
    mechanism, 173–174
    phagocytosis, 174, 175f
    quantum dots, 181–182, 182f–183f
Macropinocytosis-independent pathways, 172–173
Magnetic nanoparticles (MNPs), 32, 69, 157–159, 359
Magnetic resonance imaging (MRI), 49
Mannosylation, 149–150
Medical and biomedical imaging
    advantage, 355–356
    fluorescence-based in situ hybridization aka FISH, 356–359, 358f
    fluorescence confocal microscopy, 356, 357f
    high-resolution imaging techniques, 355–356
    mixed lineage leukemia (MLL), 356–359, 358f
    nanocarriers
        inorganic nanomaterials. See Inorganic nanomaterials
        lipid nanocarriers. See Lipid nanocarriers
    photoacoustic (PA) imaging, 367–369
        gold nanoparticles, types, 368t, 369
    photobleaching, 359
    super-resolution microscopy, 359
    ultrasound imaging, 367–369
Membrane translocation signals, 32
MEMS-based cochlear prosthesis, 268–269, 268f
MEMS microflex interconnect technology, 269
Mesenchymal stem cells, 73
Methotrexate (MTX)-magnetic nanoparticles, 134, 137f
MiconJet, 347
Microcantilevers (MCs)
    advantages, 239
    microcantilever deflection
        biochips, 244
        cancer detectors, 240–241, 242t–243t

Microcantilevers (MCs) (*Continued*)
   coronary heart diseases, 241
   mechanism, 239, 240f
   nanocantilevers, 244
   nucleotide polymorphisms, 241
   Shuttle-worth equation, 239
   Sotney's equation, 240
   surface strain, 240
Microchip reservoir, 271, 271f
MicroCor system, 347—349
Microelectromechanical systems (MEMS), 249—250. *See also* Microtechnology-based implantable devices and bionics
Microemulsification, 116
Microemulsion, 29, 134, 297
Microinjection technique, 249—250, 250f
Micro/nanogel, 31
Microneedles (MNs), 269—270, 270f
   AdminPen pen-injector device, 348f, 349
   anoDyne, 349
   coated microneedles (CMNs). *See* Coated microneedles (CMNs)
   Daytona MT Dermal Roller, 349
   designs selection, 346, 347t
   dissolving microneedles (DMNs). *See* Dissolving microneedles (DMNs)
   hollow microneedles (HMNs). *See* Hollow microneedles (HMNs)
   hydrogel-forming microneedles (HGMNs). *See* Hydrogel-forming microneedles (HGMNs)
   Imperium, 349
   MiconJet, 347
   MicroCor system, 347—349
   Micro-Trans, 347
   3M Microneedle transdermal system, 349
   SCS microinjector, 347
   self-administration, 333—334
   solid microneedles (SMNs). *See* Solid microneedles (SMNs)
   Soluvia, 346—347
   types, 333—334, 334f
   Zosano patch, 349
Microparticles
   fabrication techniques, 26—27
   free-flowing powders, 24
   functional moieties conjugation, 35. *See also* Functional moieties
   membrane-bound vesicles, 24
   microcarriers, 24
   peptide and protein therapeutics (PPTs), 150—151
   solid/small liquid droplets, 22—24
   stimuli-responsive elements, 26—27
   structures, 24, 24f
   surface functionalization, 35
   Trojan microparticles, 26
Microtechnology-based implantable devices and bionics, 253t—255t
   development of, 258—262
   drug delivery devices
      applications, 272, 273t
      capsule-like microdevices, 271—272
      implantable pumps, 269—270, 270f
      microchip reservoir, 271, 271f
      microneedles, 269—270, 270f
      polymeric microchip device, 272, 272f
      smart pills, 269—270, 270f
      solid-state silicon microchip, 271—272
      toxic effects, 269—270
   sensing systems
      artificial silicon retina (ASR) microchip, 267—268, 268f
      biomechanical endocardial sorin transducer (BEST) sensor, 267
      complementary metal oxide semiconductor (CMOS), 264—265
      ENDOCOM, 265—267, 266f
      HeartPOD, 265—267, 266f
      implantable bladder pressure sensor, 265—267, 266f
      implantable hemodynamic monitoring (IHM) device, 265
      implantable telemetric endosystem (ITES), 263—264
      intracranial pressure (ICP), 263—264, 264f
      intraocular pressure (IOP) sensors, 262—263, 263f
      intravascular pressure monitoring system, 265—267, 266f
      MEMS-based cochlear prosthesis, 268—269, 268f
      MEMS microflex interconnect technology, 269
      multiaxis bone stress sensor, 269, 270f
      piezoresistors, 262
      retinal prosthetic system, 267—268
      silicone capsule, 265—267
      wireless implantable microsystems, 264—265

Micro-Trans, 347
Mixed lineage leukemia (MLL), 356—359, 358f
3M Microneedle transdermal system, 349
Multiaxis bone stress sensor, 269, 270f
Multifunctional micro/nanocarrier, 26—27, 27f
   chemical functional groups, 35
      inorganic micro/nanocarriers. *See* Inorganic micro/nanocarriers
      lipid-based micro/nanocarriers. *See* Lipid-based micro/nanocarriers
      polymeric micro/nanocarriers. *See* Polymeric micro/nanocarriers
   types, 27—28, 28f
Multiresponsive systems, 201
Multivesicular bodies (MVBs), 174—175, 176f
Multiwall carbon nanotubes (MWCNTs), 236

N
Nafion, 235—236
Nanoelectromechanical systems (NEMS), 249—250. *See also* Nanotechnology-based implantable devices and bionics
Nanomaterials
   gene delivery, 376, 377t—379t
   nano drug delivery systems, 379—383
   properties and mechanism, 379
Nanomedicine, 376
Nanomicelles, 31, 366—367
   advantages, 48, 53—54
   Biopharmaceutics Classification System, 50—52
   clinical trial, 50, 51t
   computed tomography (CT), 48—49
   critical micellar concentration (CMC), 45—46
   drug delivery carriers, 50
   hydrophobic drugs, 50—52
   imaging tools, 48
   magnetic resonance imaging (MRI), 49
   multifunctional nanomicelle carrier, 53
   near-infrared fluorescent imaging (NIRF), 49—50
   phases, aqueous solution, 45—46
   preparation, 46—47
   properties, 53—54, 54f
   stimuli-responsive nanomicelles
      light sensitive, 53
      oxidative and reductive enzyme expressions, 53
      pH sensitive, 52
      temperature sensitive, 52
      ultrasound responsive, 53
   targeted nanomicelles, 52
   van der Walls forces, 45—46
Nanoparticles
   based medicines, 21—22, 23t
   CNS disorders, 67
   functional moieties conjugation, 35, 36t—38t. *See also* Functional moieties
   magnetic nanoparticles (MNPs), 69
   nanocarriers, 67
   particle—particle aggregation, 25—26
   peptide and protein therapeutics (PPTs), 151—152
   polymeric nanoparticles, 67—68, 68t
   solid lipid nanoparticles (SLNs), 68—69
   stimuli-responsive elements, 26—27
   structures, 25—26, 25f
   surface functionalization, 35
Nanoparticulate systems
   classification, 106—108, 108f
   endocytosis, 106
   fluorescent biological labels, 106—108
   nanomedicine, 106
   nanometer levels, 105
   nonrigid nanoparticles
      lipid-based nanoparticles, 108
      liposomes. *See* Liposomes
   rigid nanoparticles. *See* Rigid nanoparticles
   US Food and Drug Administration, 106, 107t
Nanoscaffold-coated model bioreactor, 94—95
Nanosystems
   biological sensors, 233f
      glucose sensors. *See* Glucose sensors
      microcantilevers (MCs). *See* Microcantilevers (MCs)
      multidisciplinary research, 232—233
   biomedical applications, 217—218
   carbon nanotubes (CNTs), 222
   contrast agents, 218
   dendrimers, 225—226
   diagnostic imaging
      advantages and disadvantages, 226—227, 227t
      computed tomography (CT), 230—231
      fluorescence-based optical imaging, 229
      lipoprotein delivery systems, 229—230
      magnetic resonance imaging (MRI), 227—228
      nonionizing radiation, 228—229

Nanosystems (*Continued*)
    nuclear imaging, 230
    research and clinical applications, 226—227, 228f
    silica nanoparticles, 229—230
    ultrasound/sonography, 231—232
  drug loading and functionalization, 218, 219f
  gold nanoparticles, 221—222
  interdisciplinary approach, 217—218
  iron oxide nanoparticles
    advantages, 218, 220t
    disadvantages, 219—220
    magnetic resonance imaging (MRI), 218
    physiochemical properties, 218—219
  liposomes, 223, 224f
  lysosomes, 225
  magnetic nanomicelle system, 225
  NIR organic dyes, 225
  pH-responsive nanomicelles, 224—225
  quantum dots, 220—221
  silica nanoparticles, 222—223
Nanotechnology-based implantable devices and bionics, 253t—255t
  clinical trials, 272—274, 274t
  drug delivery devices
    applications, 277, 278t—279t
    electrospinning nanotechnique, 277
    silica nanoparticle (SiNP), 280
    stimulus-responsive membrane triggering, 279, 280f
    ultrasound-stimulated titania nanotube (TNT) arrays, 279—280, 280f
  fabrication techniques, 272—274
  NEMS, benefits, 272—274
  sensing systems
    biodegradable molybdenum wires, 276—277
    gold nanogap device, 274—275
    in vivo monitoring, 275—276
    nanowires (NWs), 274—275
    piezoresistive nanomechanical membrane-type surface stress sensor (MSS), 276
    silicon sensors, 276—277, 276f
    ultrananocrystalline diamond (UNCD) thin films, 275—276
Natural polymers, 1—2, 30
Near-infrared fluorescent imaging (NIRF), 49—50
Nerve tissue engineering, 205
Neurodegenerative disorders, 60

Neurodiagnostic nanoimaging platforms, 78t
  CT imaging agents, 74—75
  monitoring events, 74
  MRI, 75
  optical imaging, 76, 77f
  optoacoustic tomography, 77
  PET, 75—76
  X-ray CT, 74—75
Nonaqueous phase separation method, 122
Nonbiodegradable polymers, 1—2, 30
Nonenzymatic glucose biosensors, 233—234
Nonionic surfactants, 46
Nonviral gene delivery system, 97—98
Nucleic acids, 33—34

O

Ocular drug delivery, 6—7, 9f
Optoacoustic tomography, 77
Organelle-targeted nanocarrier, 169—170
Organic micro-nanoparticles, 27—28
Osmotic pumps, 250, 256f
Oxidative stress—responsive nano fiber systems, 200

P

Paclitaxel-loaded phosphatidyl ethanolamine (PEG-PE) micelles, 52
Passive and active reservoir, 250, 256f
PEGylation (PEG), 147—148
Pentablock copolymers, 6
Peptide and protein therapeutics (PPTs)
  applications
    adenocarcinoma, 160—161
    cancer, 155—156
    cell penetrating peptides (CPPs), 157
    clinical trials, 157, 158t
    DHBV replication, 157
    gold nanoparticles, 159—160
    graphene CNT, 160
    magnetic nanoparticles (MNPs), 157—159
    ocular diseases, 156—157
    protein microarray technology, 160
    silver-gold nanorods, 160
    SWCNT, 160
  aquasomes, 154
  biological membranes, 147
  carbon nanotube (CNT), 152—153
  chemical modifications
    glycosylation, 148—149

mannosylation, 149−150
PEGylation (PEG), 147−148
liposomes, 153−154
in market, 146, 146t
micelles, 154−155
microparticles/microspheres, 150−151
nanoparticles, 151−152
proteolytic enzymes, 147
secondary and tertiary structures, 146
solid lipid nanoparticles (SLN), 152
Peptides, 32−33
Peristaltic pump, 250, 257f
Permeability modulation, 62−63
Phagocytosis, 174, 175f
Pharmaceutical nanocarriers, 170
Photoacoustic (PA) imaging, 367−369, 368t
Photodynamic therapy (PDT), 221−222
pH-responsive systems, 195
Poly(D,L-lactic-co-glycolic acid) (PLGA), 30
Polyethylene glycol (PEG)-coating, 307, 307f
Polymeric materials
  biodegradable polymers, 1−2
  block copolymer (BCP), 2−3
  doxorubinin, 3, 4f
  enhanced permeability and retention (EPR) effect, 2
  fluorescence diagnosis, 13−14
  glutathione (GSH) level, 3
  hyperbranched polymers (HBPs), 3
  MRI, 13
  natural polymers, 1−2
  nonbiodegradable polymers, 1−2
  ocular drug delivery, 6−7, 9f
  PET, 14
  photoresponsive drug release, 4−5, 5f
  polymer-based diagnostic agents, 2
  polymer blends, 2−3
  polymer−drug conjugates, 2, 5−6
  postpolymerization modification, 4−5
  redox-responsive drug release, 3, 4f
  SPECT, 14−15
  synthetic polymers, 1−2
  theranostics, 2
  therapeutic and diagnostic applications, 8−15
  thermoplastic aliphatic polyesters, 1−2
  tissue engineering, 7−8, 8f−9f, 10t−12t
Polymeric microchip device, 272, 272f
Polymeric microfabrication techniques
  casting technique, 249−250, 251f
  hot embossing technique, 249−250, 251f
  microinjection technique, 249−250, 250f
  stereolithography technique, 249−250, 252f
Polymeric micro/nanocarriers
  macromolecular drugs, 30
  natural polymers, 30
  synthetic polymers, 30−31
Polymeric nanoparticles, 67−68, 68t
Prodrug lipidization, 65
Protein microarray technology, 160
Proteins, 33
PuraMatrix hydrogel, 95

Q
Quantum dots (QDs), 170
  inorganic micro/nanocarriers, 31−32
  inorganic nanomaterials, 361−362, 362f
  macropinocytosis, 181−182, 182f−183f
  nanosystems, 220−221
  stem cell tracking, 90−91

R
Radiolabeled liposomes, 364−365
Radiolabeled nanoparticles, 363−364, 364t
Receptor-mediated transcytosis, 71−72
Receptor-mediated transport (RMT), 65
Reciprocating pump, 250, 257f
RhoA-mediated uptake, 173
Rigid nanoparticles, 119
  biodegradable polymeric nanoparticles. *See* Biodegradable polymeric nanoparticles

S
Salting out/emulsion diffusion method, 122, 122f
SCS microinjector, 347
Silica nanoparticles, 361, 361f
Silver-gold nanorods, 160
Skin tissue engineering, 202−203
Small interfering RNA (siRNA), 375−376
Smart pills, 269−270, 270f
Solid lipid nanoparticles (SLNs), 29−30, 68−69
  advantages, 114−115, 292−293, 293t
  antitumor effect, 117−119, 119f
  applications
    anticancer carriers, 308−310
    chemotherapy, 308
    cytotoxic drugs pose toxicity, 308
    hydrophilic and lipophilic drugs, 302
    hydrophilic anticancer actives, 310

Solid lipid nanoparticles (SLNs) (*Continued*)
    ocular administration, 306–307
    oral administration, 302–303
    parenteral route, 303–304
    polyethylene glycol (PEG)-coating, 307, 307f
    pulmonary administration, 305, 306f
    rectal administration, 305
    topical administration, 304–305, 304f
  Biopharmaceutical Classification System, 292
  brain capillary endothelial cells (BCECs), 117, 118f
  cold homogenization, 116
  components
    lipids, 293–294, 294t
    surfactants, 295, 295t
  diagnostic applications, 320–321, 321f
  disadvantages, 292–293, 293t
  docetaxel (DTX), 117, 118f
  drug-enriched core model, 116–117, 300, 300f
  drug-enriched shell model, 116–117, 300, 300f
  drug entrapment, 116–117, 117f
  drug-loading capacity, 298–299
  drug release
    etomidate, 300–301, 301f
    principles, 300
    surfactant, 302
    temperature, 301
  emulsification–diffusion technique, 298
  high-pressure homogenization (HPH) technique, 292–293. *See also* High-pressure homogenization (HPH) technique
  homogenous matrix model, 116–117
  hot homogenization, 115–116
  in vivo fate, 321–322
  lipid-based formulations, 292
  lipids and surfactants, 115, 115t
  microemulsification, 116
  microemulsion-based technique, 297
  oral administration, 295
  peptide and protein therapeutics (PPTs), 152
  solid solution model, 299, 300f
  solvent displacement technique, 298
  solvent emulsification–evaporation method, 116, 297–298
  stability, 119
    coalescence, 318
    cryoprotectants, 313–314
    crystallization kinetics, 316–317
    drug entrapment, 315
    factors, 310–311
    gelation, 315–316, 316f
    gelling tendency, 314–315
    lipid concentration, 311
    lipid transformations, 313
    lyophilization, 313–314
    matrix, 316–317
    nanostructured lipid carriers (NLC), 312
    Ostwald ripening, 318
    packing material, 311
    phospholipid stability, 318
    polymorphism, 317
    shear forces, 311
    SLNs *vs.* bulk material, 312
    spray drying, 313
    triglycerides stability, 319
  stress and strain, 119
  structures, 114, 114f
  surfactant-stabilized lipids, 114
  toxicity, 319
Solid microneedles (SMNs)
  biocompatible metals, 334, 336f
  drug formulation/transdermal drug patch, 334, 335f
  limitation, 337
  microchannels formation, 336
  permeation enhancement techniques, 336–337
  pharmaceutical applications, 334–335
Solid solution model, 299, 300f
Solid-state silicon microchip, 271–272
Soluvia, 346–347
Solvent casting method, 47
Solvent displacement technique, 298
Solvent emulsification–evaporation method, 116, 297–298
Solvent evaporation method, 121, 121f
Somatic stem cells, 85
Sonochemical synthesis, 134, 135t, 136f, 136t
Spontaneous emulsification/solvent diffusion method, 121
Spray drying, 124, 124f, 313
Spring-powered pump, 250, 256f
Stem cell therapy
  adult stem cells/somatic stem cells, 85
  cell types, 85
  embryonic stem cells, 85

nanoparticles application
  isolation, 86—89
  macromolecular delivery systems. *See* Macromolecular delivery systems
  stem cell tracking. *See* Stem cell tracking
 regenerative medicine, 85—86
 regulation of, 100
 sources, 85—86, 87t—88t
 tissue engineering. *See* Tissue engineering
Stem cell tracking
 cobalt zinc ferrite nanoparticles, 93
 endothelial progenitor cell, 91
 gadolinium-diethylene triamine pentaacetic acid (Gd-DTPA), 90
 gold nanorods, 92
 gold nanotracer-labeled mesenchymal stem cells, 91
 immunohistochemistry, 89
 iron oxide nanoparticles, 90
 macrophages, 92
 modeoxyuridine (BrdU), 89—90
 nanoscale scaffolds, 92, 93f
 polydopamine-coated gold core-shell nanoprobe, 92
 quantum dots, 90—91
 silica nanoparticles, 92
 SPIO nanoparticles, 89—90
 transfection agents, 89—90
Stereolithography technique, 249—250, 252f
Supercritical fluid technology, 124
Surface active agents, 46
Surface-enhanced Raman scattering (SERS), 362—363
Surface modification techniques, 249—250
Synchromed II micropumps, 250—252, 258f
Synthetic polymers, 1—2, 30—31

T

Thermoresponsive systems, 199—200
Tissue engineering, 7—8, 8f—9f, 10t—12t
 adipose tissue—derived progenitor cells, 94—95
 biocompatible and biodegradable nano fibers, 201—202
 3D biodegradable scaffolds, 94
 biometric scaffolds, 93—94
 bone tissue engineering, 203—204
 calcium sensors, 93—94
 cardiac tissue engineering, 204—205
 COOH-functionalized single-walled carbon nanotubes, 95—96, 97f
 extracellular matrix (ECM), 201—202
 lab-on-a-chip, 95—96
 matrix biomolecules, 93—94
 micro fluidic perfusion bioreactors, 95—96
 nanoscaffold-coated model bioreactor, 94—95
 nerve tissue engineering, 205
 niches, 93—94
 PLGA, 202
 PuraMatrix hydrogel, 95
 regenerative medicine, 94
 skin tissue engineering
  degradation rate, 202—203
  mechanical properties, 202—203
  nanofibrous membranes, 203
  scar-free regeneration, 203
 three dimensional scaffolds, 202
Transdermal drug delivery system, 208, 331
 skin structure and barrier, 331—333, 332f—333f
Transporter-mediated transcytosis, 71
Transporter-targeted prodrugs, 65—66, 66t
Trojan microparticles, 26

U

Ultrasound imaging, 367—369
Ultrasound-mediated drug delivery (USMD), 63
Ultrasound-responsive systems, 200
Ultrasound/sonography, 231—232
US Food and Drug Administration, 106, 107t, 250—252

W

Water-soluble organic solvents, 47

X

X-ray-computed tomography, 230—231

Z

Zosano patch, 349